PRIMARY CARE PSYCHIATRY

PRIMARY CARE PSYCHIATRY

DAVID J. KNESPER, M.D.

Associate Professor of Psychiatry
Director, Hospital Consultation and Neuropsychiatry Services
Department of Psychiatry
University of Michigan Medical Center
Ann Arbor, Michigan

MICHELLE B. RIBA, M.D.

Clinical Associate Professor of Psychiatry
Associate Chair for Education and Academic Affairs
Department of Psychiatry
University of Michigan Medical Center
Ann Arbor, Michigan

THOMAS L. SCHWENK, M.D.

Professor of Family Practice
Chair, Department of Family Practice
University of Michigan Medical Center
Ann Arbor, Michigan

W.B. SAUNDERS COMPANY

A Division of Harcourt Brace & Company

Philadelphia London Toronto Montreal Sydney Tokyo

W.B. SAUNDERS COMPANY
A Division of Harcourt Brace & Company

The Curtis Center
Independence Square West
Philadelphia, Pennsylvania 19106

NOTICE

Psychiatry is an ever-changing field. Standard safety precautions must be followed, but as new research and clinical experience broaden our knowledge, changes in treatment and drug therapy become necessary or appropriate. Readers are advised to check the product information currently provided by the manufacturer of each drug to be administered to verify the recommended dose, the method and duration of administration, and contraindications. It is the responsibility of the treating physician relying on experience and knowledge of the patient to determine dosages and the best treatment for the patient. Neither the Publisher nor the editors assume any responsibility for any injury and/or damage to persons or property.

The Publisher

Library of Congress Cataloging-in-Publication Data

Knesper, David J.
Primary care psychiatry / David J. Knesper, Michelle B. Riba, Thomas L. Schwenk.—1st ed.

p. cm.

ISBN 0-7216-6509-8

1. Psychiatry. 2. Primary care (Medicine) I. Riba, Michelle B. II. Schwenk, Thomas L. III. Title.
[DNLM: 1. Mental Disorders—therapy. 2. Primary Health Care. WM 400 K68p 1997]

RC454.K586 1997 616.89—dc20

DNLM/DLC 96-43966

PRIMARY CARE PSYCHIATRY ISBN 0-7216-6509-8

Printed in the United States of America.

Last digit is the print number: 9 8 7 6 5 4 3 2 1

With sincere appreciation to all of our contributing authors and reviewers who made the production of this book so rewarding. Most importantly, our sincere thanks to our patients who always help us be better physicians.

David J. Knesper, MD, Michelle B. Riba, MD, and Thomas L. Schwenk, MD

To my wife, Eileen, and my daughters, Kathy and Jenny, who patiently endured my all-too-frequent inattention and preoccupation and unselfishly gave me all the support, encouragement, and love needed to work on this project and countless others.

I also wish to dedicate this book to my parents and brother, Richard, and sister, Nancy, who have always been there for me and have always had faith in my ability to improve health and health care regardless of their misgivings about both.

Over the years I have had the continuing support and affection from my teacher, friend, and standby father, George Mayer. A physician is always being shaped; the person who first mentored me was the late Gardner Quarton, whom everyone called "Q" and whose wisdom will always be with me. A special dedication goes to each of them.

David J. Knesper, MD

To my loving and supportive family, Arty, Alissa, and Erica.

Michelle B. Riba, MD

To the people in my life who helped me find my soul as a person while I became a physician, and who taught me, as Francis Peabody first said, the importance of caring about the patient while caring for the patient—"Oz" Rothermich and David Connell, and most importantly, my wife, Jane.

Thomas L. Schwenk, MD

Contributors

MICHAEL S. ALDRICH, MD
Associate Professor of Neurology, Director, Sleep Disorders Center, University of Michigan Medical Center, Ann Arbor, Michigan
Insomnia and Sleep Disorders

NORMAN E. ALESSI, MD
Associate Professor of Psychiatry, Chief Information Officer and Director, Psychiatric Informatics Program, Department of Psychiatry and Division Director, Child and Adolescent Psychiatry, University of Michigan Medical Center, Ann Arbor, Michigan
Common Emotional and Behavioral Problems of Children and Adolescents; The World Wide Web as a Psychiatric Information Source for the Primary Care Physician

KIRK J. BROWER, MD
Associate Professor of Psychiatry, University of Michigan Medical School, Ann Arbor; Executive Director, Chelsea Arbor Treatment Center, Ann Arbor, Michigan
Alcohol and Other Drug-Related Problems

OLIVER C. CAMERON, MD, PhD
Professor of Psychiatry, Department of Psychiatry, University of Michigan Medical Center, Ann Arbor, Michigan
Essential Psychopharmacology Skills and Tools

THOMAS CARLI, MD
Clinical Assistant Professor; Director, Managed Psychiatric Services, Department of Psychiatry, University of Michigan Medical Center, Ann Arbor, Michigan
The World Wide Web as a Psychiatric Information Source for the Primary Care Physician; Guide to Self-Help Books About Primary Care Psychiatry Problems

MARIAN COHEN, MSW
Clinical Social Worker and Instructor in Behavioral Science, Department of Family Practice, University of Michigan Medical Center, Ann Arbor, Michigan
Domestic Violence and Abuse

GREGORY W. DALACK, MD
Assistant Professor, Department of Psychiatry, University of Michigan Medical Center, Ann Arbor; Chief, Mental Health Clinic, Ann Arbor Veterans Administration Medical Center, Ann Arbor, Michigan
Counseling for Behavioral Change

MARK A. DEMITRACK, MD
Adjunct Associate Professor of Psychiatry, University of Michigan Medical School, Ann Arbor, Michigan; Clinical Research Physician, Lilly Research Laboratories, A Division of Eli Lilly and Company, Lilly Corporate Center, Indianapolis, Indiana
Chronic Fatigue Syndrome and Fibromyalgia; Eating Disorders and Disordered Eating

JAMES E. DILLON, MD
Clinical Assistant Professor of Psychiatry, Director of Residency Training in Child and Adolescent Psychiatry, University of Michigan Child and Adolescent Psychiatric Hospital, Department of Psychiatry, University of Michigan Medical Center, Ann Arbor, Michigan
Common Emotional and Behavioral Problems of Children and Adolescents

ALAN B. DOUGLASS, MD
Clinical Assistant Professor; Director, Sleep Program in Psychiatry, Department of Psychiatry, University of Michigan Medical Center, Ann Arbor, Michigan
Insomnia and Sleep Disorders

GLORIA J. EDWARDS, PhD
Program Associate II, Department of Internal Medicine, Division of Hypertension, University of Michigan Medical Center, Ann Arbor, Michigan
Obesity

N. CARY ENGLEBERG, MD
Associate Professor of Internal Medicine and Microbiology and Immunology, Department of Internal Medicine, Division of Infectious Diseases, University of Michigan Medical Center, Ann Arbor, Michigan
Chronic Fatigue Syndrome and Fibromyalgia

A. E. EYLER, MD, MPH
Clinical Assistant Professor, Department of Family Practice, University of Michigan Medical Center; Adjunct Lecturer, University of Michigan School of Public Health, Ann Arbor, Michigan
Common Neurologic Disorders: Alzheimer's Disease, Parkinson's Disease Dementia, HIV/AIDS, Stroke, Multiple Sclerosis, and Epilepsy; Sexuality Issues and Common Sexual Dysfunctions: Evaluation and Management in the Primary Care Setting; Domestic Violence and Abuse

RACHEL LIPSON GLICK, MD
Clinical Assistant Professor; Director, Psychiatric Emergency Services, Department of Psychiatry, University of Michigan Medical Center, Ann Arbor, Michigan
Common Psychiatric Emergencies in the Office Setting

JOHN F. GREDEN, MD
Professor of Psychiatry and Research Scientist; Chair, Department of Psychiatry, University of Michigan Medical Center, Ann Arbor, Michigan
Major Mood Disorders

SALLY K. GUTHRIE, Pharm D
Associate Professor of Pharmacy, College of Pharmacy, University of Michigan; Associate Professor of Pharmacy, Department of Psychiatry, University of Michigan Medical Center, Ann Arbor, Michigan
Essential Psychopharmacology Skills and Tools

MILTON P. HUANG, MD
Lecturer in Psychiatry; Assistant Director, Psychiatric Informatics Program, Department of Psychiatry, University of Michigan Medical Center, Ann Arbor, Michigan
The World Wide Web as a Psychiatric Information Source for the Primary Care Physician

MICHAEL D. JIBSON, MD, PhD
Clinical Assistant Professor of Psychiatry, Department of Psychiatry, University of Michigan Medical Center, Ann Arbor, Michigan
Psychosis and Schizophrenia; Medication Fact Sheets: Patient Handouts Describing the Major Side Effects of Psychotropic Drugs

BARBARA KAMHOLZ, MD
Clinical Assistant Professor of Psychiatry, Department of Psychiatry, University of Michigan Medical Center, Ann Arbor; Chief, Hospital Consultation-Liaison Services, Ann Arbor Veterans Administration Medical Center, Ann Arbor, Michigan
Major Pain Syndromes and Chronic Pain

KEVIN B. KERBER, MD
Clinical Assistant Professor of Psychiatry, Department of Psychiatry, University of Michigan Medical Center, Ann Arbor, Michigan
Making Referrals for Psychiatric Care: Clinical Advice and Managed Care Implications

MARTHA O. KERSHAW, MD
Clinical Assistant Professor, Department of Family Practice, University of Michigan Medical Center, Ann Arbor, Michigan
Domestic Violence and Abuse

MICHAEL S. KLINKMAN, MD, MS
Assistant Professor of Family Practice, Department of Family Practice, University of Michigan Medical Center, Ann Arbor, Michigan
A "Roadmap" for Differential Diagnosis and Treatment of Mental Health Problems in the Primary Care Setting; Minor Depression

DAVID J. KNESPER, MD
Associate Professor of Psychiatry; Director, Hospital Consultation and Neuropsychiatry Services, Department of Psychiatry, University of Michigan Medical Center, Ann Arbor, Michigan
Essential Psychopharmacology Skills and Tools; Making Referrals for Psychiatric Care: Clinical Advice and Managed Care Implications; Common Neurologic Disorders: Alzheimer's Disease, Parkinson's Disease Dementia, HIV/AIDS, Stroke, Multiple Sclerosis, and Epilepsy; Guide to Self-Help Books About Primary Care Psychiatry Problems

ALAN M. MELLOW, MD, PhD
Associate Professor of Psychiatry, Director of Geriatric Psychiatry, Department of Psychiatry, University of Michigan Medical Center, Ann Arbor; Chief of Psychiatry, Ann Arbor Veterans Administration Medical Center, Ann Arbor, Michigan
Essential Psychopharmacology Skills and Tools

PATRICIA MARES MILLER, RN, MS, CS
Clinical Nurse Specialist, Psychiatric Emergency Services, Department of Psychiatry, University of Michigan Medical Center, Ann Arbor, Michigan
Guide to Self-Help Books About Primary Care Psychiatry Problems; Resource Service Catalogues Listing Numerous Handouts for Primary Care Patients; Guide to Organizations Dedicated to Specific Primary Care Psychiatry Problems; Referral Information from Mental Health Professional Associations

RANDOLPH M. NESSE, MD
Professor of Psychiatry, Department of Psychiatry, University of Michigan Medical Center, Ann Arbor; Research Associate, Institute for Social Research, University of Michigan, Ann Arbor, Michigan
Anxiety Disorders in Primary Care

THOMAS P. O'CONNOR, MD
Clinical Assistant Professor of Medicine, Department of Internal Medicine, University of Michigan Medical Center, Ann Arbor, Michigan
Psychosis and Schizophrenia

OVIDE F. POMERLEAU, PhD
Professor of Psychology in Psychiatry, and Director, University of Michigan Behavioral Medicine Program; Director, University of Michigan Substance Abuse Research Program, Department of Psychiatry, University of Michigan Medical Center, Ann Arbor, Michigan
Nicotine and Smoking

PAUL E. QUINLAN, DO
Child and Adolescent Psychiatry Fellow, Division of Child and Adolescent Psychiatry, Department of Psychiatry, University of Michigan Medical Center, Ann Arbor, Michigan
Common Emotional and Behavioral Problems in Children and Adolescents

MICHELLE B. RIBA, MD
Clinical Associate Professor of Psychiatry; Associate Chair for Education and Academic Affairs, Department of Psychiatry, University of Michigan Medical Center, Ann Arbor, Michigan
Common Psychiatric Emergencies in the Office Setting

DAVID S. ROSEN, MD, MPH
Assistant Professor of Pediatrics, Lecturer in Internal Medicine; Director, Section of Teenage and Young Adult Health, Departments of Pediatrics and Internal Medicine, University of Michigan Medical Center, Ann Arbor, Michigan
Eating Disorders and Disordered Eating

RANDY S. ROTH, PhD
Clinical Assistant Professor of Psychology in Anesthesiology, Physical Medicine and Rehabilitation; Director, Pain Management Program, Department of Physical Medicine and Rehabilitation, Associate Director, Multidisciplinary Pain Center, Department of Anesthesiology, University of Michigan Medical Center, Ann Arbor, Michigan
Major Pain Syndromes and Chronic Pain

DAVID E. SCHTEINGART, MD
Professor of Internal Medicine; Director, Obesity Rehabilitation Program, Department of Internal Medicine, University of Michigan Medical Center, Ann Arbor, Michigan
Obesity

THOMAS L. SCHWENK, MD
Professor of Family Practice; Chair, Department of Family Practice, University of Michigan Medical Center, Ann Arbor, Michigan
Major Mood Disorders

JOHN D. SEVERIN, MD
Clinical Assistant Professor of Family Practice, Department of Family Practice, University of Michigan Medical Center, Ann Arbor, Michigan
Alcohol and Other Drug-Related Problems

KENNETH R. SILK, MD
Associate Professor of Psychiatry; Associate Chair for Clinical and Administrative Affairs, Department of Psychiatry, University of Michigan Medical Center, Ann Arbor, Michigan
"Difficult" Patients

MINDY SMITH, MD, MS
Associate Professor of Family Practice, Department of Family Practice, Michigan State University, College of Human Medicine, East Lansing, Michigan
Nicotine and Smoking

MONICA N. STARKMAN, MD
Associate Professor of Psychiatry, Department of Psychiatry, University of Michigan Medical Center, Ann Arbor, Michigan
Obesity

RAJIV TANDON, MD
Associate Professor of Psychiatry; Director, Hospital Services Division, Department of Psychiatry, University of Michigan Medical Center, Ann Arbor, Michigan
Psychosis and Schizophrenia

MARCIA V. VALENSTEIN, MD
Clinical Instructor of Psychiatry, Department of Psychiatry, University of Michigan Medical Center, Ann Arbor; Staff Psychiatrist/Primary Care Liaison, Ann Arbor Veterans Administration Medical Center, Ann Arbor, Michigan
A "Roadmap" for Differential Diagnosis and Treatment of Mental Health Problems in the Primary Care Setting; Minor Depression

WILLIAM WADLAND, MD, MS
Professor of Family Practice; Chair, Department of Family Practice, Michigan State University, College of Human Medicine, East Lansing, Michigan
Nicotine and Smoking

BRENT C. WILLIAMS, MD, MPH
Assistant Professor of Internal Medicine, Department of Internal Medicine, University of Michigan Medical Center, Ann Arbor; Attending Physician, Ann Arbor Veterans Administration Medical Center, Ann Arbor, Michigan
"Difficult" Patients

MARK A. ZAMORSKI, MD
Clinical Assistant Professor of Family Practice, Department of Family Practice, University of Michigan Medical Center, Ann Arbor, Michigan
Anxiety Disorders in Primary Care

ANDREW J. ZWEIFLER, MD
Professor of Internal Medicine; Chief, Hypertension Clinic, Department of Internal Medicine, University of Michigan Medical Center, Ann Arbor, Michigan
Counseling for Behavioral Change

Foreword

The importance and timeliness of this book are underscored by the following facts.

Primary care physicians have long been in the "front lines" in the battle against psychiatric illnesses such as major depression and anxiety disorders. The reason is the prevalence of psychiatric disorders. Based on published studies, conservatively 30% of patients seeing a primary care physician do so because of a psychiatric disorder or because of a psychiatric disorder that is significantly confounding their medical illness, treatment, and response to such treatment. For example, six month mortality rates are higher following an acute myocardial infarction if major depression is present.

Beyond these basic facts of clinical life, the important role of primary care physicians in the treatment of psychiatric disorders is being expanded by the managed care movement. This is occurring regardless of whether primary care physicians want such an expanded role or whether they feel confident in their training and abilities to deal with patients suffering from these illnesses.

Unfortunately, the sum total of the formal training of primary care physicians in the diagnosis and management of patients with psychiatric illnesses is often limited to a six- to eight-week course in general psychiatry in the third year of medical school. Thus, primary care physicians have two years of clinical training in medical school and then three to five years of postgraduate training to treat 70% of their patients and perhaps two months of training for the remaining 30%. Moreover, the training they historically have received in that six to eight weeks of a traditional medical school clerkship in psychiatry often had little to do with the psychiatric conditions that they are generally expected to treat in primary care practices. Their psychiatric clerkships often are based around inpatient psychiatry rotations. Their experience then is primarily with patients whose treatment was unsuccessful in primary care and outpatient psychiatric settings. This has always seemed a curious situation to me, much as did my only rotation in pediatrics, which was on a tertiary care level oncology team. Based on that rotation, I could have erroneously concluded that pediatricians saw only terminally ill children with leukemias and other malignancies.

This situation is made worse by the fact that most doctors, being products of our culture, have been exposed for many years to all the standard myths abut mental illnesses. Thus, they enter medical schools with preconceptions and do not receive adequate training to realize that those cultural myths are just that. Imagine if physicians still entered medical school thinking that tuberculosis could be due to an underlying personality trait or that epilepsy could be the result of being "touched by the gods" and, then, received such minimal training that those misconceptions were only partially corrected.

Given the above, one can realize the importance of a book for general physicians. *Primary Care Psychiatry* presents the essential elements of the diagnosis and management of psychiatric disorders commonly seen in primary care. It benefits significantly from the fact that it has been jointly edited and written by faculty from both primary care and psychiatry from the University of Michigan.

As a result of being authored by people who work closely together, this book avoids the common "disjointedness" and "unevenness" that can occur in textbooks that are multi-authored by people who take different approaches based on their backgrounds, temperaments, and proclivities. The reader does not feel the necessity to change mindsets when going from chapter to chapter. This is particularly important since I suspect that this book will often be used as a reference guide as opposed to being read once and put away.

Also, being authored by both primary care and psychiatric physicians, "the forest or the tree" orientations that plague similar books that are written by one group or the other are avoided. This book provides the framework of the broad perspective required by general physicians, particularly given the severe time constraints they face, and at the same time provides adequate depth to be truly helpful to primary care physicians and their patients.

The careful, deliberate, and painstaking approach described by the editors in their preface has borne fruit of which they can be justifiably proud. Moreover, this approach has produced a book that will be a source of aid and comfort to the readers and their patients.

Sheldon H. Preskorn, MD

President and Medical Director
Psychiatric Research Institute
Wichita, Kansas

Foreword

Over the last two decades, a new interest in the psychiatric issues in primary care has evolved from a disparate and isolated series of essays and descriptive, epidemiologic studies and monographs[1,2] into a robust discipline in which the phenomenologic, taxonomic, and treatment variations that exist in primary care have been identified,[3] tested to some extent, and correlated with training needs and approaches.[4] Thus, one trend underlying the need for *Primary Care Psychiatry* is the large-scale production of new and tailored knowledge and skills.

At the same time, social changes concerning the care of persons with psychosocial problems have been extraordinary and pervasive. The direct payers for health care—industry and government—concluded that controlling costs of care through corporatization of management, budget control, and regulation of benefits would free funds for competition or profits. The governmental victory of the idea of smaller government also led to decreased budgets in public health programs at federal and state levels. The bottom line is shrinking budgets and tighter controls on mental health dollars and the "carving out" of mental health benefits. This means that instead of a health or managed care plan providing mental health benefits, it subcontracts them to outside companies. These companies may sometimes be efficient and of decent quality, but their profits are often made by utilizing the least costly mental health providers, none of whom can prescribe medication or have the educational background to understand the interaction of mind and body in useful depth. Also, they limit the use of psychiatrists, put the prescribing burden on primary care physicians, and create an impetus on each side to shift the effort in care to the other.[5] Recent evidence has shown that in the United States the majority of the effort and spending is on the less sick patients, and the opposite is true in Ontario, Canada, with its universal coverage.[6]

The impact of these trends is that more primary care physicians are bearing the principal responsibility for recognizing and treating straightforward common mental disorders (depression, anxiety disorders, and substance abuse) and for referring the others (psychotic disorders, bipolar disorder, nonresponsive common mental disorders). "Ever more" because we have known since the mid-70s that primary care physicians have provided the sole care for about half of those with defined mental disorders in this country.[7,8] Recently this number has been increasing. Yet, because of insufficient training in these areas, inadequate training approaches, personal and societal barriers to dealing with mental problems, and lack of reimbursement for such care in the fee-for-service sector and the corresponding pressure to spend less time with patients in the managed care sector, primary care physicians have under-recognized, under-treated, and over-avoided these problems.

At the same time, in part because of added stresses of practice and inadequate training, the relationships between mental health providers and primary care physicians have added competition to pre-existing tribal suspicion, communications problems related to different professional jargons, and different working styles. The chasm between the disciplines has grown wider as psychiatry has become more biological and primary care increasingly sees itself as the guardian of the traditions of concern for the whole patient and the biopsychosocial approach.[5]

For these reasons, this outstanding text on psychiatric issues in primary care is timely and unique. *Primary Care Psychiatry* provides, in one volume and a coherent format, extensive and detailed coverage of the mental disorders and the principal problems of living and the principal problems in special situations and difficult types of patients encountered in the primary care setting. Because the chapters are written by teams of primary care and behavioral medicine experts, they talk the talk and walk the walk of primary care, while being current with the best expert approaches.

Primary Care Psychiatry is a welcome addition to the volumes and texts that deal with these issues. *Primary Care Psychiatry* is appropriate in my view for four groups of readers: beginning students of psychiatric issues for medical providers of all types; all levels of learners in primary care; learners of psychiatry in the managed care era; and practitioners wanting an efficient and up-to-date reference source.

Primary Care Psychiatry is, to be sure, a textbook and not a training process. Training models that have changed behaviors in desirable directions integrate knowledge, skills, and attitudinal learning in an experiential program of learning.[9] Starting with the learners' issues in care, working on their difficult situations, but providing over-arching concepts, epidemiology, and evidence-based treatment approaches work best. There needs to be skilled skills teaching, consisting of practicing targeted behaviors with focused feedback, and discussion of the learners' feelings and attitudes so that they will not reject the area because of personal fear or inhibition.

Used well by readers, this unique book will prove an invaluable resource.

Mack Lipkin, M.D.

Founding President
American Academy on Physician and Patient
Professor of Clinical Medicine
Director, Primary Care
New York University Medical Center
New York, New York

References

1. Rutter M, Shaffer D, Shepherd M: A Multi-Axial Classification of Child Psychiatric Problems. Geneva, World Health Organization, 1975.
2. Lipkin M, Kupka K: Psychosocial Factors Affecting Health. New York, Praeger, 1982.
3. American Psychiatric Association. Diagnostic and Statistical Manual of Mental Disorders: Primary Care Version. Washington, DC, American Psychiatric Association, 1995.
4. Lipkin M Jr, Putnam S, Lazare A (eds): The Medical Interview: Clinical Care, Education, and Research. New York, Springer-Verlag, 1995.
5. Lipkin M Jr: Pulling together or falling apart. Prim Psychiatry 4:22–31, 1997.
6. Michels R: Improving outpatient medical care. N Engl J Med 336:578–579, 1997.
7. Hankin JR, Steinwachs DM, Regier DA, et al: Use of general medical care services by persons with mental disorders. Arch Gen Psychiatry 39(2):225–231, 1982.
8. Robins LN, Regier DA (eds): Psychiatric Disorders in America: The Epidemiologic Catchment Area Study. New York, The Free Press, 1991.
9. Lipkin M Jr, Kaplan C, Clark W, Novack DH: Teaching medical interviewing: the Lipkin model. *In* The Medical Interview: Clinical Care, Education, and Research. New York, Springer-Verlag, 1995, pp. 422–435.

Preface

Primary care physicians and clinical psychiatrists collaboratively wrote *Primary Care Psychiatry* to be highly relevant and immediately useful in the daily practice of primary care medicine. The initial decisions about content and all aspects of development, writing, and editing were the product of an intense and sustained effort between primary care physicians and psychiatrists at the University of Michigan. Consequently, the organization of *Primary Care Psychiatry* is intended to match the realities of primary care practice. For example, *Primary Care Psychiatry* begins with a "roadmap" for differential diagnosis and treatment of mental problems. This original approach derives directly from the processes of primary care practice and minimizes the use of criterion-based psychiatric diagnosis. During the typical 10 to 15 minute office visit, the busy primary care practitioner wants abbreviated diagnostic rules that cut to the core of the problem. These rules are provided wherever possible. Each chapter contains considerable practical, clinical wisdom and insight about diagnoses and treatments in specific, utilitarian terms not usually shared with primary care physicians.

"User friendly" describes another intended attribute of the book. *Primary Care Psychiatry* uses an outline format. "Take home" messages are frequent and appear in italics. While the authors were given the freedom to deviate in order to write clearly, at the same time we worked hard to give each chapter a consistent format. Our goal is to give the busy clinician the opportunity to grab information for immediate use. Another device to permit the busy clinician to grab information is the extensive use of charts and tables. The appendix material deserves special mention. We have assembled material that can be photocopied and handed to patients as a means to help them become partners in care. For example, there are "Fact Sheets" describing the essential effects and side-effects of psychotropic medications, and annotated lists of self-help books and related patient education materials.

One particularly innovative feature of *Primary Care Psychiatry* is the frequent use of dialogues or scripts that illustrate effective strategies the primary care physician can use when conducting interviews or providing patient education and supportive counseling. For example, Chapter 6, "Making Referrals for Psychiatric Care," the 'Sounds Far-Fetched to Me' strategy is one means of helping the psychotic patient to better participate in treatment and referral. In Chapter 8, "Major Mood Disorders," there are extensive scripts about what to tell the patient and family during the beginning stages of treatment and about how to explain the use of antidepressant medication.

Primary Care Psychiatry seeks to offer primary care physicians the equipment to deliver the same quality of care that would be available from a mental health specialist. To this end, all chapters were peer reviewed internally; some chapters were reviewed externally by a practicing primary care physician. We also asked our senior residents in both primary care and psychiatry to review the chapters because we wanted trainees to be able to benefit from reading our book throughout their years of practice. The material, we feel, is quite practical and useful.

It is our intention for the mentally ill to receive the same high standards of care regardless of provider or clinical setting. Accepted standards of care are uncompromised. We believe treatment-responsive mental and emotional problems should be the province of primary care. Mental health specialists should be reserved for interactive consultation and for the treatment of patients with moderate to severe illness who are unresponsive to standard initial interventions. Driven by these values and beliefs, we did our very best to assemble a responsive text.

The absence of a broad consensus about the "best" treatment for a particular mental or emotional problem has never prevented such patients from seeking care nor practitioners from providing services. Because of the relatively recent union of psychiatry with pharmacology, the specialty has somewhat more uncertainty compared with other areas of medicine. Regardless of ambiguity, clinicians usually decide to offer their patients something. Our intentions are to provide the reader-user with what is standard practice at the University of Michigan Medical Center. Recommendations approximate our medical center's consensus practice. We do not claim to have found the "best" treatment; we do give you our best thinking, wisdom, and experience in a format that minimizes equivocation. For example, our first-line medication is named along with its brand name and the specifics about dose, uptapers, and the like. Our format may allow the primary care physician to get on with the difficult job of actually treating mental illness, and, as much as possible, to be unencumbered by lots of academic "maybes" and menus of generalizations and instructions to "select one" from a lengthy list of alternative medications.

We felt that a book like *Primary Care Psychiatry* could not have been written by authors from several medical centers because of the extensive collaboration involved. Editors and authors had frequent face-to-face meetings and countless electronic mailings to hammer out our final products. During the completion of each chapter there came an uncommon sense of enthusiasm and teamwork. In the process, we have reaffirmed our conviction that patients present with a set of problems that are not sorted by specialty; it is within this context that teams of physicians working as a responsive unit will have the best chance of providing comprehensive services and improving health status.

Of course, inclusion and exclusion decisions had to be made to keep the size of the book within bounds. We have included only high frequency conditions that we believe match the substantial time constraints characterizing primary care. The availability of effective and acceptable treatments was an inclusion principle. Conditions and treatments that we believe should not be managed in primary care are identified and the exclusion rationale is explained. We omitted considerable information that is of general interest; such information is often included in textbooks for purposes of completeness, but it has little immediate clinical value.

It is our and the authors' hope and intent that *Primary Care Psychiatry* be easily available during daily patient care and that it become dog-eared and coffee-stained from frequent use.

David J. Knesper, MD
Michelle B. Riba, MD
Thomas L. Schwenk, MD

Acknowledgments

We were blessed to have the privilege of working with the many contributors to *Primary Care Psychiatry.* Despite numerous competing obligations and priorities, in very meaningful and highly individual ways, each contributor seemed to immediately understand the need for and advantages of a book that links primary care and psychiatry. Work on this book moved to the top of everyone's priority list. When we asked for volunteers to do tasks, we got volunteers. When we asked for a one-week turnaround, authors came through in under a week. Chapters were revised and then revised some more, and with each revision the contributors to *Primary Care Psychiatry* willingly took the challenge and worked harder. We were most fortunate to be able to collaborate with such a distinguished group of teachers, researchers, clinicians, and outstanding human beings.

Every chapter was reviewed, often more than once, and we acknowledge with deep gratitude the following reviewers, who gave highly detailed comments and salient critiques and provided them, often, in a matter of days: John E. Billi, MD, Gregory W. Dalack, MD, Robert D. Ernst, MD, Evan Feibusch, MD, Ernesto R. Figueroa, MD, Douglas J. Gelb, MD, Sally K. Guthrie, Pharm D, Grace Huang, MD, Sean K. Kesterson, MD, David S. Rosen, MD, MPH, Lori A. Schuh, MD, Patricia Marsh, MD, Thomas Wang, MD, Sara Warber, MD, and Donna M. Woods, MD.

A special thank you goes to Gary J. Frantz, MD, who is in family practice in Mansfield, Ohio. Whenever we needed to have a manuscript reviewed with the perspective of someone who practices outside a large metropolitan area, we could turn to Gary who would always come through with critical comments and invaluable suggestions.

Next to the text, a book's index is perhaps the most important component. Modern word processing can make it easy to build an index of key topics, but it takes experts in specific disciplines to make sure an index is useful and responsive to information needs. Drs. Kirk Brower, Michael Jibson, and Paul Quinlan volunteered to meticulously review the index, which is often a thankless task. Not so. We give our sincere thank you and our deep appreciation to these three colleagues and friends.

It has been our genuine pleasure to work with Judy Fletcher, Senior Editor for Medical Books at W.B. Saunders. She believed in the importance of our book from the moment she first read our proposal. Judy had marvelous ways of making us all decision-makers in every key aspect of the publication process. We profoundly appreciate her shepherding our book to a timely completion.

We have had the good fortune to work with Terry Helinski, who was the copy editor. Although we made every effort to give our multiauthored book a uniform format, it was Terry who gave the book real cohesion by providing important insights, suggestions, and editorial advice aimed at making the book read as if authored by a single person.

Agnes Hunt Byrne made very special contributions to *Primary Care Psychiatry.* As Project Supervisor, Agnes gave this book much of its cohesion. We will always be thankful for her many phone calls.

We are grateful for the understanding and help provided by Michael Carcel, Production Manager at W.B. Saunders. Mike, without extending the book's release date, somehow always found a way to accommodate last minute changes, additions, and modifications intended to make information current and responsive to our beliefs about our readers' expectations.

This book would not be possible without the unmentioned but critical support staff at W.B. Saunders: thank you all. We similarly acknowledge people we will come to know and who will contribute to the distribution and marketing of *Primary Care Psychiatry.*

Our sincere thanks goes to Linda Gacioch and Judy Darrow who have been so helpful in organizing psychiatry and family practice resident involvement in this project and to Blythe A. Bieber for her ongoing support and assistance.

We are indebted to Penelope Martin who has to be one of the most organized and forgiving persons on the planet. She was unbelievably effective in finding important manuscript pages, computer files, and related items for the editor who misplaced them. The book involved numerous authors, letters, electronic mail, and permissions, and Penni was remarkably capable of tracking them all and reminding us when something needed to be done. She always managed to make sense out of the most sketchy messages and even anticipated messages and tasks that were about to arrive.

Finally, we wish to thank the many people at the University of Michigan and Medical Center who, in a time of constrained resources, gave us room to remain creative and the support necessary to bring our ideas to fruition.

David J. Knesper, MD
Michelle B. Riba, MD
Thomas L. Schwenk, MD

Contents

I

Principles of Practice, Diagnosis, and Treatment

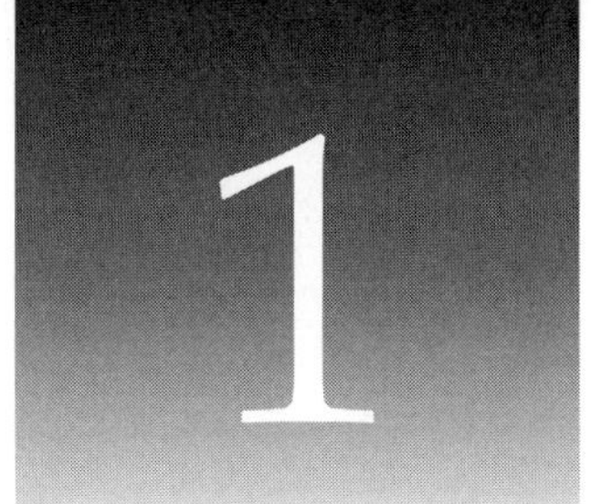

MICHAEL S. KLINKMAN, MD, MS

MARCIA V. VALENSTEIN, MD

A "Roadmap" for Differential Diagnosis and Treatment of Mental Health Problems in the Primary Care Setting

I. Introduction.

Our understanding of the epidemiology of mental health problems in the primary health care setting has grown rapidly over the past decade, but significant gaps remain. Investigators have examined the twin issues of recognition and management of mood disorders in primary care practice, with growing awareness of several significant differences between psychiatric and primary care practice.

Problem identification is far more complex in the primary care setting than in the psychiatric care setting because patients often present with ill-defined or somatic complaints that are not acknowledged as representing mental health problems. *Patient resistance* to treatment is more problematic in primary care: unlike psychiatric patients, primary care patients may not expect or desire psychosocial assistance for unrecognized mental health problems. The *process of care* is also very different between settings: the mental health problem is the sole focus of psychiatric care, whereas in primary care, clinicians often manage multiple problems simultaneously and almost never address mental health problems in isolation from other health problems. Finally, growing evidence indicates that the *range and type of mental health problems differ significantly* between settings. Most distressed patients seen in primary care may not meet the full diagnostic criteria for conditions included in the *Diagnostic and Statistical Manual of Mental Disorders, 4th edition* (DSM-IV),[1–3] and many have features of several different conditions.[4]

In the unstructured, "messy" world of primary care, clinicians may prescribe therapeutic trials of antidepressant medications without first reaching a formal psychiatric diagnosis, or they may provide brief counseling without developing a diagnostic formulation or a formal treatment plan. Clinicians may address coexisting medical or social problems as the most expeditious way to "solve" psychiatric problems, or they may choose to ignore recognized problems. They may cycle though a standard menu of treatment options (talking, counseling, prescribing antidepressant medications) for a wide range of psychiatric conditions. This seemingly unstructured approach may represent the most efficient—and effective—way to deliver mental health care in the primary care setting, where disabling but subsyndromal or subthreshold depression and anxiety are far more prevalent than their threshold DSM diagnostic counterparts.

The precise diagnostic nomenclature used in the psychiatric setting is simply not useful for most distressed patients seen in a typical primary care practice: it provides meaningful diagnostic assistance for only a small minority of patients at a high cost in terms of clinician time and effort. This chapter presents an alternative approach to the identification and management of mental health problems in the primary care setting. Using this approach, clinicians can move to the level of diagnostic specificity needed to appropriately manage patients' problems, reserving formal psychiatric diagnosis for situations in which management depends on diagnostic precision. Growing evidence indicates that primary care clinicians use just this type of sequential process to respond to suspected mental health problems.[5, 6] Examples of these abbreviated methods of diagnosis are presented in subsequent chapters of this book.

II. A stepped approach to psychiatric problems in primary care.

This approach can be illustrated as a "roadmap," or algorithm (Fig. 1–1), in which each branch implies different management or treatment. To provide efficient care, clinicians "drive" only as far as is necessary to manage the patient's problem.

The main branch in the algorithm separates "primary," "secondary," and "can't tell" mental health problems. In primary problems, the major problem is the mental health problem; in secondary problems, the patient's major problem is biomedical; in "can't tell" problems, biomedical and psychosocial issues are so intertwined that distinction is not clinically meaningful. Examples of "can't tell" conditions include addictions (substance abuse or smoking) and obesity. Subsequent chapters describe each of these major branches in more detail.

A. "Primary" mental health problem branches.

In general, the pattern of these branches resembles a simplified DSM structure, at the level of specificity needed for primary care practice.

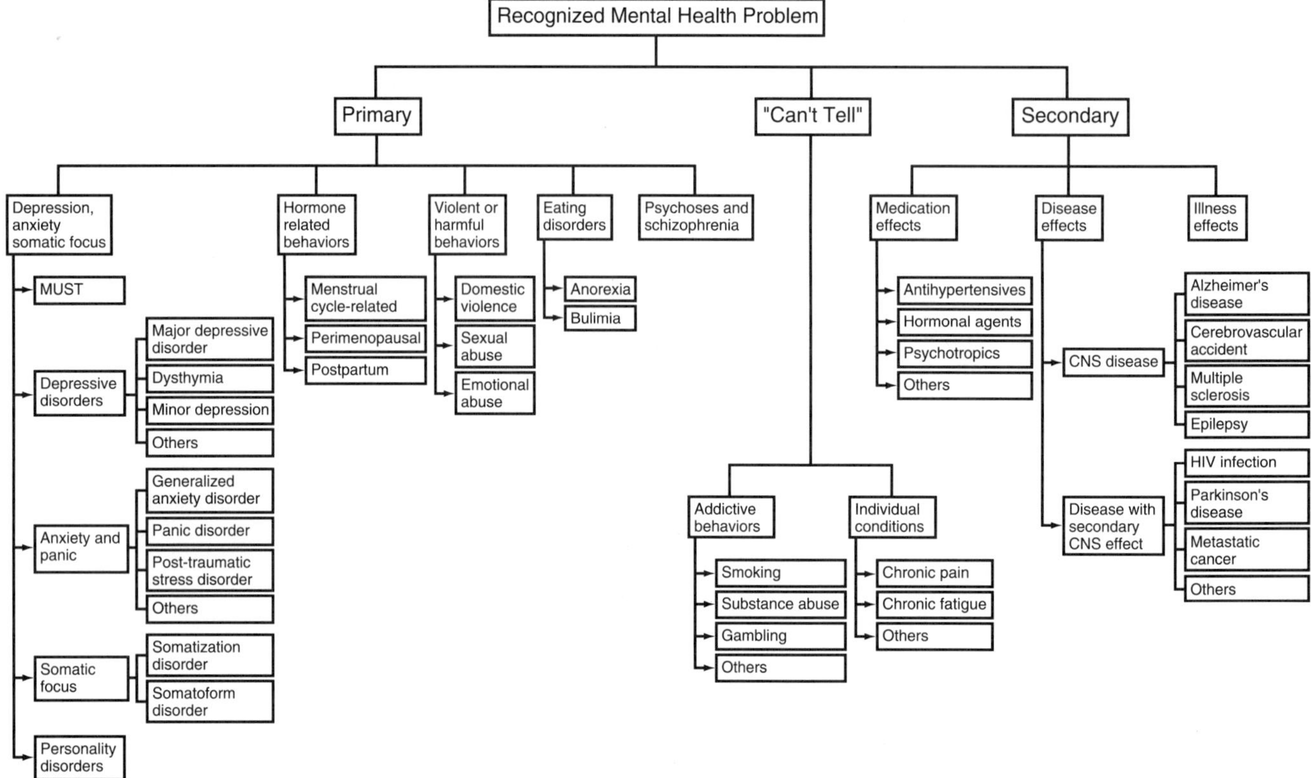

Figure 1–1
Suggested algorithm for the approach to mental health problems in primary care.

The first branch is characterized by the symptoms of *depression, anxiety,* and *somatic focus.* Subsequent branches lead to (1) **m**ultiple **u**ndifferentiated **s**ymptom **t**ypes **(MUST)**, for example, mixed presentations of anxiety, depression, and somatic focus; (2) depressive disorders, with branches for major depressive disorder, dysthymia, and minor depression, among others; (3) anxiety and panic, with branches for generalized anxiety disorder, panic disorder, post-traumatic stress disorder, and others; (4) somatization, including branches for somatization disorder and multisomatoform disorder; and (5) personality disorders.

The second branch might be labeled *hormone-related behaviors.* Secondary branches include (1) menstrual cycle–related emotional conditions, (2) perimenopausal mood disorders, and (3) postpartum mood disorders.

The third branch is *violent or harmful behaviors:* (1) domestic violence, (2) sexual abuse, and (3) emotional abuse.

The fourth main branch is *eating disorders,* with subsequent branches for anorexia and bulimia.

The fifth branch comprises *learning or attention problems,* with attention-deficit hyperactivity disorder being distinguished from other learning and/or central processing problems.

The sixth branch represents *psychoses and schizophrenia:* the absence of subsequent branches of this element reflects the limited expertise of primary care clinicians with these conditions.

B. "Secondary" mental health problem branches.

The first branch consists of *medication effects:* problems are most commonly seen resulting from antihypertensive, hormonal, and psychotropic medications. The second branch captures known *disease effects:* either (1) central nervous system disease, such as Alzheimer's disease, cerebrovascular accident, multiple sclerosis, and epilepsy, or (2) disease with secondary effects on the central nervous system, such as human immunodeficiency virus infection, Parkinson's disease, and metastatic cancer. The third main branch represents what is probably the most common secondary mental health problem, here labeled *illness effects:* the emotional response to the presence of a medical problem or disease or its consequences, either in one's self or others.

C. "Can't tell" mental health problem branches.

The first main branch of "can't tell" mental health problems includes *addictive behaviors,* such as smoking, substance abuse, compulsive gambling, and similar behavioral additions. The other branches are specific to individual conditions, such as chronic pain or chronic fatigue syndrome, and each condition requires a specialized management approach—often requiring resources beyond those available in the primary care office, as is discussed later.

III. Identification and management in primary care.

A useful way to think about the process of identification and management is to use the acronym ReACT to describe its four major steps: *re*cognize the presence of distress or a potential problem, *a*ssess the severity of the problem, *c*ategorize the problem, then *t*reat it appropriately. The following sections describe each of these steps in detail.

A. Recognize the presence of distress or problem.

This step often requires clinicians to carefully look beyond the patient's stated reason for the professional encounter or the patient's chief complaint. Recognition of distress can be a "red flag" as clinicians evaluate patient complaints; the clinician may be aware that underlying issues exist during the interactions. Is the patient simply "sick" in the biomedical sense, or is more than the expected amount of emotional distress present? Is the presenting complaint an ill-focused one that might represent a masked mental health problem? Does the primary problem of the patient seem psychosocial rather than biomedical? When this red flag appears, recognition of the problem as either primary, secondary, or can't tell facilitates further assessment. Recognition simply triggers an initial assessment of the patient's emotional condition, and development of a high level of sensitivity to emotional distress, or a high "index of suspicion" for mental health problems, is extremely important for primary care clinicians. However, attempting to reach a formal mental health diagnosis at this step is both premature and unnecessary.

B. Assess the severity of the problem.

If the mental health or emotional problem is considered secondary, as outlined earlier, the primary problem is treated first. Treatment of the primary biomedical problem often results in resolution or marked improvement in the secondary problem as well; one example of this phenomenon is the changing of anthypertensive regimens from nonselective beta blockers to angiotensin converting enzyme inhibitors in order to minimize the symptoms of fatigue and depression.

For primary mental health problems, clinicians can perform an initial triage to assess severity and to assign patients into one of three management categories. The six factors in this triage, level of distress, presence of identifiable stressor, level of impairment, duration, potential for harm, and need for specialized treatment, are sufficiently focused to allow their use during routine 10- to 15-minute office visits.

1. *Level of distress.*
   The level of patient distress is perhaps the single most important factor in the assessment and can be determined through the use of patient self-report questionnaires or ordinal scales. Some useful single questions include
   - How bad is this? (or How hard is this for you?)
   - Have you ever felt this bad before?
   - Can you cope with this, or is it unbearable?
   - On a scale of 1 to 10, in which 1 is the worst you ever felt and 10 the best, how are you feeling right now?

   Increased levels of distress often signal a more severe mental health problem.

2. *Presence of an identifiable stressor.*
   Stressful life events often result in emotional distress as well as physical illness, but the intensity of the emotional response may indicate whether distress is normative or indicative of a primary mental health problem. Screening for the presence of stressors can give valuable clues about the nature and the appropriateness of distress experienced by the patient. One or more of the following questions may be helpful:
   - Sometimes, people feel like this when they are facing a stressful situation. Have you faced a difficult situation lately?
   - Has anything stressful been going on at home or at work?
   - Have you had any setbacks recently?
   - People under a lot of pressure often have problems like this. Have you been under a lot of pressure lately?

   Most stressors fall into one of three categories: major discrete stressors, such as death, divorce, and job loss; chronic stressors, such as ongoing medical illness, marital conflict, and dysfunctional relationships with others; or minor daily stressors, such as noisy children, traffic, and work deadlines.

   Matching the level of distress to the category of the stressor can be very useful. *Distress following a major discrete stressor may be intense, but it should be temporary. Intense distress in response to minor daily stressors suggests the presence of a more severe primary mental health problem.*

3. *Level of impairment.*
   The DSM-IV[1] specifies impairment criteria for many psychiatric disorders, confirming the central importance of this factor in assessment. Impairment usually proceeds in stepwise fashion, beginning with difficulty in fulfilling one's social role, then progressing through dissatisfaction and decreased productivity in the work-

place to difficulty with self-care (e.g., meal preparation or grooming). The following questions can be used to assess the level of impairment:

- Have you missed any work or school because of this problem?
- Have you been unable to take care of your responsibilities because of how you've been feeling?
- Have you been able to take care of your own needs—fixing meals and so forth?

If the patient is not impaired, it is much less likely that a significant mental health problem is present.

4. *Duration of episode.*
Clinicians need to determine how long the problem has been present:
   - A few days
   - Two weeks
   - Three months or more
   - Years
   - "All my life"

   If the problem has been present for only a few days, there is no need to complete a full diagnostic evaluation or therapeutic intervention unless the patient is in immediate danger of self-harm. Two weeks is the arbitrary time requirement for diagnosis of many formal mood disorders. *If symptoms, particularly depressive symptoms, have been present for 3 months or more, it is likely that specific interventions, such as medication therapy or psychotherapy, are necessary.* Distress that has been present for years is unlikely to be easily treated with any modality and may signal the presence of a personality disorder.

5. *Potential for self-harm.*
The potential for self-harm must be assessed in any patient with significant distress or in whom depressive disorder is suspected. Suicidal ideation is a particularly common symptom of major depressive disorder: most such patients have at least fleeting suicidal thoughts at some time during the course of a depressive episode. Although addressing this issue may seem awkward, specific questions regarding thoughts of suicide are important to ask because discussion with a clinician may decrease the risk of suicide. These questions may help clinicians assess the potential for self-harm:
   - It sounds as though you have been feeling very distressed, and many people feel like giving up when things get really tough. Has it been so bad that you've had thoughts of hurting yourself or committing suicide?
   - When you've had these thoughts, has it been easy for you to put them out of your mind, or do you think about them a lot?
   - Do you ever feel like you might act on these thoughts?
   - Have you made a plan for how you would act? What is it?
   - Do you have what you would need to commit suicide?
   - Have you ever made a suicide attempt?

   The presence of suicidal thoughts increases the likelihood that the patient has a psychiatric disorder and should have a thorough psychiatric diagnostic interview. Patients with fleeting thoughts of suicide or self-harm or those with passive suicidal thoughts (e.g., wanting to "go to sleep forever" without a definite plan), can often be treated in the primary care setting. Those with active or frequent thoughts, intent, or a firm plan should be promptly referred for psychiatric care.

6. *Need for specialized treatment.*
For some problems, specialized management protocols have emerged as the most effective therapeutic option, particularly for addictive behaviors and other can't tell conditions. When initial assessment suggests the presence of a can't tell condition, clinicians should determine whether an effective management protocol exists, and then either provide protocol-guided care or refer the patient for such care. Examples of protocol-driven care that could be delivered in the primary care office include smoking cessation and chronic fatigue management, whereas care for substance abuse or eating disorders is likely to be beyond the capacity of most primary care offices.

C. Categorize the problem.

Based on clinicians' initial assessment, most patients can be assigned into one of three management categories: patients needing acknowledgement and talk (PAT), patients needing assessment and monitoring (PAM), and patients needing immediate intervention and treatment (PIT). As mentioned above, the "can't tell" conditions are exceptions to this general rule, and management for each is discussed separately below.

1. *Patients needing acknowledgement and talk (PAT).*
For patients in this category, distress is tolerable and is commensurate with an identifable stressor. Impairment is absent or minimal. The symptoms have been of brief duration, usually less than 3 months, and the patient denies having thoughts of self-harm. The problem does not appear to require protocol-driven management. Examples of PAT-type diagnoses are minor depression, adjustment reaction, grief reaction, premenstrual syndrome, anxiety, mild multisomatoform disorder, and irritable bowel syndrome.

2. *Patients needing assessment and monitoring (PAM).*
Patients in the PAM category are more severely impaired than those in the PAT category, and the prevalence of treatable psychiatric illness is higher in this group. Patients present with significant distress, which is often out of proportion to that expected with identifiable stressors or is in response to a chronic stressor. Impairment is often present, either in social or work role function. The problem has been present at this level for at least 2 weeks, which meets the time threshold required for diagnosis of most formal psychiatric disorders, and passive but not active thoughts of self-harm can often be elicited. These patients can also be treated in the primary care setting because specialized management protocols are not usually necessary. Examples of PAM conditions are generalized anxiety disorder, depression (not otherwise specified), major depressive disorder, dysthymia, somatization disorder, postpartum depression, and depression associated with multiple sclerosis.

3. *Patients needing immediate intervention and treatment (PIT).*
Patients in the PIT category represent a small fraction of the emotionally distressed patients seen in routine primary care practice, but diagnosis of these patients should not be missed. They often present with a high level of distress, but an event or situation that can plausibly be linked to the distress is either missing or difficult to identify. Significant impairment is present, and patients may be unable to perform meaningful work or basic self-care. Symptom duration is variable, but it is usually greater than 1 week. Patients may reveal frequent or intrusive thoughts of self-harm, sometimes accompanied by intent or plan. These patients require careful and immediate psychiatric assessment and, often, intensive psychiatric treatment. Examples of PIT conditions are severe major depressive disorder, schizophrenia, severe bipolar disorder, and psychoses.

D. Treat the problem appropriately.

Management of psychosocial problems in the primary care setting is based on two characteristics: the type of problem (primary, secondary, or "can't tell") and the management category the patient best fits (PAT, PAM, or PIT) (Table 1–1). If the problem is secondary, clinicians should treat the primary problem, then reassess the severity of the psychosocial problem. Patients with "can't tell" conditions are likely to benefit most from a specific integrated approach to management, either office-based protocol-driven (smoking cessation) or multidisciplinary (chronic pain); these patients may require referral unless the primary clinician is skilled in the appropriate protocol. Most or all patients in the PIT category are referred to mental health specialists. Patients in PAT or PAM categories can generally be managed in the primary care setting: their referral depends on clinician skill, level of comfort, and patient expectations.

1. *For patients needing acknowledgement and talk (PAT).*
No specific interventions have proved effective for the conditions included in this group; these conditions generally improve spontaneously over the course of weeks to months. Clinicians can use common-sense interventions, such as acknowledging patient distress, discussing underlying interpersonal and social issues, helping patients interpret the meaning of related somatic symptoms, normalizing feelings, and giving realistic expectations for improvement. As a rule, medications are not helpful and are not needed. Follow-up visits may be scheduled as the situa-

Table 1–1
General Approach to Management of Mental Health Problems

	Type of Problem		
Management Category	*Primary* (*e.g., major depression*)	*Secondary* (*e.g., medication effects*)	*"Can't tell"* (*e.g., chronic fatigue*)
PAT (patients needing acknowledgement and talk)	Give *supportive care:* acknowledge distress, give expectations	*Treat* primary problem	Use specific management *protocol*
PAM (patients needing assessment and monitoring)	Provide *diagnostic assessment* followed by treatment or referral	*Treat* primary problem *Reassess* severity of mental health symptoms	Use specific management *protocol;* may require *referral*
PIT (patients needing immediate intervention and treatment)	Provide *immediate diagnostic assessment* with treatment or referral	*Treat* primary problem *Assess or refer* for mental health treatment	Use specific management *protocol;* may require *referral*

tion warrants, but in treatment "drop-outs" (patients who cancel or do not come for follow-up appointments), the problems are usually resolved, and the patients probably do not need to be pursued.

2. *For patients needing assessment and monitoring (PAM).*
   A more careful diagnostic assessment is necessary for patients in the PAM category. This may require scheduling of a longer follow-up session within a week or two of initial presentation, during which a formal psychiatric screening instrument can be administered. Based on the results of the diagnostic assessment, the common-sense interventions described can be coupled with more specific counseling, psychotherapy, or medication prescription. Patients may be referred for expert treatment as deemed necessary by clinicians, based on their own levels of skill and interest in managing specific problems. These patients require more careful monitoring, and those who discontinue treatment should be pursued.
3. *For patients needing immediate intervention and treatment (PIT).*
   Patients in the PIT category require immediate diagnostic assessment, as well as careful assessment of the potential for harm to themselves or others. They should not leave the office until this process is complete. If this is not possible, or if the potential for self-harm or harm to others is high, the patients should be emergently referred for specialist psychiatric care. Specific treatment based on diagnosis should be initiated as soon as possible. Frequent follow-up is necessary, and patients who discontinue treatment should be vigorously pursued with immediate contact after missed appointments. Many of these patients require referral for psychiatric evaluation, management, or comanagement.
4. *For patients with "can't tell" conditions.*
   Two basic approaches to management for patients with "can't tell" conditions exist. For patients with addictive behaviors, such as nicotine or alcohol addiction, specific management protocols are considered to be the most effective. Clinicians with specific interest or expertise in the condition and its protocol can treat patients at the primary care site. For complex problems, such as fibromyalgia or chronic fatigue syndrome, coordinated or multidisciplinary care is the most promising approach. Clinicians can coordinate a comprehensive treatment regimen with the help of specialists, or they can refer their patients to multidisciplinary clinics or centers (e.g., a fibromyalgia clinic), if available. Specific approaches to these conditions are discussed in later chapters.

Summary

Because significant differences exist between primary care and psychiatric practice, the structured approach to psychiatric diagnosis embodied in the DSM-IV is of limited usefulness in routine primary care practice. The most efficient—and effective—primary care management strategy is pursuit of diagnostic specificity only as far as is needed for effective management of the problem.

We recommend that primary care clinicians "ReACT" when they suspect mental health problems in their patients:

1. ***Re***cognize the presence of emotional distress or a potential mental health problem.
2. ***A***ssess the cause and severity of the problem.
   If it is secondary, treat the primary problem.
   Perform initial triage by using six factors: level of distress, presence of stressor,
   impairment, duration, potential for harm, and need for specialized treatment.
3. ***C***ategorize into PAT, PAM, or PIT based on the triage.
   PAT: Patients needing acknowledgement and talk.
   PAM: Patients needing assessment and monitoring.
   PIT: Patients needing immediate intervention and treatment.
4. ***T***reat using specific treatment and follow-up based on categories and/or diagnoses.

If clinicians follow these steps, they can identify most mental health problems at the appropriate level of specificity for primary care, provide effective management for these problems during routine office practice, and accurately identify and refer patients who require specialized treatment. Subsequent chapters describe how this process can be used with specific mental health problems.

References

1. American Psychiatric Association. Diagnostic and Statistical Manual of Mental Disorders. Fourth Edition. Washington, DC: American Psychiatric Association; 1994.
2. Goldberg D. The concept of a "case" in general practice. Soc Psychiatry 1982; 17:61–65.
3. Barrett JA, Barrett JA, Oxman TE, Gerber PD. The prevalence of psychiatric disorders in a primary care practice. Arch Gen Psychiatry 1988; 45:1100–1106.
4. Von Korff M, Shapiro S, Burke JD, et al. Anxiety and depression in a primary care clinic. Arch Gen Psychiatry 1987; 44:152–156.
5. Coyne JC, Schwenk TL, Fechner-Bates S. Nondetection of depression by primary care physicians reconsidered. Gen Hosp Psychiatry 1994; 16:267–276.
6. Goldberg D. A classification of psychological distress for use in primary care settings. Soc Sci Med 1992; 35:189–193.

2

DAVID J. KNESPER, MD

OLIVER C. CAMERON, MD, PhD

SALLY K. GUTHRIE, Pharm D

ALAN M. MELLOW, MD, PhD

Essential Psychopharmacology Skills and Tools

This chapter reviews the psychopharmacology skills and tools psychiatrists use routinely. We believe that our selective review of the major psychopharmacology issues and our observations will be helpful because they are often not provided in standard psychopharmacology texts and are generally not easily available to primary care physicians.

I. Evaluation, diagnosis, and medication response.

Psychopharmacology is the treatment of mental disorders with drugs and the study of the mechanisms by which these drugs work. As with all other medical disorders, the most essential component of treating a mental disorder is accurate recognition and diagnosis. Because medication efficacy does not covary absolutely with diagnosis, lack of precision in diagnosis can sometimes lead to effective treatment. Most often, however, incorrect diagnoses lead to incorrect decisions about treatment.

A. The diagnostic and statistical manual of mental disorders.

The *Diagnostic and Statistical Manual of Mental Disorders* (DSM) system is categorical (all or none), and inclusion depends on whether or not the patient has the minimum number of symptoms for a particular diagnosis; however, in reality, atypicality in presentation is common. For example, a person who has four of the symptoms used in defining major depression would not merit the diagnosis, no matter how severely depressed he or she actually is. In such a situation, the DSM system should be used as a set of expert guidelines, and a provisional diagnosis often must be made and treatment initiated when full criteria are not met (see Chapter 1).

No rules exist for easily remembering and recognizing all of the DSM syndromes. It is wise for the clinician to commit to memory a few sine qua non rules for the most common, troublesome, or hard-to-diagnose disorders. For example, in order to merit a diagnosis of major depression, a person must have one or the other of two symptoms: *depressed mood* (obvious and easy to remember) or *markedly diminished interest or pleasure in all or almost all activities* (called *anhedonia*—not as obvious). Nonetheless, knowing to ask about these two symptoms alone can guide the primary care physician in the identification of depression. A few rules of this kind can be invaluable.

B. Medication response.

Most psychotropic drugs are effective for more than one disorder, and most disorders respond to more than one drug. For example, the tricyclic antidepressants (TCAs) were discovered in the late 1970s to be beneficial for people with panic anxiety. Although controversy initially existed about whether or not this response was due to treatment of depression, perhaps because panic represented "masked" depression, most clinicians now believe this benefit is not dependent on the presence of coexisting depression. Further, panic is responsive not only to drugs from the antidepressant class, but also (among others) to benzodiazepines, drugs that do not improve depressed mood. Thus, just as in most other branches of medicine, the doctor must not only be an expert diagnostician, he or she must also know what medications treat what disorders. Simple appellations like *anxiolytic* or *antidepressant* are marketing terms that usually do not fully describe what the drugs in question treat. This is undoubtedly true both because these drugs often have multiple pharmacologic effects and because the pathophysiologies of the various disorders they are used to treat overlap.

Once a diagnosis has been made, will medication be helpful? This question has two answers: (1) most people improve if they have a well-defined syndrome that is known to be responsive to a given medication, and (2) one never knows for sure until one tries.

Additional helpful tips include

- If drug A helped the patient before, it should help him or her again (although sometimes not quite as much).
- If drug A helped a patient's close relative who

had the same problem, it is somewhat more likely than not to help the patient too.

- If the patient's symptoms are not classic, the patient's response often *will not* be either.
- The more diagnoses the patient has, the harder he or she is to treat.
- If the patient was hard to treat before, he or she will be again.

Other factors, such as nonadherence, are also important. However, no patient should be considered non-responsive to medication until all reasonable therapies have been given fully adequate trials. If the clinician feels uncomfortable raising a dose, giving a second-line drug, or using an appropriate drug combination, the patient should be referred to a clinician who is expert at these matters. *Patients who are labeled "treatment resistant" have likely received an incorrect diagnosis and/or an inadequate program of treatment trials—not enough medication and/or therapy given for too short a time. Patients from special populations, such as the young and old or the medically ill, often respond differently than the model patient. Aids to medication decisions are listed in Table 2–1.*

II. Medical disorders presenting as psychiatric problems: Implications for psychopharmacotherapy.

Many factors affect the likelihood of a disorder's being medical rather than psychiatric (Table 2–2; see also Chapter 1). For instance, the age of onset of an illness can provide the primary care physician with important information. Many psychiatric disorders, such as schizophrenia and the anxiety disorders, have their onsets in adolescence or early adulthood, an age when people are not exactly immune to medical illnesses but when illnesses are less probable than in older individuals. Thus, a disorder associated with anxiety symptoms in someone 22 years old is much more likely to be a primary anxiety disorder than a pheochromocytoma (especially because primary anxiety disorders are so much more common in general), whereas the new onset of a complaint of anxiety in a 53-year-old person should prompt a more vigorous search for an underlying medical cause. In this era of cost containment, it is not possible to evaluate every patient for all disorders associated with a given symptom. Making probabilistic judgments and refining the judgments over time as the symptoms change or respond to treatment form the necessary approach to diagnosis.

Data concerning the association of certain medical disorders with psychiatry symptoms are tentative. Contained in Table 2–3 are listings of medical illnesses that the literature most commonly indicates are associated with presenting symptoms of depression, anxiety, and psychosis. In addition to associated medical illnesses, medication classes are listed that are believed to produce such symptoms. The table is not intended to be completely inclusive, but it does contain most of the illnesses that should be considered.

III. General guidelines for psychopharmacotherapy.

A. Dose.

An emotionally distressed patient may abruptly discontinue treatment or stop taking medication if high doses are used initially and/or doses are quickly increased at the beginning of treatment. *The patient's demand for a quick fix needs to be balanced against the reality that emotionally distressed patients are frequently unwilling to tolerate temporary medication side effects and, with the exception of the benzodiazepines and psychostimulants, psychopharmacology efficacy develops over days or weeks—rushing the process usually causes problems.* Moreover, once a patient stops taking a medication because of its side effects, it is difficult to persuade the patient to ever try that medication again. If the patient unnecessarily experiences side effects and, as a result, does not take the same medication at lower doses, a possibly effective agent is discarded without any knowledge about the medication's efficacy if it had been used less aggressively.

We advocate the "go slow" approach. The foundation for this strategy is the assertion that the manufacturer's suggested initial dosing schedule was developed for subjects who volunteer for and are accepted in clinical drug

Table 2–1
Factors to Be Considered in Medication Choice

Efficacy	Benefit to be derived when the optimum dose and treatment duration has been used
Short-term side effects	Usually occur within the first day to week; most patients will develop some, but not complete, tolerance
Long-term side effects	Includes tardive dyskinesia from antipsychotic drugs
Abuse potential	Separate from development of pharmacologic tolerance and characterized by recreational use and withdrawal symptoms when drug therapy is discontinued
Patient acceptance	Including cost (especially availability of a generic preparation)
Alternative medications	What drugs are likely to be equally effective? Which drugs have side effects that are likely to benefit a concurrent medical problem?

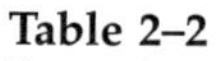

Table 2–2
Factors to Be Considered in Differentiating a Medical from a Psychiatric Disorder

Factor	Differentiating Characteristics
Age of onset	Onset in early adulthood or earlier usually favors the diagnosis of a primary psychiatric disorder.
Course and duration	Medical disorders are usually progressive and can usually be expected to develop symptoms inconsistent with a diagnosis of a primary psychiatric syndrome.
Family history	Many medical and many psychiatric disorders are familial; thus, a family history of many disorders raises the likelihood of that disorder in the proband.
Laboratory test results	Many medical disorders (e.g., thyroid disease) have characteristic laboratory findings.
Type of impairment	The clinical picture of typical associated impairments (e.g., joint pain in collagen vascular disease versus agoraphobic symptoms associated with panic attacks).
Past history	What a patient had before, he or she will likely have again.
Predisposing factors	For example, chest discomfort in an otherwise healthy 24-year-old woman is likely to be primary panic disorder, whereas the same symptoms in a 57-year-old man who has been a smoker is much more likely to have a cardiovascular origin.
Presence of stressors	Stressors are often hard to validly identify, but when they are clearly present, they are suggestive of a primary psychiatric syndrome.
Prevalence	Common things (e.g., depression) are common, whereas uncommon things (e.g., adrenal insufficiency producing only depression) are rarely seen.
Response to treatment	Anxiety-like symptoms that decrease in response to benzodiazepine treatment are less likely to be of cardiac origin than are symptoms that respond to nitroglycerin.

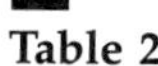

Table 2–3
Medical Disorders Thought to Cause Symptoms of Depression, Anxiety, or Psychosis

Disorder	Examples
Depression	
Anemia	Especially vitamin B_{12} deficiency—pernicious anemia
Cancer	Pancreatic, "oat cell" of the lung, ovarian, thyroid, paraneoplastic syndromes
Cardiovascular	Myocardial infarction, dysrhythmias
Chronic pain	Any form
Drug induced	Antihypertensives (methyldopa, clonidine, reserpine), levodopa, glucocorticoids, oral contraceptives, antineoplastics, sedatives, narcotics, digitalis, cimetidine, some of the antituberculous medications (see Table 2–9)
Endocrine	Cushing's syndrome, Addison's disease, hypothyroidism, "apathetic hyperthyroidism" (i.e., hyperthyroidism presenting clinically as an apathetic, slowed-down state; most common in the elderly), menopause
Infectious	AIDS, some viral syndromes (especially Epstein-Barr virus), tuberculosis, mononucleosis
Neurologic	"Pseudodementia," Parkinson's disease, stroke, temporal lobe pathology
Rheumatologic	Cerebral vasculitis (especially systemic lupus erythematosus)
Anxiety	
Cardiovascular	Any dysrhythmia, hypertension, hyperventilation, any cause of hypoxia, type A behavior pattern, mitral valve prolapse
Drug induced	Caffeine, psychostimulants, hallucinogens, steroids, sedative-hypnotic withdrawal, SSRIs (see Table 2–9)
Endocrine	Hyperthyroidism, hypoglycemia, pheochromocytoma, carcinoid, Cushing's syndrome, hypoparathyroidism, menstrual and menopausal associated disorders
Neurologic	Epilepsy, vestibular dysfunction
Other	Irritable bowel syndrome
Psychosis	
Delirium	Fluid and electrolyte abnormalities (see Chapter 3)
Drug induced	Chronic psychostimulants, hallucinogens, anticholinergics (see Table 2–9)

AIDS = acquired immunodeficiency syndrome; SSRI = selective serotonin reuptake inhibitor.

trials. Such subjects are free of known concurrent illnesses, have well-defined conditions, and have the emotional stamina to withstand placebo administration. Such patients are infrequent visitors to standard office practices. Because of these factors, we suggest strongly that the manufacturer's initial dose recommendation be cut in half or in quarter and that dosage be increased every 2 to 3 days as tolerated. For example, if the recommended starting dose of an antidepressant is 50 mg per day, therapy would be started at 12.5 mg for the first 2 to 3 days, followed by 25 mg, then 37.5 mg for a similar period thereafter; finally, at the end of 6 or 9 days, the patient is taking the manufacturer's recommended initial dose. Sometimes, such instructions do not fit on the prescription bottle or office samples are used; in this situation, it is necessary to provide the patient (and family, as appropriate) with written instructions. The patient may be told that he or she may increase the dosage faster or slower, depending on his or her side effect experience. This approach gives the patient the message that he or she has some control over both the situation and the experience of side effects and makes the patient a treatment partner.

Once the known lowest therapeutic dose is reached, it is necessary to wait for an expected effect before the dose is increased. In the case of antidepressants, an effect may not be noticed until 3 to 6 weeks have passed. If at the end of that time, there is no or minimal effect, the dose should be increased by use of the same slow increase. Intervals of slow dosage increases are repeated until one of two endpoints is reached: either the patient is improved and further gains are unlikely or the patient is intolerant of the side effects of the highest possible therapeutic dose of medication achieved by means of a slow increase in dose. Another medication trial is appropriate if further gains are thought to be likely or the patient becomes intolerant of side effects at some dose below the maximum known upper limit. For a particular patient, *a medication is judged to be ineffective only after the medication has been used at its maximum dose and for the longest time known to have resulted in a favorable response.* Because many medicines take weeks to be persuasively effective and effectiveness may become obvious only after several intervals of dose adjustment, the patient may take the medicine for months before an effect is seen. This is one of the most important reasons to be certain of the diagnosis before a psychoactive medicine is prescribed.

B. Baseline behaviors.

Target symptoms are recorded and tracked. Often, poor record keeping and an incomplete reassessment concludes that no improvement has occurred when, in fact, the patient has experienced some minimal, but favorable, changes. The importance of this assertion is illustrated by the following example and commentary.

Obviously, a medication is selected because it is expected to diminish the severity of identified target symptoms. The patient for whom a medication is prescribed returns to the office after several days of therapy, and, in the interim, many other patients have come and gone. When the patient returns and the patient record contains a short note like "patient moderately depressed; antidepressant started," the information is of little help. Although some patients can confidently say "I'm better," many are far less certain, and the practitioner needs to review a record of each original target symptom and look for changes that have occurred since the last visit. For example, if a patient is depressed and disturbed sleep is one target symptom, the doctor might best record: "every night, patient takes an hour or longer to fall asleep; wakes up at least three or four times per night and has difficulty falling back to sleep; always awake at 5:30 a.m. and cannot fall back to sleep." Emotionally distressed patients may not remember what they told the physician, and if sleep is still disturbed, the patient may simply report: "my sleep is still lousy." Yet, when sleep disturbance is reassessed in more detail, the patient may report: "Well, now that you force me to think about my sleep, I had two nights this last week when I seemed to fall asleep more quickly, and once I even woke up to my alarm!" In this case, the severity of the sleep target symptom is actually diminished, and this new state needs to be recorded. *Making the patient aware of even very small symptomatic changes gives the patient strong incentive to continue with the treatment.*

C. Gathering target symptom information.

The emotionally burdened patient is not necessarily the best source for accurate information. As the severity of mental illness increases, the quality and correctness of patient-provided descriptive information declines. Mental illness causes impaired concentration, perception, judgment, and other skills related to descriptive and explanatory accuracy. Consequently, the doctor must seek symptom descriptions from family and significant others. The following example will illustrate this point.

Continuing with our illustrative depressed patient, the doctor asks the patient, "Tell me about your appetite; have you lost or gained weight?" The patient answers, "As good as always; I always weigh the same." Depressed patients, even those with minimal apathy and social withdrawal, may ignore subtle changes. Moreover, if depression has been ongoing for some time, the patient may have so slowly acquired depressive symptoms that they are seen as normal or expected. However, when the spouse is asked, the following different description may be provided: He [or she] hasn't changed weight, but he [or she] is really less interested in food; I haven't heard a single request for a favorite dish lately; he [or she] seems to eat out of habit.

D. Medication selection.

If a medication was convincingly effective and tolerated before, it will most likely be effective again, even when newer agents are available. Older agents were discovered by chance and tend to have a lengthy profile of poorly tolerated side effects. Recent drug development strategies have yielded newer medications with a short list of better tolerated side effects. Generally, a newer agent is preferred over an older one.

A more refined medication selection decision seeks a medication with a side effect profile that might benefit any concurrent medical condition. For example, because the experience of pain is often improved by TCAs, a depressed patient with severe pain might improve the most with a well-tolerated TCA, such as nortriptyline (Pamelor). If nortriptyline is already being used at low doses for pain control, rather than add a newer antidepressant, it is reasonable to increase nortriptyline doses to therapeutic levels if a concurrent depression exists. (Unlike TCAs, at least one type of chronic pain problem, diabetic neuropathy, does not appear to benefit from selective serotonin reuptake inhibitors [SSRIs], and pain may not be very sensitive to SSRI treatment.) Table 2–4 provides a list of medical conditions and associated useful psychotropic agents. Unfortunately, no easy rules of thumb are available for the making of informed choices, and the doctor must rely on lists, which are provided at the end of this chapter.

Alcohol or other substance use confounds medication selection and associated treatment. Considerable overlap exists between symptoms of mental illness and symptoms of substance use. This confound is eliminated once substances are out of the body for weeks or months, depending on the substance. Accordingly, patients should be withdrawn from alcohol and/or other substances before beginning treatment for any suspected psychiatric diagnosis (e.g., depression). Patients claiming that a mental health problem causes them to use alcohol or other substances are best treated by substance abuse specialists.

E. Monotherapy or polypharmacy?

Polypharmacy is the concurrent use of two or more drugs, either of which can produce the same outcome. Mental conditions are best treated with a single agent to avoid having to contend with the actions and interactions of multiple medications and an unpredictable side effect profile. Given the correct diagnoses, monotherapy is expected to be effective across the entire symptom profile, whereas polypharmacy makes it impossible to identify the single agent most responsible for success or failure. Following this principle, a single antidepressant would be preferred for a patient with depression mixed with anxiety symptoms. For these reasons, we strongly discourage the use of agents that are combined and marketed as a single preparation (e.g., an antidepressant and an antipsychotic combined in a single tablet).

Not many years ago, polypharmacy was discouraged for all the aforementioned reasons. Although this is generally still true, it has become clear that some patients who do not improve on a single drug alone benefit from the use of appropriate drug combinations. Examples include augmentation of antidepressant drugs with lithium or thyroid hormone (liothyronine, or T_3) for treatment-resistant depression, addition of an antipsychotic to an antidepressant for psychotic depression, and combination of an antidepressant and a benzodiazepine for depression with substantial anxiety. Polypharmacy may be appropriate in some cases, but it should be used only when it is clearly indicated and after monotherapy has most surely failed.

Three exceptions exist to this general rule favoring monotherapy:

1. *Side effect minimization.*
   The patient may complain of side effects that are known to be temporary. For example, the SSRIs may increase arousal and activation and, consequently, may produce temporary insomnia. Under these circumstances, some clinicians prescribe a concurrent sleep-producing medication, such as trazodone (Desyrel), to be used until the patient has been taking a constant SSRI dose for 2 weeks; after this interval, it is good practice to discontinue the sleep medication. After all, sleep is a target symptom, and masking a sleep disturbance prevents a full assessment of response to antidepressant. *Sleep that remains disturbed is most often a symptom of continuing depression rather than a medication side effect.* Consequently, the doctor's appropriate response would be to increase the dose of antidepressant and consider further temporary use of a sleep aid.

   Because most psychiatric conditions are chronic or recurrent, medication management may extend over the patient's lifetime. This possibility is another reason to select a drug that best matches the patient's long-term, side effect tolerance. Sometimes, an effective agent without unpleasant side effects cannot be found. For example, some patients with manic depression can take only lithium, and unfortunately, lithium produces diarrhea in some patients.

Table 2–4
Psychotropic Drugs Useful for Common General Medical Conditions

Medical Condition	Psychiatric Drug	Comments
Agitation, especially in Alzheimer's and other dementias	Zolpidem (Ambien)	PRN or 2.5–5 mg t.i.d. as tolerated; anecdotal and author's (Knesper's) experience.
Agitation, severe restlessness, nonpsychotic	Trazodone (Desyrel)	Slow increase of trazodone dosage; watch for postural hypotension.
	Zolpidem	Zolpidem, 2.5–5 mg, may be used PRN or t.i.d.
	Buspirone (BuSpar) combined with neuroleptic (e.g., perphenazine [Trilafon])	Combination increases effect.
Arrhythmia, sustained tachycardia	Imipramine (Tofranil), other tricyclics prolong cardiac conduction time	For depressed cardiac patients. Of the tricyclics, imipramine has the most quinidine-like effect. Combined with other Type I-A antiarrhythmics, imipramine produces a paradoxic proarrhythmic effect.
Hepatic encephalopathy	Flumazenil (Romazicon)	May improve symptoms.
Nocturnal enuresis	Imipramine	25–100 mg; "nocturnal enuresis" applies to children 4–5 years of age.
HIV agitation, sleep disorder	Amitriptyline (Elavil) Trazodone (Desyrel)	Amitriptyline can be given IM (see Chapter 12).
Hypertension due to MAOI	Nifedipine (Procardia)	10–20 mg; bite capsule and swallow contents.
Orthostatic hypotension	Fluoxetine (Prozac)	20 mg for 6–8 wk may be effective for some patients who are refractory to, or intolerant of, other forms of therapy. Other SSRIs have been less studied.
Insomnia	Trazodone	Psychiatrist's first choice; monitor for postural hypotension, especially in elderly.
Migraine	Sumatriptan (Imitrex) + lithium Sumatriptan + monoamine oxidase inhibitor	Combinations may increase sumatriptan effect.
Migraine prophylaxis	Fluoxetine or other SSRI Nortriptyline (Pamelor) or other trycyclic	May be beneficial for some patients. SSRIs may cause or worsen migraines for some patients.
	Amitriptyline (Elavil) or other tricyclic Any SSRI	May benefit some patients.
Nausea	Neuroleptics Nortriptyline (Pamelor)	Chlorpromazine (Thorazine) is the most studied, but others have effect. Nortriptyline for nausea with chemotherapy.
Chronic pain	Amitriptyline Amphetamine (Dexedrine, Desoxyn) Clomipramine (Anafranil) Nortriptyline	Adjuncts to morphine; additive risk for respiratory depression and toxicity (see Chapter 15.)
Pruritis, urticara	Doxepin (Adapin)	Powerful antihistamine.
Vasovagal and carotid sinus syncope	Fluoxetine Sertraline (Zoloft)	Fluoxetine 20 mg or sertraline 50 mg for 4–6 weeks may be effective for some patients who are refractory to, or intolerant of, other forms of therapy.
Temperature elevation	Neuroleptics	Chlorpromazine is the most studied, but others have effect.
Terror, great fear of suffering (e.g., terminal cancer, ALS.)	Neuroleptics	Low dose of haloperidol (Haldol) or slow increase of molindone (Moban) dosage until desired effect or reach 100 mg/d of molindone.
Peptic ulcer disease	Doxepin	Compares favorably to traditional agents (e.g., cimetidine (Tagamet).

HIV, human immunodeficiency syndrome; MAOI, monoamine oxidase inhibitor; ALS, amyotrophic lateral sclerosis; PRN, as necessary; t.i.d., three times a day; IM, intramuscularly; SSRI, selective serotonin reuptake inhibitor.

Such patients may require the daily use of diphenoxylate-atropine (Lomotil).

2. *Augmentation.*
Augmentation (also known as combination strategy, or copharmacy) is considered when, over an extended time, a patient fails to respond or only partially responds to adequate therapeutic doses of a usually effective agent. A second drug is added in order to improve the therapeutic effect of the original agent. This strategy permits a full assessment of the potential usefulness of the original drug and may avoid another lengthy therapeutic trial in which an entirely new drug is used. For example, lithium is often used to augment an antidepressant in order to enable a person who is not responding or is only partially responding to treatment to have a more favorable mood state.

3. *Immediate symptom relief.*
Some symptoms are so incapacitating that rapid relief is desired and two agents are used. One drug is used during the initial treatment interval and only until a second drug becomes effective. For instance, panic attacks that occur many times each day may be treated with a combination of alprazolam (Xanax) and fluoxetine (Prozac). Alprazolam is usually quickly effective, but when it is used for more than 1 or 2 weeks, it produces dependence, interdose anxiety, and withdrawal symptoms. Fluoxetine causes none of these problems, but it may initially increase anxiety and requires at least a week to become effective. In this situation, alprazolam may be used for the first week or two of treatment, and thereafter the dosage can be decreased.

F. Maintenance, discontinuation, and prophylaxis.

Unless persuasive information to the contrary exists, all psychiatric conditions should be considered to be chronic, or recurrent, or both. Medical conditions like asthma, diabetes, or bowel dysmotility disorders have time and frequency courses that are quite similar to those of serious mental problems. Once a patient who has experienced a first and only episode of a mental disorder has returned to his or her normal functional state or further gains are unlikely, gains need to be maintained (i.e., maintenance therapy) by continuation of medical therapy at therapeutic doses for at least 6 months; a full year at therapeutic doses is reasonable, especially if the first episode was severe. Patients who have experienced three or more episodes of a serious mental illness should be considered for *lifetime maintenance* (i.e., prophylactic therapy). Prophylaxis also should be considered any time the episode of serious mental illness is comorbid with another serious mental or medical condition (e.g., when a depressed or psychotic patient fails to continue to take needed drugs or resumes heavy alcohol consumption).

When good reason exists for withdrawal of a psychiatric medication, abrupt discontinuation is to be avoided. A slow decrease may unmask early symptoms of the mental illness that provided the reason to use the drug in the first place. If such symptoms are unmasked, full therapeutic doses can be resumed before a full-blown illness develops. For many psychotropic agents, abrupt discontinuation has a high probability of producing a *withdrawal syndrome* that often is hard to distinguish from the original condition or that is debilitating because of an altogether different profile of symptoms. *A conservative rule of thumb is to withdraw a psychiatric medication over one quarter the number of days the drug was maintained at therapeutic levels. For example, if an antidepressant was maintained for 1 year, a slow decrease would take 3 months.*

G. Drugs are only one component of a comprehensive treatment plan.

Drug treatment is generally insufficient for a complete recovery. Usually, the onset of mental illness is associated with some stressful event in the patient's life. Any combination of counseling, skill building and training, education, social intervention, and psychotherapy is needed to deal with the emotional consequences of the acute stressful event and to give the patient new personal and social skills and a more functional and durable set of attitudes, beliefs, coping resources, and situation-response behaviors. In the treatment of depression and anxiety, for example, many nonpharmacologic techniques exist, such as cognitive behavior methods and in vivo desensitization, that have proven efficacy and potency. The patient who is able to adopt and meaningfully use a new or strengthened repertoire of strategies to more effectively deal with the consequences of medical illness and psychosocial stress is less susceptible to future emotional and behavioral dilapidation. In our opinion, *the use of behavioral change strategies is the most important part of a comprehensive treatment plan that has as its ultimate goal the prevention or minimization of the number and frequency of recurrences.*

Educating the patient, family, and significant others about the early warning signs and symptoms of relapse is critical. An educated patient can seek early intervention and thereby have the best possible chance of avoiding the worst consequences of the relapsed state.

It must also be acknowledged that in some quarters, prejudices exist against the use of medications in the treatment of mental disorders, despite the fact that their usefulness has been demonstrated beyond any reasonable doubt. The patient's welfare has to be more important than adherence or opposition to some abstract theory about how mental disorders arise or how they should be treated.

IV. What to tell the patient and family.

A. Information for the nonpregnant patient and family.

The examples in this section do not apply well to the treatment of paranoid or drug-seeking patients; they do apply to the treatment of severe mental illness in a legally competent and voluntary patient. Our approach is illustrative rather than prescriptive and allows the patient and doctor to become partners in care. Whenever possible, simple, straightforward language and explanations are used. Each point is written entirely as if the doctor were talking to the patient, family, and/or significant other.

1. *What is mental illness? What causes mental illness?*

   Mental illness is a brain disease caused by a change in brain chemistry, and right now you need a little help from chemistry, so I'm recommending you take some medicine that will help return your brain's chemistry to its usual state.

   The doctor may then go on to explain the particular disease, emphasizing the causal contributions from family history (genetics), risk factors (e.g., history of physical abuse, previous episode), and immediate past stressful events. If before the onset, the patient's own actions and behaviors made an obvious contribution, these should be acknowledged in such educational terms as "skill deficiency" caused perhaps by early personal traumas beyond his or her personal control (e.g., growing up in a family in which alcohol seemed more important than children). *The emphasis on skill deficiency (rather than on mental illness and its implications) lays the foundation for later counseling recommendations.* Obviously, patients may contribute to their own emotional difficulties, but it is important to place their actions within a larger system of inter-related events, to be optimistic about the potential for meaningful changes, and to avoid making moral judgments or statements about personality.

2. *Patient adherence.*

   Medicine we use for mental problems takes a lot longer to work than medicine we might use for, say, pneumonia. The medicine I'm recommending will go to work right away, but recovery will take some time, and it's really important for you to keep taking the medicine, even if you feel a little worse when you start. If you begin to feel a lot worse, please call me rather than stop taking the medicine.

3. *General side effects.*

   All medicines have side effects. Fortunately, there are now a lot of new medicines for mental problems that are much better tolerated than the older drugs were. The medicine I'm recommending has several common side effects.

   The doctor goes on to describe the most common and follows with:

   If you read about this medicine, you will see a long list of possible side effects that have been reported. These are much less common than the ones I mentioned. I can't go over them all. If you learn of a side effect that concerns you, let me know, and, of course, if you experience anything strange or unpleasant while taking the medicine, let me know right away.

   Many psychiatric medicines have side effects that either go away or become better tolerated over the initial phase of drug treatment. The patient should be so informed and asked to continue with the treatment through this phase.

4. *Sexual dysfunction.*

   Many psychiatric medications cause sexual dysfunction of some sort or another for a good number of patients. If you experience such a problem, you should tell me right away.

   Sometimes, the dysfunction disappears over time. Other times, remedies are used that are discussed in the later drug-specific subsections of this chapter.

5. *Alternative options.*

   It is often wise to offer the patient medication alternatives to educate and in order to gain patient compliance and cooperation. For example, the doctor might explain the differences between the SSRIs and an alternative with less potential for sexual side effects, such as bupropion (Wellbutrin). Although bupropion is largely devoid of sexual side effects, it is more stimulating, needs to be taken in divided doses separated by 6 hours, and has a higher risk for seizures (0.4%). A sustained-release form of bupropion (Wellbutrin SR) is now available (see section XIII). Of course, if the doctor has a preference or the patient is unable to participate in this fashion, the doctor should make one recommendation.

6. *Uptaper and possible switch to another medicine.*

   All psychiatric medicines are effective, but no one can predict the medicine that will best help you or whether you will experience intolerable side effects. It's important that we are truly certain that this medicine is not for you. I don't want to not use a medicine that will ultimately be helpful because of a temporary problem. So we are going to start with small doses and increase slowly; I'm going to ask you to try your very best to get through any side effects that you can stand.

7. *Duration of treatment.*

   Once the treatment begins to work, it's important to maintain success, so don't stop taking the medicine when you start to feel better. If you stop too soon, your symptoms will most likely return, and they may be tougher to treat the next time. You may need to continue taking this medicine for at least 6 months, maybe even a year or more. The good news is that some patients get so much better that they don't want to stop taking their medicine because they don't want to risk getting sick again.

B. Information for the pregnant patient and family.

Much of the information suitable for the nonpregnant patient is suitable for the pregnant patient. In addition, the following apply:

1. *Smoking and alcohol.*

Smoking, alcohol, and recreational drugs, such as cocaine, cause far more damage to the baby (fetus) than any psychiatric drug.

2. *Risks versus benefits.*

Even in the absence of reports of birth defects and changes in behavior after birth, not taking a drug has different consequences than taking a drug. We need to carefully weigh the consequences of taking and of not taking the drug and see which choice would be best.

Having said that, the doctor can use the following points to structure further discussion.

Rules of thumb and "discussion points" relevant to risks versus benefits:

a. If at all possible, avoid all drugs during the first trimester and especially during the first 4 to 10 weeks after conception, the time of highest risk for teratogenicity. If at all possible, decrease the dosage 2 weeks before estimated date of confinement (EDC). Use ultrasonography to monitor for high-probability birth defects.
b. "Use of a safe medicine does not equal use of no medicine during pregnancy."
c. "There is very little evidence that psychotropics taken during pregnancy cause behavioral problems at any point later in life; however, research about this subject is so limited that we cannot eliminate the possibility of neurobehavioral teratogenicity."
d. "We know more about older medicines because there has been more time to study them."
e. "Studies do not control for alcohol use, age, tobacco use, prenatal care, environmental toxins, and the like; accordingly, *if you are forced to assume some risk, minimize those factors under your control.*"
f. "All known psychotropics permeate the placental barrier."
g. The newborn undergoes substantial physiologic changes at a variable rate; hepatic enzyme systems are undeveloped; the concentration of drug excreted in breast milk is largely unstudied, but some quantity of drug can be assumed to appear in breast milk; *if the patient is taking psychotropics, a strong rationale must support breast feeding.*
h. "To date, the FDA has not approved any psychotropic drug for use during pregnancy or lactation."
i. *"The risks of untreated mental illness during pregnancy may be substantial.* These risks may include behaviors that limit prenatal care, are risky, lead to alcohol and/or street drug use, and result in poor mother-child attachment. *The risks from a severe behavioral disturbance are often far greater than the benefits gained by avoiding psychotropic medication."* Patients who are unlikely to use or benefit from alternatives to medication therapies (e.g., supportive counseling) are at increased risk. *Any decision has potential legal ramifications, making it essential to seek consultation when use of a high-risk drug is considered for a patient with mental illness of uncertain severity.*

Table 2–5 provides the FDA's risk categories for the common psychopharmacologic agents. We recommend that primary care physicians refer to this or similar lists during the decision-making process. Also see section XIII.

V. Answers to tough questions and fears about drugs.

A. Why does it take so long for the medicine to work?

When people have pneumonia, their chest hurts, their throat hurts, they cannot get out of bed; they are really sick. The right antibiotic goes to work right away, but it takes awhile to feel really better because the disease has done some damage to the lungs, and the body's overall response to pneumonia makes them feel sick and weak. Regardless of the antibiotic's effectiveness, time is needed to make repairs. It's the same way with medication for mental illness; there has been some "damage," and it takes time for repairs to happen, but a lot more time than pneumonia treated with antibiotics.

B. Is this drug going to control my mind?

It's really the other way around; the disease you have is changing and limiting your natural behavioral and thought patterns. The medicine returns your brain's chemistry to its natural balance. There are street drugs, like phencyclidine (PCP), that can make people do strange and very dangerous things. You're going to take some real medicine for a real medical problem.

C. Will this drug make me a walking zombie?

For this question, it is important to ask for a definition of "zombie." Most often, the reference is to the severely and chronically mentally ill who have been taking neuroleptic agents for years. The question may be answered with an educational statement. Sometimes, hangover-type symptoms or

Table 2–5
Common Psychotropic Drugs and Risk Categories During Pregnancy

Drug and Comments	Pregnancy Risk Categories				
	*A**	*B**	*C**	*D**	*X**
Alcohol >6 drinks/wk: abstinence is recommended					•
Amantadine (Symmetrel): teratogenic in animals			•		
Amphetamine (methamphetamine [Desoxyn]), dextroamphetamine (Dexedrine): neurobehavioral deficits suspected; should be avoided				•	
Anticholinergics used for side effects of neuroleptics (e.g., benzotropine [Cogentin]): caution is recommended			•		
Barbiturates, phenobarbital or barbital: not recommended				•	
Benzodiazepines: safety is not established; should be avoided; if necessary, lorazepam [Ativan] should be used as first choice					•
Alprazolam (Xanax), chlordiazepoxide (Librium), clorazepate (Tranxene), diazepam (Valium), halazepam (Paxipam), lorazepam (Ativan), oxazepam (Serax), prazepam (Centrax)			•		
Clonazepam (Klonopin)					
Estazolam (ProSom), flurazepam (Dalmane), quazepam (Doral), temazepam (Restoril), triazolam (Halcion)				•	
Beta-adrenergic blockers (e.g., nadolol [Corgard], propranolol [Inderal]): risk-benefit problem†			•		
Bromocriptine (Parlodel): risk-benefit problem†			•		
Bupropion (Wellbutrin): no human data are available		•			
Buspirone (BuSpar): no human data are available		•			
Calcium channel blockers: risk-benefit problem†			•		
Carbamazepine (Tegretol): likely teratogenic; should be avoided			•		
Chloral hydrate (Noctec): risk-benefit problem†			•		
Clonidine (Catapres): risk-benefit problem†			•		
Clozapine (Clozaril): there is limited experience with this agent		•			
Levodopa carbidopa (Sinemet): risk-benefit problem†; teratogenic in animals			•		
Lithium: risky but less risky than alternatives; suggest collaboration with a psychiatrist				•	
Methadone: suspected behavioral teratogen; should be avoided			•		
Methylphenidate (Ritalin): risk-benefit problem†			•		
Mirtazapine (Remeron): no human data are available			•		
Monoamine oxidase inhibitors: should be avoided regardless of FDA rating; teratogenic in animals			•		
Nefazodone (Serzone): no human data are available			•		
Neuroleptics: minimal risk exists; perphenazine (Trilafon) and trifluoperazine (Stelazine) pose the least teratogenic risk		•	•		
Olanzapine (Zyprexa): no human data are available			•		
Opioid antagonists: risk-benefit problem		•			
Pemoline (Cylert): no human data are available		•			
Pergolide (Permax): risk-benefit problem†		•			
Phenytoin (Dilantin): collaboration with a neurologist or psychiatrist should be suggested				•	
Risperidone (Risperdal): possibly teratogenic in one case report			•		
Selective serotonin reuptake inhibitors: limited data suggest they are safer than cyclic-tricyclics‡		•			
Selegiline (Eldepryl): risk-benefit problem†			•		
Trazodone (Desyrel): teratogenic in animals			•		
Tricyclics and cyclic antidepressants: no consistent evidence of congenital malformations or neonatal withdrawal exists; if used, nortriptyline (Pamelor) is authors' first choice					
Amitriptyline (Elavil), imipramine (Tofranil), nortriptyline (Pamelor)				•	
Amoxapine (Asendin), clomipramine (Anafranil), Desipramine (Norpramin), doxepin (Adapin), protriptyline (Vivactil), trimipramine (Surmontil)			•		
Maprotiline (Ludiomil)		•			

Table continued on opposite page

Table 2–5
Common Psychotropic Drugs and Risk Categories During Pregnancy *Continued*

Drug and Comments	Pregnancy Risk Categories A*	B*	C*	D*	X*
Valproate (Depakene), divalproex (Depakote): should be avoided				•	
Venlafaxine (Effexor): no human data are available			•		
Zolpidem (Ambien): no human data are available			•		

FDA, Food and Drug Administration.

*Pregnancy risk category A: controlled studies show no risk; category B: no evidence of risk in humans; category C: risk cannot be ruled out; category D: positive evidence of risk—may designate drugs with no safer alternatives; category X: contraindicated in pregnancy—designates drugs with substantial risk.

†Risk-benefit problem: the risks of untreated mental illness during pregnancy may be substantial; these may include limited prenatal care, risk-taking behaviors, drug use, poor mother-child attachment, and so on.

‡Recent evidence suggests that, when taken late in pregnancy, the SSRIs may increase the risk of premature delivery. These data remain controversial.

temporary side effects are of concern, and these cannot be avoided entirely. In this situation, the answer might be.

It's true that some medicine has side effects we'd rather avoid, but we get used to them. Lots of people take allergy medicine and feel sleepy for the first few days or even the first weeks of the allergy season. With time, they get accustomed to these side effects and can go about their business as usual.

If more severe side effects are being discussed:

For any serious illness, drugs may be required that make people feel uncomfortable; it's the price you may need to pay for getting better. But once you are better, there will be ways to reduce the side effects you may experience.

D. Can't I just go on a vacation or go to counseling and skip the drug part of treatment?

(It is assumed that the patient's condition is so severe that drugs are a necessary part of an overall treatment plan.)

Let's talk about these options one at a time. There is no question that removing yourself from particularly stressful circumstances will bring you some relief. You would feel *temporarily* better, but your condition is such that you likely won't feel much better, and even if you feel somewhat better, your symptoms will likely recur and may even get worse. As for the second part of your question, drugs will allow you to better participate in counseling or make use of the talking therapies. Counseling may help you make some lifestyle changes that will bring more permanent relief, and they may help you avoid any unwise and irrevocable decisions. The very best solution is to combine everything; take some time off if you can, start the medicine, and get started with a counselor.

The severity of the symptoms determines the use of a doctor's letter in support of time off work. However, *once the patient insists on an extended leave of absence, we suggest that a psychiatrist be involved.* In 1994, all employers with 15 or more employees became affected by the Americans with Disabilities Act. Part of the definition protecting individuals with a record of a disability explicitly addresses a person who is recovering from or who has recovered from a mental illness. Consequently, a reduced, less stressful workload can now be more easily combined with a comprehensive mental illness treatment plan. Both the doctor and the patient need to be informed of the provisions of this act.

E. If I tell my employer about my mental problem, will I be fired?

Unfortunately, this sort of discrimination is still with us. It is also with us for serious medical illnesses in general. For example, the patient who has had a serious heart attack may somehow be passed up for a promotion and be given less meaningful work to do. The following answer may prove to be helpful:

Your mental illness is probably already interfering with your work; you may be unaware of the symptoms your employer has noticed (and the patient has mentioned some symptoms that the doctor can list). It is better for your employer to know that you are being responsible and have a medical explanation for your performance rather than allow your employer to think that you have become lazy or unmotivated. With an explanation, your employer may be able to even help, especially if it is known that you will recover and even stay recovered (as in depression). You can tell your employer that you are taking medicine that may take some time to work. Then, your employer will know that something very helpful is being done. Moreover, the Americans with Disabilities Act specifically protects you (depending on the size of the business). Here is some reading material about the act.

VI. Medication treatments for mood and anxiety disorders.

A. Overview.

The correct diagnosis is essential because different diagnoses call for different medications and because a given diagnosis is a predictor of how a patient will respond to one medication versus another. Other important general issues follow.

1. *How much improvement to expect and with what dose of antidepressant.*
It is atypical for a patient to have all symptoms completely resolve in response to treatment, and thus this is not a reasonable goal. On the other hand, it is not appropriate to be satisfied with a response that is not substantial. As a general guideline, a patient should be at least 50%, and hopefully 75% improved, for a particular treatment program to be considered successful. All antidepressant drugs take at least 2, and sometimes as much as 6, weeks for full benefit to be realized; sometimes, patients show continued improvement even beyond the 6-week time. Further, differences exist between individuals in what constitutes a full therapeutic dose. The most reasonable approach is to assume that most patients will need full doses and that full doses should be prescribed (with a gradual increase in order to foster development of some tolerance to side effects), unless side effects abort this approach. The most common cause of treatment resistance is subtherapeutic doses. The 6-week "clock" does not start until the full dose is reached.

2. *The "neurotransmitter continuum" and antidepressants.*
All medications known to be effective in the treatment of depression affect serotonin and/or norepinephrine (by inhibiting metabolism, monoamine oxidase inhibitors [MAOIs] also affect these systems). The TCAs all affect norepinephrine; some of them have a significant effect on serotonin as well. The SSRIs, as their group name implies, have direct effects only on serotonin (although, of course, they might have secondary effects mediated through serotonin on other systems as well). Therefore, when a patient does not respond to therapeutic doses of an SSRI, it is reasonable to switch to TCA because TCAs affect neurotransmitter systems other than the serotonin system. When this substitution is made, SSRIs can raise the blood concentration of TCAs; consequently, there needs to be a washout period for the SSRI before the TCA dosage is increased.

3. *Hidden antidepressant side effects.*
Patients readily describe some antidepressant side effects—for example, excessive sedation and dry mouth. Others, patients are sometimes reluctant to mention. For example, almost all of the antidepressant drugs cause disturbances of sexual functioning, including both impaired sexual performance and decreases in libido. Because side effects are a problem by themselves and also because they contribute to nonadherence to therapy, relevant inquiry should take place frequently. Furthermore, patients themselves are not necessarily aware of some detrimental hidden effects, and these effects can be difficult for the clinician to discern as well. For example, it is difficult to determine whether a patient at risk for bipolar disorder has experienced a switch from depression to hypomania in response to antidepressant drug treatment or is just experiencing a return to baseline mood. This is especially difficult to determine when the patient has been depressed for a long time and cannot reliably discriminate between attainment of normal mood and hypomania. *Patients starting antidepressant therapy should be warned about the possibility of a switch from depression to a manic state and to contact the doctor whenever the patient or family suspects this change of mental state.*

4. *Treatment resistance.*
The major cause of resistance is lack of response to a usually effective antidepressant regimen, but other causes are equally important. These causes include incorrect diagnosis, nonadherence, and delivery of a less-than-optimal treatment regimen (e.g., a dose that is too low or, less frequently, a duration that is less than 4 to 6 weeks). When a treatment has truly failed, alternatives include medication augmentation or change to another antidepressant.

B. Medications for mood disorders.

1. *Selective serotonin reuptake inhibitors.*
Selective serotonin reuptake inhibitors have become the most popular antidepressants, partly because of their more benign side effect profile and partly because of their apparent usefulness in a wide variety of disorders, including depression, anxiety disorders, and eating disorders. There is no evidence, however, that as antidepressants, SSRIs are more effective than either TCAs or MAOIs, and some experienced clinicians believe that more severely depressed patients respond more frequently and more fully to TCAs. The first SSRI introduced in the United States was fluoxetine (Prozac), and thus there is more experience with this SSRI than with the others. Fluoxetine has a longer half-life than the other SSRIs and inhibits the metabolism of many other drugs. Therefore, when fluoxetine is combined with some other medications, the physician must determine if it is necessary to decrease the dose of the other drug (see sections IX and X). *Among the available SSRIs, inhibition of the metabolism of other drugs appears to be least likely with sertraline (Zoloft), making it a preferred agent for use in the medically ill.* Fluoxetine also has mild stimulant-like effects in some individuals; in these people, it should be administered in the morning. Other SSRIs seem to have less stimulant effect, and some are somewhat sedating (indeed, even fluoxetine is sedating in some patients). Paroxe-

tine (Paxil) has a small anticholinergic effect that may become meaningful at doses greater than the 20-mg starting dose. *An SSRI is a reasonable first-choice antidepressant in any patient who is not expected to respond specifically to some other antidepressant* (e.g., because of prior responsiveness or family history of responsiveness). Fluvoxamine (Luvox) is another SSRI that has recently appeared. It is approved by the FDA for use in obsessive-compulsive disorder, but it undoubtedly has antidepressant effects as well.

2. *Tricyclic antidepressants.*
Tricyclic antidepressants were the most commonly used antidepressants before the SSRIs were introduced in the late 1980s. Examples of TCAs are imipramine (Tofranil), amitriptyline (Elavil), desipramine (Norpramin), and nortriptyline (Pamelor). The first two agents have a tertiary amine chemical structure, and the other two have a secondary amine structure. This difference is important because the tertiary amines are metabolized to the secondary (e.g., imipramine to desipramine and amitriptyline to nortriptyline), meaning that if a tertiary amine is administered, the result is a blood level for both the tertiary and the secondary metabolite. Drugs from the secondary amine group are generally better tolerated and have a preferential effect on the norepinephrine system (whereas the tertiary group affects both norepinephrine and serotonin). Nortripyline has a therapeutic window, in which improvement correlates with blood levels of 50 to 150 ng/mL. Clomipramine (Anafranil), a drug used principally for obsessive-compulsive disorder, is a tertiary TCA.

Various laboratory tests, such as electrocardiography and liver function tests, are potentially useful before TCA therapy is begun. (The same could be said for most medications.) It could be argued that comprehensive (including defensive) medical practice dictates that such tests should always be performed; however, this does not seem practical, because of decreasing reimbursement for disputably routine tests. Furthermore, it is not necessary or appropriate. Tests should be performed when circumstances dictate (e.g., known history of cardiovascular disease, patient age of 40 to 50 years old or older), and the clinician must vigilantly determine when such circumstances are present before the initiation of medication. Additionally, should a patient's medical condition change during treatment, laboratory testing may be indicated.

Tricyclic antidepressants have many side effects. Probably the most common side effect is dry mouth. Other common effects are sedation, constipation, and orthostatic hypotension. Hypotension is probably the most common serious side effect; it leads to noncompliance, especially in the elderly. In overdose, the most serious side effect is dysrhythmia; TCAs have quinidine-like effects on the cardiac conduction system.

Like SSRIs, TCAs can be considered "broad-spectrum" psychotropic drugs and, as previously mentioned, have benefits for many disorders, including enuresis and chronic pain. The most commonly used TCA for pain is amitriptyline, but the other TCAs, such as nortriptyline, seem to be beneficial as well and are preferable for patients made uncomfortable by amitriptyline's highly sedating and strong anticholinergic effects. The TCAs with the most benign side effect profiles appear to be desipramine and nortriptyline, although desipramine has stimulant effects that are problematic especially for some patients with significant anxiety symptoms and may be the most cardiotoxic in overdose.

3. *Atypical antidepressants.*
Many antidepressant drugs introduced in the 1970s and 1980s are referred to as "atypical antidepressants" because they do not have the chemical structure of a TCA. Three are noteworthy here. First, trazodone (Desyrel) has been found to be useful as a sedative as well as an antidepressant and has gained popularity for use as a hypnotic agent both because it does not produce rapid tolerance and it is effective for a longer period of time than other sedative drugs (≥ 5 weeks). The second drug is bupropion (Wellbutrin). It is well tolerated, and it appears to be less likely to cause a bipolar patient to convert from depression to mania. Among the antidepressants, bupropion least affects sexual function. Finally, amoxapine (Asendin) has a metabolite that has antipsychotic effects, and, thus, this drug is claimed to be good for patients with psychotic depression. Like most antipsychotic drugs, amoxapine may produce symptoms of parkinsonism and related movement abnormalities as well as tardive dyskinesia. For these and related reasons, the authors recommend caution when using amoxapine.

4. *Monoamine oxidase inhibitors.*
Monoamine oxidase inhibitors are usually used as second-choice antidepressant drugs. Nonetheless, they are useful first-choice medications for appropriate patients. MAOIs seem to be particularly useful for "atypical" depression, including that with symptoms of mood reactivity, rejection sensitivity, leaden anergia (loss of energy and interest in things), hypersomnia, and hyperphagia (SSRIs are also thought to be particularly useful in this group). Although a great deal of concern exists about food-related hypertensive crises, hypotension is a less severe but much more common problem. Fur-

ther, sexual side effects are common with these drugs (approximately 20%).

5. *Venlafaxine (Effexor) and nefazodone (Serzone).* New drugs are constantly being introduced; some are very similar to drugs already available, whereas others are unique. Although some of the chemically unique drugs do not offer any novel clinical benefit, others are true advances. Two recently introduced drugs for depression are venlafaxine and nefazodone.

   Nefazodone is an antidepressant that is chemically similar to trazodone, but it has fewer side effects. It mainly affects the serotonin system, weakly blocking reuptake and functioning as an antagonist at 5-HT_2 receptors. Usual doses are 300 to 600 mg/d, and lower and higher doses are apparently less efficacious. In other words, similar to the TCA nortriptyline, this drug appears to have a therapeutic window.

   Venlafaxine is chemically unique as an antidepressant. Pharmacologically, its main effects are reuptake inhibition of both serotonin and norepinephrine. Thus, it's effect on monoamine systems is similar to that of the tertiary amine TCAs, a more broad spectrum than either the secondary TCAs (primary effect on norepinephrine) or the SSRIs (effect on serotonin reuptake). For this reason, some psychiatrists believe that venlafaxine is useful in cases in which other antidepressants have failed. Of special importance, higher-dose treatment with venlafaxine (≥300 mg/d), produces blood pressure increases. The increase is usually clinically insignificant unless the patient already has a tendency to be hypertensive.

6. *Lithium.*
   Lithium is a first-choice drug for the prophylaxis of mania and hypomania and for the acute treatment of hypomania (for full mania, the addition of an antipsychotic is usually required). Lithium has also been used for the prophylaxis of depression in patients with bipolar disorder, but its efficacy for this purpose remains controversial. Prophylactic blood levels are from 0.7 to 1.0 mEq/l, whereas levels for treatment of an active episode are 0.8 to 1.3 mEq/L. Typically, it takes at least a week, and usually 2 to 4 weeks, for benefit to occur. Lithium has a low therapeutic index, with the toxic level being only 1.5 to 2.0 times the therapeutic level, and lethal levels are 3.0 to 5.0 times the therapeutic level. Older individuals may develop confusion when given dosages at the high end of the therapeutic range. Acute toxicity is first indicated by gastrointestinal symptomatology and tremor. Indeed, mild nausea and tremor are common, even at therapeutic levels, as is increased urination (which can be specifically benefited by the diuretic amiloride [Midamor]). Long-term effects include effects on the thyroid and the kidney. Lithium can produce thyroid gland enlargement and mild hypothyroidism. Periodic thyroid-stimulating hormone determinations (every 6 to 12 months) should be obtained. Whether the effect of lithium on the kidney is detrimental is controversial. We believe that a very small number of people who receive long-term lithium therapy experience decreases in glomerular filtration rate. As with thyroid-stimulating hormone, plasma creatinine levels should be determined every 6 to 12 months, but the clinician should remember that significant damage can occur before plasma creatinine increases and that 24-hour urinary creatinine clearance is a more sensitive test of early changes.

7. *Anticonvulsants and calcium channel blockers.*
   In addition to lithium, other drugs have been found to be beneficial for bipolar disorder. For both acute treatment and prophylaxis, considerable evidence indicates that the anticonvulsant drugs divalproex sodium (Depakote) and carbamazepine (Tegretol) are beneficial and that carbamazepine may be as effective as lithium. Although it is common practice to be guided by the blood levels appropriate for use as anticonvulsants, blood levels for this use of these drugs in bipolar disorder have not been established. Although calcium channel blockers, such as verapamil (Calan), have been tried, this class of drugs has less predictable benefit for bipolar disease.

D. Treatment of side effects associated with the use of antidepressants.

Often, tolerance develops to antidepressant side effects observed at the onset of treatment. If the side effect is more than mild and tolerance does not develop, use of an alternative antidepressant is often the preferred strategy. There are standard treatments for psychotropic side effects, such as the use of various medications to control TCA-associated constipation. The recommended treatments for the other, more common, side effects follows.

1. *Anticholinergic effects of tricyclics.*
   Peripherally acting cholinergic drugs, such as bethanechol (Urecholine), have been used; these should be avoided if any chance of outlet obstruction from, for example, an enlarged prostate exists.

2. *Hypotension from tricyclics.*
   Salt supplementation and mineralocorticoids (e.g., fludrocortisone acetate [Florinef]) have also been used to treat TCA-induced hypotension, but at the risk of aggravating congestive heart failure. Yohimbine has been studied as an antidote to TCA-induced hypotension; this strategy is not standard and should be used cautiously.

3. *Sexual dysfunction.*
All too often, sexual dysfunction is a continuing complaint about antidepressant use. Bupropion (Wellbutrin) is the only antidepressant that produces almost no sexual dysfunction. This advantage has become more important because bupropion is now available for twice-a-day dosing. The new antidepressant nefazodone (Serzone) is reported to have no sexual side effects. About one third or more of patients taking SSRIs report sexual dysfunction.
If sexual dysfunction persists after about 6 weeks, counteractive therapies are sometimes useful. Yohimbine has been studied as an acute treatment for sexual dysfunction associated with TCAs and SSRIs. Yohimbine (5.4 mg) usually hastens erections about 1 hour after a dose and may consequently improve the patient's overall sexual experience; however, yohimbine often produces rhinorrhea and feelings of anxiety and can induce hypertension. Cyproheptadine (Periactin), 2 to 4 mg 1 hour before intercourse, may improve delayed ejaculation, but cyproheptadine must be used sparingly because it causes sedation and is an antiserotonin drug and can reduce the effectiveness of an SSRI. Delayed orgasm and anorgasmia may respond to amantadine (Symmetrel), given at 100 to 200 mg/d for 3 or more days. The addition of low-dose bupriopion to SSRI therapy may improve sexual performance.

4. *Lithium tremor.*
Benzodiazepines and beta blockers (e.g., 10 to 20 mg of propranolol [Inderal]) 2 to 4 times a day) have been used to control the tremor associated with lithium.

5. *Lithium polyuria.*
The diuretic amiloride (Midamor) has been used to reverse polyuria caused by lithium therapy. Amiloride therapy is started at 5 mg twice a day; at dosages greater than 10 mg twice a day, no further benefit exists.

E. Anxiety disorders.

All of the antidepressant drugs have also been demonstrated by clinical experience to be useful in the treatment of anxiety. Other drugs are also available for the treatment of anxiety. The primary drugs used are the benzodiazepines and buspirone, which are not antidepressants.

1. *Benzodiazepines.*
Benzodiazepines are very widely used as antiepileptics, muscle relaxants, sedative-hypnotics, and anxiolytics. Although some differences exist between the available benzodiazepines, primarily in metabolism and pharmacokinetics, they are all more similar than different. Concerning metabolism, the most important difference is the fact that some of the drugs—oxazepam (Serax), lorazepam (Ativan), and temazepam (Restoril)—are metabolized in the liver by low-affinity, high-capacity conjugation pathways. These pathways often remain active in various types of liver disease. Accordingly, the aforementioned agents are favored for use in individuals with liver disease, such as alcoholic damage. Unlike the antidepressants, benzodiazepines act on first administration rather than after many days of administration. Also, unlike the medications discussed so far, these drugs do not act through serotonergic or noradrenergic mechanisms. Rather, they interact with gamma-aminobutyric acid, an inhibitory neurotransmitter that is widely distributed in the brain.
A major issue in the use of benzodiazepines has been concern about the potential for abuse. It is clear that these drugs produce tolerance and withdrawal if discontinued abruptly. These problems are associated with dose and duration. Although this controversy continues, it seems clear that most people given these medications do not abuse them. Data suggest that the only clear predictor of benzodiazepine abuse is history of prior drug abuse.
The other issue concerns efficacy with long-term use of benzodiazepines. *It is well documented that people become tolerant to the sedative-hypnotic effects of these medications within 2 to 3 weeks or less. On the other hand, it appears that patients might not become tolerant to the antianxiety effects of these drugs over many months.* This finding suggests that the sedative-hypnotic and the antianxiety effects of benzodiazepines are mediated by different mechanisms.

2. *Buspirone (BuSpar).*
Buspirone is an antianxiety drug that is not a benzodiazepine. It has a benign side effect profile and seems not to have abuse potential. Buspirone's antianxiety effect seems to be mediated by actions mediated by serotonin. Because of the benign side effects, buspirone is a reasonable first-choice anxiolytic. However, many patients do not derive substantial benefit from this medication. Moreover, effects are most apparent after at least 1 to 2 months of use. Thus, clinicians should be prepared to use an alternative drug if the patient has not improved after that amount of time or if the patient is not willing to give this medication a trial of adequate duration. Buspirone has no use in alcohol withdrawal syndromes because it lacks cross-reactivity with alcohol; it also lacks cross-reactivity with benzodiazepines, and buspirone is not an anticonvulsant.

VII. Psychosis.

Psychosis is strictly defined as the presence of delusions or hallucinations, but the term may be used to describe gross impairments in thought and reality testing. Psychosis can occur as the primary manifestation of a mental disorder (as in schizophrenia), as a feature of a subtype of a disorder (as in psychotic depression), as a complication of another neuropsychiatric or medical disorder (as in psychosis complicating dementia or brain tumor), or as a manifestation of drug toxicity (as in cocaine-induced psychosis). Unlike symptoms such as depression and anxiety, which almost always produce distress and discomfort for a patient who then seeks treatment, psychosis can so distort a patient's perception of self and environment that he or she is unaware of the need for treatment. Sometimes, the patient's behavior is disruptive to those around him or her, but the patient may have no insight into this fact. Hence, the standard "therapeutic contract" used for competent patients is frequently modified for the treatment of psychotic patients, and families and other social support systems may need to be more involved than in other clinical situations.

A. Neuroleptics.

The mainstay of pharmacotherapy for psychosis lies with a group of agents called neuroleptics. These agents, which were first introduced in the early 1950s, revolutionized the treatment of severe mental disorders, particularly schizophrenia. The neuroleptics have varying chemical structures, but most share the property of significant potency in blocking the D_2 dopamine receptor, a subtype of brain dopamine receptor. Blockade of this receptor is thought to be partly responsible for both the therapeutic antipsychotic effects of these drugs (diminuition or resolution of symptoms of psychosis) and their motor side effects, extrapyramidal symptoms. Other major side effects of these drugs include orthostatic hypotension, sedation, and anticholinergic effects. With the exception of clozapine (Clozaril) noted below, all neuroleptics appear to be equally efficacious in producing antipsychotic effect, but they differ as to potency and side effects. *A rule of thumb that is useful in prescribing this class of drugs is as follows: the low-potency agents, such as chlorpromazine (Thorazine) and thioridazine (Mellaril) are effective in the 200 to 600 mg/d range and are more sedating, more anticholinergic, more likely to produce orthostatic hypotension, and less likely to produce extrapyramidal symptoms, whereas the high-potency agents, such as haloperidol (Haldol) and fluphenazine (Prolixin) are effective in the 2 to 20 mg/d range and are less sedating, less anticholinergic, less likely to produce orthostatic hypotension, and more likely to produce extrapyramidal symptoms.* Agents of midrange potency are intermediate in their side effect profiles. We suggest the practitioner become familiar with the use of at least one high-potency and at least one low-potency agent and one in the midrange. For example, perphenazine (Trilafon) is effective in the 8 to 24 mg/d range; trifluoperazine (Stelazine) is effective in the 10 to 40 mg/d range. Many neuroleptics are available in tablet and liquid forms, and some are available in parenteral forms. Oral dosing is most commonly used for in-patient and out-patient treatment. Fluphenazine and haloperidol are available in long-acting parenteral depot formulations for use in patients receiving maintenance therapy and/or for those for whom long-term compliance may be a problem.

1. *Principles of neuroleptic therapy.*
   Because neuroleptics have significant (and in the case of tardive dyskinesia, potentially irreversible) side effects, it is of utmost importance that these agents be used only when indicated. With very few exceptions, *they should be used only if the presence of psychotic symptoms has been established.* Neuroleptics are sometimes used nonspecifically for their antiagitation properties.

   In the initiation of therapy, the physician must remember that as with antidepressant agents, the *full antipsychotic benefit may not be obtained for days to weeks, but the major side effects occur more acutely after dosing.* This fact may be used to advantage in the case of sedating (low-potency) agents when they are used in psychosis with severe agitation. Neuroleptics can produce significant anticholinergic and cardiovascular side effects that may be of serious consequence, particularly in the elderly. *Low-dose haloperidol (Haldol) is arguably the safest of the neuroleptics for use in the medically ill elderly.*

   The half-life of all the neuroleptics is long enough to allow a single daily dose to be effective; however, if both therapeutic effects and side effects are to be more evenly distributed, it is often desirable or necessary to prescribe neuroleptics in divided doses. Because the major side effects of neuroleptics are dose dependent, patients should be treated with the minimum effective dose. Plasma levels are generally of no use in routine clinical practice because *plasma levels are not correlated well with clinical response. Objective clinical monitoring of target symptoms continues to be used for the assessment of drug efficacy.*

2. *Management of neuroleptic-induced side effects.*
   The major extrapyramidal side effects of neuroleptics include the following.
   a. *Acute dystonia.*
      This reaction typically occurs in the musculature of the head and neck, producing a torticollis-like picture, but it can occur with other muscle groups. This reaction occurs most commonly in young men in the first few days of treatment with a high-potency neuroleptic, such as haloperidol. The treatment is immediate parenteral administration of an anticholinergic agent, such as 2 to 4 mg benztropine (Cogentin), intramuscularly or intravenously, or 50 mg of diphenhydramine (Benadryl), intramuscularly or intravenously; the response is immediate. This reaction usually indicates an overall

sensitivity to the extrapyramidal side effects of neuroleptics, and so continued treatment usually requires the aforementioned strategies.

b. *Akathisia.*
This is a syndrome of subjective motor restlessness, characterized by inability to sit or stay in the same position for an extended time. *When severe, akathisia can be confused with the agitation that may be part of the psychotic syndrome, rather than understood as a side effect of the therapy.* Akathisia often responds, like other subacute extrapyramidal symptoms, to dosage reduction and/or anticholinergic therapy. In addition, low doses of beta-blocking agents, such as 10 to 30 mg of propranolol (Inderal) three times a day or 40 to 80 mg/d of nadolol (Corgard) given as a single dose, or short-acting benzodiazepines such as 1 mg of lorazepam (Ativan) three times a day can be effective in cases in which anticholinergic agents are minimally effective. None of these agents affect other extrapyramidal symptoms.

c. *Parkinsonian signs and symptoms.*
Typical symptoms are coarse tremor, rigidity, and bradykinesia, all similar to those seen in idiopathic Parkinson's disease. These side effects can be managed by dosage reduction, switching to a lower-potency agent or addition of an anticholinergic agent, such as 1 to 2 mg of benztropine (Cogentin) twice a day or 1 to 3 mg of trihexiphenidyl (Artane) three times a day. In some cases, the prodopaminergic agent amantadine (Symmetrel) at 100 mg two or three times a day will relieve neuroleptic-induced parkinsonian side effects; however, this agent may also worsen psychotic symptoms.

d. *Tardive dyskinesia.*
This is a long-lasting movement disorder that occurs in 10% to 20% of patients who receive neuroleptics for more than 1 year, although it can occur after briefer periods of therapy. *Unlike other extrapyramidal symptoms, TD is equally likely to occur with low-potency and high-potency antipsychotics.* TD can include a variety of abnormal involuntary movements of the mouth, trunk, and extremities. The risk of developing TD is increased with increasing duration of therapy, neuroleptic dosage, and age of patient. Although previously thought to be permanent, even after drug discontinuation, evidence now indicates that *many patients experience a remission of TD symptoms if neuroleptics can be discontinued, particularly early after the development of TD.* No proven efficacious treatment exists for established TD; hence, we make the strong recommendation to use neuroleptics only when they are clearly indicated and in minimum effective dose. Neuroleptic therapy in chronic psychotic illnesses, such as schizophrenia, may need to be continuous; for many other indications (e.g., mania, psychotic depression, behavioral disturbance in dementia), it is important to continue neuroleptic therapy for only as long as is indicated, so as to reduce the risk of TD.

e. *Neuroleptic malignant syndrome.*
This is a rare but potentially life-threatening idiosyncratic side effect of neuroleptic therapy. It can occur under any circumstances, but it is *most likely in young men receiving high doses of high-potency agents.* The syndrome is characterized by muscle rigidity, fever that may be high, autonomic instability, and fluctuating levels of consciousness. Associated laboratory findings include (most commonly) creatine phosphokinase level increases as well as increases in hepatic transaminase levels, leukocytosis and myoglobinemia and myoglobinuria, that may be associated with acute renal failure, especially in patients who are also dehydrated. Mortality can be as high as 30% in untreated or inadequately treated cases, but it is lower with adequate treatment. Treatment includes discontinuation of neuroleptics and aggressive supportive fluid, body temperature, and cardiovascular management. Agents that have been used successfully to treat this syndrome include the dopamine agonist bromocriptine (Parlodel) beginning at 2.5 mg orally three times a day and increasing as tolerated to 5 to 10 mg orally three times a day; even higher doses have been recommended for more severe neuroleptic malignant syndrome. Treatment may include the concurrent use of the skeletal muscle relaxant dantrolene (Dantrium) starting at 1 to 3 mg/kg/d, orally or intravenously in four divided doses; hepatotoxicity is more likely at dosages exceeding 10 mg/kg/d. However, dosages of dantrolene for this indication have not been well established. For additional symptomatic relief, an intermediate-acting benzodiazepine like lorazepam (Ativan) may be added to this protocol.

f. *Other neuroleptic-induced side effects.*
These effects include hyperprolactinemia, photosensitivity that usually requires routine use of sunscreen for affected patients, and benign pigmentation of the retina, cornea, lens, and conjunctiva. *However, doses of thioridazine (Mellaril) greater than 800 mg/d produce pigmentary retinopathy and irreversible degenerative changes and potential blindness; thioridazine should never be used at dosages greater than 800 mg/d.*

B. Atypical neuroleptics: clozapine (Clozaril) and risperidone (Risperidal).

Over the past decade, there has been increasing effort to develop agents with antipsychotic properties but lacking extrapyramidal side effects. All these drugs are "atypical" because of their lower incidence of disabling extrapyramidal symptoms. Clozapine is the first of these new agents to become available in the United States.

Clozapine has a low incidence of extrapyramidal symptoms (including TD); this is thought to arise from its low affinity for brain D_2 dopamine receptors, unlike the typical neuroleptics. Clozapine's antipsychotic effects appear to arise in part from its actions on other dopamine and serotonin receptor systems in the brain. In addition to clozapine's lack of motor side effects, in doses ranging from 200 to 900 mg/d, *clozapine has been shown to be effective in reducing psychotic symptoms in about one third of schizophrenic patients who have not responded to traditional neuroleptic therapy.* Common dose-related side effects of clozapine include sedation, orthostatic hypotension, sialorrhea, and often significant anticholinergic symptoms. Seizures can occur at therapeutic doses but are more common at higher doses. Patients may experience transient high fevers, unrelated to neuroleptic malignant syndrome, that remit with continued clozapine use. The use of clozapine has been limited by its capacity to produce bone marrow suppression and potentially life-threatening agranulocytosis in 1% to 2% of treated patients, necessitating weekly blood count monitoring throughout the course of treatment. Because of this serious side effect, clozapine is recommended for use only in patients with unmanageable extrapyramidal symptoms or in patients with schizophrenia that is refractory to standard neuroleptic therapy. Recently, *low-dose clozapine (12.5 to 75 mg at bedtime) has become the treatment of choice in patients with Parkinson's disease for the management of frightening hallucinations caused by levodopa-carbidopa (Sinemet) therapy.*

Another atypical neuroleptic, risperidone (Risperdal) has recently been approved for use in the United States. It is an effective antipsychotic in dosages from 2 to 8 mg/d, and it appears to have a lower incidence of extrapyramidal symptoms than typical agents of comparable potency, such as haloperidol. It is not associated with bone marrow toxicity. Unlike clozapine, in psychotic patients, risperidone has not been shown to have superior efficacy to that of standard neuroleptics. Risperidone has a tendency to cause postural hypotension, but it has no significant anticholinergic side effects. When it is used cautiously in the elderly, preliminary reports suggest that risperidone may be a helpful antipsychotic agent at doses of 0.25 to 2.0 mg at bedtime. However, because it is newly marketed, risperidone is more expensive than most other antipsychotics, and its usefulness for primary care patients remains to be fully explored.

VIII. Psychopharmacology in the elderly: Special considerations.

A. Overview.

Psychopharmacologic treatment of older patients requires an understanding of the biology of aging as well as the social factors related to aging. Psychotropic agents are among the most commonly prescribed class of drugs in the elderly, and most are prescribed by primary care practitioners. In general, most psychiatric disorders in the elderly seen in primary care are as amenable to pharmacotherapy as those in younger patients. The psychiatric complications of dementia are usually treatable pharmacologically (see Chapter 12).

Although significant morbidity and mortality can result from inappropriate use of psychotropic agents, equally bad outcomes can result from nontreatment or undertreatment of geropsychiatric illness (including suicide in the elderly depressed and poor outcomes from comorbid medical illnesses). Hence, it is important to adequately diagnose and vigorously treat drug-responsive psychiatric syndromes, even in the very old. However, as with any drug therapy, psychotropic drugs in elderly patients must be prescribed with special caution, and *lower dosing should be used in older patients for all psychotropic drug classes.* Research on antidepressants indicates that all ages appear to respond to the same blood levels. Therapeutic blood levels appear to be the same in the elderly as in younger patients. Because of slower metabolic rates in elderly patients, lower doses tend to produce higher blood levels, making it is wise to reach these blood levels by a slower uptaper using smaller incremental doses.

B. Side effects.

Compared with younger patients, the elderly are more sensitive to such side effects as sedation and central and peripheral anticholinergic effects. Decreased baroreceptor sensitivity makes the elderly vulnerable to orthostatic hypotension. Cardiovascular side effects are common. Changes in the central nervous system increase risk for neuroleptic-induced extrapyramidal side effects and delirium. Reduced bowel motility predisposes to constipation and impaction. Aging heavily affects these phenomena. Accordingly, pharmacokinetics and pharmacodynamics play a large part in the elderly patient's responsivity to drug therapy.

C. Age-related changes in pharmacokinetics (drug handling by the body).

1. *Increase in total body fat relative to total body water.*
   At age 25, fatty tissue is 20% of body weight; at age 70, the figure is 35%. The

vast bulk of psychotropic agents are fat soluble, and in the elderly such agents distribute more widely and more slowly and tend to accumulate. Consequently, *medication effects may be delayed, and side effects may begin later than anticipated.* Water-soluble agents (e.g., lithium) have higher peak postdose plasma concentrations.

2. *Decrease in hepatic metabolism, particularly oxidation.*
   This change may lead to decreased dose requirement and prolonged half-life for most major psychotropic drug classes: antidepressants, neuroleptics, and benzodiazepines. However, because hepatic conjugation reactions are less affected by aging, the benzodiazepines so metabolized—*lorazepam (Ativan), oxazepam (Serax), and temazepam (Restoril)—are recommended for use in the elderly because their half-lives are unaffected and their accumulation is reduced.* Nevertheless, lower doses of these agents are recommended in the elderly because of this population's increased sensitivity to the pharmacologic effects that occur with aging.

3. *Decreased creatinine clearance and renal excretion.*
   Because lithium is cleared by the kidneys, the decreased clearance of lithium carbonate requires a reduction in dose. TCAs have water-soluble metabolites, and reduced renal clearance increases the risk of cardiac arrhythmias and other cardiotoxic effects that may be caused by these metabolites.

D. Age-related changes in pharmacodynamics (proximate drug effects on the body): Common problems.

1. Cognitive dysfunction secondary to central anticholinergic side effects can be caused by declines in cholinergic neurotransmission resulting from aging. Dementia is an additional risk factor. Highly anticholinergic antidepressants (e.g., amitriptyline [Elavil]) and neuroleptics (e.g., thioridazine [Mellaril]) should be avoided.

2. Orthostatic hypotension from tricyclic antidepressants.

3. Sedation from benzodiazepines.

4. Extrapyramidal side effects from neuroleptics.

E. Polypharmacy.

The number of prescribed drugs is directly proportional to age in most treatment settings, and the probability of adverse drug reactions is proportional to the number of prescribed drugs, in terms of both the interactions with disease states and the drug-drug interactions that can occur. Common examples of drug-drug interactions relevant to treatment of the elderly are:

1. Thiazide diuretics, nonsteroidal anti-inflammatory drugs, and angiotensin-converting enzyme inhibitors increase lithium blood levels by decreasing lithium excretion.

2. Theophylline decreases lithium blood levels by increasing lithium excretion.

3. Fluoxetine (Prozac) and all other SSRIs may increase blood levels of hepatically metabolized drugs by inhibiting hepatic microsomal metabolism. Among the SSRIs, sertraline (Zoloft) appears to be the least inhibitory.

4. Sedative effects of antidepressants, benzodiazepines, opioid analgesics, antihistamines, and so on are generally additive.

5. Hypotensive effects of TCAs add to those of antihypertensive drugs.

F. Nonadherence (noncompliance) and its treatment.
Nonadherence can take several forms in the elderly:

1. *Underadherence.*
   Patients take too little or none of prescribed drug. This can occur because of side effects (that may not have been discussed with the physician), memory difficulties, disbelief in the benefits of treatment, or lack of finances to purchase drugs. These tendencies are worsened by depression, psychosis, or other mental disorders. Transportation is also often a problem.

2. *Overadherence.*
   Patients may take too much of a prescribed drug (e.g., benzodiazepines) or may take additional drugs not prescribed (from previously prescribed medications or even a spouse's medication!).

3. *Dysadherence.*
   Patients may take medication but use the wrong or a misunderstood regimen.

4. *Treatment.*
   Adherence issues should be anticipated and addressed when medicines are prescribed. Medication actions and side effects should be explained clearly, and an assessment should be made of the context in which the patient will be taking the medication.

Does the patient live alone? Is another person responsible for the patient's medications? What are the patient's finances? Are there previously prescribed medicines in the patient's house? The prescribed regimen should be as simple as possible because *regimen complexity is a major factor in nonadherence.*

IX. Essential psychopharmacology for drug-drug interactions.

This section describes changes in the pharmacokinetic properties of psychotropic drugs. Altered pharmacokinetics can be attributed to accompanying physiologic changes in renal or liver disease, pregnancy, or obesity. This section also provides a fairly extensive list of drug-drug interactions, their expected effects, and the most appropriate corrective actions to be taken. When faced with a situation in which the pharmacokinetics of a drug are likely to be altered, primary care physicians use the information in this section to make informed decisions about whether it is wiser to do nothing, to alter drug dose, or use an alternative medication. The principles covered in this section are relevant to all drug therapy, not just psychotropic drug therapy.

A. Pharmacokinetics versus pharmacodynamics.

The term *pharmacokinetic* relates to the concentration of drug in the body and factors such as absorption, distribution, and clearance that regulate concentration (i.e., what the body does to the drug). The term *pharmacodynamic* relates to the relationship between the drug and its actions in the body, such as interactions at a receptor site (what the drug does to the body). Thus, pharmacokinetically based drug-drug interactions are mediated by one drug's alteration of the plasma concentration of the other drug, which may or may not result in a clinically significant change in the effect of one or both of the drugs involved. Pharmacodynamically based drug-drug interactions are mediated by one drug's alteration of the effect of the other drug at the site of effect, not necessarily involving any change in plasma concentration; for example, an MAOI like phenelzine (Nardil) when combined with meperidine (Demerol) produces a profile of often lethal physiologic changes called the *serotonin syndrome.*

B. Pharmacokinetic principles in psychoactive drug therapy.

Terms commonly used to describe pharmacokinetic principles follow:

1. *Clearance (CL).*
   Clearance refers to the volume of plasma from which the drug is removed per unit of time, such as liter per hour or milliliter per minute.

2. *Volume of distribution (V_d).*
   This measure is a proportionality constant rather than an actual physical space within the body; V_d relates the concentration of drug in the blood to the amount of drug that is elsewhere in the body at the same time. V_d is measured in units of volume such as milliliters or liters.

3. *Elimination half-life ($T_{1/2}$).*
   This measure refers to the time required to eliminate half of the drug from the body; *approximately four to five $T_{1/2}$'s are required either to eliminate most of the drug (97%) from the body after the drug is stopped or to reach a steady state blood concentration of drug in the body once a drug regimen is begun.*

   The pharmacokinetic parameter that is most familiar to most clinicians is $T_{1/2}$, but half-life is a composite parameter that is related to both V_d and CL in the following manner:

$$T_{1/2} = \frac{0.693\,(V_d)}{CL}$$

Changes in $T_{1/2}$ are produced by changes in V_d or CL. The physiologically based parameters (CL or V_d) can each inversely affect the $T_{1/2}$. All these parameters are summarized in Table 2–6.

C. Pharmacokinetic principles: practical information.

An application of pharmacokinetic principles can provide clinicians with practical information such as the following:

1. *Half-life.*
   Because it takes four to five $T_{1/2}$s for a drug to reach steady state or to be eliminated from the body, therapeutic effects and drug-drug interactions have a predictable time course. For example, the combination of fluoxetine (Prozac) and desipramine (Norpramin) results in significant increases in desipramine's blood concentration. Because the $T_{1/2}$ for norfluoxetine, the major active metabolite of fluoxetine, is 10 days, it takes 40 to 50 days before the total extent of this inter-

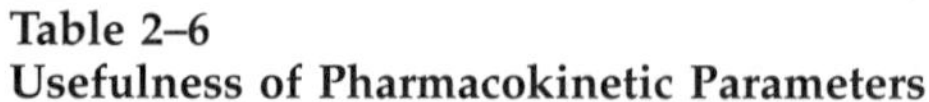

Table 2–6
Usefulness of Pharmacokinetic Parameters

Parameter	An Important Determinant of:
Clearance	Average blood concentration at steady state Peak and trough drug concentrations Elimination $T_{1/2}$
Volume of distribution	Peak and trough drug concentrations Elimination $T_{1/2}$
Elimination half-life ($T_{1/2}$)	How long it takes to get to steady state How long it takes to eliminate most drug from the body

action is evident, and *it is prudent to wait 40 to 50 days before switching from fluoxetine to desipramine or any TCA*. $T_{1/2}$ values can be found in the *Physicians' Desk Reference*.

2. *Average plasma concentration at steady state.*
When a drug has a narrow therapeutic index, that therapeutic range must be maintained because the steady state plasma concentration is assumed to correlate strongly with the concentration at the site of effect. Accordingly, knowledge of the plasma drug concentration is helpful before dosage adjustments are made. Once a patient has received a medication by use of a constant dosing regimen for four to five $T_{1/2}$s a steady state is reached. The therapeutic window for nortriptyline (Pamelor) is 50 to 150 ng/mL, and $T_{1/2}$ is about 24 hours. Consequently, *it is appropriate to wait 4 to 5 days after a dosage adjustment before determining nortriptyline's blood concentration.*

3. *Peak and trough drug concentrations.*
The peak and trough plasma concentrations of a drug are important determinants of possible toxicity or accumulation for some drugs that are administered intermittently. Use of the psychotropic drugs does not require monitoring of peak and trough plasma concentrations because the drug effects generally do not seem to correlate well with either of these values. Lithium is an exception; some patients who achieve high peak lithium plasma concentrations may be particularly prone to gastrointestinal side effects, and a *sustained-release formulation of lithium, which results in lower peak lithium concentrations, may alleviate this problem.*

4. *Effects of different physiologic conditions on the pharmacokinetics of drugs.*
Most drugs are eliminated via hepatic metabolism or renal clearance. Most psychotropic drugs are eliminated via hepatic metabolism. The major exception to this rule is lithium, which is eliminated entirely via renal clearance.

Table 2–7 describes how certain physiologic conditions might affect the pharmacokinetics of psychotropic drugs. It is important to realize that dosing changes may be necessary in a particular patient for either pharmacokinetic or pharmacodynamic reasons and that a change in blood level does not always cause a clinically significant change in response.

Table 2–7 lists a series of altered physiologic states. For each physiologic state, a model drug has been chosen to illustrate changes that may take place. These changes in pharmacokinetics associated with a model drug are identified by the capital letters *A* to *J* at the top of each column and are described in the following text. (*A* through *J* below corresponds to *A* through *J* in Table 2–7.) In some cases, no data are available about psychotropic drugs, so other example drugs have been chosen to illustrate how changes in the physiologic state may alter pharmacokinetic parameters.

A. *Renal dysfunction on renally cleared drugs.* Drugs that are primarily cleared renally and undergo minimal hepatic metabolism are not common in psychiatry. However, lithium exhibits this profile. Renal dysfunction has a profound effect on lithium pharmacokinetics. A decrease in renal function causes a decrease in lithium clearance (because it is virtually 100% cleared by

Table 2–7
The Effects of Physiologic Changes on Pharmacokinetic Parameters

Variable	Renal Dysfunction	Hepatic Dysfunction	Aging	Pregnancy	Obesity
Renally cleared drug example	*A (e.g., lithium)*	*B (e.g., lithium)*	*C (e.g., lithium)*	*D (e.g., aminoglycosides)*	*E (e.g., aminoglycosides)*
Clearance	↓	↔	↓	↑	↑
Volume of distribution	↔	↔ or ↑	↑ or ↓	↑ or ↔	↑ or ↔
Elimination half-life	↑	↔ or ↑	↑	↓	↔ or ↓
Dose requirement	↓	↔	↓	↑	↑
Hepatically cleared drug example	*F (e.g., TCAs)*	*G (e.g., TCAs)*	*H (e.g., TCAs)*	*I (e.g., TCAs)*	*J (e.g., diazepam or lorazepam)*
Clearance	↔	↓ or ↔	↔ or ↓	↑ or ↔	↔ or ↑
Volume of distribution	↔	↔ or ↑	↑ or ↓	↑	↑
Elimination half-life	↔	↑ or ↔	↔ or ↑	↑	↔ or ↑
Dose requirement	↔	↔ or ↓	↔ or ↓	↑ or ↔	↔ or ↑

For each physiologic state, a "model" drug has been chosen to illustrate changes that may occur and is placed at the top of each column. In some cases, no data are available on any of the psychotropic drugs, so other agents (e.g., aminoglycosides) have been chosen to illustrate changes in pharmacokinetic parameters.

↔, no change; ↑, increased; ↓, decreased; TCAs, tricyclic antipressants.

the kidneys). *Because CL determines the average plasma concentration at steady state, as the CL decreases, a dosage reduction is required.*

B. *Hepatic dysfunction on renally cleared drugs.* Lithium is also used as the model drug in this instance. Patients suffering from hepatic dysfunction generally do not require an alteration of lithium dose. However, *in a patient with such severe hepatic dysfunction that renal blood flow is affected, lithium dose may need to be decreased.* The V_d may increase in a person who develops ascites; this increase in V_d does not require an alteration of dose but it would result in an increase in lithium elimination $T_{1/2}$.

C. *Aging effects on renally cleared drugs.* The effects of aging on lithium pharmacokinetics are predictable. *Because renal function decreases with age, the CL of lithium decreases as a person ages, and the dose of lithium needs to be decreased.* Both increases and decreases in the V_d of lithium may occur with aging, but the CL changes generally overshadow the importance of any changes in the V_d, and the elimination $T_{1/2}$ can be expected to increase with age.

D. *Pregnancy effects on renally cleared drugs.* Lithium therapy is usually avoided during pregnancy, and no information regarding the pharmacokinetics of lithium in pregnancy is available. However, the aminoglycoside antibiotics are also cleared exclusively by the kidneys, so they are used as the model of renally cleared drugs in pregnancy. An increase in V_d and a marked increase in glomerular filtration rate occur in the later stages of pregnancy. These changes result in *an increase in CL and a decrease in elimination $T_{1/2}$ in pregnant patients; these phenomena may necessitate an increase in aminoglycoside dosage.*

E. *Obesity effects on renally cleared drugs.* Lithium pharmacokinetics have not been evaluated in obese patients. Aminoglycoside antibiotics serve as the model for a discussion of the effects of obesity on renally cleared drugs. Generally, the magnitude of the changes in pharmacokinetics depends on the magnitude of the obesity. Increases in both the V_d and the renal CL are seen in the morbidly obese (two times the ideal body weight). These changes may result in no change in $T_{1/2}$, but *an increase in the required aminoglycoside dose may result from the increase in renal CL.*

F. *Renal dysfunction on hepatically cleared drugs.* The TCAs are used as a model for hepatically cleared drugs; however, most antipsychotics and the newer SSRIs exhibit similar pharmacokinetic characteristics. Plasma steady state concentrations of TCAs are not usually altered by the presence of renal failure. However, TCAs are biotransformed into various metabolites, and some are cleared renally. Metabolite concentrations are not readily available from most clinical laboratories. Based on blood levels of the parent drug, dose adjustment would not appear to be necessary. Nevertheless, *TCA toxicity has been reported in renal dysfunction, so patients with renal failure should be monitored closely for any clinical signs of TCA toxicity.*

G. *Hepatic dysfunction on hepatically cleared drugs.* Again, the TCAs serve as the model. Severe hepatic dysfunction is likely to decrease the clearance of hepatically cleared drugs. The effects of less severe hepatic dysfunction are not well characterized. *With severe liver dysfunction, lower doses of TCAs (or any drug) are indicated.* No guidelines exist for dose adjustments in the hepatically compromised patient. For this reason, a combination of plasma monitoring (if available) and clinical evaluation is prudent policy.

H. *Aging effects on hepatically cleared drugs.* The dose of TCAs may require a decrease during aging. The principle reason for this is not pharmacokinetic, but pharmacodynamic. The effects of aging of TCA pharmacokinetics are conflicting. There may be a decrease in CL in some patients. Although several studies have not shown any significant difference in CL with aging, the definition of "elderly" varies from study to study, and those studies that have evaluated healthy elderly persons are less likely to find changes.

I. *Pregnancy effects on hepatically cleared drugs.* As discussed earlier, TCAs are relatively safe to use in pregnancy. For example, nortriptyline (Pamelor) is a reasonable antidepressant to prescribe during pregnancy. *A woman after week 20 of pregnancy requires 1 to 6 times the dose of nortriptyline that she would need if she were not pregnant. This general rule applies to all TCAs.* The necessary increase in dose is likely to be caused by an increase in CL, which may be caused by either a decrease in plasma protein binding or an increase in enzyme metabolic activity or a combination of both during pregnancy.

J. *Obesity effects on hepatically cleared drugs.* Pharmacokinetic parameters of TCAs have not been evaluated in obesity. Benzodiazepines are also primarily hepatically cleared and are used as the model in this section. However, the effects of obesity on the pharmacokinetics in benzodiazepines that are oxidatively metabolized (e.g., diazepam [Valium] and most other benzodiazepines) are different than those in benzodiazepines that are conjugated (e.g., lorazepam [Ativan], oxazepam [Serax], and temazepam [Restoril]). The V_d increases in both cases, but the CL of conjugated benzodiazepines increases in obese individuals, whereas the CL of oxidatively metabolized benzodiazepines is not changed. Consequently, *the dose of lorazepam, but not the dose of diazepam, may have to be increased in obese persons.* Also, the half-life is likely to increase in persons taking diazepam, but not in those taking lorazepam.

D. The role of blood levels.

1. Blood or plasma levels are most helpful when the therapeutic index of a drug is narrow and the therapeutic range of the drug in question is relatively well defined. Most psychotropic agents are administered primarily on the basis of clinical response. However, in some situations, knowledge of the blood level of a psychotropic agent is necessary or helpful. *When maintenance blood levels of psychotropic drugs are checked, blood should be drawn 12 hours after the previous dose and before another dose is taken.*
   a. Lithium blood levels must be monitored.
      (1) Lithium has a very narrow optimal therapeutic range (0.8 to 1.3 mEq/L), and high blood concentrations are associated with severe toxicity.
      (2) If the patient is taking a stable therapeutic dose of lithium, blood levels should be obtained when lithium levels have achieved steady state. Because $T_{1/2}$ for lithium averages about 24 hours in persons with normal renal function, most people achieve steady state in 4 to 10 days; consequently, blood levels are obtained about 4 to 5 days after a dosage change. In cases of suspected overdose, lithium blood levels should be obtained as soon as possible.
      (3) Other situations in which lithium blood levels should be checked include the following:
         - If a recent change in renal function has occurred.
         - If a patient complains of signs of lithium toxicity, such as nausea, vomiting, diarrhea, or tremor, or if the physician notes confusion in an older patient who is taking lithium.
         - If a patient has been recently placed on a low-sodium diet, or if a drug that may interact with lithium has been added to the medication regimen (e.g., a thiazide diuretic or any other diuretic that works primarily on the distal renal tubule, a nonsteroidal anti-inflammatory drug, theophylline, or an angiotensin-converting enzyme inhibitor).
   b. If the patient is showing a therapeutic response to the TCA, there is little reason to obtain a blood level. Although the therapeutic range for most TCAs has not been well defined, therapeutic ranges for imipramine (Tofranil), desipramine (Norpramin), and nortriptyline (Pamelor) are reasonably well established. The therapeutic range for nortriptyline is 50 to 150 ng/mL, and desipramine's range is greater than 150 ng/mL. Because imipramine is partially metabolized to desipramine in the body, the imipramine therapeutic range includes both drugs; the imipramine level should be added to the desipramine plasma level, and this combined level should be greater than 150 ng/mL. Determinations of TCA plasma concentrations are available from most laboratories.
   c. Obtaining a TCA blood level may be especially helpful in the following situations:
      (1) Patients who are neither responding to the TCA nor complaining of side effects may not be taking the medication as prescribed. Checking a blood level could help identify these circumstances.
      (2) About 5% to 10% of people of northern European descent metabolize TCAs very slowly because of their genetic phenotype; consequently, they may develop toxic blood concentrations while taking doses of TCAs that are within the normally accepted therapeutic dosage range. Someone who complains of many TCA side effects while receiving a relatively modest dose of TCA might be a slow metabolizer of the drug, and a blood concentration determination helps establish this.
      (3) Because TCAs can be fatal when taken in an overdose, a blood level for TCAs should be obtained in all cases of suspected TCA overdose.

X. Important drug-drug interactions.

A. Examples.

Drug-drug interactions are likely to be clinically significant only when a new drug is added or deleted from a stable medication regimen. Such interactions may be pharmacokinetically based (e.g., drug A increases or decreases the CL of drug B, resulting in an increase or decrease in blood levels of drug B). Drug-drug interactions may also be pharmacodynamically based (e.g., drug A increases or decreases the effect of drug B, or together they cause a toxicity, but drug A does not alter the pharmacokinetics of drug B). Table 2–8 describes both pharmacokinetic and pharmacodynamic drug interactions. More comprehensive lists of reported drug interactions can be found in any drug interactions reference book; we attempt here to list only the most clinically significant interactions that involve psychotropic drugs.

B. Cytochrome P_{450} system.

Two major types of metabolic reactions are responsible for the biotransformation and elimination of a drug. Phase I metabolism involves transformation reactions via hydroxylation, reduction, dealkylation, or hydrolysis. Many of the phase I reactions are mediated by the mixed-function oxidase system that is composed of multiple forms of the cytochrome P_{450} (CYP450)

Text continued on page 40

Table 2–8
Pharmacokinetics and Pharmacodynamics-Based Drug-Drug Interactions with Psychotropic Drugs

Interacting Drug	Drug Added to Regimen	Mechanism of Interaction	Resulting Effect	Appropriate Action
Alprazolam (Xanax)	Fluoxetine (Prozac)	Inhibition of alprazolam clearance	Increase in sedation	Decrease alprazolam dose.
Alprazolam	Fluvoxamine (Luvox)	Inhibition of alprazolam clearance	Increase in sedation	Decrease alprazolam dose.
Alprazolam	Nefazodone (Serzone)	Inhibition of alprazolam clearance	Increase in sedation	Decrease alprazolam dose.
Benzodiazepines Lorazepam (Ativan) Oxazepam (Serax) Temazepam (Restoril)	Oral contraceptives	Induction of clearance of benzodiazepines cleared by conjugation	Decrease in anxiolytic or hypnotic effect	May need to increase benzodiazepine dose.
Benzodiazepines Diazepam (Valium) and most others	Oral contraceptives	Inhibition of clearance of benzodiazepines cleared by oxidation	Increase in anxiolytic or sedative effect	May need to decrease benzodiazepine dose.
Buspirone (BuSpar)	Trazodone (Desyrel)	Pharmacodynamic interaction	"Serotonin syndrome" (see text)	One case report only; combination is probably safe, but use caution and monitor the patient closely.
Caffeine	Fluvoxamine	Inhibition of caffeine clearance	Caffeine toxicity; decrease in seizure threshold	Decrease caffeine intake.
Carbamazepine (Tegretol)	Fluoxetine	Inhibition of carbamazepine clearance (also decrease in clearance of active carbamazepine metabolite)	Increase in carbamazepine blood levels; confusion, ataxia	Decrease carbamazepine dose; monitor both blood levels and clinical effect; monitor metabolite (epoxide) levels if possible.
Carbamazepine	Valproic acid, divalproex (Depakene; Depakote)	Inhibition of carbamazepine metabolite (10-11-epoxide) clearance	Confusion, ataxia; maybe normal carbamazepine levels but increased epoxide metabolite levels	Decrease carbamazepine dose, if clinically indicated.
Clozapine (Clozaril)	Lithium (Eskalith)	Pharmacodynamic interaction	Neuroleptic malignant syndrome; delirium, dyskinesia	This combination is sometimes used without problem; use caution and monitor patient closely.
Clozapine	Tricyclic antidepressants (TCAs) Imipramine (Tofranil) Amitriptyline (Elavil) Doxepin (Sinequan) Clomipramine (Anafranil) Nortriptyline (Pamelor) Desipramine (Norpramin)	Pharmacodynamic interaction	Delirium, possibly from the combined anticholinergic properties of both drugs	Use caution and monitor the patient closely; many patients may tolerate this combination without any problem; slowly increase doses of both agents.

Hypothesized interaction: Cyclosporine (Sandimmune)	Nefazodone	Inhibition of cyclosporine metabolism	Renal dysfunction	May need to decrease cyclosporine dose.
Dextromethorphan (Robitussin DM)	Fluoxetine	Inhibition of dextromethorphan clearance	Confusion, delirium	Avoid using this combination if possible; otherwise, monitor patient closely.
Diazepam	Fluvoxamine	Inhibition of diazepam clearance	Increase in anxiolytic or sedative effect	May need to decrease diazepam dose.
Haloperidol (Haldol)	Carbamazepine (Tegretol)	Induction of haloperidol clearance	Decrease in therapeutic response to haloperidol	May need to increase haloperidol dose.
Haloperidol	Lithium (Eskalith)	Pharmacodynamic interaction	Delirium, a "neurotoxic" reaction; incidence of this reaction is likely to increase with age	Use caution and monitor the patient closely; this combination is often used safely; if there is a neurotoxic reaction, consider switching haloperidol to a benzodiazepine or a different neuroleptic.
Haloperidol	Paroxetine (Paxil)	Pharmacodynamic interaction	Delirium	There are several case reports; this combination may be tolerated without problem in many patients; use caution and monitor the patient closely.
Levodopa (Sinemet and others)	Bupropion (Wellbutrin)	Pharmacodynamic interaction	Agitation, nausea and vomiting; as the dose is increased	Possibly due to the combined dopaminergic effects of both drugs; use caution. Monitor the patient closely. This combination is often used safely.
Lithium	ACE inhibitors Enalapril (Vasotec) *Hypothesized interaction:* Captopril (Capoten) Quinapril (Accupril) Ramipril (Altace) Benzapril (Lotensin) Fosinopril (Monopril) Lisinopril (Prinivil, Zestril)	Decrease in renal clearance of lithium	Lithium toxicity; increase in lithium blood levels	Monitor lithium blood levels and decrease lithium dose if necessary.
Lithium	Carbonic anhydrase inhibitors Acetazolamide (Diamox) *Hypothesized interaction:* Methazolamide (Neptazane) Dichlorphenamide (Daranide)	Increase in renal clearance of lithium	Decrease in lithium blood levels, possibly a decrease in response to lithium	May need to increase lithium dose.

Table continued on following page

Table 2–8
Pharmacokinetics and Pharmacodynamics-Based Drug-Drug Interactions with Psychotropic Drugs *Continued*

Interacting Drug	Drug Added to Regimen	Mechanism of Interaction	Resulting Effect	Appropriate Action
Hypothesized interaction: Lithium	Diuretics acting on the distal renal tubule metolozone (Mykrox, Zaroxolyn) Chlorthalidone Indapamide (Lozol)	Decrease in renal clearance of lithium	Lithium toxicity; increase in lithium blood levels	May need to decrease lithium dose
Lithium	Haloperidol	Pharmacodynamic interaction	Delirium, a "neurotoxic" reaction; incidence of this reaction is likely to increase with age	Use caution and monitor the patient closely; this combination is often used safely; if there is a neurotoxic reaction, consider switching haloperidol to a benzodiazepine or a different neuroleptic.
Lithium	Methylxanthines Theophylline Aminophylline Caffeine	Increase in renal clearance of lithium	Decrease in lithium blood levels, possibly a decrease in response to lithium	May need to increase lithium dose; if caffeine intake remains stable, no changes are likely to be necessary, but if caffeine intake is significantly increased or decreased, the lithium dose may need adjustment.
Lithium	NSAIDs Ibuprofen (Motrin) Naproxen (Naprosyn, Alleve) Indomethacin (Indocin) Diclofenac (Voltaren) Piroxicam (Feldene)	Decrease in renal clearance of lithium	Lithium toxicity; increase in lithium blood levels	Monitor lithium blood levels and decrease lithium dose if necessary.
Lithium	Sodium	Increase in sodium intake increases lithium clearance; conversely, decrease in sodium intake (low-sodium diet) decreases lithium clearance	With increased sodium, lithium levels decrease; with decreased sodium, lithium levels increase, possibly causing toxicity	If patient is given a low-sodium diet, the lithium dose will have to be decreased; if patient receives salt tablets or any other large sodium load (e.g., some antibiotics) the lithium dose may need to be increased.
Lithium	Thiazide diuretics Hydrochlorothiazide	Decrease in renal clearance of lithium	Lithium toxicity; increase in lithium blood levels	Decrease lithium dose.
Lithium	Thioridazine (Mellaril)	Pharmacodynamic interaction	Symptoms of lithium toxicity	Usually a safe combination; use caution and monitor the patient closely.
Lithium	Thiothixene (Navane)	Pharmacodynamic interaction	Symptoms of lithium toxicity, extrapyramidal symptoms	Usually a safe combination; use caution and monitor the patient closely.
Loxapine (Loxitane)	Lorazepam (Ativan)	Pharmacodynamic interaction	Delirium and respiratory depression	Several case reports; often this combination can be given safely; use caution and monitor the patient closely.

Metoprolol (Lopressor)	Fluoxetine *Hypothesized interaction:* Paroxetine	Decrease in clearance of metoprolol	Marked bradycardia, hypotension	May need to decrease metoprolol dose.
Midazolam (Versed)	Erythromycin *Hypothesized interaction:* Nefazodone	Decrease in clearance of midazolam	Sedation, long-lasting and severe	Decrease midazolam dose.
Molindone (Moban)	Paroxetine	Possible decrease in clearance of molindone	Increased incidence of extrapyramidal symptoms	Decrease molindone dose.
Monoamine oxidase inhibitor (MAOIs) Phenelzine (Nardil) Tranylcypromine (Parnate)	Decongestants Pseudoephedrine (Sudafed) Phenylpropanolamine Ephedrine These agents are present in just about any OTC sinus or decongestant preparation	Pharmacodynamic interaction	Hypertensive crisis	Avoid using this combination; strokes and death have been reported.
MAOIs Phenelzine Tranylcypromine	Dextroamphetamine (Dexedrine) Phentermine (Ionamin) *Hypothesized interaction:* Cocaine Any other stimulant	Pharmacodynamic interaction	Hypertensive crisis	Avoid using this combination; strokes and death have been reported.
MAOIs Phenelzine Tranylcypromine	Dextromethorphan (Robitussin DM, many other cough syrups; see text)	Pharmacodynamic interaction	Serotonin syndrome	Avoid using dextromethorphan in any patient receiving monoamine oxidase inhibitors; this interaction could be lethal.
MAOIs Phenelzine Tranylcypromine	Meperidine (Demerol)	Pharmacodynamic interaction	Serotonin syndrome	Avoid using this combination; this interaction could be lethal.
MAOIs Phenelzine Tranylcypromine	Metoprolol	Pharmacodynamic interaction	Bradycardia	Usually a safe combination; use caution and monitor the patient closely.
MAOIs Phenelzine Tranylcypromine	Selective serotonin reuptake inhibitors (SSRIs) Fluoxetine Fluvoxamine Sertraline (Zoloft) Paroxetine	Pharmacodynamic interaction	Serotonin syndrome	Avoid using this combination; this interaction could be lethal.
MAOIs Phenelzine Tranylcypromine	Other antidepressants Imipramine Amitriptyline Doxepin Clomipramine Nortriptyline Desipramine Venlafaxine (Effexor)	Pharmacodynamic interaction	Serotonin syndrome	Occasionally, these drugs have been combined safely; usually, there is no need to combine these agents; especially problematic is *clomipramine,* which is the most likely TCA to cause a fatal interaction of this type. Avoid venlafaxine.

Table continued on following page

Table 2–8
Pharmacokinetics and Pharmacodynamics-Based Drug-Drug Interactions with Psychotropic Drugs *Continued*

Interacting Drug	Drug Added to Regimen	Mechanism of Interaction	Resulting Effect	Appropriate Action
MAOIs Phenelzine Tranylcypromine	Tryptophan	Pharmacodynamic interaction	Serotonin syndrome	Avoid using this combination.
Morphine	Cimetidine (Tagamet)	Decrease in clearance of morphine	Respiratory depression, delirium, possibly lethal	Either decrease the morphine dose or avoid the combination if possible.
Nifedipine (Procardia, Adalat)	Naltrexone (Trexan, ReVia)	Pharmacodynamic interaction	Delirium	Use with caution and monitor the patient closely.
Paroxetine	Molindone (Moban)	Pharmacodynamic interaction	Extrapyramidal symptoms	Molindone can cause extrapyramidal symptoms when used alone; but these symptoms may be exacerbated by paroxetine; use caution and monitor the patient closely.
Phenytoin (Dilantin)	Fluoxetine	Decrease in phenytoin clearance	Phenytoin toxicity, confusion, possibly seizures, increase in phenytoin blood levels	Avoid the combination of these two drugs; if combination cannot be avoided, monitor phenytoin levels closely.
Phenytoin	Meperidine	Pharmacodynamic interaction	Seizures	Avoid this combination; other analgesics can be safely used.
Pimozide (Orap)	Fluoxetine	Possible decrease in pimozide clearance	Bradycardia, pseudoparkinsonism, delirium	Either decrease pimozide dose or avoid the combination of these two drugs.
Propranolol (Inderal)	Haloperidol	Pharmacodynamic interaction or possible decrease in propranolol clearance	Hypotension, cardiopulmonary arrest	Usually a safe combination; use caution and monitor the patient closely; avoid administering either haloperidol or propranolol by intravenous route if they are both going to be used.
Propranolol	Maprotiline (Ludiomil)	Pharmacodynamic interaction	Delirium	Use with caution and monitor the patient closely.
Selegiline (Eldepryl)	Cimetidine	Decrease in selegiline clearance	Conversion of selegiline from a monoamine oxidase B–specific-enzyme inhibitor to a nonspecific monoamine oxidase A and B inhibitor	May need to decrease selegiline dose.

Selegiline	Indapamide	Pharmacodynamic interaction	Erythema multiforme, angioedema	One reported case; this may have been an idiosyncratic reaction; nevertheless, if the combination is used, use caution and monitor the patient closely.
Selegiline	Meperidine	Pharmacodynamic interaction	Delirium	Use this combination with caution; if it can not be avoided, then monitor the patient closely; consider choosing a different analgesic.
Selegiline	SSRIs Fluoxetine Fluvoxamine Sertraline Paroxetine	Pharmacodynamic interaction	Confusion, ataxia, delirium, erratic changes in blood pressure	This combination has been used safely; however, it is still prudent to monitor patients receiving this combination; because selegiline specifically inhibits only one of the two monoamine oxidases, this interaction does not appear to be as serious as the MAOI + SSRI interaction with phenelzine or tranylcypromine.
Terfenadine	Carbamazepine (Tegretol)	Pharmacodynamic interaction	Delirium	Use with caution and monitor the patient closely.
Terfenadine Hypothesized interaction: Astemizole (Hismanal) Cisapride (Propulsid)	Ketoconazole (Nizoral) Erythromycin Itraconazole (Sporanox) Hypothesized interaction: Nefazodone Fluvoxamine	Decrease in terfenadine, astemizole, or cisapride clearance	Syncope; QT interval prolongation; associated with serious cardiac events, including death; cardiac arrest and ventricular arrhythmias, including torsades de pointes	Owing to the potential severity of this interaction, avoid these combinations of drugs; if a nonsedating antihistamine is necessary, loratadine (Claritin) may be substituted.
Theophylline Aminophylline Caffeine	Fluvoxamine	Decrease in clearance of methylxanthines	Theophylline toxicity, including confusion and possible seizure; increases in theophylline blood levels	Decrease the dose of theophylline; determine how much coffee is ingested daily and warn patients of the potential for caffeine toxicity.
Thioridazine (Mellaril)	Propranolol	Pharmacodynamic interaction	Pigmentary retinopathy	High doses of thioridazine alone can cause this adverse effect, which can result in loss of vision; if this combination is used, a relatively low dose of thioridazine should be maintained and the patient should be monitored regularly by an ophthalmologist.

Table continued on following page

Table 2–8
Pharmacokinetics and Pharmacodynamics-Based Drug-Drug Interactions with Psychotropic Drugs *Continued*

Interacting Drug	Drug Added to Regimen	Mechanism of Interaction	Resulting Effect	Appropriate Action
Thioridazine	Paroxetine	Possible decrease in thioridazine clearance	Delirium	Decrease thioridazine dose.
Triazolam (Halcion)	Nefazodone Fluvoxamine	Decrease in triazolam clearance	Increased and prolonged sedation	Decrease triazolam dose.
TCAs Imipramine Amitriptyline Doxepin Clomipramine Nortriptyline Desipramine	Cimetidine	Decrease in clearance of TCAs	Increased sedation, possible confusion or delirium; QT prolongation and other cardiac arrhythmias, possibly seizures	Decrease dose of TCA or substitute another histamine$_2$-blocking agent, such as ranitidine.
TCAs Imipramine Amitriptyline Doxepin Clomipramine Nortriptyline Desipramine	Fluoxetine Paroxetine Fluvoxamine To a lesser extent: Sertraline	Decrease in clearance of TCAs	Increased sedation, possible confusion or delirium; QT prolongation and other cardiac arrhythmias, possibly seizures	Decrease dose of TCA (sertraline has less of an effect, but the dose may still require decrease).
TCAs Imipramine Amitriptyline Doxepin Clomipramine Nortriptyline Desipramine	Phenytoin (Dilantin)	Increase in clearance of TCAs	Decrease in antidepressant response	May need to increase the dose of TCA.

Valproic acid, divalproex (Depakene, Depakote)	Aspirin	Large doses of aspirin displace valproic acid from plasma protein binding sites; aspirin apparently also decreases metabolic clearance of valproic acid	Valproic acid toxicity; possibly sedation, GI upset, or confusion	May need to decrease dose of valproic acid.
Valproic acid, divalproex (Depakene, Depakote)	Carbamazepine	Increase in clearance of valproic acid	Decrease in valproic acid levels, possibly a decrease in response	Monitor valproic acid blood levels; may need to increase dose of valproic acid.
Valproic acid, divalproex (Depakene, Depakote)	Erythromycin	Decrease in clearance of valproic acid	Increase in valproic acid levels, possibly sedation, GI upset, or confusion	Monitor valproic acid blood levels; may need to decrease dose of valproic acid.
Valproic acid, divalproex (Depakene, Depakote)	Fluoxetine	Decrease in clearance of valproic acid	Increase in valproic acid levels, possibly an increase in sedation, GI upset, or confusion	Monitor valproic acid blood levels; may need to decrease dose of valproic acid.
Warfarin (Coumadin)	Valproic acid, divalproex (Depakene, Depakote)	Valproic acid displaces warfarin from plasma protein binding sites, but it does *not* appear to alter metabolic clearance of warfarin	Transient increase in PT/INR	This interaction is likely to result in a transient increase in PT/INR, which may last for several weeks; ultimately, the dose of warfarin that is required will be the same as before the addition of valproic acid.
Warfarin	Fluvoxamine Fluoxetine Sertraline Paroxetine	Possible decrease in clearance of warfarin	Increase in PT/INR	May need to decrease the dose of warfarin. Most likely to occur with fluvoxamine.

ACE, angiotensin-converting enzyme; GI, gastrointestinal; INR, international normalized ratio; NSAID, nonsteroidal anti-inflammatory drug; OTC, over the counter; PT, prothrombin time; TCAs, tricyclic antidepressants.

isoenzymes. Phase II metabolic biotransformation generally involves the conjugation of a parent drug or drug metabolite (from phase I) with an endogenous substance like glucuronic acid, sulfate, or glycine. These conjugation phase II reactions often have a prior phase I metabolic step, and they usually render a drug or its metabolite more water soluble and, thus, more easily eliminated in the urine.

Cytochrome P_{450} enzymes exist primarily in the liver and are also located elsewhere in the body (e.g., kidney, lungs, intestine, and brain). At least eight different families of CYP450 isoenzymes have been found in humans, and each of these may exist in several different forms or subfamilies. Isoenzymes responsible for much of the biotransformation of drugs in humans include CYP450-3A3/4, 1A2, 2E1, 2D6, 2A6, 2B6, and 2C. (*CYPnXm* is the general format for naming cytochrome isoforms. For example, CYtochrome P_{450} may be further specified by n, the gene family member; X, the gene subfamily letter; and m, the gene number). Specific drugs alter the metabolism of other drugs by either induction (i.e., increasing the production of isoenzymes) or inhibition of the activity of individual isoenzymes. However, most drugs are metabolized by means of multiple isoenzyme pathways, such that inhibition or induction of one pathway may have a negligible effect on overall drug clearance. Drugs like cimetidine (Tagamet) inhibit several different CYP450 isoenzymes. Accordingly, such drugs are more likely to cause a wide range of clinically significant drug interactions when added to a pre-existing drug regimen than are drugs that inhibit only one specific isoenzyme. Several psychotropic drugs are CYP450 enzyme inhibitors (e.g., SSRIs, phenothiazines, and valproic acid), whereas carbamazepine is the only commonly used psychotropic that has significant enzyme-inducing activity. Although our knowledge about the specific isoenzyme inhibition profiles of the newer psychotropics is rapidly increasing, information is more incomplete about the biotransformational pathways of the older hepatically metabolized drugs. For example, fluoxetine (Prozac) is known to inhibit CYP450-2D6, 3A3/4, and 2C, but similar information is lacking about many older antidepressants. Moreover, much of the current ideas are based on results from experiments that are difficult to extrapolate to the human being.

Enzyme inhibition and induction reactions are particularly important when the affected drug has a narrow therapeutic index (e.g., phenytoin [Dilantin]). Lists are available of the known isoenzyme inhibition profiles for each psychotropic agent; however, because our understanding of these profiles is incomplete, it is more practical to simply list the significant drug-drug interactions that have been reported as well as to issue warnings in special cases in which the probability of interactions is high, according to current isoenzyme theory. Comprehensive lists of reported drug interactions are available in texts like those listed at the end of the chapter. Table 2–8 lists those interactions that are common to primary care practice.

C. Warnings about monoamine oxidase inhibitors.

Because MAOIs are occasionally prescribed by psychiatrists, MAOIs are found in primary care. The two nonspecific (i.e., they nonspecifically inhibit both monoamine oxidase A and monoamine oxidase B) MAOIs available in this country that are prescribed for psychiatric disorders are phenelzine (Nardil) and tranylcypromine (Parnate). One reason that these medications are used infrequently is because of their unfavorable drug interaction profile. When given in conjunction with interacting drugs, MAOIs can precipitate one of two severe pharmacodynamic interactions:

1. *Hypertensive reaction.*
   This reaction is characterized by large increases in blood pressure, throbbing headache, nausea, and diaphoresis. In its most severe form, this reaction results in stroke and death. Because certain foods may produce this reaction, the primary care physician must give the patient dietary restrictions when prescribing phenelzine or tranylcypromine or any other nonselective MAOI. Aged cheese most commonly interacts with MAOIs; this combination has resulted in deaths, and patients taking MAOIs must be instructed to avoid aged cheese. Lists of other dietary restrictions can be obtained from nutrition services or drug information services in most hospitals or from pharmacies in the out-patient setting.

2. *Serotonin syndrome.*
   The severity of the serotonin syndrome varies, but this syndrome is characterized by central nervous system excitation, restlessness, confusion, muscle rigidity, increased tendon reflexes, flushing, diaphoresis, hyperpyrexia, respiratory depression, coma, cardiovascular shock, and death.

3. *Cold or cough products.*
   Almost any over-the-counter cold or cough product contains at least one drug that interacts adversely with MAOIs. *The only safe medication that can be given for a cold is an antihistamine (e.g., diphenhydramine [Benadryl] or chlorpheniramine [Chlor-Trimeton]) that is not combined with a decongestant or antitussive. For coughs, codeine can be used, but dextromethorphan should be avoided.* For severe pain, morphine can be used, but *meperidine (Demerol) must be avoided.*

   Table 2–9 lists some of the OTC cold or cough remedies that are SAFE to use with MAOIs.

Table 2–9
Antihistamines that Can Be Safely Combined with Monoamine Oxidase Inhibitors

Generic Name	Trade Name
Brompheniramine	Dimetane (not Dimetapp)
Chlorpheniramine	Chlor-Trimeton (not Chlor-Trimeton 12-Hour Relief or Chlor-Trimeton 4-Hour Relief)
Clemastine	Tavist or Tavist-1 (not Tavist-D)
Diphenhydramine	Benadryl (not Benadryl Decongestant Kapseals/tablets), Benylin syrup (not Benylin Decongestant liquid)
Triprolidine	Actidil (not Actifed)
Promethazine	Phenergan (not Phenergan VC)

XI. Adverse neurobehavioral effects of common medical drugs.

Adverse effects or *side effects* are unwanted results of drug action that are often unrelated to therapeutic effects. In contrast, *allergic reactions* are entirely unexpected and are often serious. Compared with the expected duration of a drug's use, clinical trials are relatively short and are designed to allow discovery of the more common side effects in preparation for marketing. For this reason, new side effects are reported years after a drug has been introduced, making it necessary for the clinician and the patient to be vigilant. Moreover, postmarketing surveillance is imperfect, making judgment of the frequency of particular side effects difficult, and the existence of drug-induced psychiatric symptoms is often overlooked or unreported.

A wide variation exists in the symptoms of drug-induced changes in mental state. It is easy to recognize disorientation and confusion, but most patients report having less dramatic states, such as mood instability and increased irritability. Such nonspecific symptoms may be drug induced, a situational response or the first signs of a mental disorder. Generally, adverse effects occur at the start of treatment; however, some common long-acting drugs, like diazepam (Valium), are associated with discontinuation syndromes that may be so delayed that the relationship to the responsible drug is hard to identify. For these and related reasons, it is possible to argue that under-reporting or over-reporting happens. Regardless, many drugs seem to be capable of producing psychiatric symptoms.

Table 2–10 lists medical drugs that are commonly believed to cause psychiatric symptoms. *The Medical Letter on Drugs and Therapeutics* provides a more comprehensive list. Therefore, nonstandard drugs (e.g., hallucinogens) and well-known withdrawal syndromes (e.g., cocaine withdrawal) or physiologic reactions (e.g., insulin hypoglycemia) are not listed. Rather than identify all agents suspected of causing such reactions, we have attempted to keep our list short in order to increase its utility.

XII. Psychotropic drugs useful in medical conditions and medical drugs useful for neurobehavioral states.

Medical and psychiatric illness are frequent partners, and when both are present, selecting the best psychotropic can be a challenge. Meeting the challenge is made easier by a knowledge that there are

1. Psychotropic drugs that may benefit a medical condition (see Table 2–4).
2. Medical drugs that may benefit a psychiatric condition (Table 2–11).

Of the two tasks, the most difficult is selecting a psychotropic drug for a medical patient with a psychiatric illness. Psychotropic drugs that benefit medical conditions have the desired psychiatric therapeutic effect and have a side effect profile that most benefits the medical illness. For example, the antidepressants doxepin (Adapin, Sinequan) and trimipramine (Surmontil) are potent histamine-2 blockers. For a patient with peptic ulcer disease and depression, either of these two agents is a good choice (see Table 2–4).

The reverse situation is also encountered, although much less frequently. For example, propranolol (Inderal) might be a good choice for a patient with both hypertension and stage fright. Likewise, captopril (Capoten) might be a good medication for a patient with hypertension who is prone to depression (Table 2–11). On the other hand, methyldopa (Adomet) would be an unwise choice for the control of hypertension in a patient with a history of depression (see Table 2–4).

Tables 2–4 and 2–11 are designed to stimulate thinking; these tables are not designed for prescriptive use. Anyone considering using one of the strategies suggested by either table needs to consult more specific literature before applying the strategy to a specific patient.

XIII. Guide to newly released psychotropics.

A. When, if ever, should a primary care physician administer a newly released psychotropic?

Because knowledge about new psychotropic drugs is always limited, we recommend strongly that great caution be used when administering newly released psychotropic drugs. Prior to administration, advice should be obtained from a knowledgeable and objective psychiatrist who has considerable experience with a new agent. Potentially dangerous drug interactions are often unknown at the time of release. For example, when fluoxetine (Prozac) was first released, its interactions with MAOIs were unknown. People died from the serotonin syndrome produced by this combination. The mixture of any selective serotonin inhibitor (SSRI) with any MAOI is contraindicated.

Some concerns remain unresolved until years after a drug's release. For example, the SSRIs

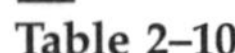

Table 2–10
Adverse Neurobehavioral Effects of Common Drug

Drug	Adverse Effect
Albuterol (Proventil, Ventolin)	Hallucinations, paranoia
Amiodarone (Cordarone)	Movement disorders, minor tremor and possible dyskinesias, myoclonus, hemiballism
Anabolic steroids	Irritability, rage, affective instability, suicidality
Anticholinergic drugs	Delirium
Asparaginase (Elspar)	Confusion, paranoia, depression
Baclofen (Lioresal)	Affective instability, hallucinations, nightmares, paranoia; especially with abrupt discontinuation
Benzodiazepines	Memory impairment, especially in elderly with compromised CNS
Beta blockers, lipophilic Metoprolol (Lopressor) Propranolol (Inderal) Others	Depression; hydrophilic variety less likely to cause this (e.g., atenolol [Tenormin], sotalol [Betaspace])
Calcium channel blockers Diltiazem (Cardizem) Nifedipine (Procardia) Verapamil (Calan)	Manic and hypomanic states
Cimetidine (Tagamet)	Agitation, confusion, depression, especially in elderly; ranitidine (Zantac) causes fewer neurobehavioral side effects
Contraceptives, oral	No convincing relationship to depression
Cyclobenzaprine (Flexeril)	Anticholinergic delirium
Cycloserine (Seromycin)	Confusion, psychosis, depression
Cyproheptadine (Periactin)	Reversal of SSRI effect
Glucocorticoids, ACTH	Affective instability; occurs in more than 5% of patients taking >60 mg/d of prednisone
Indomethacin (Indocin)	Delusions, dissociations, hallucinations, paranoia, hypomania, especially in elderly
Ketamine (Ketalar)	Hallucinations (common finding)
Ketoconazole (Nizoral)	Hallucinations (one report)
Meperidine (Demerol)	Postoperative delirium, avoid in elderly
Methyldopa (Aldomet)	Depression, especially with prior history
Methysergide (Sansert)	Agitation, depression, depersonalization
Metoclopramide (Reglan)	Acute dystonic reactions due to neuroleptic properties, tardive dyskinesia
Nifedipine (Procardia)	Depression, especially in elderly
Oxymetazoline (Afrin)	Anxiety, insomnia, hallucinations, mostly in children
Procaine (Novocain)	Panic attacks, especially with pre-existing panic disorder
Prochlorperazine (Compazine)	Acute dystonic reactions due to neuroleptic properties, tardive dyskinesia
Reserpine (Serpasil)	Depression when large doses are used (>0.5 mg/d), nightmares
Selegiline (Eldepryl)	Becomes a traditional MAOI at >10 mg/d
Sulindac (Clinoril)	Bizarre behavior, illusions, especially in elderly
Thiethylperazine (Torecan)	Acute dystonic reactions due to neuroleptic properties
Tocainide (Tonocard)	Agitation, psychosis, terror, delirium, depression
Triazolam (Halcion)	Memory impairment, anterograde amnesia, especially in elderly
Trimethobenzamide (Tigan)	Acute dystonic reactions due to neuroleptic properties
Trimethoprim-sulfamethoxazole (Bactrim, Septra)	Psychosis, depression, disorientation
Vincristine (Oncovin)	Hallucinations, especially at high doses

ACTH = adrenocorticotropic hormone; CNS = central nervous system; SSRI = selective serotonin reuptake inhibitor.

have been available for nearly a decade, but data are just becoming available about their potential effects during pregnancy and lactation. Recent evidence suggests that when taken late in pregnancy, fluoxetine and other SSRIs may increase the risk of premature delivery. These data remain controversial.

B. Advice about bupropion sustained release (Wellbutrin SR), mirtazapine (Remeron), and olanzapine (Zyprexa).

Since the submission of *Primary Care Psychiatry* to the publisher, three new drugs were released and a fourth is at the door. In addition to the

Table 2–11
Medical Drugs Useful for Common Neurobehavioral States

Psychiatric Condition	Medical Drug(s)	Comments
Agitation, especially in Alzheimer's and other dementias	Zolpidem (Ambien)	PRN or 2.5–5 mg t.i.d. as tolerated; anecdotal and author's (Knesper's) experience
Akathisia	Beta blockers (atenolol [Tenormin], betaxolol [Kerlone], metoprolol [Lopressor], nadolol [Corgard], propranolol [Inderal])	Most effective are betaxolol and propranolol.
Anticholinergic side effects, peripheral (e.g., constipation, urinary hesitancy)	Bethanechol (Urecholine)	Urinary retention is best treated by switching to nonanticholinergic drugs and avoiding UTIs.
Anxiety disorder, generalized; performance anxiety (e.g., stage fright)	Beta blockers (atenolol, betaxolol, metoprolol, nadolol, propranolol) and benzodiazepines	Propranolol combined with clonazepam (Klonopin) is especially synergistic; propranolol is the most effective for performance safety.
Attention-deficit hyperactivity disorder	Amphetamine (Dexedrine, Desoxyn), clonidine (Catapres)	Combination more effective than single use.
Depression	Captopril (Capoten)	Reserved for concurrent hypertension and depression; adjunct to traditional antidepressant.
	Bromocriptine (Parlodel)	Reasonably effective. Useful adjunct to traditional antidepressants.
	Methimazole (Tapazole)	May have antidepressant effect.
Diabetes insipidus, lithium-induced	Amiloride (Midamor)	Monitor lithium levels.
Mania, bipolar disease	Calcium channel blockers (diltiazem [Cardizem], nifedipine [Procardia], verapamil [Calan])	For patients unresponsive to traditional agents; diltiazem and verapamil are the most studied.
Schizophrenia; maybe psychosis in general	Bromocriptine (Parlodel)	Combine with a traditional neuroleptic.
Tardive dyskinesia (TD)	Vitamin E	Likely effective in early TD as prophylaxis for elderly starting long-term neuroleptic therapy.

PRN = as necessary; t.i.d. = three times a day; UTI = urinary tract infection.

above general advice, we offer the following thoughts about these new agents:

1. *Bupropion sustained release (Wellbutrin SR).* Sustained release bupropion is the first available sustained release antidepressant. Sustained release preparations have the advantage of smoothing out the overall side-effect experience, and, indeed, this appears to be true for bupropion sustained release. Additional advantages over the immediate release product are a dose 150 mg twice a day and a risk of seizure equivalent to that of other antidepressants. Nevertheless, until we know more, use is contraindicated for patients with seizures or at risk for seizures (e.g., patients with eating disorders).

2. *Mirtazapine (Remeron).* Mirtazapine's efficacy probably is similar to other available antidepressants. Use in primary care populations is limited because of reports of agranulocytosis, estimated maximum is 3.1 cases per 1000 patients; excessive somnolence; and weight gain.

3. *Olanzapine (Zyprexa) and sertindole (Serlect).* Olanzapine follows clozapine (Clozaril) in what will be a series of atypical antipsychotics that are designed to minimize extrapyramidal disorders and to better treat negative psychotic symptoms (e.g., social withdrawal). Sertindole (Serlect) may be the next available agent. At this time, these agents cannot be recommended for routine use in primary care. Olanzapine is most "clozapine-like" but, unlike clozapine, olanzapine appears to be unassociated with agranulocytosis. On the down side, patients on high-dose olanzapine appear to be at some increased risk for hepatotoxicity. Sertindole can prolong the cardiac QT interval, and patients taking sertindole have died, likely because of adverse cardiac events.

4. *Venlafaxine extended release (Effexor XR).* This repackaged product will likely be the second sustained release antidepressant on the market. The advantage is once-a-day dosing and likely adverse-effects minimization.

Resource

The Pharmaceutical Research and Manufacturers of America (PhRMA) lists company programs that provide free drugs to physicians whose patients could not otherwise afford them. The PhRMA Directory of Prescription Drug Assistance Programs may be obtained by writing to PhRMA, 1100 Fifteenth Street, NW, Washington, DC, 20005 or by calling 1-800-PMA-INFO. Unlisted companies should be contacted directly; they are sometimes willing to provide the physician with free medicines for disadvantaged patients.

Suggested Reading

Altshuler LL, Cohen L, Szuba MP, et al. Pharmacologic management of psychiatric illness during pregnancy: Dilemmas and guidelines. Am J Psychiatry 1996; 153:592–606.

American Psychiatric Association. Diagnostic and Statistical Manual of Mental Disorders, 4th ed. Washington, DC: American Psychiatric Association; 1994.

Ayd FJ, Jr. Lexicon of Psychiatry, Neurology, and the Neurosciences. Baltimore: Williams & Wilkins; 1995.

Ciraulo DA, Shader RL, Greenblatt RI, et al (eds): Drug Interactions in Psychiatry. 2nd ed. Baltimore: Williams & Wilkins; 1995.

Cohen LJ. Principles to optimize drug treatment in the elderly: Practical pharmacokinetics and drug interactions. Geriatrics 1995; 50(Suppl. 1):S32–S40.

DeVane CL. Fundamentals of Monitoring Psychoactive Drug Therapy. Baltimore: Williams & Wilkins; 1990.

Dubovsky SL. Psychotherapeutics in Primary Care. New York: Grune & Stratton; 1981.

Hyman SE, Arana GW, Rosenbaum JF. Handbook of Psychiatric Drug Therapy, 3rd ed. Boston: Little, Brown & Co.; 1995.

Jefferson JW, Marshall JR. Neuropsychiatric Features of Medical Disorders. New York: Plenum Publishing Corp.; 1981.

Kane JM, Lieberman JA (eds.). Adverse Effects of Psychotropic Drugs. New York: Guilford Press; 1992.

Krishnan KRR, Steffens DC, Doraiswamy PM. Psychotropic drug interactions. Prim Psychiatry 1996; 3:21–45.

Salzman C (ed.). Clinical Geriatric Psychopharmacology, 2nd ed. Baltimore: Williams & Wilkins; 1992.

Schatzberg AF, Nemeroff CB (eds). Textbook of Psychopharmacology. Washington, DC: American Psychiatric Press; 1995.

Schiffer RB, Klein RF, Sider RC. The Medical Evaluation of the Psychiatric Patient. New York: Plenum Publishing Corp.; 1988.

Silver PA, Editor. Psychotropic drug use in the medically ill. In: Wise TN (ed). Advances in Psychosomatic Medicine. Vol. 21. Basel, Switzerland: S. Karger; 1994.

Stoudemire A, Fogel BS, Gulley LR, et al. Psychopharmacology in the medical patient. In: Stoudemine A, Fogel BS (eds). Psychiatric Care of the Medical Patient. New York: Oxford University Press; 1993.

Zelnik T. Depressive effects of drugs. In: Cameron OG (ed). Presentations of Depression: Depression in Medical and Other Psychiatric Disorders. New York: John Wiley & Sons; 1987.

3

RACHEL LIPSON GLICK, MD

MICHELLE RIBA, MD, MS

Common Psychiatric Emergencies in the Office Setting

Unsafe, unusual, or disruptive thoughts and behaviors underlie all psychiatric emergencies. The keys to handling these situations in the office setting are to keep the patient and others, including the clinician, safe; to recognize the potential underlying medical causes; and to make an appropriate disposition or referral. *This chapter provides strategies that can be used in the event of an emergency.* Possibly, the worst mistake would be to say, "This could not happen to me."

I. Agitation, threats, violence, and weapons.

Agitation is a state of increased mental and motor activity. The agitated patient may be threatening, and agitation often precedes violence. In the primary care office setting, agitation must be rapidly assessed, and interventions must be quickly made. If verbal interventions do not calm the patient, he or she should be immediately transferred to a more contained environment (either a medical or psychiatric emergency room or a mental health crisis center).

A. Diagnostic overview/epidemiology.

Certain patient populations are predisposed to agitation and violence. Diagnosis, history, and demographics should all be considered in assessments of the potential for violence.

1. Many diagnoses are associated with agitation and violence.
   a. *Delirious patients* can be agitated and violent (see section VI).
   b. *Psychotic patients* can be agitated and violent, regardless of the underlying cause of the psychosis (see section V).
   c. *Substance-abusing patients* can become agitated, especially when they are intoxicated or when they are in a withdrawal state.
   d. *Patients with brain disease,* especially those with global, frontal, or temporal lobe pathology, may be prone to frustration, unpredictability, agitation, and violence.
   e. *Patients with personality disorder,* particularly those with paranoid, antisocial, and borderline personality, may act out aggressively.
2. Historical factors to consider in assessments of the risk of violence include a history of violence. This is the best predictor of violence if the patient has been in his or her current mental state before. (In patients who are delirious or psychotic for the first time, lack of a violent history has no predictive value.) In addition, exposure to violence, including a history of child abuse, is a risk factor.
3. Demographic factors associated with violence include age, sex, and socioeconomic factors. Young males (aged 15–24 years) are more likely to be violent.

   Individuals who are without social support, poor, uneducated, or members of minority groups experiencing racial injustice are also more likely to be violent.

B. Warning signs of potential assault.

People do not usually strike out violently against health care providers without warning. Assaults are usually preceded by a period of tension buildup. During this time, the patient gives many clues to the impending attack, including the following:

1. Hyperactivity: pacing or any other increase in motor activity is cause for concern.
2. Loud, angry, or profane speech.
3. Increased muscle tension (e.g., clenched jaw or fists, rigid posture, fixed facial expression).
4. Posture that suggests anger or tension (e.g., sitting on the edge of a chair or gripping the arms of a chair).
5. Intoxication.
6. Suspiciousness or guarded speech or behavior, including increased startle response.
7. Angry, irritable, or anxious affect.
8. Breathlessness, tachycardia, diaphoresis, or visibly pulsating temporal arteries.

9. Uncooperativeness with requests.
10. Door slamming, chairs toppling, or property destruction.
11. Carrying of weapons or grabbing of objects that can be used as weapons.
12. Verbal or physical threats.
13. The clinician's own response to the patient. If a patient makes the clinician feel anxious, he or she should trust these feelings and be alert to possible danger. The clinician should watch carefully for other warning signs noted here and be sure that help is close by.

C. Management of the agitated or violent patient.

1. The clinician should approach the patient in a particular way.
   a. Try to approach the patient at an angle rather than head-on. Never approach the patient from behind.
   b. Keep your distance. The paranoid patient, in particular, needs more personal space than is typical in order to feel safe.
   c. Do not touch an agitated patient, particularly if he or she is paranoid.
   d. Take a nonthreatening stance. Stand at a slight angle rather than directly facing the patient. Stay at least a leg's length away from the patient so that you cannot easily be kicked, grabbed, or struck. Keep your feet slightly apart, one in front of the other, to ensure better balance and the ability to move away quickly, if necessary.
   e. Keep your hands at your side so that they are visible and also readily available to fend off a blow. Do not put them in your pockets or behind you, because the psychotic or paranoid patient may fear that you have a weapon. Do not cross your arms, because this stance can be perceived as threatening.
   f. Eye contact is good, so do not be afraid to look at the patient as you speak with him or her; however, intense staring is perceived as threatening.
   g. Leave the office door open while you talk with the patient. Both you and the patient should feel that there is easy access to the door (see 3a below).
2. The clinician should use certain verbal interventions.
   a. Remain calm. Do not respond emotionally, because this causes increased tension and greater chance of violence.
   b. Use formal titles, such as "Mr." or "Ms.," rather than the patient's first name, to convey respect.
   c. Reassure the patient that your main goal is to help him or her. Show concern.
   d. Tell the patient that violence is not acceptable, and that you cannot help him or her if you are frightened.
   e. Allow the patient to verbalize why he or she is angry or frightened.
   f. Do not confront; rather, work with the patient. Be open to what the patient requests. Give the patient reasonable choices, such as "If you can calm down now we can talk now. Otherwise, I'll have to come back to talk to you in a little while when you are calmer."
   g. Use verbal limit-setting techniques, such as telling the patient that he or she needs to sit down to talk because pacing or standing over you makes you uncomfortable. Agitated patients fear losing control, and seeing that you are willing to take control and set limits can be comforting and controlling.
   h. Some patients respond better to a person of one sex or the other. For example, a staff member of the opposite sex may be particularly calming if the patient has fears of a homosexual attack. If the patient is not responding and calming with your verbal interventions, you could ask a staff member of the opposite sex to try to intervene.
   i. If available, a family member or friend of the patient may be able to help calm the patient or provide important data.
3. The clinician should be aware of his or her surroundings.
   a. Note exits. The best situation is for both you and the patient to be able to exit the room without tripping over the other, but if the room is not designed in a way that makes this possible, be sure that you are positioned in a manner that allows you to escape easily.
   b. If any objects that can be used as weapons (e.g., letter openers, paperweights, needles, furniture that can be lifted) are readily available, be aware of their location in relation to the patient. You can use some objects, such as pillows and light pieces of furniture, to protect yourself. Be aware of their whereabouts as well in case they are needed.
   c. If a confrontation is taking place in an area where other patients are present, such as the waiting area, you should consider asking them to leave.
4. Use a show of force—there is safety in numbers. While you meet with the patient, have all available staff join you to show that enough other people are around to keep the patient in control.
5. The clinician should not hesitate to call for help.
   a. Have a prearranged system (e.g., panic buttons that signal staff, a specific phone message, such as "Can you ask Dr. Smith to join us?") for signaling your staff that you need emergency help.

b. If someone is agitated and exhibits behavior that is escalating, staff should immediately call security or the police.
c. If a patient becomes loud while in a closed office with a staff member, other staff members should know to knock, enter, and check on the safety of the situation.

6. The clinician should offer medications to help calm the patient if you have them readily available. Give these orally. Do not attempt to give injections unless the patient is appropriately restrained.
   a. A neuroleptic, such as haloperidol (Haldol), 5 to 10 mg by mouth (PO), is most helpful in the treatment of the paranoid or psychotic patient. It is available in an oral liquid form that can be mixed with syrup; this form is more rapidly absorbed than pills. Anticholinergic prophylaxis against dystonic reactions should be administered in some patient populations. Patients at high risk for dystonic reactions include young men, particularly African-American men. Benztropine (Cogentin), 1 mg PO, could be offered with the haloperidol.
   b. Benzodiazepines, such as lorazepam (Ativan), 1 mg, can also be used. These should be avoided, however, if the patient is already intoxicated. Rarely, but more often in patients with brain abnormalities resulting from such conditions as dementias, retardation, and head trauma, *the benzodiazepines can cause a paradoxical increase in agitation. Benzodiazepines (e.g., 1 to 2 mg of lorazepam given intramuscularly [IM]) may be used in combination with neuroleptics (e.g., 2 to 5 mg of haloperidol IM) for their combined sedative effects.* Lorazepam and haloperidol may be mixed in the same syringe so than one intramuscular injection may be given.

7. If the patient wants to leave and the clinician is unable to hold him or her with verbal intervention, the clinician should not try to physically restrain the patient. In settings where security or other staff trained in the safe restraint of patients is available, this resource should be used. If not, the agitated patient should be allowed to leave, and the local police should be notified if risk to the patient, specific others, or the community at large is thought to exist.

D. Evaluation of the agitated patient.

If the patient calms with verbal intervention, the clinician may evaluate the situation further. If the patient does not calm, the clinician should get help and the patient should be transferred to a safer place where restraint and seclusion are possible, such as a hospital emergency department.

1. The clinician begins with a screening mental status examination. In talking with the patient to calm him or her, the clinician may begin to understand whether the patient is experiencing intoxication, psychosis, paranoia, confusion, or just plain anger. Important aspects of the mental status examination are the patient's behavior toward the clinician, psychomotor movement, speech, and thought process. Any previous history of similar episodes that the patient or other informants can provide would be useful.

2. If the patient is intoxicated, the clinician performs a screening examination to check for head trauma, acute abdomen, or other injuries. Breathalyzers and blood or urine toxicology screens can be useful if the substances involved are unknown. The clinician ensures that the patient has a safe place to "sleep it off." *The clinician does not try to make recommendations for treatment while the patient is intoxicated.* The clinician arranges a follow-up time so that the problem can be discussed in greater depth.

3. *If the patient is psychotic, the clinician attempts to determine whether the psychosis is new.* If the patient has no known psychiatric history, particularly if the patient is older, medical and neurologic causes of the changed mental status must be investigated. A psychiatric disposition is needed if no medical cause can be found (see section V).

   If the patient has a known psychiatric history and the clinician suspects that the current agitation is a manifestation of that, the appropriate psychiatric consultation is sought.

4. If the patient is confused and has a fluctuating level of consciousness, the clinician considers a diagnosis of delirium, and works aggressively to determine the underlying cause. Such patients usually require medical admission to ensure their safety from violence and self-harm as well as from the medical underlying condition (see section VI).

5. If no evidence of a mental status abnormality is present, the clinician may need to warn the patient that the clinician and his or her office staff will not tolerate out-of-control behavior. Although the clinician would be available to talk to the patient in the future, if the patient is angry enough to be frightening, he or she will be asked to leave. If the patient makes threats, is assaultive, or destroys property, the clinician will bring legal charges against the patient.

   Patients who behave this way often have an underlying personality disorder, and a psychiatric consultation may be helpful. Suggesting a psychiatric consultation to an already angry patient is not easy. A statement such as "I am not a psychiatric expert so I wonder if a psychiatrist or counselor could help us understand how you cope with your anger" might work. If the patient refuses referral, the clinician may still benefit from discussing the case with a psychiatric colleague.

E. Counseling and caregiver assistance.

Educational intervention is possible once the acute situation has passed. The family of a delirious patient can be reassured that the violent tendencies will disappear once the underlying condition is corrected. The family of the psychotic patient, as well as the patient, can be educated to watch for early warning signs of decompensation.

The intoxicated patient can be told about the risks of drinking or using substances on future behavior and can be encouraged to get help with his or her problem. His or her family can be warned about the potential for violence when the patient is using the substances and can be given information about alcoholism or substance abuse and the community resources that are available.

The patient with personality disorder can be taught that he or she is responsible for his or her actions.

F. Special situations.

1. Threats against the clinician or his or her staff or family should be taken seriously. Local law enforcement agency can provide advice on how to handle these situations. Psychiatric involvement may be necessary for assessing the dangerousness of the situation. *Patients may be banned from the office or clinic as long as they are not abandoned clinically. Clinicians can discharge the duty to continue to treat the patient by sending a registered letter explaining that the clinician can no longer see the patient and suggesting alternative places to seek care.* For example, the clinician could suggest that the patient call the local medical society for referrals. In these situations, the clinician may need to document in the patient's chart a consultation with a colleague about the situation.
2. If the clinician is confronted with a weapon, experts recommend the following actions:
   a. Look the patient in the eye calmly.
   b. Move slowly and deliberately.
   c. Speak in a natural tone of voice.
   d. Assume that the patient is in control, and tell him or her so.
   e. Keep talking in a reassuring voice.
   f. People who carry weapons often feel helpless and frightened. Requesting that the weapon be given up immediately may heighten these feelings. Instead, asking the patient why he or she feels the need for a weapon, and then explaining that you want to help but do not feel that you can really listen to the patient or examine him or her while the patient has a weapon because it frightens you, often leads to voluntary disarmament.
   g. People are often injured when weapons change hands. If the patient volunteers to give up the weapon, do not take it directly from him or her. Instead, ask that he or she leave it on the table, a chair, or the floor, from where security personnel can safely remove it.
   h. Do not threaten verbally or try to physically disarm a patient with a weapon. This sort of action usually just triggers assaults.
   i. If the patient refuses to give up the weapon, get out of the situation as quickly as you can and get trained help. In this situation, panic buttons in places where a clinician can push them inconspicuously to signal the need for help can be invaluable.

Case Study

Mr. Jones, a 27-year-old divorced, unemployed man comes to the clinic and requests to be seen, although he does not have an appointment. His first visit with his new doctor was last week. At that time, he requested "tranquilizers for my nerves." The physician noted a slight tremor, somewhat increased blood pressure and pulse, and abnormal liver function results. Because alcoholism was suspected, the doctor refused to give the patient tranquilizers and instead suggested an alcohol treatment program. The patient became furious and stormed out of the office.

Today, while waiting to be seen, Mr. Jones tells the patient sitting next to him in the waiting area "I'm going to kill that doctor," and shows him a knife he is concealing. The other patient does not know what to do, because he is afraid of being the target of anger himself if he warns the physician. As soon as Mr. Jones is called into the examination room, the other patient, however, reports what Mr. Jones said to him to the receptionist, who in turn tells the nurse. The nurse tells the receptionist to call the police and request assistance; at the same time, she heads to the room where the doctor is meeting Mr. Jones.

Meanwhile, the doctor sees that Mr. Jones appears angry and agitated. He smells of alcohol and is clenching his fists and jaws. She realizes that she is frightened and notes that she can easily leave the room without walking close to Mr. Jones. She elects to do so just as the nurse knocks, opens the door, and asks her to come quickly because there is an emergency down the hall. They leave Mr. Jones sitting in the examination room until the police arrive; then, they all approach him together. The police transport Mr. Jones to a local emergency room, where he can sober up safely and then be assessed for dangerousness.

It is decided by the doctor and staff that the patient cannot be cared for safely in the clinic. A letter to this effect with some referral options is sent to the patient. All staff are notified of this decision. The clinic's lawyer is consulted about obtaining a restraining order should the patient attempt to return.

II. Assessing dangerousness: suicidal ideation and actions

It is important for primary physicians to recognize and assess the suicidal patient. *Data show that 75% of all patients who commit suicide see their primary physician within 3 months of killing themselves, and 50% of patients who attempt or complete suicide have seen a physician during the previous week.*

A. Diagnostic overview/epidemiology.

Certain patients are at greater risk for attempting suicide than the general population. Risk factors are based on diagnosis, history, current life stresses, and demographic and socioeconomic factors (Table 3–1).

1. *Diagnostic factors.*
   a. *Psychiatric illness.* The risk of suicide in the mentally ill is about 10 times higher than that in those who are not mentally ill, and 90% of patients who attempt suicide have a major psychiatric disorder.
      (1) Major depression. This is the diagnosis most commonly associated with suicide. Half of all patients who commit suicide are depressed.
      (2) Alcohol and/or drug dependence.
      (3) Psychosis.
      (4) Delirium.
      (5) Personality disorders, particularly antisocial and borderline.
      (6) Postpartum psychiatric disorders.
   b. *Medical illness.* Risk of suicide is increased in patients with medical illness.
      (1) Chronic pain.
      (2) Chronic illness.
      (3) Recent surgery.
      (4) Terminal illness, including acquired immunodeficiency syndrome and cancer.

Table 3–1
Suicide Risk Factors

Psychiatric diagnosis
Major depression
Alcohol and/or drug dependence
Psychosis of any etiology
Delirium
Personality disorder (borderline and antisocial)
Postpartum psychiatric disorder
History of suicide threats or attempts
Family history of suicide or attempts
Male
Older
White
Single, widowed, separated, divorced
Living alone, especially if recent loss or separation has occurred
Unemployed
Urban dweller
Chronic or terminal medical illness
Chronic pain
Access to a gun
Lack of willingness to acknowledge need for help

2. *Historical factors.*
   a. A *history of suicide attempts* is a strong risk factor. Up to half of successful suicide victims have made a prior attempt.
   b. Patients with a *family history of suicide or suicide attempts,* particularly in close relatives, are at higher risk for suicide.
3. *Demographic factors.*
   a. *Sex:* although women attempt suicide 3 to 4 times more often than men, men are 2 to 4 times more likely to be successful.
   b. *Age:* suicide rates tend to increase with age. For men, they peak at age 75 years, whereas for women, the peak is at about age 60. The rate of suicide in adolescents and young adults has risen recently, but it is still lower than that in older adults.
   c. *Race:* whites commit suicide more often than African Americans or Hispanics.
   d. *Marital status:* those who are single, widowed, separated, or divorced are more likely to commit suicide than are those who are married.
   e. *Living alone* is strongly associated with suicide, particularly in the first year after the loss of a significant other.
   f. The *unemployed and unskilled* are at higher risk for suicide.
   g. Those who live in *urban areas* are at higher risk for suicide than are those who live in rural settings.
   h. Those with *access to guns* may be at higher risk for suicide.

Note: Suicide risk factors are based on statistical information derived from population studies. In an individual patient, suicidal ideation must be evaluated, when appropriate, regardless of the number of risk factors that are apparent. *The presence of risk factors might increase concern about a patient's safety, but the absence of risk factors does not negate the need for assessment or concern.*

B. Assessing and Referring the Suicidal Patient

It is never wrong to ask a patient about suicidal thoughts, regardless of the situation. If the clinician believes a patient is depressed, or if a patient has just been given "bad news," the clinician should ask about suicide. If a patient conveys a sense of hopelessness, the clinician should ask about suicide. By asking about suicide, the clinician will not put the thought of self-destruction into the head of a patient who has not considered the option. Most suicidal patients, in fact, are ambivalent about their suicidal thoughts and feel relieved that someone is willing to discuss the issue.

If a patient has made a suicide attempt or admits to suicidal ideation, the clinician must first attend to the patient's safety. The suicidal patient should not be left alone during the evaluation, or if he or she must be left alone, it should be in seclusion or restraint, away from any objects that could be dangerous.

1. *Assessment and referral of the patient who has made a suicide attempt.*
   Although most patients who have made a suicide attempt are seen in an emergency room rather than in an office setting, occasionally, a patient may first seek assistance from his or her primary care provider.
   a. Determine whether the patient is medically stable and whether transfer to an emergency setting is necessary.
   b. If transfer is needed, make sure that the patient is constantly observed so that his or her escape or further acts of self-harm are prevented.
   c. If the patient refuses transfer to an emergency setting that you deem medically necessary, transfer can be made against the patient's will because acts of self-harm activate commitment procedures in all states (see section IV).
   d. If the patient is stable medically, an initial suicide assessment can begin. Questions to consider include the following:
      (1) How dangerous was the method used? Assess the patient's understanding. For example, most patients think aspirin and acetaminophen must be relatively safe in overdose because they are available without a prescription.
      (2) Did the patient really want to die, or was he or she just trying to get attention? If so, why?
      (3) How likely was rescue? Did the patient take a mixture of drugs and alcohol and then go into the woods, where it was unlikely that anyone would find him or her, or did the patient take an overdose at home while others were there or expected?
      (4) Was the suicide attempt planned or impulsive?
      (5) Did the patient do such things as get his or her personal and financial affairs in order, write a farewell note, or stop the mail?
      (6) After the attempt, is the patient sorry or relieved to still be alive?
      (7) Does the patient still want to die?
      (8) Is the patient psychotic or delirious? (see sections V and VI)
      (9) Is the patient at all hopeful about the future?
      (10) Has anything changed in the patient's situation to give him or her more hope now than when he or she made the attempt?

   All patients who have made a suicide attempt should be referred to a mental health professional for assessment. Such patients at high risk are those:

   - Who have made a potentially lethal attempt.
   - Who had little chance for rescue.
   - Whose acts were impulsive.
   - Who still wish to die.
   - Who are delirious or psychotic.
   - Who are without hope.
   - For whom nothing has changed.

   (If emergency psychiatric referral is not available, see section II.C.)

   When the clinician refers a patient who has made a suicide attempt and is still at risk for further attempts, the clinician should ensure that the patient will get to the consultation with a mental health professional safely. If family or friends are available, seem reliable, and are willing to take the patient, they can be asked to help if the patient is cooperative and willing to go. If the patient is reluctant to go for the assessment; if the patient is agitated, psychotic, uncooperative, or alone; or if others feel uncomfortable transporting the patient, he or she should travel by ambulance or police.

2. *Assessment and referral of the patient with suicidal ideation.*
   If the clinician finds that a patient has been contemplating suicide, he or she should ask the following questions:
   a. How much is the patient thinking about suicide? Is it an occasional thought that he or she is able to put out of his or her mind easily, or is it a constant thought?
   b. Does the patient think that he or she might act on the suicidal ideation?
   c. Has the patient planned how he or she would commit suicide?
   d. Is the patient's plan plausible? Does he or she have the means to carry it out?
   e. Has the patient practiced the plan?
   f. Does the patient have access to weapons, particularly guns?
   g. Is the patient psychotic or delirious? (See sections V and VI.)
   h. Does the patient feel that there is any hope for the future?

   The clinician should consider referring all patients with suicidal ideation for psychiatric evaluation. (If emergency psychiatric referral is not available, see section II.C.) Those who think of suicide constantly, have intent and a plan that is lethal, have access to guns, are psychotic or delirious, and have no hopes or plans for the future are at especially high risk and should be referred emergently. As mentioned earlier, the clinician should make sure the suicidal patient will get to the psychiatric assessment safely. In addition, if the clinician believes that a patient is dangerous to himself or herself, commitment laws can be used to require the patient to get a psychiatric evaluation, even if he or she refuses. The clinician may even keep some commitment forms in his or her office (see section IV).

The clinician should not hesitate to notify family or significant others if he or she believes a patient is at risk for attempting suicide. They may be able to assist in getting the patient to the appropriate help, and often they are as worried as the clinician is about the patient but have not known how to get help. *The clinician may choose to contact family even if the patient asks the clinician not to. Despite rules about confidentiality, if the clinician believes the patient is truly a danger to himself or herself, the clinician should act to protect the patient.* The clinician would be much better able to defend himself or herself in a lawsuit over breach of confidentiality than in one over wrongful death or injury if the patient does make a suicide attempt. The clinician should carefully document why he or she has decided to contact family against the patient's wishes.

C. Treatment and disposition of the suicidal patient.

In most settings, the primary care provider can refer the suicidal patient to a psychiatric setting for treatment and decision making about disposition. For clinicians practicing in a setting where referral to a psychiatric setting is not possible, a brief summary of the continued management of such cases follows.

1. If the patient has few or no risk factors, says that he or she does not want to die, feels control over the suicidal impulses, and feels some hope knowing that help is available, the patient may be sent home *if* a family member or friend is willing to stay with the patient until a full psychiatric assessment can take place. Sometimes, education about depression and the fact that it makes one feel hopeless but is very treatable can provide sufficient support such that hospitalization is not necessary. *Arrangements should be made for any guns or potentially lethal medications to be removed from the patient's home.*
2. If the patient has no social supports to be mobilized, wants to die, feels hopeless even when assured that help is available, has made a particularly lethal attempt or has a lethal plan in mind, is psychotic, or is severely depressed, hospitalization should be arranged immediately. Hospitalization may be on a voluntary basis if the patient agrees, or it may need to be on an involuntary basis. If the clinician works in a setting that lacks easy psychiatric assistance in emergencies, the clinician should know what psychiatric hospitals are available and how to access beds at these facilities on both a voluntary and an involuntary status. These patients must be kept safe and undergo constant observation, seclusion, or restraint so that they cannot leave or hurt themselves while awaiting transfer to a psychiatric facility.
3. If the clinician is unsure about the need to hospitalize a particular patient, the patient should be hospitalized. (The clinician should be on the safe side in these potentially lethal situations.)
4. The clinician should carefully document his or her discussions with the patient as well as the clinician's reasons for the decision of hospitalization. The clinician should be sure to document all the facts leading to his or her conclusions.
5. Sometimes, the clinician may believe that the patient's disposition is not clear-cut. Likely scenarios might be that the patient and family argue persuasively that instead of hospitalization, an alternate plan could be developed that would keep the patient safe. The clinician may agree that hospitalization is not necessary but that some risk for suicide still exists. The clinician may then want to work out a plan, or "contract for safety." Under such an arrangement:
   a. Certain family members are designated to stay with the patient around the clock.
   b. The patient states an explicit, practical, and acceptable plan for what he or she shall do if more serious feelings of self-harm start intruding (e.g., go directly to the emergency room).
   c. The patient explains who he or she shall call (e.g., call you, call a friend who has agreed to be available to take the call).
   d. Arrangements are made for keeping the patient busy and in meaningful contact with supportive human beings. *A suicidal patient should not return to an unchanged environment, with nothing to do and no one to talk to.*
   e. Arrangements are made for an intensive follow-up treatment plan, to begin the very next day and for shortly thereafter. The follow-up plan includes frequent outpatient appointments, pre–agreed on criteria for psychiatric hospitalization, and other appropriate elements tailored to the individual patient's problems.
   f. Safety contracts are either written or verbal. Some psychiatrists insist that the contract be written and signed by the patient and the significant others who are immediately available. A written contract emphasizes the importance of "keeping one's word" to stay safe. Moreover, a written document serves to help the patient see the arrangements so that if he or she starts to waver, the contract can be read again and remembered. Of course, written contracts are not legal documents, so they do not have much medical-legal value.

An element of risk always exists for the patient, the responsible family members, and the doctor when such contracts are made. *Contracts are best initiated when the practitioner knows the patient and has had some previous experience with the reliability of the patient. Contracts with patients and families whom the doctor does not know are most risky. The authors of this chapter do not recommend that safety contracts, written or unwritten, be used in general primary care practice;* we provide the aforementioned guidelines for practitioners who have had extra training for working with suicidal patients.

D. Special situations involving suicide assessment.

1. *The intoxicated patient.*
Patients who threaten or attempt suicide while intoxicated present a special problem. *Psychiatric assessment for involuntary hospitalization must be performed when a patient is sober.* Often, the patient who is suicidal when drunk or under the influence of drugs is no longer suicidal once he or she is sober. However, the patient remains at risk, especially when using substances.
If a patient comes to the clinician's office intoxicated and suicidal, he or she should be transported to an emergency room, where he or she can be monitored and kept safe until sober. At that time, a psychiatric assessment should take place. If the patient is still suicidal, psychiatric hospitalization should be pursued. If the patient is no longer suicidal, the patient and the patient's significant others should be educated about the potential danger of drug use, and substance abuse treatment should be strongly encouraged.

2. *The patient who has made multiple attempts or gestures.*
Usually, the patient who makes repeated suicidal threats, gestures, or attempts has the diagnosis of borderline personality disorder (see Chapter 4). These patients can be difficult to manage and can use suicidal gestures manipulatively. All threats, gestures, or attempts, no matter how often they occur, need to be taken seriously and assessed. Any primary caregiver providing ongoing care to a patient with borderline personality disorder should have continuing contact and consultation with the patient's psychiatrist.

3. *The patient who reports suicidal thoughts or a suicide attempt by phone.*
Patients who call to report that they are suicidal or have just made an attempt also present a special problem. If the clinician believes the patient is truly at risk, the clinician must help the patient get appropriate help.
The clinician should ask to speak to a family member if one is present with the patient and should enlist the family member's help in getting the patient to either medical or psychiatric help. If no one is with the patient, or if family is unable or unwilling to help, the clinician should find out where the patient is and send an ambulance or the police. The clinician should try to stay on the phone until help arrives.
If the patient is calling from an unknown location and refuses to give his or her whereabouts, the physician should attempt to trace the call so that the police can be dispatched. If the patient hangs up before the clinician can determine his or her location, the clinician should notify the family of the situation and his or her concerns in the hope that they will know the patient's whereabouts.
Clinicians with questions about any of these procedures should contact their psychiatric consultant or local community mental health organization. These mental health professionals would be able to illustrate how commitment procedures are begun, if this is necessary, and may also have other resources, such as outreach teams, that can be used.

Case Study

A 62-year-old woman whom the clinician has been treating for chronic back pain calls and says that it is urgent that she speak to the clinician. During the telephone call, the patient begins to cry, and it is hard to understand her. Her speech is slurred, and the clinician wonders if she has been drinking. She says that she has been unable to sleep, and if someone does not do something to take away her pain "right now," she will kill herself. The clinician knows from her history that when she was a young adult she had difficulty with alcohol and that she had once made a suicide attempt by driving her car off the road, but this event occurred many years ago. She has been sober and reported attending Alcoholics Anonymous meetings during the past 8 years.

The clinician asks her how she will kill herself, to which she replies "I'll blow my f . . . ing brains out." The clinician asks if she has a gun, and she laughs and says that her husband's loaded gun is sitting on her lap. The clinician communicates a desire to help her with her pain and with how bad she is feeling. The clinician asks the patient if her husband is there to drive her to the hospital. She says that he is at work "where he always is," and says that she does not want him involved. Then, she hangs up, saying "you're going to call him anyway."

The clinician immediately notifies the local police of the situation, and a police car is dispatched. The clinician also calls the patient's husband, who works only a few minutes from their home. Both the police and her husband arrive at the same time and discover her sitting by the phone crying and clutching the gun. She surrenders the gun and is taken to a local emergency room for evaluation.

III. Assessing dangerousness: threats against others.

Based on case law that began in the 1970s with the Tarasoff case in California (Tarasoff v. Regents of the University of California, 17 Cal.3d 425, 551.2d 334, 131

Cal Rptr. 14 [1976]), *psychiatrists and other mental health professionals in all states now have an obligation to warn or protect potential victims of their patients. In some states, this obligation is extended to other health care providers as well.* Laws governing this duty vary from state to state. In general, either a warning to the potential victim or victims and/or the appropriate police authorities or hospitalization of the patient is required.

If the clinician has reasonable cause to believe that a patient is a threat to others, based on his or her behavior or words, the clinician should ask about homicidal ideation. If this characteristic is present or if the clinician remains concerned even if the patient denies having homicidal ideation, the clinician should immediately seek psychiatric consultation. If the patient is suffering from a mental illness that is leading to the threats or threatening behavior, hospitalization should be sought. If no mental illness is present and there is an identifiable victim (meaning that the person's identity is known or can be easily determined), that person must be warned according to the procedures determined by that state. In this circumstance, the clinician's duty to warn and protect the potential victim supersedes patient confidentiality.

If the clinician practices in an area without access to immediate psychiatric referral, he or she must carefully document the reasons for his or her actions in these cases. The clinician should consider discussing the case with colleagues and should document these consultations. In addition, the clinician should inform the patient that the clinician is obligated to warn the patient's intended victim and/or the local police.

Case Study

The brother of Mrs. Smith, a patient Dr. Jones has known for several years, comes to Dr. Jones for a consultation. He says that it has been a long time since he has had a physical examination and that he wants Dr. Jones to be his doctor. As he speaks, Dr. Jones can find no evidence of any mental status abnormality, except that he seems tense and angry. He is not psychotic, and he denies having symptoms of depression. He admits to "probably drinking more" than he should in general, but he is not intoxicated. His vital signs and physical examination are unremarkable.

As Dr. Jones completes the assessment, the patient asks for a referral to a psychiatrist. Dr. Jones asks him why, and he hesitates at first, then appears angry and says "My brother-in-law just screwed me out of a lot of money." When Dr. Jones reflects that the patient seems very angry about this, he says, "I'm going to kill the bastard, and I want it to be on my record that I saw a psychiatrist right before I did it!" Dr. Jones explains to the patient that although he is happy to refer him to a psychiatrist so that he can learn to deal with his angry feelings, his seeing a psychiatrist is unlikely to change any of the legal ramifications he would face if he acted on his threat, because he sees no evidence of mental illness. Furthermore, Dr. Jones explains that he has a legal obligation to warn the patient's brother-in-law and the police of his threat. The patient storms out of Dr. Jones's office. Dr. Jones calls the Smith home and warns Mr. Smith of the threat. He is not surprised, saying "He has said things like this before." Dr. Jones also notifies the local police, who indicate that they have been called by others about threats in this particular family. Dr. Jones carefully documents the patient's behavior and his own actions.

IV. Involuntary hospitalization.

Each state has its own laws concerning involuntary hospitalization or commitment to psychiatric facilities. In general, these laws allow involuntary hospitalization for a brief period of time (72 hours to 10 days), until a court hearing is held, *if* there is imminent danger to the patient or others or if the patient's inability to care for himself or herself is present *in the setting of mental illness.*

Specific procedures, paperwork, and rules as to who makes the decision about involuntary hospitalization vary from state to state. In most states, any physician can make the initial decision to initiate the process.

If the clinician has access to immediate psychiatric consultation, mental health professionals should make these decisions. If psychiatric evaluation is not readily available, the clinician should know his or her state's laws on involuntary hospitalization, as well as how to access this service, if needed. Typically, the local community mental health organization or department of social services are able to provide assistance.

V. Acute psychosis.

Acute psychosis, the development of psychotic symptoms, including hallucinations, delusions, and disorganized thinking, which has developed over hours to days, is a medical and psychiatric emergency. The acutely psychotic patient is often anxious, scared, or paranoid, usually exhibits poor insight and judgment, and is often prone to violent or dangerous behavior.

A. Diagnostic overview/epidemiology.

Psychosis is a symptom, like fever. It is not a diagnosis. The first step in the assessment of acute psychosis is determination of its cause. Psychosis can have many causes, some of which are serious or even life threatening.

1. *Potentially life-threatening causes of psychosis.*
   a. Hypoglycemia.
   b. Meningitis or encephalitis.
   c. Decreased oxygen to the brain.
   d. Hypertensive encephalopathy.
   e. Wernicke's encephalopathy.
   f. Intracranial bleeding.
   g. Drug withdrawal or intoxication.
2. *Other medical causes of psychosis.*
   a. Metabolic disorders (e.g., hyperglycemia, hyponatremia).
   b. Neurologic disorders.
   c. Nutritional deficiencies.
   d. Industrial exposures.

3. *Drug-related causes of psychosis.*
   a. Intoxication.
   b. Withdrawal states.
   c. Toxic reactions to prescribed drugs.

4. *Psychiatric causes of psychosis.*
   a. Schizophrenia or schizophreniform disorder.
   b. Brief psychotic disorder.
   c. Mood disorders, including bipolar illness and psychotic depression.
   d. Schizoaffective disorder.

For specific causes, the reader may refer to a standard medical or psychiatric textbook.

B. Management of the acutely psychotic patient.

The first step in the successful assessment of the acutely psychotic patient in the office setting is the safe management of his or her behavior and probable inability, or at least difficulty, cooperating with the examination.

1. If the patient is agitated or extremely paranoid, he or she may need to be transferred from the clinician's office to a hospital emergency department so that an assessment can be safely performed. Transfer by ambulance is probably the safest method; even if the patient seems very trusting of family members or friends who are willing to take him or her to the hospital, newly psychotic patients can be unpredictable, and this characteristic may be dangerous.

2. Even psychotic patients who are initially calm may become agitated, threatening, or violent (see section I).

3. If the patient is accompanied by a family member or friend whom he or she trusts, that person may remain with the patient during the interview and examination.

4. If the patient is alone, a trusted family member or friend may be called in order to be present while the assessment is taking place. This person can give support to the patient while giving the clinician additional historical data and assisting in treatment planning. If the patient is alone, very close observation should be provided, perhaps by a staff member who stays with the patient.

5. The clinician's staff should be aware of the fact that the clinician is dealing with a potentially volatile patient. They should be ready to assist with a show of force or a call to security or police, if necessary.

6. The clinician should focus the history and physical examination and should ask simple, one-answer questions. The clinician should explain what is needed but avoid long discussions or arguments.

7. Patient stimulation should be decreased. Patients should wait in an examination room rather than the waiting area.

8. The clinician should explain to the patient exactly what he or she is doing during the physical examination.

9. The clinician should set limits without making the patient feel more threatened or scared. *The patient should be given reasonable options. For example, if the patient refuses to leave the waiting area, the clinician could offer to see him or her in the consultation room or the examination room, whichever he or she chooses.* If the patient refuses to have blood drawn, he or she should be given the option of having the blood drawn in the clinician's office or at the hospital, but the patient should be firmly informed that the blood needs to be obtained.

10. The clinician should try to avoid giving medications in the acute setting, at least until a specific cause of the psychosis is either suspected or confirmed. If a pharmacologic agent is needed in order to keep the patient calm enough to examine, a small amount (0.5 to 1 mg) of lorazepam (Ativan) can be given, either PO or IM. If the clinician is concerned about intoxication or the medical effects of a benzodiazepine, a small amount of a high-potency neuroleptic that is usually safe in medically unstable patients, such as haloperidol (Haldol), 2 to 5 mg PO or IM, may also be used. Prophylaxis for dystonic reactions (e.g., benztropine [Cogentin] 1 mg PO twice daily) should be considered if haloperidol is used in a patient who is at high risk for these reactions; however, most prophylactic agents are highly anticholinergic.

C. Evaluation of the acutely psychotic patient.

Once the clinician has ensured his or her safety and the safety of the patient and others in the area, the assessment can begin.

1. *Vital signs* should be checked immediately. Abnormalities can help the clinician begin to narrow the extensive differential diagnosis. Although agitated or frightened patients may have slightly increased pulse and/or blood pressure, markedly abnormal values are notable.

2. A rapid *physical examination* to screen for head trauma (or other trauma), neck rigidity, and funduscopic or other neurologic abnormalities should follow. The chest and abdomen should be examined, and whether or not the patient looks physically ill or has poor coloring should be noted after the initial neurologic screening.

3. The *history* of the psychotic symptoms should also be obtained. Depending on how disorga-

nized or cooperative the patient is, the clinician may have to obtain most of the history from family or friends. In addition to pinpointing the start of symptoms and whether they are related to any medication, other drug use, or physical symptoms, the clinician should ask about premorbid psychiatric symptoms, drug abuse, alcohol abuse, over-the-counter medication use, and family psychiatric history. *For medical/legal reasons, all psychotic patients should be asked about suicidal and/or homicidal thoughts.*

4. The *mental status examination* (part of which has already been performed if the patient has been determined to be psychotic) should include notation of the level of consciousness, appearance, behavior, speech, orientation, and attention.
   a. Fluctuating level of consciousness suggests delirium (see section VI).
   b. Inattention may suggest a medical or neurologic abnormality, although hallucinating patients may appear inattentive to you while they are responding to internal stimuli.
   c. Disorientation is unusual in the psychiatrically ill and suggests a medical or neurologic explanation for the psychosis.
   d. Visual, olfactory, and tactile hallucinations are less common in primary psychiatric illness than are auditory hallucinations. The presence of hallucinations other than auditory should raise the clinician's suspicions of medical or neurologic abnormalities.

5. Certain *laboratory tests* should be performed in all acutely psychotic patients, including
   a. Complete blood count, including differential and mean corpuscular volume.
   b. Glucose level.
   c. Electrolyte levels.
   d. Blood urea nitrogen and creatinine levels.
   e. Drug screen, alcohol level.
   f. Urinalysis.

   Depending on the patient presentation, past medical history, and physical examination, it may also be appropriate to check
   a. Arterial blood gases.
   b. Chest x-ray study.
   c. Electrocardiography.
   d. Calcium, magnesium levels.
   e. Thyroid-stimulating hormone and free thyroxine levels.
   f. Liver function tests, including aspartate transaminase and bilirubin levels.
   g. Computed tomography or magnetic resonance imaging of the brain.
   h. Electroencephalography.
   i. Lumbar puncture.
   j. Erythrocyte sedimentation rate; tests for lupus.
   k. Serum test for syphilis.
   l. Human immunodeficiency virus antibodies.
   m. Others: cortisol, ammonia, ceruloplasmin, vitamin B_{12}, and folate levels, heavy metal screen.

D. Treatment of the acutely psychotic patient.

1. If a medical cause for the psychiatric symptoms is found, it should be treated. Sometimes, a low dose of an antipsychotic drug, such as 2 mg of haloperidol (Haldol) once or twice a day, may be necessary for short-term use, until underlying medical issues resolve or medications causing the symptoms are cleared from the body. Psychiatric consultation should be obtained to assist with the choice of medication and dose.

   If the patient is suicidal or homicidal, or if he or she has been engaging in dangerous behavior, either psychiatric hospitalization (see section V.D.3) or medical hospitalization with *suicide precautions, such as 24-hour on-site staff monitoring, should be arranged.*

2. If no medical cause can be found and a primary psychiatric problem is suspected, the patient should be referred to a psychiatrist for diagnostic evaluation and treatment. If the patient is agitated, threatening, violent, or suicidal, or if he or she has no social supports or if those who are supportive feel that they cannot care for the patient, he or she should be hospitalized (see section IV).

   If a patient is calm and cooperative and has family or friends to watch over him or her, hospitalization may not be needed. If treatment must be begun because psychiatric consultation is not immediately available, haloperidol, 5 mg twice daily (or its equivalent), may be used. Regardless of the underlying psychiatric diagnosis (major depression with psychotic features, mania, or schizophrenia), the initial treatment of the psychotic symptoms is antipsychotic medication.

   A more sedating (less potent) neuroleptic, such as thioridazine (Mellaril) 50 mg PO every 4 to 6 hours as needed, may be required, depending on the patient and the situation. The more sedating neuroleptics usually do not cause acute dystonic reactions but may cause hypotension; therefore, anticholinergics (e.g., benztropine) should not be used with the sedating neuroleptics. Prophylactic anticholinergics (benztropine [Cogentin], 1 mg PO twice daily) should be used in patients at high risk for dystonic reactions when the more potent neuroleptics, such as haloperidol, are used. Low doses of benzodiazepines may be added to the neuroleptic regimen in order to calm or sedate the patient. Once a psychiatrist has assessed the patient, a more definitive treatment plan can be formed.

3. In a few situations psychiatric hospitalization is appropriate, even though a medical cause for the mental status symptoms is found. In these situations, medical hospitalization is not needed to treat the underlying problem, and the patient cannot be treated as an outpatient. For example,

patients who are intoxicated with phencyclidine (PCP) or a hallucinogen might require a brief psychiatric hospitalization until their psychotic symptoms resolve.

E. Caregiver assistance.

Educating the caregiver or caregivers about psychosis is important, particularly if the psychotic patient is to be sent home. Family or significant others need to know that the patient's behavior may be unpredictable, that the patient may be out of touch with reality, and that the patient should be watched carefully. They should be told that any dangerous behavior or talk should prompt the patient's rapid return to a medical setting for further treatment and possible hospitalization.

Explaining to the family (and the patient) that the basis of the symptoms is medical and should resolve with treatment is very reassuring. If the clinician suspects a primary psychiatric disorder, stressing that treatment is available and that the patient has not brought the symptoms on himself or herself can be helpful.

Case Study

A 33-year-old single woman is brought to her doctor by her roommate. She had been seen by the physician the week before because of an increase in her asthma symptoms. Steroid therapy was started, and her breathing improved, but over the past 3 to 4 days, her roommate noticed that the patient seemed withdrawn, distracted, and "not quite herself." Early this morning, the patient awoke her roommate, saying, "You have to get up to see this. There are some baby raccoons in the living room!" The roommate went to see what the patient was talking about, but she saw nothing. Even now, in the doctor's office, the patient reports that she sees "a mother cat and three cute kittens" in the corner.

The patient has no psychiatric history and no family psychiatric history. She seems only puzzled, but not terribly distressed, by the hallucinations. She is cooperative but asks if her roommate can stay for the examination.

She is awake, alert, and oriented, and her attention and concentration are grossly normal. She does not appear physically ill. Vital signs and neurologic and physical findings are normal, except for some minimal wheezing. A complete blood count and electrolyte, blood urea nitrogen, creatinine, and glucose levels are obtained and are all normal. Urinalysis is normal, and a urine drug screen is negative.

Given the fact that symptoms started several days after steroid therapy began and that the patient has normal neurologic findings, her physician elects to taper the steroid therapy and to treat her asthma in an alternative way. He explains to both the patient and her roommate that steroids can sometimes cause a reaction like this, and that the hallucinations should go away once she is no longer taking the prednisone. He asks how safe the patient feels and whether she is feeling frightened. She says that she is not, so although he tells her that there are medications she could take to try to get rid of the symptoms more rapidly, he does not recommend these at this time, and if the symptoms become bothersome, this strategy can be reconsidered.

He also explains to her roommate that acutely psychotic patients need to be watched for dangerous thoughts or behavior. Because the roommate works during the day and is unable to stay with the patient, the physician contacts the patient's parents, who live 2 hours away; explains what has happened; and asks if they could have their daughter stay with them for a few days. The parents agree to this and meet their daughter and her roommate at their apartment to drive their daughter to their home.

The doctor stays in telephone contact with the patient, and with a rapid steroid taper, her symptoms resolve. When she is seen in follow-up a week later, her mental status is back to normal, and the physician advises her and her parents that she can return to her apartment and resume her normal activities.

VI. Delirium.

Delirium is an acute state of cerebral dysfunction. It is often confused with psychosis because psychotic symptoms may be part of the syndrome of delirium. Delirium is usually *transient* and *reversible*. It has an *acute* or subacute onset and is manifested clinically by a wide range of *fluctuating* mental status abnormalities, including

1. Global cognitive impairment in
   Thinking
   Memory
   Perception
2. Decreased attention.
3. Change in the level of consciousness.
4. Agitation or decreased motor activity.
5. Disturbances in the sleep-wake cycle.

The presence of delirium suggests a serious medical problem. Delirious patients are quite ill and need rapid assessment. Patient safety is of paramount importance because of mental status changes and consequent poor judgment.

A. Diagnostic overview/epidemiology.

1. *Causes of delirium.*
   Various medical and neurologic problems can cause delirium.
   a. Some causes of delirium are life threatening and must be ruled out immediately. Table 3–2 lists these emergent causes of delirium.
   b. Other, less emergent, problems that must also be treated can cause delirium. These are listed in Table 3–3.

Table 3–2
Differential Diagnosis for Delirium: Emergent Items (WHHHHIMP)

Wernicke's encephalopathy or withdrawal
Hypertensive encephalopathy
Hypoglycemia
Hypoperfusion of central nervous system
Hypoxemia
Intracranial bleeding or infection
Meningitis or encephalitis
Poisons or medications

Adapted from Wise MG, Brandt GT. Delirium. In: Yudofsky S, Hales R. The American Psychiatric Press Textbook of Neuropsychiatry. Second Edition. Washington, DC: American Psychiatric Press; 1992.

c. Almost any medication, including over-the-counter medications, can lead to delirium, especially if they are taken in much larger quantities than prescribed. It would be prudent for the clinician to review all the medications, including the specific quantities, used by the patient with delirium. Further, it is often useful to ask a patient's family member to bring in all the patient's pill bottles for the clinician to review. Clinicians may be surprised to see the multiple pill bottles, many outdated medications, and duplicate prescriptions that patients may have, especially if the patients are seeing more than one physician for their care.

2. *Clinical features of delirium.*
   a. Prodromal symptoms of delirium include anxiety, irritability, restlessness, and disrupted sleep.
   b. A fluctuating course, with periods of mental status clearing, is a hallmark of delirium.
   c. All patients with delirium have difficulty paying attention and are easily distracted. It may be difficult for them to complete a thought or idea.
   d. Patients with delirium have altered arousal and psychomotor abnormalities. They can be hyperactive and vigilant, or hypoactive and sleepy. Mixed states also occur, and a given patient may experience fluctuations from one state to another.
   e. Sleep-wake disturbance is common in delirium. Often, these patients are awake and agitated at night and sleep during the day.
   f. Impaired immediate and recent memory is common. Patients often do not remember episodes of delirium or may have only fleeting memories of when they were confused.
   g. Disorganized thinking and impaired speech occur in some patients.
   h. Disorientation is common, although not necessary to the diagnosis.
   i. Altered perceptions are also common and can often be mistaken for an underlying psychiatric problem. Because of perceptual abnormalities, patients can develop delusions and hallucinations. Visual hallucinations may occur, and auditory and tactile disturbances are often illusionary in nature (e.g., a noise is misinterpreted to be a gunshot, or intravenous tubing brushing against an arm is believed to be a snake).
   j. Neurologic abnormalities in delirium include dysgraphia, dysnomic aphasia, constructional abnormalities, and motor abnormalities. The electroencephalogram shows either diffuse slowing or low voltage; fast activity occurs in hyperactive, agitated patients.
   k. Emotional disturbances that may accompany delirium are anxiety, panic, fear, anger, sadness, depression, and apathy.

Table 3–3
Differential Diagnosis for Delirium: Critical Items (I Watch Death)

Infectious
Withdrawal
Acute metabolic abnormalities (e.g., hyperglycemia, hyponatremia)
Trauma
Central nervous system pathology
Hypoxia
Deficiencies (e.g., thiamine)
Endocrinopathies
Acute vascular injuries or accident
Toxins or drugs
Heavy metals

Adapted from Wise MG, Brandt GT. Delirium. In: Yudofsky S, Hales R (eds). The American Psychiatric Press Textbook of Neuropsychiatry. Second Edition. Washington, DC: American Psychiatric Press; 1992.

3. *Populations at risk for developing delirium.* Although delirium is possible in any patient, certain populations appear to be at higher risk for developing delirium. In the outpatient setting, the clinician is most likely to see the following populations.
   a. The elderly. *In geriatric patients, delirium is sometimes the first clue that something is medically wrong. For example, confusion is often the first sign of a serious urinary tract infection* because changes in temperature and white cell count may not be present. It is not clear why this is the case, but it is probably caused by a combination of factors. The elderly are more likely to have structural brain abnormalities or dementia. They have decreased ability to metabolize medications and tend to be taking several. Their sleep patterns often change, and they have visual or hearing impairments that can add to confusion.
   b. Patients with any kind of pre-existing brain abnormality, especially dementia.

c. Patients who abuse drugs and are prone to withdrawal states.
d. Patients with acquired immunodeficiency syndrome.

In hospital settings, other risk groups are burn patients and patients who have undergone open heart surgery.

4. *Differential diagnosis of delirium.* Delirium is most difficult to distinguish from dementia and psychosis. Dementia is usually longstanding and nonfluctuating. Psychotic patients are rarely disoriented, and they usually have a clear sensorium.

B. Management of delirium.

Delirious patients are usually critically ill. The first step in managing delirium is recognizing it. Then, the object of care should be safe management of the patient's behavior and confusion, while rapid assessment to determine the underlying cause of the mental status changes takes place.

1. The key to recognizing delirium is to pay attention to the patient's mental status. Patients who exhibit fluctuating levels of consciousness, decreased attention, or disorientation should be considered delirious until proven otherwise. Sometimes, delirium is subtle and is not detected except by a vigilant clinician. Some fairly sensitive, easy, neuropsychiatric tests can be performed in the clinician's office in order to test for dysgraphia and dysnomia; these tests include clock drawing or writing or asking the patient to name simple objects. Also, attention and concentration can be tested by asking the patient to name the days of the week or months of the year backward.

2. Remembering that the delirious patient is critically ill and suffering from an acute organ failure (in this case, the failure of the brain), the clinician may need to transfer the patient from the office to a hospital setting as quickly as possible. This measure both facilitates the work-up and helps ensure safety. For safety reasons, the clinician should consider transferring the patient by ambulance rather than having him or her travel by family car.

3. Delirious patients may become agitated or threatening. They can easily harm themselves or others, either intentionally, because they perceive a threat or have psychotic symptoms, or accidentally, because of confusion (see section I).

4. As discussed in the section on care of the psychotic patient (see section V), when dealing with a delirious patient, the clinician should keep interactions simple, realize that an accurate history may need to be obtained from others, set limits without making the patient feel threatened, and always keep the safety of the clinician, the patient, and others in mind.

5. The clinician should try to avoid administering medications in the acute setting, at least until a definitive diagnosis is made. If agitation is putting the patient or others at risk, however, the patient may need to be medicated. Haloperidol (Haldol) is the agent of choice. It may be given in doses of 0.5 to 1 mg PO or IM, in an office setting. Intravenous administration is not recommended in the outpatient setting, because of reports of arrythymias with this mode of administration, although the delirious patient whose heart is being monitored in an inpatient setting is often best treated with the titration of intravenous haloperidol. Haloperidol, 0.5 to 1 mg PO or IM, may be given with a small amount of benzodiazepine (e.g., lorazepam [Ativan] 0.5 to 1 mg PO or IM) in order to potentiate its sedative effects. Administration of prophylactic anticholinergics (e.g., benztropine [Cogentin]) should be avoided in delirious patients until the clinician is sure that anticholinergic toxicity is not part of the presenting problem.

   If alcohol or sedative-hypnotic withdrawal is believed to be the cause of delirium, the treatment of choice is benzodiazepine therapy.

C. Evaluation of the delirious patient.

The delirious patient must be rapidly assessed, particularly for life-threatening causes of the confusion.

1. *Vital signs* should be assessed, and a focused *physical examination* should be performed immediately.

2. A *history,* which may need to be obtained from others, should include the course of the symptoms, associated complaints, medication and drug use (including over-the-counter drugs), and possible exposures to toxins.

3. *Laboratory evaluation* should at least include electrolyte, glucose, blood urea nitrogen, creatinine, and calcium levels; liver function tests; complete blood count; sedimentation rate; drug screen; medication blood levels (if appropriate); arterial blood gases; urinalysis; electrocardiogram; and chest x-ray study.

   Additional blood tests, computed tomography or magnetic resonance imaging of the brain, lumbar puncture, and electroencephalography may also be needed. Electroencephalographic findings can suggest the presence of delirium if the diagnosis is not clear from the clinical presentation.

D. Treatment of delirium.

The medical cause of the delirium must be treated. Most delirious patients require hospitalization, both for treatment of the underlying problem and for management and safety. *Psychiatric hospitalization is not appropriate for the delirious patient.* Psychiatric consultants can help manage behavior problems in the medically hospitalized delirious patient.

E. Prevention of delirium.

The primary care provider can play a role in the prevention of delirium by being aware of predisposed patient populations, knowing what drugs can cause delirium and avoiding these whenever possible, and minimizing polypharmacy.

F. Counseling and education.

Delirium is very frightening. Patients often understand their misperceptions to represent danger and may be very suspicious, even of loved ones. They may be so confused that they do not recognize family or close friends. The use of orienting devices, such as large clocks, calendars, or family pictures, is often helpful. The entire situation is, however, quite disturbing to both the patient and those who care about him or her. To the extent that it is practical, explaining what delirium is to both the patient and the family members is vital; the goal is to try to reassure both the patient and the family.

Case Study

A 74-year-old woman is brought to the clinician's office by her daughter. Her daughter explains that when she called her mother this morning, as she does each day, she noticed that her mother sounded "funny." When she had spoken to her mother the previous afternoon, her mother had sounded fine, but when her mother answered the phone today, she sounded confused. She did not seem to recognize her daughter's voice, sounded frightened, and did not know what day it was.

Because the patient's daughter is able to keep her calm, the clinician decides to begin the work-up in his office. The patient has no psychiatric history. She is in remarkably good health. She has mild hypertension, which is diet controlled, and hypothyroidism, for which she takes thyroxine. Her daughter reports that her mother does not drink alcohol and that she does not take any other medications (including over-the-counter medications) as far as she knows.

The patient seems to trust her daughter but is very suspicious of the clinician, despite the fact he has been her doctor for 23 years. When he asks her where she is, she looks about and seems confused and says that she thinks she is in her living room. She has no idea of the year or month, which is far different from her baseline. The clinician asks her to draw a clock face, which she is unable to do. He also asks her to sign her name and notes a deterioration in her usual neat penmanship. While the clinician is preparing to examine the patient, a metal instrument drops in the hallway outside the room. This seems to frighten the patient. She says to her daughter, "See, we are at war. I can hear the gunshots. We should take cover."

Her neurologic and physical findings are unremarkable. Her vital signs are notable for a temperature of 100.8°C, a pulse of 102, and a blood pressure of 110/60 mm Hg (a decrease from her usual 130/80 mm Hg). Given her vital signs, the clinician suspects that she may have an infection. Laboratory tests are ordered and include electrolyte, glucose, and calcium levels; liver function tests; complete blood count with differential; urine toxicology screen; urinalysis; thyroid tests; electrocardiogram; and chest x-ray study. While results are pending, the clinician arranges for the patient to be admitted to the hospital for further evaluation and treatment. The clinician explains to the patient and her daughter that sometimes an underlying infection, or another problem, can cause the changes in thinking that she is experiencing, and that although further tests and treatment will have to be performed, he believes that her mental state is temporary and will resolve as soon as the exact cause is found and treated. The clinician sends her by ambulance for better monitoring on the way to the hospital.

Urinalysis reveals a urinary tract infection, which cultures confirm. Gradually, after several days of antibiotic treatment and hydration, the patient's mental status returns to normal.

Summary

The salient messages from this chapter are as follows:

1. Be prepared to handle psychiatric emergencies.
2. Be attentive to changes in mental status in your patients and recognize suicide risk, psychosis, and delirium.
3. Know the general issues regarding civil commitment in your state.
4. Document facts and your decision-making process appropriately.

Preparation is essential to coping with a psychiatric emergency and must occur at several levels:

1. You should talk with your staff about this possibility so that a heightened awareness exists.
2. You should have good communication with your staff about anything unusual that is observed regarding your patients.
3. You may need structural changes in your office, such as warning buttons, emergency telephone numbers readily available. Additionally, internal codes should be set up among you and your staff.
4. If you work alone, you may want to discuss such issues with office neighbors in order to set up a system of protection.
5. You should consider office drills that you and your staff could rehearse for various types of psychiatric emergencies. What would you do, for example, if someone began throwing furniture or medical equipment? What would be your reaction if someone walked into an examining room and pulled a gun?
6. Finally, the most important point is that the identified patient, patients in the waiting room, your staff, and you come to no harm by the end of the incident.

As to acute changes in mental status that manifest as psychosis, suicidal ideation or intent, or delirium, these possibilities should be considered as part of the differential diagnosis. Many clinicians believe that these problems are seen only in an emergency department or that these conditions are treated on inpatient units of hospitals. The problem with this reasoning is that the clinician may, in fact, be the first person to recognize the problem and will then need to transfer the patient to the hospital or manage the situation in some other way. The triage may be in the form of voluntary hospitalization or involuntary commitment. The issues addressed in this chapter are not easy ones. They are difficult for the patient, the family, the office staff, and the physician.

Suggested Reading

Blumenreich PE, Lewis S. Managing the Violent Patient: A Clinician's Guide. New York: Brunner/Mazel; 1993.

Hilliard JR. Manual of Clinical Emergency Psychiatry. Washington, DC: American Psychiatric Press; 1990.

Hyman SE, Tesar GE. Manual of Psychiatric Emergencies. Third Edition. Boston: Little, Brown & Company; 1994.

Kaplan HI, Sadock BJ. Pocket Handbook of Emergency Psychiatric Medicine. Baltimore: Williams & Wilkins; 1993.

Wise MG, Brandt GT. Delirium. In: Yudofsky S, Hales R (eds). The American Psychiatric Press Textbook of Neuropsychiatry, Second edition. Washington, DC: American Psychiatric Press; 1992, pp. 291–310.

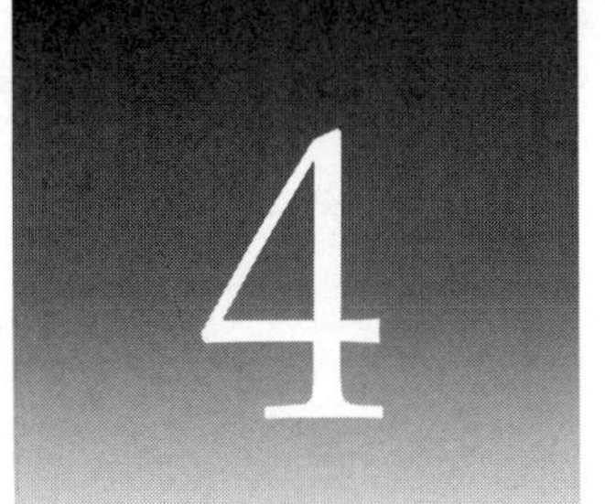

BRENT C. WILLIAMS, MD, MPH

KENNETH R. SILK, MD

"Difficult" Patients

Many types of primary care patients can be "difficult." The reasons for the difficulty are sometimes obvious—for example, distress from family discord, resulting in poor medication compliance. Often, however, the physician or the patient becomes exasperated with the course of care without a clear understanding of why or how to improve the situation. Instead, the physician may be unusually annoyed or angry with the patient or his or her family; the physician may make extra appointments, do special favors, or engage in other exceptional duties for the patient that are uncommon for the physician or the physician's practice; or the office staff may have an unusually strong (usually negative) reaction to the patient.

Case Study

Ms. F. is a 39-year-old white woman who has seen you, her primary care physician, four times over the past 8 weeks. She has come to the office with a urinary tract infection, abdominal pain, back pain, headaches, and other complaints. Her demeanor is generally demanding, she frequently remarks that other physicians do not know what they are doing, and she usually rejects or does not follow the management plans suggested. She frequently contacts the physician before or after office hours for minor complaints, and she often calls for appointments stating that she needs to be seen that day. When she calls, the physician usually feels a combination of disappointment, anger, apprehension, and frustration. The office staff is aware of the physician's feelings about this patient, and they find her difficult as well.

Many difficult patients present a challenge because their problems, although couched in terms of physical complaints or expectations of particular services from the primary care provider, are rooted in psychological factors. Thus, even the best efforts of the physician who treats these patients through medical means often end in failure; the treating physician experiences failure and rejection, feelings that probably parallel some of the patient's own feelings. The goal of this chapter is to enable the primary care physician to identify and manage psychological issues that occur in encounters with the difficult patient. Early recognition and appropriate management of the difficult patient can improve care, minimize unnecessary testing, improve efficiency, and decrease frustration for the primary care physician.

This chapter focuses on two broad types of difficult patients—*somatizing patients* and *behaviorally disruptive patients. Somatization* can be defined as the expression of emotional discomfort and psychosocial stress in the physical language of bodily symptoms.[1] Because not all somatizing patients have previously diagnosed comorbid or primary psychiatric conditions, recognition of this phenomenon can be difficult.

Disruptive patients are those who are demanding of attention and are self-centered, paranoid, or aggressive in their interpersonal style. Most disruptive patients meet or come close to meeting diagnostic criteria for personality disorder. The emphasis in this chapter, however, is on the general recognition of the psychological roots of some forms of disruptive behavior and the development of effective management strategies rather than on the precise diagnostic labeling of personality disorders or their subtypes.

By following a step-by-step approach, the primary care physician can avoid much frustration in interactions with these types of difficult patients. A general approach is outlined in Figure 4–1.

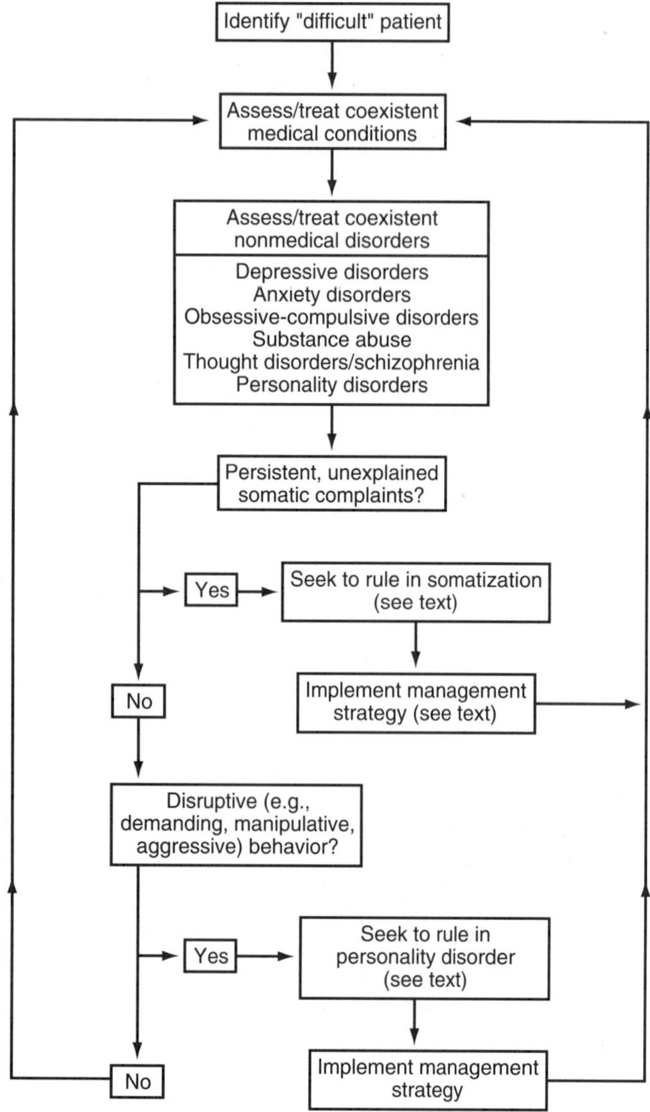

Figure 4–1
Systematic approach to the "difficult" patient.

The Difficult Somatizing Patient

I. Identifying difficult patients.

Effective management of demanding, frustrating, or manipulative cases requires early recognition of the possible psychological roots of the problems and attempts to identify clues to the psychological diagnosis. Failure to develop a causal explanation or a working hypothesis results in ineffective management and a growing sense of frustration and failure for both the patient and the physician.

A. Physician clues to psychological or social causes of "difficulty."

1. *Annoyance or distress* when the patient's name appears on the daily schedule or when the patient calls the physician on the telephone.
2. *Anger* toward the patient during interactions, which may result from the physician's belief that all of his or her suggestions are being rejected by the patient while the patient continues to complain.
3. *Difficulty terminating interviews,* with new complaints regularly offered at the end of the interview.
4. *Frustration* at not being able to eliminate patient's symptoms or decrease his or her distress (i.e., cure the patient), thus intensifying the physician's feeling of helplessness.

B. Patient behaviors suggestive of psychological or social, rather than purely biomedical, difficulties including the following:

1. *Demanding behavior,* in which the physician is expected to respond immediately to complaints, even for minor ailments, or in which a "cure" is sought for vague, nonspecific complaints.

2. *Overly emotional or dramatic behavior* (often referred to in psychiatry as "histrionic") that leads to cognitive experience as well as physical experience on the part of the patient and perhaps presentation of an ailment or ailments that far exceed what would be expected in most patients. Although the behavior or presentation is presented in an overly emotional or dramatic way, it has a shallow quality as well.
3. *Confusing presentation* in that symptoms change, are vague, or do not fall into a pattern of known illnesses or syndromes.
4. *Quick movement from one complaint to another,* in which the patient replaces an old complaint with a new one or suddenly switches to a discussion of family or relationship issues without completing the discussion of the original complaint.

Other symptoms suggestive of a psychological origin are included in Table 4–1.

II. Assess/treat coexistent medical conditions.

Even if certain behaviors suggest the presence of a psychological origin for the patient's complaints, the physician must appropriately consider and evaluate possible organic causes. Because the likelihood of physical illness is no less among somatizing or disruptive patients than among the general population, the physician must maintain vigilance through the *history* and *physical examination,* and do basic tests (e.g., blood chemistries and blood counts) when necessary. Although the patient's presentation and interpersonal style can be indicative of underlying psychological issues, the physician should not prematurely dismiss the possibility of an actual medical illness merely because clues to a probable psychological origin of the complaints are present.

The physician must also consider the potential role of *prescribed medications* as the cause of symptoms. In addition, the patient may exhibit drug-seeking behavior (e.g., analgesics, especially narcotics and psychoactive medications, in patients with chronic pain).

Table 4–1
Clues to Psychogenic Symptoms

Clinical presentation: the symptom(s)

Symptoms that **do not make** much **clinical sense.** Symptoms appear unusual, inconsistent, even bizarre and may change from visit to visit. Even if they don't change, they **do not improve despite treatment.**

Many doctors probably have been consulted about a variety of symptoms; the patient may have **had a number of procedures, operations, and diagnostic evaluations** over the years, such as gallbladder, exploratory laparotomy, and nerve entrapment.

The symptom may have occurred or **presented** itself **at a time** of acute **psychological distress,** though the **patient denies** the **significance of the stress.**

Psychological issues: the person/patient

Presentation with one of two personality styles is common:
(a) an **hysterical style** that is dramatic, vague, quite emotionally labile and reactive or quite suggestible, or
(b) an **inability to express affects** or feelings verbally (alexithymia).

The **patient does not think** that **the symptom has** anything to do with a psychological state or that it has any **psychological meaning.**

The patient and/or family may have had a **history of psychiatric illness** such as a mood disorder, schizophrenia, or substance abuse.

III. Assess/treat coexistent nonmedical conditions.

The presence of coexistent psychiatric disorders is common in somatizing or disruptive patients. Common coexistent diagnoses that require therapy are *major depressive disorder, generalized anxiety disorder, panic disorder, alcohol abuse,* and *obsessive-compulsive disorder.* Some difficult patients demonstrate easily recognizable *personality disorders.* Patients with known (or suspected) personality disorders should always be evaluated for these treatable comorbid psychiatric disorders, which are more prevalent in those with personality disorder than in the general population. Other psychiatric disorders are often difficult to discriminate in patients with personality disorders, and the assistance of a psychiatrist, either for consultation or treatment, may be needed.

The primary care physician should screen for the presence of these disorders. The identification and diagnostic criteria for many of these disorders are discussed in other chapters in this book. Although diagnosing these psychiatric disorders is often not easy, in primary care practice, in recent years, many screening instruments have been devised to assist the primary care physician in this task. These include the CAGE questionnaire and Michigan Alcohol Screening Test (MAST)[2] for alcohol abuse; Centers for Epidemiological Study—Depression (CES-D) and Beck Depression Inventory[3] for depression; and Prime-MD (Primary Care Evaluation of Mental Disorders)[4] for anxiety disorders, depression, eating disorders, somatization, and alcohol abuse. The CAGE and the CES-D are included in the appendix to this chapter.

In general, screening instruments for psychiatric disorders should be used in patients for whom the clinician has a suspicion of psychiatric disorder or severe psychological distress, so that the potentially large number of false-positive results is minimized. *Psychiatric screening tools are not diagnostic.* Patients whose screening results are positive for psychiatric disorders should be further evaluated for specific disorders.

IV. If persistent, unexplained physical complaints are a significant part of the clinical picture, evaluate further for *somatization.*

A. Definitions and diagnostic features of somatization.

1. Somatization is the *expression of emotional discomfort and psychosocial stress in the physical language of bodily symptoms.*[1]
2. Somatization disorder may be defined as a polysymptomatic disorder beginning before the age of 30 years and extending over a period of years; it is characterized by a combination of pain, gastrointestinal, sexual, and pseudoneurologic symptoms that cause the patient to take medications or seek medical attention. In the United States, it has been believed to be primarily (or exclusively) a disorder of women.
3. *Somatization is common among primary care patients.* Patients meeting the criteria for somatization disorder (as many as 5% of family practice patients) represent a severely affected subset (perhaps as few as 6%) of all somatizing patients. More common are patients with persistent, unexplained somatic complaints for whom no explanatory cause can be found after appropriate investigation but who do not meet criteria for somatization disorder. In this sense "[somatization is] not a diagnostic category of patients, but rather a generic term referring to a set of experiential, cognitive and behavioral features exhibited by patients who may have a variety of psychiatric [and medical] diagnoses."[5] Explicit diagnostic criteria for somatization other than those for somatization disorder have not been developed, because of the heterogeneity of somatizing patients and because of the large overlap of psychiatric and medical conditions between somatizing and nonsomatizing patients.
4. Somatization is more than the presence of persistent, unexplained (or disproportionate) somatic complaints. It also involves the way or ways in which the patient interprets his or her symptoms and his or her relationship with the medical system (Table 4–2). The presence of several characteristics listed in Table 4–2 should help the clinician determine the presence of somatization while maintaining appropriate vigilance for physiologic disease.

B. Epidemiology.

1. As many as 60% of primary care patients recurrently present with somatic symptoms that are an expression of psychosocial distress.[6]
2. An estimated 10% to 30% of primary care patients have somatic complaints for which no adequate physical cause can be detected.[7]

Table 4–2
Clinical Features Useful in Diagnosing Somatization

The persistence of one or more somatic complaints without a demonstrable physiologic basis (or whose severity is disproportionate to known physiologic processes) after appropriate investigation and one or more of the following:

- *Pain* is a common complaint.
- Bowel and cardiorespiratory complaints are common.
- Head, neck, abdomen, and chest are common body regions affected.
- The gastrointestinal, musculoskeletal, and central nervous systems are the organ systems most frequently implicated.
- Usually, *multiple symptoms* from several different organ systems wax and wane over long periods.
- The patient has great concern over the *authenticity,* meaning, and etiologic significance of symptoms.
- The patient has fear of disease and profound *disease conviction,* and proposals about psychological factors are frequently rejected.
- The body is the subject of preoccupation and fascination.
- Symptoms are experienced *in response to life events* and situational stressors.
- The self is viewed as *afflicted and suffering,* and the greatest accomplishment has been to endure misery.
- There is a *relentless search for medical care* and an extensive history of prior medical care.
- *Previous contact with physicians is characterized negatively,* in which the patient reports that his or her symptoms were not being taken seriously.

Adapted from Mabe PA, Jones LR, Riley WT. Managing somatization phenomena in primary care. Psychiatr Med 1990; 8:117–127.

3. More than 50% of patients with psychiatric problems present initially with somatic complaints.[6]

C. Stepwise approach to the evaluation of somatization.

Once the presence of somatization is strongly suspected (e.g., through the presence of several characteristics listed in Table 4–2), a systematic approach to evaluation should be undertaken.

1. *Does the patient have somatization disorder?* If multiple somatic complaints in different organ systems have been present without a known organic basis and the complaints began before the age of 30, somatization disorder should be suspected (see section IV.A.2 for definition).
2. *Can the patient's complaints be attributed to a physiologic disorder or disorders?* Diagnostic evaluation of somatic complaints must be individualized.
   a. To the extent that the following characteristics are present with respect to complaints or symptoms, less diagnostic work-up is necessary:
      (1) Characteristics listed in Tables 4–1 and 4–2.
      (2) Long duration of symptoms (years).
      (3) Multiple organ systems or body areas involved.

(4) Shift over time.
(5) Negative results of initial diagnostic evaluation.

b. Extensive or repeated medical work-ups of the recurrent somatizing complaints should be avoided. After initial negative diagnostic results, physicians may be tempted to repeat or intensify diagnostic work-up of complaints that are likely to be based on somatization in order to reassure the patient with negative test results. Although no specific rule or criteria exist that determine how much or how little work-up is sufficient, the decision needs to be based on an understanding of the patient's previous medical history as well as his or her history of unsubstantiated medical complaints in combination with how well the current symptoms or complaint picture fits a bona fide medical illness. *Diagnostic work-up of complaints known (or strongly suspected) to be based on somatization has no demonstrated reassurance value to the patient and is unlikely to alter behavior and complaint patterns.*[5]

c. After initial diagnosis, further diagnostic evaluation should generally be based on symptoms that have one or more of the following characteristics:
(1) *Unusually severe, persistent, or new symptoms* (for patients with a relatively stable symptom complex). "Tincture of time" is often the best diagnostic aid; many complaints shift over time, rendering diagnostic work-up beyond patient history and physical examination unnecessary. Watchful waiting, with brief encounters that emphasize pertinent history and targeted physical examination, is essential to the appropriate diagnostic work-up in somatizing patients.
(2) Accompanied by *objective findings* on physical examination or diagnostic test results.
(3) Suggestive of *medical diseases with reasonable* (e.g., >10%) *prior probabilities.*

3. *Does the patient have coexistent psychiatric illness(es),* especially those that are likely to respond to specific therapy?

The types of psychiatric illnesses listed in section III are common in somatizing patients (Table 4–3). For example, patients with three or more complaints of chronic pain have a 50% to 70% likelihood of having major depressive disorder.[8] Early identification and treatment of these and other psychiatric disorders is crucial to effective management of cases of somatization.

4. *What conditions or features characterize the somatic complaints that could help with the designing of a management strategy?*[1]

a. What *associated emotional problems* are present (e.g., anger, dependence, inadequate ego development, diminished self-esteem, guilt)?

b. What *role do the symptoms play* in the patient's life (pattern of use of medical services, family dynamics, use of illness to cope with interpersonal conflicts and stressful life events [medical illness being the only legitimate way to say "I'm tired" or "I'm overwhelmed"])?[9]

c. What is the patient's *"explanatory model"* (personal beliefs) about the illness? In other words, what are the causes, personal effects, mechanism of action, best forms of therapy, and most ideal outcomes of the illness (Table 4–4)?

Fully evaluating the nature and psychosocial context of somatization is a time-consuming process and should occur over several (three to six) visits. Attempting to accomplish these goals in a single visit leads to irritation and frustration.

Table 4–3
Psychiatric Illnesses Common Among Somatizing Patients

Major depressive disorder
Generalized anxiety disorder
Panic disorder
Alcohol abuse
Abuse or dependence on prescription or nonprescription drugs
Obsessive-compulsive disorder

Adapted from Brown FW, Golding JM, Smith GR. Somatization disorder: Psychiatric comorbidity in primary care. Psychosom Med 1990; 52:445–451.

D. Management.

Although most current recommendations (and limited data) relate to management of somatization disorder rather than to somatization in general, the following management strategies should be applied to the care of somatizing patients.[10]

1. **Set reasonable therapeutic goals.**

The key word is *reasonable.* The demanding na-

Table 4–4
Questions That Elicit the Patient's Illness Model

1. What do you think has caused your problem?
2. Why do you think it started when it did?
3. Do you have any idea about how your sickness works or about what is going on in your body right now?
4. What kinds of therapies have you received in the past, and which ones helped the most?
5. What are your goals for therapy, especially if we are not able to relieve your symptoms completely?
6. How has your sickness affected your daily activities? Are there activities that you used to do or would like to do that you do not do now?
7. Is there any specific illness that you fear you might have? What do you fear most about your illness?

Adapted from Kleinman AM. Explanatory models in health care relationships. In: Health and the Family. Washington, DC: National Council for International Health; 1975, pp. 159–172.

ture of these patients and the physician's negative feelings may lead her or him to feel guilty or ineffective, resulting in a desire to "cure" the patient or set other unrealistic goals. The strong wish to cure may result from an equally strong wish to never see the patient again. Reasonable therapeutic goals include:

a. *Decreased use of medical time and attention* (office or emergency department visits at first, and eventually phone calls).
b. *Improved functional capacity or social function.* Functional capacity is the ability of the patient to perform social, role-defined, and occupational tasks; social functioning relates to interpersonal style and interaction. A valuable goal is for the patient to relate better to people in areas outside his or her physical complaints, that is, to lead as normal a life as possible, despite the somatic complaints.
c. *Avoidance of unnecessary tests, referrals, and procedures.* Although this sounds easy, these patients are very demanding, and it may become easier to perform the test rather than to repeatedly see them in the office or listen to them on the phone with the same complaints. Explaining why the physician is unwilling to perform tests, prescribe medications, or make referrals can be difficult. Suggested statements include

   "The results of all the tests we've run have been normal. I'm not sure what the cause of your pain is, but I've run all the tests that I think need to be done right now. I doubt that further testing (or procedures or referrals) will give us any new information. We can always consider other tests in the future, but I think we need to just watch your symptoms for a while."

   A productive discussion might follow about the value of a trial of safe symptomatic therapy or of a limited (one or two visit) referral for a second opinion regarding further diagnostic tests.
d. *Avoidance of polypharmacy,* especially opiate analgesics and benzodiazepines. This is an important caveat. Attempts may be made to assuage the complaints with medications, but many patients may be covertly depressed (a relative contraindication for opiates or benzodiazepines), and the risk of overuse, abuse, or overdose of medications is increased in somatizing patients.
e. *Periodic monitoring for biological illness.* The somatizing patient runs the same risk of any person of developing a bona fide medical illness.
f. *In the treatment of somatizing patients, "cure" is rarely a realistic goal, but moving toward a decrease in use of medical resources and an improvement in interpersonal functioning should be the objective.*

2. **Use appropriate management strategies.** Few controlled trials exist to guide the practitioner in methods that have demonstrated efficacy in improving the subjective or behavioral consequences of somatization. Recommendations for management follow.
   a. *Treat underlying psychiatric conditions that are likely to respond to therapy* (see Table 4–3).
   b. *Center care around a single provider who provides regular, brief follow-up that includes pertinent physical examination.* At each visit, a period of open-ended questioning ("What's that like for you?" "Tell me more." "What else?" "How are things going in general?" "Has your life been more stressful than usual?" "Are you having stress not related to your physical problems?") and active listening should be followed by a brief physical examination of symptomatic areas.

      Before leaving the primary care physician's office, the patient should know the time of the next regularly scheduled appointment.

      Follow-up should be brief (e.g., 10 to 20 minutes) and may be via telephone.
   c. *Establish a therapeutic relationship.* This is not a simple matter with a patient who is consuming a great deal of the physician's time and energy and with whom he or she may be quite annoyed and angry. Such a patient may resist any inquiry into areas affecting him or her other than the somatic complaints. Key steps in establishing a therapeutic relationship with somatizing patients are listed in Table 4–5).
   d. *Establish appropriate therapeutic goals jointly with the patient.* Goals should be specific and realistic (e.g., decreasing medications, formulating an exercise plan) and written down, if necessary. Asking the patient what he or she would like to accomplish is crucial to helping the patient accept responsibility for his or her well-being and to strengthening the therapeutic alliance.
   e. *Follow-up should be scheduled regularly* (every 1 to 4 weeks), independent of symptom status. There should be as little linkage as possible between the patient's experience of symptoms and physician visits.
   f. *Refer for physical therapy or to a pain clinic if necessary, but the referral should be brief* (one to three visits). Emphasize that referral is NOT dismissal. Be willing to admit that the referral may not be helpful but may be worth the try.
   g. *Consider psychiatric referral if*
      (1) The patient threatens to harm himself or herself or others. If the patient has a history of previous self-harm, referral is definitely indicated.
      (2) The patient requests psychiatric referral.
      (3) A serious psychiatric disorder is likely to be present. If a patient has a psychotic condition, such as psychotic depression, referral is definitely indicated. In these instances, the patient may reveal bizarre somatic delusions ("There are animals

Table 4–5
What to Tell the Patient and Family: Establishing a Therapeutic Relationship with Somatizing Patients

1. *Acknowledge that the symptoms are real for the patient.* The patient experiences real discomfort, even if there is no "physical" reason for the discomfort.
"Of course your pain is real, and an important problem for us to solve."
"Even if we can't find a reason for your problem it does not mean that it isn't real."
2. *Accept the problem as somatic,* avoiding the implication that the difficulty is "all in the patient's head." This is the patient's reality, and he or she will not see you as an ally if you refute his or her reality. This often includes giving the patient's symptoms a "medical" diagnostic label. However, this does not mean that all hints at possible psychological contributions should be avoided.
"I think your pain is from muscular tension (or costochondritis, or bowel spasm)." (Follow with 5–10 seconds of silence. Psychosocial determinants of the symptom or symptoms should be pursued only if the patient spontaneously mentions or queries a possible connection.) or "Sometimes stress, known or unknown, may play a significant role in problems such as yours." (Again follow with 5–10 seconds of silence.)
If a somatic interpretation of the symptom is undesirable or unsuccessful, the best alternative is to simply state, "I don't know what's causing your symptom," followed by 5–10 seconds of silence.
3. *Maintain positive regard and empathy.*
"That much (or type of) pain must be difficult to live with." (Follow with 5–10 seconds of silence, with focused attention on patient's response.)

Adapted from Kaplan C, Lipkin M, Gordon G. Somatization in primary care: Patients with unexplained and vexing medical complaints. J Gen Intern Med 1988; 3:177–190.

eating out my insides") or frank paranoid ideation ("These headaches are caused by the x-ray machine that my neighbor shoots me with all day").

(4) The primary care physician has difficulty managing his or her own reactions to the patient.
(5) The primary care physician needs assistance with diagnostic or therapeutic management.

Brief psychiatric consultation with specific recommendations to the primary physician consistent with those in sections IV.D.2 and IV.D.4 has been shown to decrease health care utilization and increase physical functioning in somatizing patients.[11]

3. **Set limits.**
It is often necessary to set explicit limits on the context, frequency, duration, and goals of contact with the patient. Strategies for setting limits and suggested phrases for establishing those limits follow.
   a. Specify the length of appointments.
   "Our appointments are 20 minutes long. If we have more to discuss than we can accomplish in 20 minutes, we will need to schedule another appointment."
   b. Near the end of the visit, ask whether other issues are on the patient's mind.
   "I see we have only a few minutes left. Is there anything else you'd like to discuss?"
   If *substantial new complaints* are raised, schedule another visit to discuss them.
   c. *Set agendas for particular visits* when possible.
   "Hmmmm. That type of pain must be very troubling. Let's focus our next visit on your arm pain. Do you want me to schedule an office visit for that or should we discuss it on the phone on Wednesday at 4?"
   "What one or two things should we focus on at your upcoming visit?"
   d. *Set specific times when you are available by telephone,* except for emergencies. If the patient consistently labels non–life-threatening complaints as emergencies, specify that emergencies must be handled through emergency services, not your office. Also suggest to the patient that when events are scheduled rather than seen as emergencies, then you will be able to devote sufficient time to discussing the problem. Because of your busy schedule, unscheduled contacts often are too brief to accomplish much.
   It may be helpful to try to have a nurse establish a relationship with the patient as well. Then, the nurse might be able to handle some of the telephone calls and may help decrease the patient's dependence on the physician.
   e. If patients demand interventions (tests, medications, referrals) you deem unnecessary, *explicitly but politely state limits on your own behavior* (i.e., what you are and are not willing to do for the patient). Clearly stated, firm limits on what the patient can expect from you, although often greeted with anger, can be crucial to establishing an effective therapeutic alliance. For most patients, such differences in expectations of the physician's behavior can be successfully resolved.
   For example, you might state, "I can prescribe medication x at y dosage, in keeping with the goals we've set. I will not be able to prescribe this medication at higher doses, because I believe that therapy would be more harmful than helpful to you. In this context, we will be able to continue working together in other ways (implies continued commitment on the part of the physician) to get you feeling better." Or, "I am very conservative in using medications. I like to change only one medication at a time and to keep dosages of all medications as low as possible."
   Patient threats (e.g., to seek care elsewhere or to sue), which are often attempts at manipulation, should be met *nondefensively,* as you convey your intent to offer the patient neither

more nor less than your best medical judgment.

"You are certainly free to change primary physicians. If you'd like to transfer your care, I'll communicate all relevant medical information to your new physician. After that, I'll be unable to be your physician" (followed by 5 to 10 seconds of silence). (If the issue is not resolved immediately or the patient continues to threaten to leave) "Let me know what you decide; we can discuss it at our next visit if you choose to keep it." (A follow-up appointment is scheduled.)

4. **Follow these suggested steps during each clinical visit with somatizing patients.**
   a. *Spend 3 to 5 minutes in active, open-ended listening.* Focus on considering symptom complexes that suggest a need to screen for diseases; do not follow-up on every symptom.
   b. *Ask the patient what is on his or her mind,* and what he or she wants to accomplish during the visit. If the list is too long, then the physician should say that the list is quite long and should ask what things the patient considers most important.
   c. Briefly *query main complaints,* followed by *brief physical examination* of relevant areas.[12, 13]
   d. *Discuss the meaning of the symptom or symptoms* (see Table 4–4), allowing patient to voice his or her own explanations and concerns. The discussion often involves offering a medical diagnosis.
   e. *Agree on specific objectives for the next visit.* If possible, the patient should initiate the management plan. Objectives should be as benign as possible, for example stretching exercises, daily walks, and symptom logs. Other valuable objectives include decreases or adjustments in medications.
   f. *Schedule the next visit to precede the likely development or exacerbation of symptoms.*

E. Limits of the primary physician.

Somatizing patients can be among the most frustrating and time-consuming in primary care. Frank recognition of the degree and sources of frustration for the physician allows effective coping strategies to be developed. Sources of physician frustration and suggested coping strategies follow.

1. *Concern that a serious medical diagnosis* is being overlooked (see Table 4–1). Some discomfort is inevitable (and desirable).
2. *Discouragement over the lack of "cure."* Appropriate goal-setting is important.
3. *Anger* over the patient's apparent tendency to undermine his or her own progress, such as by requesting or demanding help, yet rejecting suggestions as to the cause or "cure" for symptoms, either overtly or by bringing up new complaints before closure is brought on the current complaint. This pattern and the physician's anger can be used as a diagnostic aid in somatization. It is important to remember that the patient's somatizing is not occurring simply to annoy the physician. Often, the physician may ask "Why is the patient doing this to me?" Of course, these patients are not doing anything to anyone; this is simply the way they are.

   Setting limited goals and minimizing interpretive statements or physician-directed suggestions for improvement of symptoms help to defray this anger.
4. *Fear of malpractice.* Few data exist that describe the litigious propensity of somatizing patients. Our own experience suggests strongly that somatizing patients rarely bring legal claims, although some frequently discuss doing so, often as an attempt to manipulate the physician's behavior. The best approach to preventing litigation is to have an alliance with the patient wherein the patient feels that the physician takes his or her complaints seriously and respectfully. Documentation is, of course, important.
5. *Excessive strain on physician and staff emotions and time.* Physicians may consider *"rotating" care,* such as on a 6- or 12-month basis, with another colleague to avoid this problem.

   Joint care of somatizing patients with a psychiatrist or psychologist can help maintain a manageable care load for each provider while fostering interchange and improving the monitoring of somatizing patients. It is also an opportunity to share the workload with respect to the patient as well as the sense of frustration about the patient with another caregiver.

The Difficult Disruptive and Personality Disordered Patient

I. If disruptive (e.g., manipulative, demanding, aggressive) behavior is present, the patient may be suffering from a *personality disorder.*

The somatizing patient may or may not be disruptive. Patients who bring forth strong negative feelings in the practitioner are not necessarily disruptive even though they may be difficult. Most somatizing patients are more difficult or annoying than disruptive. Disruptive patients, however, intrude on physicians' practices and, in turn, even on their lives. They may intrude because they are directly demanding of treatment or attention beyond what appears to be reasonable; they may threaten either harm or legal action to practitioners if they are not attended to immediately or in the manner in which they seem to feel is appropriate for them; they may act aggressively or threaten aggression; or they may repeatedly engage in self-harmful acts through self-mutilation or suicide threats or attempts. The behavior of disruptive patients can often be viewed as manipulative; that is, they can appear to be or actually be designed to elicit a specific response without directly requesting the response; in fact, the patient may appear surprised when the response occurs or deny that such a response was wished for in the first place.

Many disruptive patients have an underlying personality disorder. Although the diagnosis of personality disorder is often very difficult to make and all disruptive patients do not necessarily have a personality disorder, a substantial overlap between the two can exist. Although no pathognomonic signs exist that would assure the diagnosis of a personality disorder, many clues would strongly point to a putative diagnosis of a personality disorder (Table 4–6).

Table 4–6
Clinical Features Common in Patients with Personality Disorder

I. **A persistent pattern of experiencing feelings internally and manifesting behavior externally that deviates from the norm of the individual's culture.** These patterns can be seen in the following areas:
   A. *Cognition*—the ways that the individual perceives and understands himself or herself and others, i.e., refers to how the patient thinks and his or her cognitive processes, including delusions, hallucinations, paranoid ideation, and strange and/or unusual thoughts about self or others.
   B. *Affect*—the range, lability, intensity, and appropriateness of expression of feelings, i.e., how steady and consistent the patient's feelings are, how quickly these feelings change, and how concordant the feelings are with the content of the thought or the social situation.
   C. *Interpersonal functioning*—the ways in which the individual interacts in interpersonal situations; is the patient self-centered, aggressive, cooperative, friendly, hostile, demanding, contrite, shallow, or attention seeking?
   D. *Impulse control*—the ability to delay gratification, especially as demanded by the social situation, as well as the ability to consider the consequences of a possible decision or action before putting it into effect.

II. **The patterns appear rigid and inflexible across many situations and cause impairment of functioning across those social and occupational situations.** Rigid and inflexible refers to the inability to modify or change one's behavior based on the social situation and the needs of others.

III. **The pattern appears stable and of long duration beginning in either adolescence or early adulthood.** Thus, the physician should be able to appreciate that the particular pattern of difficulties is not something that is acute but is longstanding, even if it has only recently been brought to attention. A person may have a stable pattern of chronic instability, and patients with borderline personality disorder are often referred to as "stably unstable."

IV. **The pattern cannot be traced to another psychiatric or medical disorder.**

Adapted from the American Psychiatric Association. Diagnostic and Statistical Manual of Mental Disorders. Fourth Edition. Washington, DC: American Psychiatric Association. Reprinted with permission, Copyright 1994.

A. Definitions and diagnostic features.

Personality disorders do not universally lead to disruptive behavior, but they are manifested by an enduring pattern of interpersonal and behavioral dysfunction, often perceived more readily by people who interact with the individual with the personality disorder than by the individual.

B. Epidemiology of personality disorders.

1. Epidemiologic studies of personality disorders are limited. Studies reveal a prevalence of between 2% to 15% in community samples, but most such studies have restricted the estimates to only one personality disorder—antisocial personality disorder.[14]

2. Abnormalities of personality that are severe enough to meet the criteria for a personality disorder are found in 5% to 8% of primary care patients who display conspicuous psychiatric signs and symptoms.[15, 16]

C. Difficulties in making the personality disorder diagnosis in the primary care setting.

1. Personality disorder is a lifetime disorder that represents persistent inflexible maladaptive functioning over a long period of time (see Table 4–6); in the office, the practitioner has only a cross-sectional, time-limited view of the patient's functioning.

2. Patients with personality disorder have a difficult time viewing their behavior as abnormal. Their symptoms, which usually manifest themselves in disordered interpersonal functioning, are seen by them as ego-syntonic, i.e. as legitimate and normal reactions and behaviors given the situation. Often, the people who live with or who regularly interact with the patients with the personality disorder experience the distress. One of the people who regularly experience the stress of the disordered interpersonal interactions may be the primary care practitioner and his or her office staff because of the demanding, threatening, and potentially aggressive interpersonal style of the patient.

3. Patients with personality disorder externalize, that is, they blame others or the world for their difficulties. This characteristic differs from paranoid patients, who believe that people are deliberately plotting against them to cause them

harm. In externalization, patients have a strong tendency to blame others for the patients' own difficulties without believing that other people or the world are deliberately plotting against them. Rather than feeling outright paranoia, these patients may feel as though they are always being dealt the bad card, that nothing good ever comes their way, or that the world is generally an unfriendly, nonsupportive, nonvalidating place. Thus, in a manner similar to that of the somatizing patient, patients with personality disorder are very difficult to engage regarding issues of their behavior and/or their possible referral for psychiatric or psychological treatment.

Case Study

Mr. J., a 22-year-old single man with a very poor work record, sees his physician, complaining of chronic unhappiness and unfair treatment at the hands of his bosses. He says that he has begun to drink too much because his bosses are driving him crazy. He was recently fired from his job as a security guard in a motel because he had been found sleeping repeatedly during the night shift, the shift he was assigned to. He says that he also went to school during the day and saw no reason why he could not take a nap after he had completed his rounds and checked out all the posts in the motel and found everything quiet. When the suggestion is made that perhaps his employer had not been very eager paying him to sleep, he suddenly becomes very angry and accuses the doctor of being no different from the many bosses he has encountered; the doctor simply wants things understood his own way without any concern for the patient or the patient's own point of view. The patient storms out of the office, yelling back at the doctor as he goes through the waiting room, slamming the door behind him.

D. Arriving at the diagnosis of the disruptive patient with or without a probable personality disorder.

Personality disorder in the disruptive patient should be suspected when:

1. The patient evokes a *strong negative reaction* in the treating physician or in the office staff or the treating physician finds himself or herself spending a lot of time outside of the scheduled appointment time thinking about the patient and trying to figure out some reasonable way to manage the patient.
2. The *annoyance* that the patient evokes is not because of his or her physical complaints or tendency to somatize. Rather, it is *the manner in which these patients interact with the physician and the staff* that evokes the strong negative reaction.
3. The patient appears very "raw" in the process of making, as well as keeping, appointments. The physician and the staff labor under the impression that if the patient does not get his or her way, a serious problem could arise, which could take the form of anger, rage, sudden exiting from the office with the implicit threat of self-harm or litigation, sudden withdrawal into sullen silence, or other maneuvers that evoke anxiety and even fear in the physician.

E. Treatment and management of disruptive patients.

1. As with any putative psychiatric diagnosis, *other medical diagnoses and substance abuse and drug (prescription, nonprescription, and street) reactions* must be ruled out.
2. Patients with personality disorder or other forms of disruptive behavior may have *comorbid psychiatric disorders.* However, the primary interpersonal symptoms and interactions and reactions are not thought to be a result of the other psychiatric disorder but are thought to be primarily related to persistent disruptive patterns of interpersonal interactions.
3. *No standardized pharmacologic treatments* exist for personality disorder or for particular aspects of disruptive behavior that are not attributable to other psychiatric or organic disorders (See item 2 above). To clarify, manic or hypomanic patients may be demanding, emotionally labile, or aggressive in appearance or behavior. Intoxicated patients or patients with acute organic brain disease or dementia may appear in a similar way. Depressed patients may be withdrawn and negative and may appear to be passive-aggressive or persistently noncompliant when in fact they are hopeless and demoralized. If the primary care physician believes that the disruptive patient is in need of psychotropic medications, then a referral to a psychiatrist is probably called for.
4. Disruptive patients (with or without a bona fide diagnosis of personality disorder) are very difficult to treat in a primary care setting, particularly because of the strong negative reactions they evoke in the physician and the treating staff. Nonetheless, *they need to be treated in the primary care setting.* For that reason, even if medications are not called for, there may still be a need to *refer to a psychiatrist* or other mental health professional or to consult with a mental health professional about the interpersonal management of these patients (see item 7 below). Certainly, the primary care physician should feel free to discuss openly with another medical colleague, perhaps a psychiatrist, his or her frustrations and conflicts that are occurring in the treatment.
5. Disruptive and/or personality disorder patients

also may have bona fide medical problems. The physician should stay in close contact with the individual providing the psychiatric or psychological treatment.

6. *Extreme caution is advised in the prescribing of benzodiazepines and narcotics* to patients with personality disorder because these medications are known to disinhibit behavior in a person who already shows poor behavioral control.

7. Core management techniques are similar to those for somatizing patients.
   a. *Setting reasonable therapeutic goals.* These therapeutic goals should not only involve attempts to decrease the utilization of office time, staff time and energy, and other resources but they should also involve attempts to decrease the affective reactions of physician, office staff, and patient. In other words, how can the physician work with the patient so that the patient understands that the office staff and the physician are busy and cannot always immediately attend to the patient's perceived needs.

      "As you can see, we are very busy here, and although we try to make sure that everyone is seen as soon as possible, we also need to make judgments as to who should be seen immediately and who can wait. We also realize that when people have a problem, they may at times think the problem is more serious and more in need of immediate treatment than we do, and I would be happy to discuss those situations with you. But when you yell at the office staff or get angry with them, that only creates a situation where they may be less likely to want to help you. After all, they are only human."

      "As you know, I am very busy, and when I end my day, I like to go home and not be bothered except in a real emergency. I know you feel that when you get ill that it is really an emergency, but in truth, most times, as you can see, the problem has turned out to be a lot less of a problem than you first thought."

      The key to these conversations is to be able to resist becoming annoyed or angry even if the patient refutes everything the physician says or interrupts or denigrates the physician (or his or her staff). If all else fails, the physician may have to resort to the following statement, delivered in a calm voice:

      "Well, I understand how you see it, but nonetheless, this is how this office and my practice operate. And although we will be happy to continue to treat you, we can do that only if you understand and behave in a way that matches how we practice. If you continue to feel that you need something different or something more, we will try to refer you elsewhere, although it is my impression that most physicians would agree with me on these issues."

      These types of discussions can lead to a decrease in the disruptive behavior, although the decrease may not be permanent. If after a period of reasonable behavior, the disruptive behavior resumes, then, once again, statements similar to those outlined earlier must be made. At this point, the physician can also credit the patient with the past success and emphasize that appointments have gone better and that while the patient was less demanding, aggressive, or threatening, many of his or her complaints were successfully met. Thus, the goal should be to decrease, even temporarily, the strong affective atmosphere surrounding the patient.
   b. *Treating underlying psychiatric disorder,* if present.
   c. *Providing the opportunity for the patient to work with one specific care provider* in the office. This strategy may or may not work for either the patient or the chosen provider, but it nonetheless needs consideration. In any practice of more than one physician, some practitioners may find some behavior less troublesome or offensive than do other practitioners, and a meeting of the group should be held to try to agree on a designated provider for a difficult patient. The patient, perhaps, especially if he or she has previously demanded shifting to a different provider, needs to be recruited in the effort to identify a specific provider within the practice.

      "You have already worked with many of the doctors here, and although I know that you have, at times, not always been happy with them, I believe that it would be best to assign you to one of them. I wonder if you had a particular one in mind. (Pause for an answer.) We think that Dr. Jones would work well with you, and Dr. Jones agrees to try to see if things can work out between you and her. Also, we are trying to assign certain patients to certain doctors over an extended period of time, so if you agree, which I hope you will, then we will not change Dr. Jones, even if you are unhappy with her. We think that in the long run, it may be better for your care and for the running of the office that you plan to continue working with Dr. Jones for at least the next 2 years."

      If the patient refuses or if the patient agrees and then changes his or her mind and demands to see a different doctor, then the physician can introduce a version of the statement in 7a above, which begins with

      "Well, I understand how you see it, but nonetheless, this is how this office and my practice operate. And although we will be happy to continue to treat you . . ."
   d. *Attempting to establish an effective therapeutic relationship with the patient.* This may be very difficult, especially with a patient who is con-

stantly devaluing or demeaning of you or your office staff or copractitioners. Nevertheless, some sort of understanding of the nature and scope of the relationship is needed between the patient and the physician; otherwise, the disruptive patterns will continue. Often, the limit-setting approach, if presented without anger or before both parties are completely frustrated, can lead to a nascent, weak, but nonetheless workable relationship. Patients may be willing to acknowledge and appreciate straightforwardness on the part of the physician especially if the patient was raised in an environment in which people were not forthcoming, were manipulative, or were exploitative.

e. *Setting limits* and informing the patient as to how the office operates (the availability of office personnel, the payment policies, the telephone policies, and the proper decorum and respect of the patient for the physician and of the physician for the patient) (see 7a above). Limit setting that decreases the chaos in the office regarding the patient may be a very reasonable therapeutic goal. Specific behaviors, such as aggression (real or implied), repeated self-harm or suicide attempts, chronic substance abuse, or paranoia, may need to be addressed specifically.

(1) *Aggression.* The patient needs to be told specifically that threats of violence to others or damage to the office will not be tolerated.

"We need to provide an environment in which everyone can feel safe. The things you have been saying, as I am sure that you know, have people scared, and I cannot allow that to go on. That behavior needs to stop. If you cannot stop it, then you need to go elsewhere. Also, although it does not make me happy to say this, I want you to know that we have a policy of informing the police and pressing charges or billing people for damages when necessary."

(2) *Repeated self-harm or suicide attempts.* The patient needs to know that the physician considers the patient's safety to be paramount. Also, at this point, a psychiatric referral is mandatory.

"I cannot continue to work with you under these conditions. Obviously, you are very distressed, and I think it is essential that you go and speak with a psychiatrist. I have worked before with Dr. Smith, and I am sure that he could be helpful to you, and I regret to say this, but I must make this a condition of my continuing to see you for your medical and other problems."

(3) *Chronic substance abuse.* Suggested approaches for this situation follow.

"I know that you continue to use street drugs. It is impossible for me to keep up with all the medical problems that can occur from using those drugs. You need to stop, and I will expect you to stop or to seek help from others in a program to help you stop. In the future, I will test your urine for drugs and alcohol, and if you cannot stop or do not seek additional help, then I will need to recruit your spouse (parent) in helping you to get the assistance you need."

(4) *Paranoia.* Although this situation can seem to be overwhelming, in which the physician may fear that addressing the problem may lead to even greater paranoia, it nonetheless also needs to be addressed in a straightforward manner.

"I know that you feel that people are out to harm you, and at times, I think you include me among those who are trying to harm you. When you feel that way, we need to talk about it. Also, sometimes, small doses of medications (antipsychotics) can help 'take the edge off' your suspiciousness, and I would be most grateful if you would be willing to try this medication."

8. *Assisting and perhaps managing office staff.* Some staff members are able to tolerate difficult patients better than others, and these individuals should be on call to handle the patient's calls and complaints. Also, office and other staff may need to have a forum wherein they can freely and without criticism express their feelings and reactions to the patient. The frequency of meetings of the forum may vary; when feelings are running high and much commotion and consternation exists about the patient, then such a forum should take place. All people who are involved with the patient should be present, and it may need to be held over lunchtime, and the staff may need to be paid overtime. This is a small cost to ensure a safe and friendly working environment for all concerned, including patient consumers. Also, if the physicians try to deal more effectively with the patient, as presented in item 7 above, then the staff will feel that the physicians are trying to protect and preserve their dignity and the dignity of the practice. These behaviors on the part of the physician can serve as a good model for the office staff as well. If a forum takes place, it may be the physician's role to express his or her frustrations with the patient first; this may then create a climate and set the tone for the meeting whereby people (1) feel free to express their own frustrations and (2) work together to develop creative solutions.

9. *Having a psychiatric consultant work with the office staff.* All staff, including the primary care physician, may need to be educated about the diffi-

culties these patients cause and the uncomfortable feelings they provoke.

Summary

The somatizing patient and the disruptive patient (with or without a personality disorder) present a major common problem for the primary care physician. The physician, the patient, or both, can become exasperated with the course of care without always having a clear understanding of why, or of how the situation can be improved. It is not only the physician who may be unusually annoyed or angry with the patient and his or her family—the office staff may have an unusually strong (usually negative) reaction to the patient as well. Ultimately, the treating physician may experience failure, rejection, or rage—feelings that probably parallel some of the patient's own feelings. Early recognition and appropriate management of the difficult patient can improve care, minimize unnecessary testing, improve efficiency, and decrease frustration for the primary care physician.

This chapter has focused on two broad types of difficult patients, somatizing patients and behaviorally disruptive patients. Although somatizing patients express emotional discomfort and psychosocial stress in the physical language of bodily symptoms, disruptive patients are demanding of attention and are self-centered, paranoid, or aggressive in their interpersonal style. Most disruptive patients meet or come close to meeting diagnostic criteria for a personality disorder.

What is important to remember about the effective treatment of these patients is that the treatment may need to be focused more on issues of management than on prescribing medications or on diagnosis and therapy of specific somatic complaints. Recognition of one's strong feelings about a patient can lead to planned interpersonal interventions that can diminish anger and help office staff, patients, and physicians feel more effective and empowered and lead to more appropriate use of time, resources, and energy by all those involved.

References

1. Kaplan C, Lipkin M, Gordon G. Somatization in primary care: Patients with unexplained and vexing medical complaints. J Gen Intern Med 1988; 3:177–190.
2. Kitchens JM. Does this patient have an alcohol problem? JAMA 1994: 272:1782–1787.
3. Mulrow CD, Williams JW, Gerety MB, et al. Case-finding instruments for depression in primary care settings. Ann Intern Med 1995; 12:913–921.
4. Spitzer RL, Williams JBW, Kroenke K, et al. Utility of a new procedure for diagnosing mental disorders in primary care: The PRIME-MD 1000 study. JAMA 1994; 272:1749–1756.
5. Mabe PA, Jones LR, Riley WT. Managing somatization phenomena in primary care. Psychiatr Med 1990; 8:117–127.
6. Katon W, Ries RK, Kleinman A. The prevalence of somatization in primary care. Compr Psychiatry 1984; 25:208–215.
7. Kallner R. Somatization: Theories and research. J Nerv Ment Dis 1990; 178:150–160.
8. Brown FW, Golding JM, Smith GR. Somatization disorder: Psychiatric comorbidity in primary care. Psychosom Med 1990; 52:445–451.
9. Bass C, Benjamin S. The management of chronic somatization. Br J Psychiatry 1993; 162:472–480.
10. Margo KL, Margo GM. The problem of somatization in family practice. Am Fam Physician 1994; 49:1873–1879.
11. Smith GR, Rost K, Kashner TM. A trial of the effect of a standardized psychiatric consultation on health outcomes and costs in somatizing patients. Arch Gen Psychiatry 1995; 52:238–243.
12. Smith GR. Effectiveness of treatment for somatoform disorder patients. Psychiatr Med 1991; 9:545–558.
13. Smith RC. Somatization disorder: Defining its role in clinical medicine. J Gen Intern Med 1991; 6:168–175.
14. Oldham JM. Personality disorders: Current perspectives. JAMA 1994; 272:1770–1776.
15. Casey PR, Dillon S, Tyrer PJ. The diagnostic status of patients with conspicuous psychiatric morbidity in primary care. Psychol Med 1984; 12:673–681.
16. Casey PR, Tyrer P. Personality disorder and psychiatric illness in general practice. Br J Psychiatry 1990; 156:261–265.
17. Lipkin M Jr. Psychiatry and medicine. In: Kaplan H, Sadock B, Editors. Comprehensive Textbook of Psychiatry. 5th Edition. Baltimore: Williams & Wilkins, 1987.
18. American Psychiatric Association. Diagnostic and Statistical Manual of Mental Disorders. Fourth Edition. Washington, DC: American Psychiatric Association; 1994.

APPENDIX

CAGE Questionnaire*

1. Have you ever felt you ought to **C**ut down on your drinking?
2. Have people **A**nnoyed you by criticizing your drinking?
3. Have you ever felt bad or **G**uilty about your drinking?
4. Have you ever had a drink first thing in the morning to steady your nerves or get rid of a hangover (**E**ye opener)?

Positive response to two or more questions associated with Positive Likelihood ratio of 2 to 7.† Therefore, persons with two or more positive responses should be investigated for alcohol abuse or dependence.

*Ewing JA. Detecting alcoholism: the CAGE questionnaire. JAMA 1984;252:1905–1907.
†Kitchens JM. Does this patient have an alcohol problem? JAMA 1994;272:1782–1787.

Center for Epidemiologic Studies/Depressed Mood Scale (CES-D)

Patient's Name ______________________ Date __________

Using the scale below, indicate the number which best describes how often you felt or behaved this way DURING THE PAST WEEK.

1 Rarely or none of the time (less than 1 day)

2 Some or a little of the time (1–2 days)

3 Occasionally or a moderate amount of time (3–4 days)

4 Most or all of the time (5–7 days)

DURING THE PAST WEEK:

____ 1. I was bothered by things that usually don't bother me.

____ 2. I did not feel like eating; my appetite was poor.

____ 3. I felt that I could not shake off the blues even with help from my family or friends.

____ 4. I felt that I was just as good as other people.

____ 5. I had trouble keeping my mind on what I was doing.

____ 6. I felt depressed.

____ 7. I felt everything I did was an effort.

____ 8. I felt hopeful about the future.

____ 9. I thought my life had been a failure.

____ 10. I felt fearful.

____ 11. My sleep was restless.

____ 12. I was happy.

____ 13. I talked less than usual.

____ 14. I felt lonely.

____ 15. People were unfriendly.

____ 16. I enjoyed life.

____ 17. I had crying spells.

____ 18. I felt sad.

____ 19. I felt that people disliked me.

____ 20. I could not get "going."

Interpretation: A total score of 22 or higher is indicative of depression when this scale is used in primary care.

5

GREGORY W. DALACK, MD

ANDREW J. ZWEIFLER, MD

Counseling for Behavioral Change

I. Introduction.

All medical practitioners would agree that much of medical care requires the active participation of the patient in order for a positive outcome to be achieved. An intervention in an acute or a chronic condition involves an agreement between the doctor and the patient that the patient will begin to perform certain behaviors and cease performing others. The health care provider already knows, for example, about the importance of weight reduction in decreasing cardiovascular risk, improving control of diabetes mellitus, and preventing damage to weight-bearing joints. Other obvious examples of issues that can be targeted for behavioral intervention include cessation of smoking, moderation of alcohol consumption, and management of stress. It is also possible to consider other important behaviors which may come out of the treatment relationship. For example, compliance with prescribed medication can be seen as an important health behavior.

Sometimes, the patient already appreciates the relationship between risk factors, health behaviors, and health outcomes. The patient comes to the physician for help in addressing a problem that has not yet yielded to the patient's efforts to control it. At other times, the physician is surprised that patients are unaware of problems that could be addressed in a behavioral program.

Many obstacles often separate the physician and the patient from an action plan to address health risks. These include

- Physicians' doubts about people's ability to change.
- Physicians' doubts that behavioral change will have any real impact on health outcomes.
- Physicians' difficulty finding the time they think is necessary to work with someone who is interested in changing a perhaps lifelong behavior.
- Physicians' fear that they do not know what to do, even if they have the time and inclination to try.

In this chapter, we provide information about the rationale of counseling for behavioral change; describe an approach to counseling patients who are at different stages of readiness to accept the need for, or initiate, a behavioral program; and provide examples of the approach in specific situations.

II. Rationale.

A. Behavioral change has an impact on health outcomes.

Considerable evidence suggests that changing health behaviors has a salutary effect on health outcomes. Studies have examined the differential impact of interventions in enhancing adherence to exercise programs, in improving outcome after the diagnosis of significant coronary disease, and in reducing pain and disability of chronic arthritis. An extensive body of literature examines the relationship between hostility and coronary artery disease risk and prognosis, and recent evidence links depressive illness and poor prognosis after myocardial infarction.

Physicians are practicing at a time when economic forces support the common-sense approach of identifying and reducing risk factors in order to limit the development or progression of serious medical conditions. *The challenge, ultimately, is to consider the individual patient whom the physician may perceive as more or less unable to change, and to recognize that counseling for behavioral change is worthwhile.*

B. Every patient has the capacity to change behavior.

Both the physician and the patient must be responsive to the idea that behavioral change is possible, meaningful, and important in achieving an optimal health outcome. One important aspect of this is accepting the reality that change, if it occurs, typically occurs slowly; the process of behavioral change often does not start with the first intervention. Undoing a long-term (potentially lifelong) behavior or set of behaviors requires adaptations not only to act differently but also to develop and adapt to psychological and emotional perspectives on the real or perceived consequences of the change. A heavy smoker who is trying to quit must reckon with many issues beyond nicotine withdrawal, including the loss of a powerful (if less than optimal) coping tool, the loss of a social activity, the loss of a mood or weight regulator, and the loss of an "on-demand" pleasurable experience. Indeed, many smokers, intent on quitting for health reasons and armed with the nicotine patch and a heightened sense of motivation, are often unable to achieve the goal or understand why they cannot, unless they have considered the ramifications of not smoking. Rapid changes in health behaviors occur only when dramatic circumstances make the consequences of the status quo painfully clear. For example, exhortations from physicians to quit smoking are most effective when they are delivered in the cardiac intensive care unit after the patient has suffered a myocardial infarction. *Our goal is to develop approaches to counseling for behavioral change that are effective at an earlier point in the course of the condition or illness.*

Both patients and their clinicians may assume that failure to change indicates a lack of commitment to change or a frank inability to alter behavior. Such a line of thinking leads to an early frustration and a rapid waning of creative efforts to assess and address problematic health behaviors. All physicians have struggled with the obese patient who is "unable" to lose weight, or the heavy smoker who "refuses" to quit smoking, despite the physician's advice; eventually, perhaps, the reminders about the health risks of obesity or smoking become less frequent, and physicians settle into a disappointed acceptance of the futility of change.

1. *The most important first step to successful counseling for behavioral change is examination of the physician's own beliefs about the potential of others to change their behaviors.*

   There is no point in trying to understand and apply behavioral counseling techniques unless the physician believes that his or her patients have the capacity to recognize and change targeted health behaviors. Different patients clearly require different levels of guidance and support from the physician, depending on their individual needs.

2. *After that, the fundamental role of the physician is to help patients do the following:*
   - Identify problematic health behaviors.
   - Make a commitment to change them.
   - Develop feasible, achievable action plans to make changes.
   - Retain the gains made.
   - Promptly resume modified action plans after setbacks.

III. Beginning.

Patients come to the physician with different levels of awareness about health problems. Some have no notion that they have a medical condition or are unaware that behaviors under their control have contributed to the cause or worsening of their situation. For some patients, this lack of awareness is due to a true lack of knowledge; for others, it is a suppression of knowledge that they have but are unable or unwilling to access (denial). *It is usually safe to begin with the assumption that the patient is at worst, unaware, or at best, ambivalent about the need for change.* By definition, the issues and motivations driving his or her behavior are complex and incompletely understood. This is particularly true in situations in which patients demonstrate an understanding of the need for change and express a willingness to change, but are unable to do so. Clearly, if the change were easy for them, they would have achieved it before discussing it with you.

The initial assessment is important for ascertaining how well patients understand their condition and how motivated they are to change it. One model that can be used to determine where patients are on the change continuum is that developed by Prochaska and DiClemente.[1] These "stages of change" are a useful construct in the planning of behavioral counseling. Like any other growth process, moving through the stages of change entails achieving critical milestones in the early steps before moving on to the later stages. Trying to get an early-stage patient to initiate behaviors characteristic of the later stages is futile and potentially destructive. Such a strategy leaves the patient feeling unable to overcome a problem that could be completely amenable if it were fully understood.

In the initial assessment, patients are likely to present in one of two stages of change described by Prochaska and DiClemente.

A. Precontemplation stage of behavioral change.

In this stage, the patient is not considering the need for change and often does not see himself or herself as having a problem. As a result, patients are unlikely to present for help with a specific problem. The physician may identify an important health behavior issue during a routine examination or during a visit for the purpose of addressing another problem. Sometimes, a friend or family member recognizes the problem and wants the physician's help in convincing the family member to address it.

1. *Giving advice and assistance in undertaking a behavioral program is generally futile at this juncture.*

   A mismatch exists between the patient's motivational level and the intervention. Such patients are often labeled "unmotivated" or "noncompliant" as a consequence of the clinician's misunderstanding that mismatch.

2. *The approach to the precontemplator calls for providing information and raising awareness about the problem.* Only then can the patient consider the possibility of making a change.

B. Contemplation stage of behavioral change.

Raising awareness and providing information typically leave the patient in the contemplation stage. This stage is marked by the patient's ambivalence about the issue. With heightened awareness comes recognition that a problem may exist, alternating with doubt about whether there is really any cause for all the fuss. Patients presenting for help are often in the contemplation phase. Their ability to express the need for change and then dismiss it can exasperate the practitioner, whose goal is to enhance the movement toward, and the motivation for, change. The techniques of motivational interviewing can be very useful in this phase to move the patient to the next phase.

1. *The physician should give himself or herself the opportunity to hear and understand the obstacles to change experienced by the patient.* This initial step is perhaps the most important one in establishing an atmosphere of trust with that patient; this trust facilitates an open assessment of target health behaviors and behavioral change over the course of the treatment relationship. Part of the task in this early assessment is to gauge the patient's knowledge of his or her situation and the patient's motivation for change. Like any interactive process, this assessment can be influenced by what the physician says and how the physician says it to the patient. A more confrontational approach ("you must know that smoking and working 15 hours a day can't be good for you") quickly closes off informative communication from the patient.

2. *The initial assessment requires a good deal of reflective listening* and occasional verbal prompts, with open-ended questions geared to enable an understanding of the complexity of the patient's struggle. *As a rule of thumb in these situations, the physician should not ask three questions in a row.* Repeated questioning from the physician stifles the free flow of information from the patient and results in the obtaining of bits of information without a full understanding of the patient. A more thoughtful approach may mean that one or two visits may be required for the physician to fully understand the patient's point of view.

Case Study

Mr. A. is a 48-year-old man who presents with symptoms consistent with a mild anginal syndrome. He owns his own business and puts in long hours to ensure its success. He would describe himself as "driven" and stressed at times but feels that his stress is "part of the job." He smokes because he feels smoking helps him relax, often eats on the run, and has little time for leisure activities. This has led to some unhappiness at home with his wife and children, who feel that he is often short-tempered and liable to vent on them the frustration he feels about suboptimal work from his employees.

Physician: What is your understanding of your condition?

Patient: I guess you are telling me I have heart disease. You know, my father died of a heart attack when he was 53. I don't want that to happen to me, but I'm not sure how to avoid it. I couldn't bear the thought of leaving my family before my time.

Physician: I understand you are worried. What do you understand about your risks for heart disease?

Patient: Yeah, I know smoking isn't supposed to be good for me. I have tried to quit, even chewed the gum for a while, but it was no use. My wife says I am working myself into an early grave.

Physician: Smoking is a serious health risk for heart disease and other conditions. Are there any others?

Patient: I'm not sure. I probably don't eat right. I used to jog when we first got married, but who has the time now? There's too much to think about with the business.

Physician: You feel under a lot of pressure.

Patient: You bet. I can't depend on anyone at work. Unless I check over everything myself, I don't feel comfortable that things are being done right. Sometimes, I'll be running around the factory floor yelling instructions to the workers, and I'll get that pressure feeling in my chest. Then I get real scared.

Physician: It seems you have an idea that some of the things you do make you more likely to have heart disease or feel chest pain. We can talk about ways to address these issues and try to gain greater control over them.

In this vignette, Mr. A. has some knowledge about the relationship between his actions and his condition. There is even the suggestion that he has contemplated the consequences of not addressing his health behaviors. Mr. A. is relatively early in his transit through the contemplation phase. Others may be more clearly in the precontemplation phase. How does the physician increase the patient's knowledge and motivation to change?

3. *The techniques of motivational interviewing*[2] can be used to move patients toward behavioral change. Several premises should be kept in mind.
   a. *The patient is the agent of change.* True, the clinician has considerable influence on the facilitation or limitation of change, but the patient ultimately carries out the plan. As a result, the patient should have a great deal of freedom and responsibility to develop the plan with guidance from the physician.
   b. *People tend to identify and face problems that they understand.* Target behaviors or health problems should be defined and described, as much as possible, in relationship to the problems that the patient brings up. This strategy capitalizes on the patient's sense that a gap exists between his or her health goals and his or her current state. Presenting all the general reasons the patient should decide to lose weight, begin exercising, or take prescribed medications is less effective than linking the rationale

to the patient's perspective ("You realize that many things increase your risk for a heart attack. You have also said that it is important to you to be around to see your children grow up. Certainly, addressing some of the risks would help you do that. What do you think the next step should be?"). *Using the patient's issues and concerns as a reference point makes it more difficult for the patient to dismiss the advice or underplay the significance of the health concern.*

c. *The patient should be given enough control.* Allowing the patient considerable control over the focus of the behavioral work and the content of the action plan ("What do you think the next step should be?") increases the patient's investment in the process and increases the likelihood that the patient actually follows through.

IV. Developing the plan.

Mr. A. demonstrates some recognition of behavioral health risks but sounds relatively pessimistic about his own ability to address them. Other patients have identified target behaviors and present to the physician asking for help addressing the concerns or assistance in figuring out why their ongoing efforts are not successful. Once the patient is contemplating change, what can the physician do to move him or her beyond recognition of problems to making a commitment to addressing them?

A. Determination stage of behavioral change.

Prochaska and DiClemente[1] refer to this next stage as the *determination* phase. At this point, ambivalence has been at least partially overcome, and the patient is cognizant that change is needed. It often seems that the determination phase is available for only a brief period of time and that the person either moves ahead to take action or reverts back to the ambivalence of contemplation. The patient may signal determination to act directly (e.g., "I think I have to do something about this") or indirectly by no longer arguing the no-change side of ambivalence. Focusing on the patient's concerns (medical, psychological, or social) as he or she has presented them enables the physician to encourage the patient to take the next step.

Case Study

Ms. B. is a 38-year-old beautician who is moderately obese and has a family history of diabetes and hypertension. She has been upset by the fact that her father was recently incapacitated by a stroke. She wants advice about preventing a similar occurrence in herself. Her attempts at weight reduction in the past have been unsuccessful.

Physician: *Are you aware of the relationship between body weight and the risk of stroke?*

Patient: *I guess people who are overweight can have strokes. My dad has been heavy for years.*

Physician: *Yes. Excess weight can increase the risk of both high blood pressure and diabetes, and they can both lead to strokes. What do you think we should do about this?*

Patient: *I know I need to lose weight. It isn't like I haven't tried. It just seems so impossible for me.*

Physician: *It sounds like you have been frustrated when you tried to lose weight in the past. What kinds of things did you try to do?*

Patient: *I tried a "no meat" diet for a while. Once, I tried a diet where I had to drink eight glasses of water a day. None of it was any fun.*

Physician: *And it sounds like none of it led to any weight loss. I understand that you are concerned about the health risks you face by being overweight. I also understand how frustrated you feel when you work hard to lose weight and don't succeed. What do you think the next step should be?*

Patient: *I don't know. You're the doctor. Tell me what to do.*

Physician: *I am sure I don't know exactly what you need to do. Ultimately, we want to come up with a plan that you think can work for you. I would be happy to help you with that. I can tell you a few things that have worked for other people, as well as some pitfalls others have fallen into when they tried to lose weight. Sometimes, people go on severe diets, hoping to lose lots of weight fast. They forget that such diets are very difficult to sustain and don't address the longer-term issue of maintaining oneself at a lower weight.*

Patient: *I think that was part of my problem.*

Physician: *For some people, rather than rushing ahead to a diet, a useful first step is to keep a diary of the food they eat over a week or two. It's important to be completely honest about what you record in the diary so that you have a complete picture of what you eat and when you eat it. Then, we can go over it to get a sense of your eating habits and discuss what kind of weight reduction program might work best. Does the idea of keeping a food diary make sense to you?*

Patient: *I guess so. Sometimes, I feel that I eat more when I feel bad. Could I jot down how I am feeling when I eat?*

Physician: *Absolutely, the more information we have, the better our plan will be. Let's plan on meeting in 2 weeks to review your diary.*

B. Action stage of behavioral change.

Once the patient has made the determination to act, the physician and patient begin to develop an action plan that makes sense for the patient and would possibly be carried out. This work leads to the *action* stage. At this critical step, the patient takes the steps necessary to effect a change. If the action plan has been conceived and developed with the patient and consists of reasonable goals, appropriate follow-up, and support, the chances of success are enhanced. This step, like every other, has pitfalls for the physician as well as for the patient. By this point, the physician has worked for some time to get the patient to commit to making a change.

1. *Resist temptation.* The physician may feel the need to rush in and provide the determined patient with a behavioral change program that the physician thinks is ideal. The patient is the ultimate arbiter of whatever program he or she chooses (regardless of whether it is "best" for him or her). To challenge the patient's role risks pushing the patient back to greater ambivalence (e.g., "that sounds too hard. . . , perhaps I'm not as bad off as I think") and engages the physician in a debate about whether change (the physician's side) or status quo (the patient's side) is preferable.
2. *Remember the prize.* Long-term change is a long-term goal and takes considerable investment by both the physician and the patient in a realistic and gradual plan. The intermediate steps are, indeed, intermediate and are not the basis on which the physician's success or the patient's motivation can be judged, as long as momentum is building toward the end goal.
3. *Remain realistic.* It is important to recognize, and even tell the patient that *success on the first attempt to make changes is rare.* Emphasize the idea of using each unsuccessful experience to learn more about oneself and apply it to the next effort to change.

C. How to help patients develop an action plan.

Many approaches can help patients develop an action plan.

1. *Encourage and affirm.* Some patients need only basic encouragement and affirmation in order to proceed with a realistic plan that they have devised.
2. *Reframe extreme goals.* Other patients have a plan with inappropriate or improbable goals ("remove all stress from my life"; "lose 50 pounds in 3 months"). They need help to redefine their program and establish a realistic time frame so that lasting change is accomplished.
3. *Maintain the focus on desired outcomes.* For most patients, the physician's work consists of developing with them a plan that is reasonable and achievable in terms of the patients' commitment and past experience. Despite patients' determination to make a change, they often discover (or rediscover) their ambivalence and resistance to change as they work to establish an action plan. Here, the effort is to focus the patients again on the reasons that are important to them for contemplating the change.
4. *Circumnavigate roadblocks.* In addition, the physician may work with the patient to reframe unrealistic or extreme expectations (which make change appear impossible) and recast them into smaller steps. Therefore, the patient's concern that he or she may have no time for exercise might be met with a review of why exercise was identified as an important step by the patient and a reminder that acceptable exercise regimens come in many forms. Suggesting more feasible forms of exercise may work or may provide the patient with another opportunity to argue with the physician by dismissing these suggestions as unworkable. Rather, the physician should consider reflecting the issue back to the patient. ("It is true that exercise does take some time and commitment, although perhaps not as much as you fear. What possibilities have you considered? Are there other alternatives which might work?") In this case, advice may be offered, particularly if it is solicited by the patient. *The emphasis is on providing the patient with a menu of possibilities (this limits the likelihood of rejection) and encouraging the patient to make the choice ("Here are some ideas that have worked for other people. Do any of these make sense for you?").*
5. *Use tools.*
   a. *Daily log.* As suggested in the second vignette, an initial, helpful intervention might consist of having the patient keep a log of activity related to the behavior in question. For a weight loss program, this record might be a careful and complete log of meals consumed for 1 or 2 weeks. For stress reduction, this record might be a thought and feeling inventory in which anxious or angry thoughts are jotted down along with the time of day and event or activity going on at the time. In this way, both the physician and the patient can begin to recognize the patterns that are characteristic of the behavior. Often, the mere act of making the behavior explicit by writing it down leads to a decrease in its expression. Further efforts to change the behavior can be tailored to the information culled from the record. Continuing to keep the diary during and after behavioral changes are made also permits close follow-up of deficiencies in the plan. Sometimes, a slip may be preceded by a reversion to old habits, as indicated in the diary. At other times, a relapse cue that had not been considered is noted as the precipitant to a reversion to the old behavior.
   b. *Behavioral contract.* It is also often helpful to have the patient develop and even sign a contract that details the reasons for making the change and describes the concrete long-term goals of the behavioral change. This can be referred to by the patient when commitment wavers or when new exigencies stimulate ambivalence.

D. Patients who set minimal goals.

Sometimes, patients set goals that the physician feels are not optimal. For example, an overweight patient may talk about a minor reduction in caloric intake, or a heavy smoker may propose cutting back a few cigarettes a day.

Be patient: it is important to consider the potential value and importance of such a step toward the long-term goal. If patients can achieve such goals, they demonstrate a level of commitment, maintain positive control over the process, and can evaluate whether the first step is adequate in achieving their long-term goal. Indeed, to the patient who cannot conceive of totally giving up cigarettes, the physician might present the possibility of delaying smoking each cigarette for 5 minutes after the first thought of having one; the effect would be to demonstrate that the patient could survive for short periods without cigarettes and to diminish the number of cigarettes smoked during the day.

V. Following through and following up.

Ultimately, the patient who has undertaken a plan to effect some behavioral change has demonstrated motivation. *Arrival at this stage, however, does not mean the end of the counseling effort.*

A. The maintenance stage of behavioral change.

If a motivated patient has worked with the physician to carry out all the preceding steps to as full an extent as possible and is committed to working on the myriad obvious and subtle changes that are entailed in long-lasting behavioral change, the *maintenance* stage of change is more likely to proceed smoothly. This ideal situation is not typical.

1. *Setbacks are common.* Patients may have an incomplete view of what change means: "I put some projects on hold last month to free up some time to exercise. Now, I'm getting pressure to get back to work . . . haven't I done enough?" The action plan may not have been completely considered, the early changes might provoke ambivalence once again, or the patient may have difficulty maintaining the gains as life circumstances and stressors change. In this maintenance phase, the same techniques of listening reflectively, interviewing motivationally, and engaging the patient in the process are continued.

2. *Relapse cues are subtle and pervasive.* When the patient returns to the old behavior, the work of the maintenance stage is to
   - Acknowledge the demands and difficulty of making a change.
   - Underscore the reasons for the change.
   - Help the patient identify and learn how to respond to the risks for returning to the previous behaviors.

   Stable, long-term maintenance of behavioral change eventually indicates that the relapse risk is not significant, not because the patient has overcome the temptations, but because the new behavior patterns are now so accepted and habitual that considerable effort must be expended to relapse.

3. *Despite all of our best efforts, a return to old ways (relapse) occasionally occurs.* To be sure, maintenance is often not achieved on the first trip through these stages. More often, patients return to the previous behavior and then must consider beginning the process over again. Most patients will view relapse as a failure; *part of our effort is to reframe relapse as an opportunity to learn more about the factors driving the behavior that is targeted for change.*
   - The patient's ambivalence may have been greater than acknowledged.
   - An unrecognized trigger may have been revealed.
   - The patient's reliance on others or a weakness in the patient's support system (family, friends, coworkers) may be recognized.

B. Changing long-term, valued behaviors is hard work.

Like any other new skill, behavioral change must be practiced; setbacks provide new opportunities to learn. The goal of treatment in the face of a (minor or major) relapse is to minimize the demoralization and help the patient move decidedly back toward contemplating change once more.

VI. The primary care provider's role.

A. Be a partner in care with patient.

Throughout this chapter, the physician has been referred to as a major participant as patients work to achieve behavioral change. Almost without exception, particularly with patients making a first attempt to address health behaviors, this should be the rule. No one is more uniquely suited to apply the information the physician has collected about the patient and to establish the precedent of a relationship that will evolve over time and will address a variety of goals.

B. Make resources available.

Patients come to the physician seeking information, and there are numerous sources that the physician can use. Self-help books or information pamphlets and videos are often good sources of information beyond the physician's initial discussion with the precontemplator and the contemplator. Sources of information that have been used and found to be useful by other patients are especially good. The bibliography of this chapter also lists books that the physician may consult for more in-depth treatment about such topics as motivational interviewing and stages of change. Readers interested in becoming more involved in providing any sort of behavioral treatment (e.g., relaxation therapy, cognitive-behavioral interventions, nutritional counseling) should consider books and training seminars or a period of apprenticeship with a practitioner skilled in the specific area.

C. Remain involved.

Some practices are designed in such a way that other office staff are available to provide specific treatment and follow-up after the physician has developed the action plan with the patient. In these cases, it is important that the patient sees all of these individuals as part of the treatment team led by the physician rather than feeling that the physician has "disposed" of the problem by referring the patient.

D. Use specialist expertise.

It is also important to consider how and when specialist expertise is needed in a particular area.

1. *General considerations.* The physician needs to decide whether he or she will treat the problem directly, obtain a consultation for additional expertise, or refer the patient elsewhere for treatment. How such a process is handled with the patient can make the difference between helping the patient reach his or her behavioral goals or engendering a sense of futility about change.
2. *Problem cases.* For example, patients who have unusual difficulty in making gains in an ostensibly reasonable behavioral program often, have other difficulties (e.g., undiagnosed psychiatric conditions) that make treatment of the first issue more complicated. For example, the comorbidity of major depression in cigarette smokers and those with cardiovascular disease is high (1.5 to 3 times higher than in the general population). An episode of major depression may complicate an attempt to quit smoking or may render a patient with heart disease less able to develop and sustain a dietary and exercise plan.

Case Study

Mr. C. is a 55-year-old factory worker who has recently been found to have borderline hypertension. He and his physician agree to attempt to control his blood pressure with weight reduction, salt restriction, and exercise. They complete their behavioral contract during one visit.

Physician: So, are you clear about the diet and exercise plans?

Patient: Yes, I am pretty sure I can handle it.

Physician: How long do you think it should be before you come back to see me?

Patient: Let's give it a month. I'll know by then if I can handle things.

Visit 2 (30 minutes' duration 1 month later)

Physician: How did things go?

Patient: So-so. My wife helped me cut back on extra salt. We use very little of it at home, and she's got me bringing lunch in from home almost every day. I've cut way down on the fast food. I haven't lost any weight yet.

Physician: But it sounds like you and your wife have made some important progress regarding salt intake. It's great that she is supporting you in this. Part of the weight loss program was your diet, the other was exercise. How is that going?

Patient: Not quite as well. My wife is really into aerobics and I thought I could try it with her. I really hated it. I have been too busy to try anything else.

Physician: Okay, what other things can you consider?

Patient: I was thinking that I could try to walk more, use the stairs instead of the elevator, that kind of thing.

Physician: Sure, I think that would make a fine start. Do you think you can do those things regularly?

Patient: Yeah, I have to move a lot between floors at work. If I only take the stairs, I probably would do 10 or more flights a day. My wife has been after me to take a walk with her after dinner, too.

Physician: Fine. Keep up the good work on the salt restriction and let's see how the exercise program goes in another month.

Visit 3 (30 minutes duration 1 month later)

Patient: I have to admit that I surprised myself. Taking the stairs at work was tough at first, but I stuck with it. Even the younger guys are too embarassed to take the elevator when they are with me.

Physician: Great. How about the diet?

Patient: OK. My wife and I are trying to keep the salt low. We are even paying attention to cutting back on fats and cholesterol.

Physician: You know, your weight is down a couple of pounds. That may be the first sign of payoff for your work. Even your blood pressure is down a bit. Let's have you come back for a blood pressure check with the nurse practitioner in about 1 month, and I'll see you in 2 months. Sound good?

Visit 4 (30 minutes duration 2 months later)

Physician: I see your blood pressure and weight continued to improve at the check-up last month. How do you feel?

Patient: I was doing okay, but the factory was shut down for the past few weeks, so I am off my exercise regimen. I guess I need to try to walk more at home.

Physician: I wouldn't be too hard on yourself. Not exercising for the past few weeks doesn't mean you have undone all the good work of the past few months. You've made good progress so far, and this sounds like a temporary setback. When do you go back to work?

Patient: Probably next week.

Physician: Okay. Let's see if you can get back to your stairs at that point. Come in for a blood pressure check next month, and I'll see you the month after that.

Visit 5 (30 minutes' duration 2 months later)

Physician: By the look of your weight and blood pressure, I'd guess you are back on track.

Patient: Yes, and I feel pretty good about it.

Physician: Let's talk about aiming for a little bit lower target weight and discuss the time frame to get you there.

Visits 6 to 10 (over the next 18 to 24 months)

In the early stages, these visits focus on determining the difficulties in adhering to the regimen and reinforcing the positive outcomes (weight, blood pressure). In the maintenance phase, the effort is to establish a long-term but varied diet and exercise program that is acceptable and effective. Positive reinforcement for the maintenance of weight and blood pressure is offered, ideally at every visit. Setbacks are framed as learning opportunities to fine tune the long-term program.

Summary

Counseling for behavioral change is a challenging opportunity that requires a variety of biomedical and interpersonal skills. It can be applied to the most common situations (e.g., compliance with a medication regimen) and to the more complex situations (e.g., dietary, exercise, and stress-reduction interventions for patients with coronary artery disease). This counseling is an implicit, if unrecognized, part of all medical contacts. The physician's decision to develop his or her skills can have an enormous impact on the well-being of patients, as well as enhance the physician's own professional satisfaction with his or her work.

References

1. Prochaska JO, DiClemente CC. Transtheoretical therapy: Toward a more integrative model of change. Psychother Theory Res Pract 1982; 19:276–288.
2. Miller WR, Rollnick S. Motivational Interviewing. New York: The Guilford Press; 1991.

Suggested Reading

Frasure-Smith N, Lespérance F, Talajic M. Depression following myocardial infarction: Impact on 6-month survival. JAMA 1993; 270:1819–1825.

King AC, Taylor CB, Haskell WL, et al. Strategies for increasing early adherence to and long-term maintenance of home-based exercise training in healthy middle-aged men and women. Am J Cardiol 1988; 61:628–632.

Lorig KR, Mazonson PD, Holman HR. Evidence suggesting that health education for self-management in patients with chronic arthritis has sustained health benefits while reducing health care costs. Arthritis Rheum 1993; 36:439–446.

Ornish D, Brown SE, Scherwitz LW, et al. Can lifestyle changes reverse coronary heart disease? The lifestyle heart trial. Lancet 1990; 336:129–133.

Williams R, Williams V. Anger Kills. New York: Harper Collins Publishers; 1993.

6

KEVIN B. KERBER, MD

DAVID J. KNESPER, MD

Making Referrals for Psychiatric Care: Clinical Advice and Managed Care Implications

I. Introduction.

In order to effectively use all the information contained in *Primary Care Psychiatry,* the primary care physician (PCP) must understand his or her role in the total system of health care providers. Even the most skilled clinician must understand how to use the expertise of others, including conferring with a colleague, referring a patient to a specialist for treatment, and referring a patient for other types or levels of care, such as intermediate or full in-patient psychiatric programs. Specific referral skills are needed in every delivery system. Managed care systems have some additional requirements that may change the role of the PCP in the treatment of mental disorders. Health care is increasingly being delivered by economically linked systems or networks of care providers, both individual and institutional. An effective appreciation of one's role and function in that network is essential for the well-being of both the patient and the physician. PCPs often become frustrated when they find that they do not have the same freedom to refer for psychiatric services under managed care that they traditionally have had under other systems. This chapter aims to provide information on how to improve making psychiatric referrals at a clinical and procedural level appropriate to managed care systems. Definitions of some common managed care terms are listed in the glossary at the end of this chapter.

II. Strategies and Scripts for Overcoming Patient Resistance to Psychiatric Referral.

Some patients resist the recommendation from their PCP to obtain psychiatric services. The following strategies may motivate these patients. Each strategy is illustrated by an example of a physician's discussion with a patient—a script. These are general strategies; most chapters contain a specific section on "what to tell the patient and family," and these sections should be reviewed for a more specific script.

A. Collaborative care.

It is our routine practice to ask patients in your situation to get an opinion from Dr. Wilson. She and I have *worked together many times* under similar circumstances; she is a part of our care team, and her advice and recommendations have always proved helpful. Dr. Wilson is a psychiatrist who works with medical patients.

Primary care physicians and their patients are well served by a psychiatrist who functions as a member of the care team. One successful arrangement is for the psychiatrist to share the office suite with a group of primary care doctors. The psychiatrist's schedule and work style can be made to accommodate occasional interruptions so that a patient may make psychiatric contact before leaving. Often a handshake and a 5 minute discussion will cement a psychiatric referral. Similar arrangements permit the primary care doctor to obtain immediate telephone consultation while the patient is in the doctor's examination room.

B. Good news.

The news is all good. We have performed a series of very appropriate tests. I am really pleased to be able to tell you that your liver, kidneys, heart, lungs, and every organ system we checked is in good shape. I can't find any disease that could account for your problems. It is helpful to recognize that patients with your symptoms often have *stress-related conditions.* Even better news is that these conditions usually respond to psychiatric treatment. The first step is to get a psychiatric evaluation. I work with Dr. Wilson, and I would like you to see her.

When using this or any of the other strategies described, *it is critical for the primary care physician to remain involved.* Here is one way of making this point:

Of course, I haven't performed every possible test there is, but I have performed even more than the standard tests and examinations. Dr. Wilson is a medical doctor, and she may uncover something I have missed. Dr. Wilson and I will stay in contact and see how we can all be *partners in your care.*

When the patient is seen by Dr. Wilson, she should deliver the same "good news" message. Of course, this means that the primary care physician and the psychiatrist need to discuss their common introduction to psychiatric referral. A consistent, common message helps to cement the referral, and patients find such consistency very reassuring.

C. Just like another test.

There are no tests that I can substitute for a psychiatric evaluation. We have no means for testing your blood or scanning your brain that can tell me if you have, for example, a medical depression. Going to a psychiatrist for an evaluation is just like getting another test. And this test doesn't even hurt.

The "another test" strategy is one more method of making the psychiatric evaluation a routine part of medical practice. The referring primary care doctor wants simply to know the results, and once obtained, the doctor will see the patient for a return visit to discuss the results. *A return visit to the primary care doctor is often an essential element of this strategy.* At the return visit, the doctor should discuss the psychiatrist's findings and recommendations just as he or she would discuss the results of any test or evaluation. A responsive psychiatrist's report describes the rationale for subsequent steps in language that can be shared with the patient.

D. Leave no stone unturned.

I want to find out what's wrong and in the process I don't want to overlook any possible explanation. I want to leave no stone unturned. Sometimes, emotional factors can contribute to, and even cause, symptoms such as yours. *It would be irresponsible of me not to check out this possibility.* I want to be the best doctor I know how to be. I'd like you to see Dr. Wilson, a psychiatrist, who may provide us with answers we would otherwise not have.

This strategy is yet another version of the "another test" strategy.

E. Just like taking a course.

I really think counseling will be helpful. Seeing a counselor is like taking a course in skill development. *The subject is what's bothering you and what skills you need to improve or develop* to make your situation better. Your life experiences haven't really prepared you for what's going on now, and so you need a short training program.

Using this strategy assumes that the primary care doctor is convinced that the patient problems are, in part, related to interpersonal, situational, adjustment, or social issues for which counseling is a useful strategy. The doctor avoids presenting counseling as a cure; counseling is a means of improving a situation. Generally, *counseling* is a more neutral and acceptable term than either *psychotherapy* or *therapy,* which tend to be mysterious and even frightening to patients.

F. Reduce excessive disability.

Of course, anyone would be emotionally upset with your (chronic) illness. I've seen a lot of people in your situation, and your reaction is more intense than is typical, and such a reaction will make your symptoms worse than necessary. I'd like you to see a psychiatrist. *Being referred doesn't mean you are weak or not coping.* You are doing the very best you can. *Every illness has a unique relationship to a patient;* the response to illness is often somewhat out of the patient's control. You, for example, have very little control of your temperature; temperature is part of the illness. Patients often make the mistake of thinking they know the right way to experience an illness. There is no right way or no wrong way; there is only your way. Our goal is to make you more comfortable. Do you really care how we reach that goal? There is a real good chance that seeing a psychiatrist and getting psychiatric medicine will reduce your disability to more tolerable levels.

Depression with the dementia of depression (i.e., pseudodementia), Alzheimer's disease with depression and/or delusions, and terminal illness with severe anxiety are example problems for which the excessive disability strategy is appropriate. The key to making this strategy work is to find motivational words that do not blame the patient for his or her emotional and mental problems.

G. Sounds far-fetched to me.

I certainly am not in a position to say I know what is really happening to you. I do know that you are convinced that your neighbors are recording your conversations with your wife and listening in on your telephone calls. Stranger things than that have happened to others. What I do know is that these sorts of strange things don't usually happen, and I can't understand why your neighbors would want to do this to you. *This whole business sounds pretty far-fetched to me.* I don't go out and investigate these things; I'm just a doctor. As your doctor, I do know that experiences like you describe are caused sometimes by a disease, and I want to run some tests to be certain you are not sick. In these situations, I think it best if we get Dr. Wilson's opinion, too. Dr. Wilson is a psychiatrist whom I trust and have worked with before on problems similar to yours.

Initial neutrality is a standard way to deal with psychosis. Usually, there is no reason to agree or disagree or in any way challenge—at least at first. When patients express what you believe to be false beliefs, treat them with respect and try to work within the medical model. If the patient's family is not already involved, they should be. The PCP should make a sincere statement about how distressed the patient must feel. The PCP should be on the side of truth; the PCP and the patient simply must discover what is the real truth. Often, the patient may accept antipsychotic medication as a temporary way to help cope with the situation. "The medicine I'm recommending works on disease; it will not change what is real." Of course, psychosis is a medical emergency and must be evaluated as described in other chapters.

III. Working in a Managed Care Climate.

The current move toward managed care involves some fundamental changes in financial incentives and control over how services are provided. These changes have been especially marked in mental health service delivery, mostly because the reimbursement for these services is often "carved-out" by contract between a *health maintenance organization* (HMO) and a *center for diagnosis and referral* (CDR). A CDR is a type of managed care organization that specializes in mental health management and controls referrals and utilization in a system that is separate from medical-surgical operations.

These systems have many crucial implications for the PCP, involving finances, referrals, legal liabilities, and insurance benefit design. Six major points are discussed in this section, and case studies are provided.

A. Gatekeeping: Controlling when and where patients are referred.

An essential element of most managed systems is control over referral to specialty services. The PCP performs this gatekeeping for most medical-surgical referrals. In some systems, the PCP also controls referrals for mental health treatment. The more common arrangement, however, involves "carving out" gatekeeping responsibility for mental health to a CDR that specializes in managing those services. Typically, these specialist companies are entirely separate from the HMO that contracts with them. Authorization for care must be obtained from the CDR if the care is to be paid for by the HMO. A trend toward "carve-ins," in which the mental health gatekeeping is brought back to the HMO, seems to be underway. *In either case, the patient or the PCP must contact the mental health managers to seek authorization or referral for mental health problems.* This is true for both out-patient and in-patient services. The PCP can, of course, treat the mental health problem himself or herself but usually does not receive additional payment from the mental health capitation fund and does not, therefore, draw on the separately defined mental health insurance benefits (see section III-C).

B. Different types of managed care insurance.

The type of insurance the patient has may determine how referrals may be made. In general, the greatest restrictions on referral are in HMOs, fewer restrictions are in preferred provider organizations, and few or no restrictions are in indemnity plans. Point-of-service plans combine these three types into a trilevel set of options, in which, for any given service, the patient can choose which option he or she wishes to use. In general, the cost to the patient is lowest when care is sought from the HMO and the PCP. Cost is somewhat higher when care is received from a preferred provider organization specialist without a primary care referral and is much higher still when care is received outside the system altogether on an indemnity basis. Figure 6–1 illustrates these relationships.

HMO	PPO	Traditional Indemnity
Option 1	Option 2	Option 3

Point of Service Plans

← Greater ability to control costs

Greater freedom to choose where care is received →

← Fewer out-of-pocket expenses

Figure 6–1
Costs and freedom of choice in different types of insurance. HMO, health maintenance organization; PPO, preferred provider organization.

Note in Figure 6–1 the fundamental inverse relationship between the ability to control costs (for both the insurer and the patient) and the patient's freedom of choice over referral. This relationship will likely continue to have a powerful effect on the shaping of the constraints and choices of care delivery, even though it is misunderstood by many patients and physicians.

Assuming that the PCP is not the gatekeeper for mental health, he or she has the freedom to make referrals for only the preferred provider organization (PPO) and indemnity options. Within an HMO, he or she may need to defer to the referral of the CDR if the care is to be paid for by the HMO. Similarly, in a trilevel point-of-service plan, the PCP may be free to make referrals for options 2 and 3, though some point-of-service plans eliminate those options for mental health treatment, leaving only option 1. When only option 1 exists for mental health, the point-of-service plan is no different from an HMO, since payment for mental health services will occur only if it is authorized by the gatekeeper, just as in an HMO.

Case Study

For instance, Mrs. C., a patient with a history of a major depressive episode several years before, comes to the PCP requesting referral to the psychiatrist who treated her then, Dr. Jones.

Once the PCP has assessed and understood the clinical issues involved, the PCP must determine what, if any, restrictions the patient's insurance will place on the PCP's referral. If, like many physicians, the PCP has patients who have many different types of insurance, the PCP should not expect that he or she will always remember how a given insurance controls its referrals. The PCP or one of his or her staff may need to contact the insurer or keep records of whether a mental health specialist gatekeeper exists or whether a panel of psychiatric specialists exists to whom the PCP may refer freely. *Using this information appropriately is very important because failure to conform to needed procedures may lead to denial of payment for the services and a very unhappy patient.*

In the case of the aforementioned patient, if the patient wishes to use HMO benefits, the PCP must refer her to the CDR (and hope that Dr. Jones is on the provider panel used by them). If the patient wishes to use a PPO benefit, then the insurer pays for treatment by Dr. Jones only if he is on the preferred provider panel. If the patient has an indemnity insurance, then the PCP's referral may have no payment consequences, and Mrs. C. and Dr. Jones must determine if the insurance will reimburse for his treatment.

C. Benefit limits for mental health treatment.

Unlike the insurance benefits available for the treatment of most medical-surgical conditions, benefits for the treatment of mental health problems are explicitly limited by most managed care companies. Such limitations, in fact, began as dollar-defined limits in traditional indemnity insurance. Most HMOs, for example, limit in-patient mental health treatment to a maximum of 30 to 45 days per year and out-patient visits to a maximum of 20 to 35 per year. In addition, the benefit for substance abuse treatment usually includes days for detoxification, residential treatment, and a maximum of 20 to 35 outpatient visits. Although these benefits are sufficient for most patients, some patients have needs that exceed the benefits that are available, especially for out-patient services. Often the patient receives authorization for a number of days or visits that fall well below the maximum upper limit. In addition, copayments for mental health visits may be higher than for routine doctor visits.

Primary care physicians may be affected in many ways by these factors. *The lower copayment alone motivates some patients to prefer to receive their antidepressant medication from their PCP rather than from a psychiatrist.* Patients may also prefer that arrangement if they are also receiving psychotherapy from a nonphysician in the hopes that they can save all the available mental health out-patient benefits for the psychotherapy while obtaining psychotropic medication from the PCP. Alternatively, patients may see a psychiatrist until the mental health benefit is exhausted and then wish to return to the PCP for continued prescription of psychotropic medication.

These arrangements, however, are not necessarily undesirable. PCPs need to be aware of pressures from patients and others to participate in such treatment arrangements. PCPs need to carefully assess the possible risks and benefits of accepting such treatment responsibilities.

Case Study

Ms. K., a patient with dysthymic disorder (i.e., subthreshold depression, depressive neurosis) and borderline personality disorder, has been receiving psychotherapy from a psychologist and medication from a psychiatrist. Unfortunately, she has just used the last of the 20 visits available from the mental health benefit. She wishes to continue with the psychologist and is prepared to pay for this service herself. She calls her PCP requesting that the PCP assume her medication management from the psychiatrist.

The PCP calls the psychiatrist for information about the patient's problems and management. The PCP learns that the patient has benefited from antidepressant medication but continues to have frequent lability of mood, especially in response to interpersonal conflicts or disappointments. At those times, she usually becomes suicidal and has made many suicide attempts over the years, although usually using means of low lethality. In addition, she engages in parasuicidal behavior, in which she does not really expect to die but which involves making superficial cuts on her arms and legs. Although she functions well in numerous areas, she is often in conflict with her caretakers, sometimes managing to be both demanding and rejecting at the same time. Should the PCP accept responsibility for psychotropic medication management?

First, the perspective and recommendations of both the psychiatrist and psychologist should be sought. Do they think the patient can be safely comanaged by you and the psychologist? Does the psychologist sound like someone who will be a reliable collaborator and communicator with the PCP? Comanagement of any patient requires a good deal of mutual understanding, communication, and time. However, the patient in question clearly raises further problems. How will the suicidal ideation and behavior be dealt with? Even if the busy PCP decides that the psychologist should be the one who deals with these crises, this decision does not reduce the burden very much. This is true both because the PCP may need to be involved in medication adjustments or additions and because, given current malpractice standards, the physician may still be found liable if the psychologist errs and a poor outcome results. This is so for many reasons, including the presumption that the physician has "ultimate" responsibility for the care and is also likely to be a better financial target.

Even if, in this case, it is felt that the suicidal crisis can be dealt with through comanagement, there is another reason to suspect that comanagement with the PCP is not a good idea. The patient's interpersonal difficulties and tendency to be demanding and hostile may make the therapeutic alliance very unreliable, especially given the complexities of comanagement. Patients with borderline personality disorder often engage in splitting (seeing one of the comanagers as all good and the other as all bad), and this perception can make effective comanagement impossible. The psychologist or psychiatrist should be able to tell the PCP whether this is a risk or whether the patient would be able to build an effective working alliance.

D. Continuum of care.

Managed care companies also try to reduce health care costs by developing alternatives to traditional in-patient services. In mental health treatment, the demand for alternatives to hospitalization has encouraged development of partial hospital, intensive out-patient, home care, and other case management alternatives. This broad continuum of care will probably exist in only highly evolved managed and capitated systems. Areas where a preponderance of traditional fee-for-service payment still exist may still have only basic in-patient and out-patient services. Given that under such payment systems in-patient services are typically more profitable than out-patient services, there are likely to be more hospital beds than are really needed, with a corresponding tendency to hospitalize patients who could have been treated as out-patients.

As indicated earlier, the referrals to higher levels of care are usually made by the CDR. PCPs, like many psychiatrists, tend to rely too quickly on hospital admission in order to deal with acute problems in patients. Trouble and conflict may result if the PCP recommends hospitalization to the patient but the behavioral health gatekeepers feel that intensive out-patient care is sufficient. Both the physician and the patient may experience frustration that their expectations were not fulfilled. With such a patient, the PCP may need to talk to the behavioral specialist and express the PCP's views on the need for hospitalization before making a firm recommendation to the patient.

Criteria for the use of intermediate programs, such as intensive out-patient treatment and partial hospitalization, vary from area to area, depending on the design and the staffing of the programs. Criteria for in-patient programs vary somewhat less, although they change according to the type of alternative services available. Figure 6–2 describes the most common levels of psychiatric care.

The delivery of cost-effective care depends on a system's ability to match patient need with the least restrictive and least costly level of care. As a result, the most care is delivered in the out-patient setting. The general aim of the treatment is to return the patient to his or her previous baseline level of feeling and functioning. The continuum of care needs to function in both "step-up" and "step-down" directions because changes in clinical need require more or less intensive levels of care. Referral for more intensive treatment is not determined by the diagnosis alone but by the severity of the illness and the intensity of the services needed for safe and effective treatment.

Figure 6–2 lists one possible hierarchy of level of care. Some levels of care are more typical of mental health treatment, others of substance abuse. Selected criteria for in-patient admission are listed below. Two crucial points are relevant to these criteria: (1) the criteria apply only if the problem behavior is a result of a psychiatric condition (assaultive behavior by someone with antisocial personality disorder is not sufficient), and (2) the criteria apply only if the problem cannot be dealt with at a less intensive level of care.

1. *Mental health in-patient services* may be authorized if a patient meets any of the severity of illness or intensity of service criteria.
   a. *Severity of illness.*
      (1) A *suicide attempt* of serious intent.
      (2) Current *suicidal ideation with a plan, intention to act, and lethal means.* A patient without clear intention to act may need to be hospitalized if there is also impulsivity, hopelessness, substance abuse, or lack of positive social supports.
      (3) Recent development or worsening of *significant self-mutilation* or other behavior that places the patient or someone else, (e.g., a child) in significant danger.
      (4) Actual *assaultive behavior* or threats of assault with means and intention to cause significant harm to another person.
      (5) *Severe psychiatric symptoms* (e.g., depression, disorientation, psychomotor agitation or retardation, mania, hallucinations, and delusions) that interfere with the patient's ability to take care of himself or herself or to endanger others.
   b. *Intensity of services.*
      (1) Need for *24-hour observation and control* to protect self and others from harm.
      (2) Need to *closely monitor actual or potential medication side effects* while initiating or modifying medication regimen.
      (3) Need for *a complex treatment plan* that includes many types of treatment intervention and requires careful supervision and observation because of the severity of the patient's illness (such as may occur after failed out-patient treatment of an eating disorder).
      (4) Need for close and continuous observation for *diagnostic and treatment planning pur-*

More restrictive →				Less restrictive
In-patient admission	Nonmedical residential or crisis admission	Partial hospitalization	Intensive out-patient treatment with or without domiciliary care (provision of minimally supervised housing)	Out-patient therapy

Figure 6–2
Levels of psychiatric care.

poses in a severely ill patient (in whom this cannot be achieved at a less intensive level of care).

2. *Alcoholism and substance abuse* treatment planning depends crucially on assessment of dependence and risk of withdrawal symptoms. This topic is well covered in Chapter 17.

   In-patient treatment can cover a range of services, from detoxification to residential rehabilitation. Regarding detoxification, although the management of mild-to-moderate withdrawal symptoms can sometimes be performed on an out-patient basis, it sometimes requires a more intensive medical setting. By contrast, residential programs typically treat patients who either did not need detoxification or have completed it. Therefore, their staffing and structure may be less medically oriented and, as a result, less expensive.

   In-patient or residential services may be indicated if a patient meets any of the following severity of illness or intensity of service criteria.

   a. *Severity of illness* criteria require a pattern of alcohol or drug dependence with psychosocial difficulties, expressed by one of the following:
      (1) Ongoing abuse of alcohol or substances in a manner that may cause *clear and imminent harm* to the patient.
      (2) *Marked decline in* social, family, occupational, or educational *functioning.*
      (3) *Significant suicidal ideation or actual attempt,* especially when associated with impulsivity, hopelessness, or potentially lethal means.
      (4) *Failure to establish abstinence in an out-patient treatment program* despite solid effort and involvement of the patient.
      (5) *Likelihood of significant withdrawal symptoms,* especially involving alcohol, sedatives, multiple substances, or past history of withdrawal difficulties.

   b. *Intensity of services.*
      (1) Needs *close and continued supervision of detoxification* (patient has past history of seizures or delirium when withdrawing) and/or, for example, needs more than 30 mg four times a day of oxazepam (Serax) or cannot reliably follow a medication regimen that requires four times daily dosing.
      (2) Needs structured, *drug-free environment* to establish abstinence.
      (3) Needs *close supervision* because of suicidal or homicidal ideation.

E. Utilization review and the appeal process.

Utilization review (UR) is one of the most fundamental and widespread features of managed care. It attempts both to control the tendency of clinicians to increase treatment costs and to reduce the variability in treatment methods observed in so much of medicine. UR may be the feature of managed care that arouses the strongest opposition. It is often believed that UR is concerned only with reducing costs, not with improving quality. Reviewers sometimes appear unqualified and may themselves have incentives to deny care rather than to ensure its appropriateness.

Unfortunately, these perceptions are often accurate and reflect the still early stage of development of managed behavioral health care. Because these changes in the health care marketplace are employer and insurer driven, this situation may not improve until employers are convinced by research data that sometimes more expensive care may be of higher quality and may make a difference to them and their employees in terms of better health outcomes. Thus, there is a growing demand for treatment outcome studies in order to document effectiveness and value. *It may be less expensive in the long term to provide more intensive and more expensive mental health services earlier rather than later.*

Utilization review for levels of care more intensive than out-patient usually requires precertification and concurrent review and may require retrospective review as well. That is, in a managed system, before a clinician can refer a patient to intensive out-patient, partial hospital, or in-patient programs, authorization for admission must be obtained from those responsible for UR, such as the CDR. Concurrent review refers to the assessment, at intervals during the hospital stay, of the continued need for that level of care. Retrospective review usually involves examination of the medical record to determine if documentation exists of the clinical problems in order to justify that level of care. If such documentation is not found, payment for services may be denied. Many managed care organizations use explicit criteria for each level. UR ideally tries to maximize the cost-effectiveness of treatment by matching patients to the needed level of treatment intensity, to use no more restrictive and expensive means than necessary, and then to move the patient smoothly to less intensive levels of care as his or her condition permits.

It is essential that the PCP appeal UR decisions that he or she feels are incorrect or dangerous. Any of the following reasons may motivate UR appeal:

1. Advocate for the patient and assure that the HMO will pay for needed care.

2. Motivate institutional review of procedures and criteria used in UR.

3. Protect oneself from liability if poor patient outcome may result.

   If a UR representative tells a physician that no more in-patient days will be authorized for the hospitalized patient and the physician simply accepts this and discharges the patient, then he or she alone may be found liable should the patient, for example, commit suicide after discharge. The physician should at least appeal to a second-level (usually physician) reviewer. Appeals can be made further, to the managed care company's medical director, or, ultimately, to its board of directors. Managed care companies are more likely to also be found liable if they exercise a great deal of control over the physicians' practice, pay them a salary, or otherwise treat them more like employees than independent contractors. It appears that managed care companies are increasingly being held responsible for clinical outcomes of their UR decisions. This may eventually lead to improved and more responsible UR processes. *The essential point for clinicians is that even if a managed care company denies payment for a given service, the clinician is still responsible for delivering needed care and may be liable if he or she fails to do so.* Clinicians should request information about the appeals process and be prepared to appeal a decision as far as is possible if they feel that the patient is being put at significant risk.

F. **Treatment in primary care versus referral to a mental health specialist.**

In many managed systems, a relatively low percentage of the insured population seeks care through the CDR or the behavioral health provider panel. In some HMOs, this number can be lower than 5%. By contrast, epidemiologic studies suggest that significant psychiatric morbidity occurs at a rate several times that. Many PCPs report that perhaps 40% of their patient volume is related to somatizing or psychological problems.

This information suggests two things: (1) much psychiatric morbidity goes unrecognized and unaddressed and (2) a great deal of mental health treatment is performed in the PCP's office. This second point is reflected in the fact that PCPs write far more prescriptions in total for psychotropic medications than do psychiatrists. When this situation occurs in a capitated system, especially one with a behavioral health carve-out, many important considerations exist.

1. Whenever a behavioral health capitation is separated or carved out from the PCP capitation, a conflict can occur. Uncertainty may exist over who should provide the mental health treatment and from whose capitation fund payment should come. In general, *if the PCP provides the treatment, then it is not paid for from the behavioral health capitation fund.*

2. Because in the more competitive managed care markets, the behavioral health capitation may be only 3% to 4% (or even less) of the total health care dollar, behavioral specialists usually provide care only or mostly to the more severe or complex cases. *Mental health service providers may also provide brief consultation to PCPs who continue to treat the patient.*

3. Many clinical problems exist in a gray or boundary zone between psychiatry and primary care. These problems include attention deficit disorder, some sexual dysfunctions, psychological consequences of medical problems, chronic pain, sleep disorders, toileting problems in children, and neuropsychological dysfunctions, among many others. All these problems can be dealt with by the PCP and the mental health system. Obviously, no single policy creates sharp boundaries in all those areas. In general, these problems are dealt with by the PCP if the nonpsychiatric portion of the problem is of primary importance or occurred before the onset of psychiatric symptoms. Thus, minor psychological adjustment problems in a patient reacting to a new diagnosis of diabetes are usually dealt with by the PCP. If the psychological reaction becomes a moderate-to-severe major depressive disorder, referral to a psychiatrist is probably a good idea. Eventually, health care systems will have PCPs and mental health specialists working side by side, for example, in the same clinic.

4. When the primary care physician is operating under capitation, a conflict of financial interest exists between the CDR and the PCP. *Cost shifting* can occur as each group tries to shift clinical responsibility to the other. Because mental health capitation is usually small relative to the actual incidence of psychiatric problems, the PCP will need to provide some mental health treatment. Where this threshold should lie varies from one HMO to another. Disputes should be taken to the HMO for resolution.

Glossary

Authorization—a process whereby the gatekeeper (either the primary care physician [PCP] for medical-surgical services or the mental health case managers at the center for diagnosis and referral [CDR]) approve a particular service to be paid for by the insurance plan or health maintenance organization (HMO).

Capitation—a contractual arrangement whereby the case manager (either the PCP or the CDR) accepts a negotiated dollar amount to pay for all needed services for the patient population enrolled with them by the insurer. This amount is usually paid monthly for every such person enrolled (e.g., $3.50 per member per month for behavioral health services). *This represents a prospective shift in insurance risk from the insurer to the case managers.*

Carve-out—the separate contracting of responsibility for the management of the mental health and substance abuse benefit to a CDR that specializes in this. It is usually contracted on a capitated basis and involves giving the CDR gatekeeping responsibility for referral, authorization for care, and case management.

Case management—a process in which persons seeking treatment are matched with types of care in order to achieve satisfactory and cost-effective patient outcomes.

Center for diagnosis and referral—an agency that accepts responsibility for managing the mental health and substance abuse benefits for an insurance company or HMO. This arrangement is usually made on the basis of capitation, which means that the CDR needs to control costs by various means, including control over referral and authorization for services.

Fee-for-service—a traditional method of payment in which physicians and hospitals are paid up to a defined amount for each service rendered. *This payment is retrospective and places all insurance risk with the insurer, not with the provider of care (unlike in capitation).*

Gatekeeper—a function performed by the primary care physician in most HMO and point-of-service plans, in which the PCP must provide initial care and authorize referrals for specialty services. Specialty care not authorized by the PCP is not paid for by the HMO.

Health maintenance organization—an organization that provides (internally or through contracts with care providers) a basic set of health care benefits to an enrolled population of individuals within a defined geographic area in return for a negotiated, prepaid monthly premium. Four different types of HMOs exist: independent practice association, staff model, network model, and group model. These differ according to how physicians are employed or contracted and how they are paid.

Indemnity—a traditional fee-for-service insurance system in which covered services are paid retrospectively with little or no utilization review and no gatekeeper or authorization process.

Insurance risk—an insurance company collects premiums for a population of enrollees and then must pay for all covered medical care for that population. The company holds financial risk because the care expenses may exceed the collected premiums, and the company thereby loses money. This insurance risk may be passed along prospectively to a group of physicians, a medical center, or a CDR on the basis of capitation. If they spend more delivering care to the population of patients so covered than they received in capitation dollars, then they lose money. *This reverses the incentives to deliver care quite dramatically from traditional fee-for-service work, in which care providers make more money the more services they deliver.* It is not true, as is sometimes said, that capitation motivates care providers to deliver *no* care. Disaster would certainly result if that were done. It does motivate them to provide only the most cost-effective care.

Point-of-service plan—a type of insurance that offers members a three-level choice for each type of service being sought. Option 1 involves using the PCP for treatment and referrals, just like in an HMO, and is lowest in cost to the patient. Option 2 uses the preferred provider organization (PPO) option and requires an intermediate degree of cost-sharing by the patient. Option 3 is essentially an indemnity option and is the most expensive to the patient but offers freedom to choose a care provider outside the HMO and PPO. Many point-of-service plans limit mental health and substance abuse benefits to only option 1.

Preferred provider organization (PPO)—a panel of preferred providers of health care that is established by contract with an insurance company. Costs to the patient are lower if they use the services of a physician who is a member of a designated PPO. If services are sought outside the PPO (on an indemnity basis), then the patient usually pays a significantly higher copayment.

Utilization review or management—a process that reviews the medical necessity and appropriateness of health care, with the goal of achieving efficiency and cost-effectiveness. The review may be prospective (e.g., before admission to the hospital), concurrent (during the treatment episode), or retrospective.

Suggested Reading

Barrett JE, Barrett JA, Orman T, Gerber P. The prevalence of psychiatric disorders in a primary care practice. Arch Gen Psychiatry 1988; 45:1100–1106.

Feldman TL, Fitzpatrick J, Editors. Managed Mental Health Care: Administrative and Clinical Issues. Washington DC: American Psychiatric Press; 1992.

Galanter M, Kleber HD, Editors. Textbook of Substance Abuse Treatment. Washington DC: American Psychiatric Press; 1994.

Katon W. The epidemiology of depression in medical care. Int J Psychiatr Med 1987; 17:93–112.

Katon W, von Korff M, Lin E, et al. Distressed high utilizers of medical care: DSM-III-R diagnoses and treatment needs. Gen Hosp Psychiatry 1990; 12:355–362.

Lazarus A. The role of primary care physicians in managed mental health care. Psychiatr Serv 1995; 46:343–345.

II

Specific Neuropsychiatric Disorders

7

MARCIA V. VALENSTEIN, MD

MICHAEL S. KLINKMAN, MD, MS

Minor Depression

I. Overview.

Clinicians and researchers agree that minor depression is one of the most commonly encountered problems in primary care. Approximately 5% to 10% of primary care patients have a major depressive disorder (MDD), but almost twice as many primary care patients have significant depressive symptoms that do not meet the criteria for major depression.[1]

Although there is general agreement that minor depression is extremely common, there is less consensus about its definition. Minor depression has been used to describe (1) all depressive disorders other than MDD; (2) specific, but differently defined, subthreshold depressive disorders; and (3) nonspecific clusters of depressive symptoms.

This chapter uses the broadest definition of minor depression and describes a general approach to patients presenting with depressive symptoms.

II. Different perspectives on depression.

1. *Depression as a continuum.*
   Physicians may find it useful to think about depression and depressed patients in three ways. Physicians may think of depressed patients as falling along a *continuum* of illness severity. Patients with the fewest, mildest, or briefest depressive symptoms are at one side of this continuum, while those with more severe depressive symptoms of longer duration fall near the other end. *Depressed patients are considered to have syndromes that differ in severity but not in quality.*

2. *Depression as a set of "depressive disorders."*
   Physicians may also view depression "categorically." *Patients with depressive symptoms are considered to suffer from numerous different depressive disorders, with clear diagnostic boundaries.* Clinicians using the categorical approach are concerned with reaching the "correct" depressive diagnosis because this is considered an essential step in establishing patient prognosis, understanding the etiology of the illness, and planning effective treatment. Clinicians are thinking categorically when they diagnose MDD, dysthymic disorder, or adjustment disorder with depressed mood.

3. *Depression as a "vulnerability and lifetime process."*
   Physicians may also take a third perspective, viewing depression as a longitudinal process rather as an isolated event or a series of events. *Clinicians with this perspective view depressed patients as having enduring physiologic and psychological processes that make them susceptible to depressive illnesses at times of stress.* Physiologic or psychological "vulnerabilities" are enduring traits; *depressive disorders* are unstable manifestations of these traits at times of environmental stress.

   Highly vulnerable individuals develop clinical disorders as the result of mild stressors or no stressors, whereas less vulnerable individuals require high levels of stress before they succumb to a depressive illness. At any point in time, a patient with a propensity to depression may be asymptomatic, have depressive symptoms, or meet criteria for a threshold depressive disorder. The level of symptomatology depends on life circumstances and intervening biologic processes, such as aging or concurrent medical illness. Within this framework, *minor depression could represent the only clinical disturbance that an individual manifests, or it could be the prodrome or partial resolution of a more severe depressive illness.*

A. Practical uses of different views of depression.

Clinicians are most effective when they move flexibly between the different perspectives on depression. The *dimensional* or *continuum* approach is useful in the initial assessment of the depressed patient: it allows clinicians to develop immediate management strategies and to determine the need for further diagnostic work-up. The dimensional approach is also valuable when patients do not have depressive diagnoses with clear and specific treatments.

The *categorical* or *diagnostic approach* helps clinicians decide how moderately or severely depressed individuals should be treated. Finally, longitudinal perspectives of patients' symptoms and vulnerabilities provide information on both treatment of particular episodes and plans for future management.

B. Specific versus nonspecific management.

Some depressive disorders have clear, specific, and effective treatments, but many do not. Depressive syndromes that fall short of meeting criteria for *Diagnostic and Statistical Manual* (DSM) depressive disorder, as outlined in the DSM-III, DSM III-R, and DSM-IV, generally *do not* have specific treatments. Some of the depressive disorders that do meet threshold diagnostic criteria also do not have specific treatments.

Research efforts primarily have focused on developing and studying treatments for threshold depressive disorders (disorders that meet DSM diagnostic criteria). This approach has been helpful to mental health clinicians, who regularly treat patients with threshold disorders.

Primary care physicians treat a different patient population than do mental health clinicians; this population includes many individuals with depressive syndromes that have not been extensively addressed by mental health researchers and for which specific treatment approaches have not been developed. As a result, general practitioners often find that nonspecific management strategies are the interventions of choice for their patients.

Primary care physicians need to recognize and manage all symptomatic depressive syndromes. However, they need only diagnose those disorders that have specific treatment recommendations.

III. Why minor depression is important to recognize.

A. Minor depression results in significant disability.

Patients who meet the criteria for depressive disorders and patients who only have depressive symptoms have functional limitations that equal or surpass those arising from other common medical illnesses.[2] Physical, social, and role functioning are compromised as much by depressive symptoms as by diabetes, hypertension, chronic lung conditions, gastrointestinal conditions, or arthritis. Patients with depressive symptoms spend more days in bed than do patients with most other chronic medical conditions.

B. Minor depression may result in suicidal behavior.

Approximately 40,000 to 50,000 completed suicides occur in the United States per year. Most individuals who commit suicide suffer from a depressive disorder. Patients with a MDD are at the greatest risk for suicide; 15% of patients with MDD who require hospitalization die by their own hand.

Individuals with minor depression have a lower relative risk for suicide attempts or completions than do individuals with MDD; however, on a population basis, patients with minor depression make more suicide attempts than do patients with major depression. The larger numbers of patients with minor depression result in larger numbers of suicide attempts, despite a lower individual risk. As a result, *primary care physicians often deal with suicidal thoughts, behaviors, and attempts in patients who do not meet the criteria for MDD.*

Forty percent to 50% of patients who commit suicide see their primary care physicians within a month of dying. Twenty-five percent of patients who commit suicide see their general practitioners within a week of suicide. Recognizing both patients with full depressive disorders and those with subthreshold depressive syndromes gives the primary care physician an opportunity to intervene.

C. Minor depression results in increased medical utilization.

Primary care patients with depressive disorders and depressive symptoms use two to three times as many medical services as do primary care patients without depression. They visit their physician more often and undergo more diagnostic tests. Increased utilization increases total medical costs.[3]

IV. Improving the recognition of depressive disorders.

Recognizing depressive syndromes is not necessarily easy. Most patients with a depressive illness or symptoms do not come to the physician complaining about emotional distress. Instead, patients say they have pain or complain about other somatic symptoms.[4] Seventy-two percent of patients who eventually receive a psychiatric diagnosis from their family doctor first present with bodily complaints.

A. Carefully evaluate somatic complaints.

1. *Look at the type of somatic complaints made by the patient.*
   a. *Look for somatic symptoms that are reliably part of the depressive syndrome: sleep difficulties, appetite changes, and decreased energy levels.* The presence of any of these somatic symptoms is an indication that more time must be spent probing for a depressive disorder.
   b. Look for somatic complaints that are not considered part of the depressive syndrome per se

but regularly occur in patients with a depressive disorder. Depressed individuals often complain of dizziness, diffuse systemic malaise, and pain. Headaches and low back pain are particularly common complaints. Physicians in every specialty hear of symptoms that may indicate the presence of a depressive disorder. In primary care settings, the physician hears them all (Table 7–1).

2. *Look at the number of somatic complaints made by the patient.*
Remember that the *more* physical symptoms a patient has, the more likely he or she is to have an anxiety or depressive disorder. A recent study showed that 2% of patients who presented with zero to one physical complaint, 44% of patients who presented with six to eight physical complaints, and 60% of patients who presented with nine or more physical complaints had a mood disorder.[5]
If no physical explanation exists for the patient's somatic complaints, the association with a mood disorder is even stronger. *Multiple physical complaints greatly increase the likelihood of a mood disorder, and multiple* ***unexplained*** *physical symptoms increase the likelihood of a depressive disorder still further.*

B. Consider the use of screening questionnaires.

Many screening questionnaires have been used in primary care settings. Most of these screens are self-administered and can be completed by the patient in fewer than 10 minutes in the waiting room. Screening questionnaires for depression are easily added to the existing review of systems used by many practitioners (Table 7–2).

Self-administered questionnaires screen for distress and depressive symptoms and alert the clinician to the need for a more complete psychosocial assessment. Approximately 15% to 30% of primary care patients have questionnaire scores that indicate high levels of distress.

Clinicians need to remember that high scores on self-rating instruments do not mean that patients meet the criteria for DSM depressive disorders; many patients with significant levels of distress on these questionnaires do not meet the threshold criteria for DSM disorders. Fifteen percent to 30% of primary care patients are significantly distressed on the self-rating questionnaires; only 5% to 10% of primary care patients qualify for major depression or dysthymic disorder based on structured psychiatric interview. Investigators have suggested using higher "cut-off" scores in primary care clinics if physicians wish to use these instruments as indicators of threshold depressive disorders.[6]

Recently developed instruments, such as the Primary Care Evaluation of Mental Disorders (PRIME-MD), combine self-administered patient questionnaires with physician-administered

Table 7–1
Common Presenting Complaints from Depressed Patients in Specialty and Primary Care Clinics

Specialty	Common Complaints of Patients with Depression
Otolaryngology	Tinnitus
Orthopedics	Chronic low back pain
Infectious disease	Chronic fatigue
Obstetrics and gynecology	Premenstrual syndrome
Pediatrics	Abdominal pain
Gastrointestinal	Irritable bowel
Rheumatology	Muscle aches and tenderness (fibromyalgia)
Primary care	All of the above

Table 7–2
Commonly Used Screening Instruments in Primary Care Settings

Instrument	Description
Screens for Distress and Depressive Symptoms, Severity Scales without Diagnosis	
Beck Depression Inventory	21 items with 4 statements each. Emphasis on cognitive symptoms of depression. Suggested cut-off for higher-risk populations is 10 or more. Use a higher cut-off score of 16 points in general medical settings.
Zung Self-Rating Depression Scale	20 items, rated by how much of the time each depressive symptom is present. Suggested cut-off score is 55.
General Health Questionnaire	12, 28, or 30 questions. Suggested cut-off score is 5.
Center for Epidemiologic Studies Depression Scale	20 items that measure mood state and neurovegetative symptoms during the preceding week, with scores between 0 and 60. Usual cut-off is 16. Suggested cut-off is 27 points in a medical population to reduce false-positive results.
Screens for Psychiatric Diagnosis, No Severity Rating	
Symptom Driven Diagnostic System for Primary Care (SDDS-PC)	16-item screening tool, followed by diagnostic interview modules.
Primary Care Evaluation of Mental Disorders	26-item patient questionnaire, followed by a 12-page clinician evaluation guide, divided into 5 diagnostic categories. Clinical Evaluation Guide (CEG) can be used flexibly. Rules in or out a psychiatric diagnosis, rather than giving a score.

structured interviews. These instruments are designed for use by primary care physicians and make the diagnostic criteria for depressive disorders readily accessible.[7, 8] The PRIME-MD helps clinicians make or rule out psychiatric diagnoses but does not give symptom severity ratings.

C. Maintain a high index of suspicion.

Depressive disorders and depressive symptoms are the *most common* medical problems in general practice, occurring in about 10% to 25% of the clinic population. Hypertension, the second most common medical illness in primary care, occurs in about 6% of the clinic population.

A busy primary care practitioner with a patient load of 25 to 30 patients per day should, on average, make the diagnosis of major depression about two times per day and note minor depression and depressive symptoms in another three to four patients per day.

V. Initial assessment.

Busy clinicians have approximately 15 minutes to devote to each patient in their clinics. Once practitioners have identified the patients who are presenting to their clinics with depressive symptoms, they need to have efficient strategies for evaluating the patients and deciding on initial management plans.

Completing a full diagnostic interview for depressive disorders and determining a preliminary management plan require more than 15 minutes. Structured interviews designed for primary care physicians, such as the PRIME-MD, permit the formulation of psychiatric diagnoses by DSM criteria in about 8 to 11 minutes; however, these instruments *do not* obtain additional information needed for treatment planning, such as information about the patient's living situation, family relationships, and personal resources. An interview that elicits sufficient information for both a diagnosis and a treatment plan takes approximately 30 to 60 minutes.

Obviously, family physicians cannot and need not schedule a 45-minute session with every patient who presents to their offices with depressive symptoms. We suggest using the "roadmap" for psychiatric disorders (see Chapter 1) for efficient evaluation of patients, and then directing one's time and efforts toward treating patients who will benefit from specific interventions.

This section briefly reviews the roadmap for mental health problems as it applies to depression. The roadmap helps the clinician identify patients with time-limited depressive symptoms who need only reassurance and education, patients who would benefit from closer monitoring and diagnostic evaluation, and patients with depressive disorders requiring specific interventions.

Patients with depressive symptoms should be assessed along the following dimensions:

- Level of distress.
- Presence of an identifiable stressor and severity of the stressor.
- Impairment.
- Duration of episode.
- Potential for self-harm.

Assessment along these dimensions allows providers to predict the likelihood of threshold depressive disorders, determine the need for a full diagnostic evaluation, and decide how soon the diagnostic evaluation needs to be completed. Providers can then make adjustments in their schedules to allow for more extensive evaluations of patients who are likely to benefit from further intervention.

A. Level of distress.

Increasing levels of patient distress signal an increasing likelihood of threshold depressive disorders. Patient distress and severity of depressive symptoms also correlate with response to antidepressants or specific psychotherapies.[9]

Distress can be expressed either as a dysphoric psychological state or as an uncomfortable set of somatic symptoms; the severity of distress can be assessed through the use of self-report questionnaires or patient interviews.

Clinicians may want to ask patients questions such as

- How bad are you feeling?
- Have you felt like this before?
- If you were rating how you were feeling now, with "1" reflecting the most depressed and anxious that you have ever felt and "10" reflecting your happiest, most serene mood, how would you rate your feelings of the past week?
- Do you feel you can cope, or is this unbearable?

We have found that the use of an informal ordinal scale (asking the patient to rate themselves on a 1 to 10 scale) to be especially helpful in our clinical work. A recent study found that asking one question of patients—"How depressed or anxious have you been over the past 6 months?"—and having them respond on an ordinal scale was an effective way of screening for depressive and anxiety disorders.[10]

B. Presence of an identifiable stressor.

Life stressors can produce either temporary distress or full depressive disorders. Clinicians need to obtain information about the presence or absence of identifiable stressors in their patients' lives and about the severity of these stressors in order to determine the likelihood of a threshold psychiatric disorder and to plan for appropriate interventions.

Some patients supply information about recent stressors without prompting, but other patients need to be asked specifically about recent adverse events.

We routinely ask the following questions:

- Sometimes people develop symptoms like this when they are facing a stressful situation. Have you faced a difficult situation lately?

- Has anything stressful been going on at home or at work?
- Have you had any setbacks recently?

The primary care physician may find it helpful to think about stressors as falling into three categories:

1. *Major discrete stressors,* such as deaths, divorces, and job losses.
2. *Chronic stressors,* such as ongoing medical illnesses and marital conflict.
3. *Minor daily stressors,* such as noisy children, heavy traffic, and work deadlines.

Distress following a major discrete stressor may be intense, but it should be *temporary.* Patients without a concurrent psychiatric disorder begin to adapt after an adverse event, and their distress levels decline. Even in the face of bereavement, an event considered to be one of the most severe stressors, some adaptation and reduction in distress is expected within 2 months.

Prolonged high levels of distress, even in the presence of a severe major stressor, should alert the clinician to the possibility of a concurrent depressive disorder.

Chances of developing a depressive illness increase after a major stressor. Patients who have experienced the recent loss of a parent are 20 times more likely to develop a major depression in the next month than are individuals who have not suffered a recent loss.[11]

The primary care provider should proceed with a full diagnostic evaluation if patient distress levels remain high for more than 2 months after a discrete stressor, or if patients have significant functional impairment.

High distress levels may also occur in response to *chronic stressors.* Once again, although these stressors are ongoing rather than one-time events, a reasonable degree of patient adaptation can be expected.

Many primary care patients are dealing with stressors imposed by chronic medical illnesses. These stressors, such as physical limitations, pain, and lifestyle changes, are often ongoing. Although physicians expect patients to have moderate to high levels of distress immediately after a new diagnosis or restriction of their activities or diet, they should also expect that patients will find ways to cope with these losses and find alternative activities that interest and please them. Patients should not continue to react with high levels of distress to an established problem.

High levels of distress lasting longer than 2 to 3 months in response to ongoing stressors should prompt the physician to proceed with a full diagnostic evaluation.

Patients are often chronically stressed by ongoing interpersonal conflicts. Many patients tell the physician of marital difficulties, problems with other family members, or difficulties with coworkers. Some patients are in constant crisis, with new problems arising in their relationships each month.

Patients who are in chronically stressful relationships are often not only the recipients of untoward events but also partial contributors to the occurrence and perpetuation of these events. These patients have an increased risk of depressive disorders and may also have a higher incidence of other psychiatric illnesses, such as personality disorders.

Finally, some patients have high levels of distress in response to *minor stresses or no identifiable stressors* at all. These patients are very likely to have a psychiatric disorder and should undergo careful diagnostic screening.

Patients who react to minor stressors with high levels of distress or develop clinically significant distress without provocation may have a recurrent affective illness. Patients with recurrent depression often have their first depressive episodes in response to major stressors; however, as their illnesses progress, minor stressors begin to precipitate depressive episodes as well. Physicians need to identify and treat these patients.

Patients with personality disorders may also respond to minor problems or setbacks with high levels of distress. These patients have a limited ability to alter their customary ways of coping. As a result, they fail to respond flexibly to problems and challenges in their lives, and they develop symptoms with stressors that other individuals weather by using more diverse or flexible coping strategies.

The physician must pay careful attention to individuals who develop depressive symptoms in response to only minor stressors or no identifiable stressors. They are likely to have a threshold psychiatric disorder that may require intervention.

C. Impairment.

Most of the DSM-IV depressive disorders include impairment criteria, often worded as follows: "The symptoms cause clinically significant distress, or impairment in social, occupational, or other important areas of functioning."

Impairment usually proceeds incrementally as depression increases. Milder depressive disorders often begin with problems fulfilling social roles. Patients may start turning down invitations for dinner or may telephone friends less frequently or not at all. Patients with a more severe depressive disorder begin to have problems at their jobs, starting with dissatisfaction with job requirements and coworkers and progressing to decreased productivity and absenteeism. Problems with self-care, such as failing to prepare dinners or to keep up with grooming or hygienic needs, usually indicate a very severe depressive disorder.

Patients with mild social impairment may not have a greatly increased chance of meeting criteria for threshold depressive disorders. However, patients who are experiencing difficulties on the job or are having other functional limitations need a full diagnostic evaluation.

The following questions, which are also described in Chapter 1, help determine if the patient has impaired functioning.

- Have you missed any work or school?
- Have you been unable to take care of other responsibilities because you were feeling depressed?
- Have you had a problem getting along with other people?
- Have you been unable to take care of your own needs?

If the patient has no impairment in his or her life, threshold depressive disorders are unlikely. If the patient has impairment in several spheres of his or her life, threshold depressive disorders requiring specific interventions are likely to be present.

D. Duration.

As part of their initial evaluations, physicians need to determine how long a patient's symptoms have been present. Patients qualify for a threshold psychiatric or depressive diagnoses only when symptoms have been present for at least 2 weeks.

Physicians might find it useful to ask whether the depressive symptoms have been present for

- A few days.
- Two weeks.
- Three months.
- Years.
- "All the patient's life."

If a patient's symptoms have lasted only a few days, a full evaluation is not necessary unless the patient has a significant personal past history of a depressive disorder.

If the patient's depressive symptoms have lasted for at least 2 weeks, several threshold depressive disorders might be present, including major depression. The minimum time requirement for the diagnosis of common threshold depressive disorders and the proposed time criteria for several "subthreshold" disorders are given in Table 7–3.

In addition to indicating the likelihood of depressive disorders, the duration of depressive symptoms gives the physician a first indicator of the probability of the patient's response to treatment. *Patients who have had symptoms of major depression for 3 months or longer are unlikely to respond to placebo or nonspecific interventions; they need antidepressant treatment or psychotherapy. Patients who have been depressed for years are unlikely to respond to placebo and are also less likely to respond fully to specific treatment with antidepressants or psychotherapy.*[12] Referral to a psychiatrist may be indicated in these situations.

Determining the duration of depressive symptoms allows primary care practitioners to identify quickly patients who may meet the criteria for threshold depressive disorder and to refer patients who are likely to have refractory disorders. Patients who have been ill for years often require more complicated and time-consuming interventions than the primary care practitioner can provide and may be more appropriately treated in a specialty mental health clinic.

E. Suicidal ideation.

Suicidal ideation is a common symptom of depression, occurring in about 2.6% of all patients seen in general medical settings in the course of a year.[13] Any patient with depressive symptoms should be assessed for suicidal thoughts.

Suicidal ideation may be passive or active, chronic or new, fleeting or insistent. The physician should ask directly about the presence or absence of suicidal thoughts.

The following inquiries may be helpful:

- It sounds as if you have been feeling very distressed. During the time that you have been feeling so badly, have you had any thoughts of hurting yourself? Have you had any thoughts of committing suicide?
- When you have suicidal thoughts, are you able to put them out of your mind and go on with your other activities, or do you find yourself dwelling on these thoughts?
- Do you feel that you might act on your thoughts of hurting yourself?
- Have you made any plans to kill yourself?
- Do you have a way to kill yourself?
- Have you made a suicide attempt?

Patients give a range of responses to these inquiries, including having no thoughts of death or suicide, wishing to die, feeling that they would be "better off dead"; having fleeting thoughts of killing themselves; having frequent or persistent suicidal thoughts; planning to kill themselves; and recently attempting to kill themselves. The presence of suicidal thoughts greatly increases the likelihood of a psychiatric disorder; all patients with these thoughts should undergo a diagnostic interview.

Patients with passive suicidal ideation or fleeting suicidal thoughts can generally be assessed and treated within the structure of a primary care clinic. Patients who have frequent suicidal thoughts, plans, or intent should receive prompt referral to psychiatric services. *Patients with persistent suicidal thoughts should be seen within a few days by a mental health specialist, and patients with intent or plan of suicide should be seen that same day for urgent psychiatric evaluation.*

Practitioners should ask any patient with depressive symptoms about suicidal thoughts, even if the patient does not meet criteria for a threshold depressive disorder.

Table 7–3
Number and Duration of Symptoms Required for Common Depressive Diagnoses

Diagnosis	Required Duration of Symptoms	Number of Required Symptoms
Major depression	2 wk	5 of 9 depressive symptoms, must include depressed mood or diminished pleasure
Dysthymia	2 y	2 depressive symptoms, must include depressed mood
Personality disorder	Pervasive pattern beginning by early adulthood	Depressive symptoms may be present but are not required
Minor depression (proposed, subthreshold)	2 wk	2 depressive symptoms but less than 5 depressive symptoms, must include depressed mood or diminished pleasure
Recurrent brief depression (proposed, subthreshold)	Multiple short episodes occurring every month for 12 mo	5 of 9 depressive symptoms
Mixed anxiety-depression	1 mo	Depressed mood plus 4 depressive or anxiety symptoms

VI. Initial management strategies.

Clinicians who have assessed depressed patients for levels of distress, presence of stressors, functional impairment, symptom duration, and suicidal ideation are ready to begin management. Initial management may include (1) nonspecific measures for less severely ill patients, (2) scheduling of a diagnostic evaluation for moderately ill patients, or (3) emergent referral for severely ill patients. Clinicians may find the following categorization (see Chapter 1) to be helpful in formulating a treatment strategy.

A. Patients needing acknowledgment and talk.

This first management category includes people (1) who have distress levels that are commensurate with an identifiable stressor, (2) who have had symptoms for less than 2 weeks, (3) who are still functioning in their family roles and at work, and (4) who are not suicidal.

These patients do not qualify for any depressive diagnosis, not even the subthreshold diagnosis of "minor depression." Instead, these individuals are considered simply "patients with depressive symptoms."

Although patients with depressive symptoms constitute an important public health problem and are commonly seen in primary care settings, *no specific interventions* have proved to be of benefit. Their depressive symptoms usually remit spontaneously over the course of several weeks to months, although some patients go on to develop full depressive disorders.

The primary care physician should recognize these patients and monitor for the development of threshold disorders. *Nonspecific clinical management is the only intervention required.*

Clinical management of cases of depressive symptoms should generally include

- Acknowledging patients' distress.
- Discussing pertinent interpersonal and social issues.
- Normalizing the patients' experience and giving an expectation of improvement.
- Reattributing somatic symptoms.
- Educating patients about symptoms or problems that should prompt them to return for further treatment.
- Scheduling the patient for a follow-up visit in the next month.

Patient education is a very important component of this management strategy. Clinicians need to educate patients with depressive symptoms about threshold depressive disorders. Patients with depressive symptoms are four times more likely to develop a first-onset major depression within the next year than are patients without depressive symptoms.[14] These patients do not require specific psychotherapeutic or pharmacologic interventions at the time of the initial assessment, but they do need to know when specific interventions would be indicated.

A follow-up appointment allows the physician to be sure that the patient's depressive symptoms have subsided and also gives time for additional patient education. However, the patient may cancel or not show for this scheduled follow-up visit. Patients with depressive symptoms do not necessarily have to be pursued if they fail to return for their follow-up appointment. Many of these patients will have improved and no longer feel a need for treatment. Physicians may choose to wait for these patients to return to the clinic, when this seems appropriate.

B. Patients needing assessment and monitoring or immediate intervention.

The second and third patient management groups are discussed together. Patients in these broad management groups have (1) high distress levels that have not been precipitated by a new stressor within the previous 2 months, (2) symptoms that have lasted at least 2 weeks, and (3) impaired functioning in their social or work roles. Patients in these categories may also have suicidal ideation. All of these patients need a full diagnostic evaluation.

Patients without persistent suicidal thoughts and with no impairment that threatens safety do not require emergency care; however, they do require additional physician time. The family physician may choose not to complete a comprehensive psychiatric assessment at the time of the patient's initial visit. Psychiatric assessments take time, and patients often present with somatic complaints and medical problems that need to be addressed. These patients can be scheduled to return within the next few days into a 30- to 45-minute appointment for a thorough evaluation.

Patients who have more than passive suicidal ideation or impairment that threatens their safety need immediate intervention. These patients have an *extremely high likelihood* of psychiatric disorder and require a diagnostic evaluation that same day, either from their family physician or a mental health professional.

Patients who meet this description and do not come to their scheduled evaluations should be pursued. Clinicians cannot assume that these patients have failed to appear because they were feeling better. Studies have shown that up to 60% of patients in treatment for major depression stop coming for treatment even when their symptoms are unimproved.

VII. Continued evaluation of moderately ill patients.

A. Categorical/diagnostic assessment.

Patients with moderate depressive symptoms and functional impairment lasting 2 or more weeks need a categorical or diagnostic evaluation.

Completing a formal diagnostic interview and making a DSM diagnosis allow primary care physicians to tap the psychiatric literature for treatment and management strategies. Since the publication of the DSM-III in 1980, psychiatric researchers primarily have investigated treatments for specific diagnostic groups. Several depressive disorders are reliably diagnosed and have clear, evidence-based treatments. Clinicians and patients benefit when these disorders are identified, and treatment plans include tested and proven interventions.

The differential diagnosis of patients with moderately severe depressive symptoms for 2 weeks includes

1. Mood disorder due to a general medical condition.
2. Substance-induced mood disorder.
3. Major depressive disorder.
4. Dysthymic disorder.
5. Adjustment disorder with depressed mood.
6. Depression not otherwise specified.
   a. Minor depressive disorder.
   b. Recurrent brief depression.
   c. Mixed anxiety-depressive disorder.
   d. Premenstrual dysphoric disorder.
7. Bipolar disorder.
8. Personality disorders (borderline, histrionic, and dependent) at times of stress.

Most depressive diagnoses are defined by the presence of a specific number of depressive symptoms, in different combinations, for specific lengths of time. Table 7–4 lists depressive symptoms commonly used in making depressive diagnoses, and Table 7–3 lists the number of symptoms and the length of time that symptoms must be present for the patient to qualify for a diagnosis of threshold depressive disorder. Table 7–3 also includes the newly operationalized criteria for subthreshold depressive disorders. The subthreshold disorders are included in the DSM-IV appendix as research criteria sets.

The DSM-IV or the DSM-IV-PC *(Diagnostic and Statistical Manual of Mental Disorders for Primary Care),* a manual designed specifically for use by primary care physicians, may be useful additions to the office library. These references contain all the diagnostic criteria for depressive and other psychiatric disorders.

Alternatively, physicians may choose to use one of the diagnostic interviews that have been designed for primary care providers, such as the PRIME-MD or the Symptom Driven Diagnostic System (SDDS) for Primary Care, in order to reach an appropriate diagnosis.

B. Depressive disorders with specific treatments.

This section briefly describes threshold disorders with specific treatments. These depressive diagnoses are useful in organizing clinicians' thinking about patients and in enabling access to the psychiatric literature on patient prognosis and treatment. *Clinicians should make efforts to diagnose these disorders when present.*

1. *Mood disorder due to a general medical condition.*

Table 7–4
Depressive Symptoms Used in the Making of Depressive Disorder Diagnoses

Depressed mood	Concentration difficulties
Loss of pleasure	Feelings of worthlessness or guilt
Sleep disturbance	Psychomotor retardation or agitation
Appetite disturbance	Low self-esteem
Low energy levels	Feelings of hopelessness
Suicidal ideation	

a. *Description.* Approximately ½ to ⅔ of primary care patients have a medical illness in addition to their depressive illness. In some of these patients, medical illnesses directly precipitate the mood symptoms. The DSM-IV diagnosis of *mood disorder due to a general medical condition* refers to a depression that is the "direct physiological consequence of a general medical condition."

Minor depressive syndromes may develop as a reaction to chronic medical illnesses and the limitations and discomforts that these disorders cause. However, patients who develop mild depressive syndromes as reactions to medical illnesses are classified as having adjustment disorders rather than mood disorders due to a general medical condition.

b. *Treatment.* Mood disorders that are the direct physiologic consequence of a medical condition are addressed by treatment of the underlying medical illness. The depressogenic effect of several illnesses, including hypothyroidism, vitamin B_{12} deficiency, pancreatic cancer, multiple sclerosis, Parkinson's disease, and Alzheimer's disease, is well described. The primary care physician should treat reversible conditions, such as hypothyroidism or vitamin B_{12} deficiency, and allow sufficient time to elapse for the intervention to affect mood symptoms. Improvement in depressive symptoms may take several weeks to months.

Depressive symptoms that are the result of nonreversible or only partially treatable conditions, such as Alzheimer's disease and Parkinson's disease, are often alleviated with antidepressants. In these cases, physicians may wish to use antidepressants for depressive syndromes of lesser severity, under the assumption that remission of depressive symptoms with time in nonreversible neurologic conditions is unlikely without intervention (see Chapter 12).

2. *Substance-induced mood disorder.*

a. *Description.* Depressive symptoms and depressive disorders may develop as a result of *substance use.*

One of the most common causes of depressive symptoms is alcohol misuse. Approximately 12% of the general United States population abuses alcohol, making alcohol abuse one of the most common mental disorders. The prevalence of alcohol problems in general medical settings is even higher, with about 20% to 30% of patients in primary care settings having some problem with alcohol use. Patients who are severely dependent on alcohol and present for detoxification often have marked depressive symptoms.

Commonly prescribed medications, such as glucocorticoids, anabolic steroids, and levodopa, can also cause depressive symptoms. Case reports have implicated many other prescription medications; these reactions to medications may be idiosyncratic to the patient (see Chapter 17).

b. *Treatment.* Most depressive symptoms secondary to alcohol misuse disappear rapidly with detoxification and abstinence. Two to 3 weeks of abstinence may be needed before all depressive symptoms resolve. After several weeks of abstinence, the physician can determine whether the patients have depressive disorders that are independent of their alcohol abuse.

Depressive symptoms secondary to prescription medications also remit with drug discontinuation. Physicians should note the temporal relationship between the initiation of any new prescription medications and the occurrence of depressive disorders. If the physician suspects a relationship between a new medication and the emergence of a depressive syndrome, temporary discontinuation of the new medication can prove both helpful and diagnostic.

3. *Major depressive disorder.*

Major depression is the most extensively studied depressive disorder presenting in the primary care setting. The clinician should take care to diagnose _all_ patients with major depression who present to his or her office. The reliability of this diagnosis is high, and effective treatments exist for this disabling and sometimes lethal disorder. Chapter 8 includes an extensive discussion of major depression in the primary care setting.

4. *Dysthymic disorder.*

a. *Description. Dysthymic disorder* is often included under the rubric of "minor depression," or "nonmajor depression." However, this disorder is a threshold depressive disorder that has been part of the psychiatric nomenclature since 1980. Dysthymic disorder has been the subject of a growing body of literature, and the epidemiology, prognosis, and treatment of this syndrome are gradually becoming better understood. Dysthymic disorder is relatively common in primary care settings. The Epidemiologic Catchment Area study showed the lifetime prevalence of dysthymia to be approximately 3.1%; the National Comorbidity Study showed lifetime prevalence of dysthymia to be 4.8% in men and 8.0% in women.[15]

Although dysthymic disorder is symptomatically less severe than major depression, with fewer and less severe symptoms required for diagnosis (depressed mood plus two additional depressive symptoms), the stringent duration criterion of 2 years makes this a disorder with a low placebo response and a poor long-term prognosis. Two years after the diagnosis of dysthymic disorder, only 39% of patients are in remission. The Medical Outcomes Study found that dysthymic patients had the poorest initial functioning as well as the poorest prognosis of all patients with a mood disorder.[16]

Dysthymia is often accompanied by other psychiatric conditions: 70% to 75% of dysthymic individuals also meet the criteria for a second psychiatric disorder. Patients with dysthymic disorder are more likely to have a concurrent personality disorder than are patients with major depression, with up to 60% qualifying for personality disorder diagnosis.[17]

Many individuals with dysthymic disorder go on to have MDD: 10% of patients identified with dysthymic disorder develop MDD within a year. Patients with both dysthymic disorder and MDD are less likely to achieve full remission and more likely to have frequent episodes than are individuals with MDD alone.

b. *Treatment.* Antidepressants can be helpful for patients with dysthymic disorder, and a trial of antidepressant medication should be given to most patients who meet the criteria for dysthymia.

The response rates to antidepressants are less than those seen in patients with MDD; approximately 50% of patients with dysthymic disorder respond to pharmacologic treatment, compared with approximately 65% to 75% of the patients with MDD. Both tricyclics and fluoxetine (Prozac) have been shown to be effective treatments for dysthymic disorder.[18]

Pharmacologic therapy for dysthymic patients should begin with a serotonin reuptake inhibitor because these patients are more likely to find the side effects of these medications to be tolerable and are more likely to comply with treatment. Dysthymic disorder is a chronic illness, and prolonged treatment with an antidepressant may be needed; patients may find even mild side effects to be unacceptable when taking medication for long periods of time.

Less is known about the efficacy of psychological treatments for dysthymic disorder. Most of the published psychotherapy trials for dysthymia have been uncontrolled. Several of these trials have suggested benefit from interpersonal therapy or cognitive behavioral therapy; one controlled trial showed benefit from marital therapy.

Controlled trials have clearly demonstrated that cognitive behavioral therapy and interpersonal therapy is of value in the treatment of MDD. By inference, a case can be made that these psychotherapies should also be tried in dysthymia. Indeed, given the high incidence of comorbidity of dysthymia with MDD, the clinician is often treating both disorders simultaneously.

In summary, the primary care provider who has diagnosed dysthymic disorder should proceed with an antidepressant trial. The practitioner should also engage the patient in supportive problem solving during clinic visits and should assist the patient in tapping resources to alter environmental stressors. If the patient has an incomplete recovery after 8 to 12 weeks of treatment, he or she should be referred for formal interpersonal or cognitive-behavioral psychotherapy.

C. Depressive disorders without specific interventions.

Diagnosing the following disorders does not clearly benefit either clinicians or patients. We have included brief descriptions of these diagnostic entities for completeness and to allow interested clinicians to stay abreast of the developing literature on mild depressive syndromes. *Clinical management of these cases is determined by factors other than diagnosis and is described at the end of this chapter.*

1. *Adjustment disorder with depressed mood.*

a. *Description. Adjustment disorder* is not defined in terms of its symptomatology, as are the other depressive disorders in the DSM-IV; instead, this disorder is defined by its etiology—as an emotional and behavioral syndrome resulting from a stressor. Adjustment disorder is a residual category for "presentations that are in response to an identifiable stressor and do not meet the criteria for another specific threshold disorder." The patient's symptoms must be in "excess of what would be expected" from the experienced stressor or must result in functional impairment.[19]

Adjustment disorder is a common diagnosis in outpatient settings, but studies show poorer inter-rater reliability for this disorder than for other psychiatric disorders. Poor inter-rater reliability may result from problems in defining the precipitating stressor or in deciding whether symptoms are in "excess of what would be expected."[19]

As mentioned earlier, some individuals are clearly more disposed to develop symptoms in response to stressors than are others. These differences in stress vulnerability may be the result of the underlying biology of the individuals or the result of life circumstances.

The psychiatric literature suggests that psychotherapeutic interventions are likely to be helpful for patients with adjustment disorder, although few controlled trials of psychotherapy in this disorder exist. *Suggested treatment approaches include brief therapies that focus on developing alternative, adaptive coping strategies and dynamic therapies that look at the meaning that the adverse event has for a particular patient. Stress management and relaxation techniques may also be tried.*

Antidepressants are usually not needed.

However, if patients' symptoms are severe or longstanding, or if there is a positive family or personal history of depression, antidepressants should be considered. If the physician decides to prescribe antidepressants, a full discussion of the relative benefits and risks of the medication should occur.

2. *Depression not otherwise specified.*
Depression not otherwise specified is the DSM-IV diagnosis for all patients not meeting the criteria for MDD, dysthymic disorder, adjustment disorder with depressed mood, or adjustment disorder with mixed anxiety and depressed mood.

These patients may have too few depressive symptoms to qualify for a diagnosis of MDD, symptoms for too short a period of time to qualify for MDD or dysthymic disorder, or symptoms that are not clearly related to a psychosocial stressor, as required for adjustment disorders.

Four proposed subsyndromal disorders, previously categorized simply as depression not otherwise specified, have been included in the DSM-IV appendix as research criteria sets: minor depressive disorder, recurrent brief depression, mixed anxiety-depressive disorder, and premenstrual dysphoric disorder.

a. *Minor depressive disorder.*

(1) *Description. Minor depressive disorder* has been defined in many different ways in the research literature. The DSM-IV research criteria for this disorder specify that patients have *two to four depressive symptoms* lasting for 2 or more weeks. DSM-IV also specifies that one of these symptoms must be depressed mood or lack of pleasure or interest. *Minor depression has the same duration criteria as major depression but requires two to four rather than five depressive symptoms.*

Minor depression results in poor marital functioning and increased absence from work. Patients with minor depression are as likely as those with major depression to seek treatment for their symptoms, although they more often go to a family physician or lay counselor than a mental health specialist. Elderly patients may be more likely to develop minor depressive disorders, possibly because of an increased incidence of concurrent medical illnesses in this population.[20]

(2) *Treatment.* Very little literature exists on the treatment of minor depressive disorder. There has been one randomized controlled trial showing that short-term behavioral group therapy can be helpful in this disorder.

b. *Recurrent brief depression.*

(1) *Description. Recurrent brief depression* has the same symptomatic criteria as MDD, requiring five of nine depressive symptoms. However, in recurrent brief depression, the depressive symptoms do not last 2 weeks and thus do not meet the minimum *duration* criterion for major depression. The research criterion for recurrent brief depression stipulates episodes of at least 2 days but less than 2 weeks. Patients also must experience *repeated episodes* of depression, with at least one depressive episode a month for a year. *Patients with this disorder have depressive symptoms* ***comparable in severity*** *to major depression but for shorter time periods and at more frequent intervals.*

Recurrent brief depression is relatively common in primary care settings, with a prevalence of 9.9%. Suicide attempts occur frequently in these patients, 23.3% of patients with this disorder make a suicide attempt at some point during their illness. This rate is comparable to the rate of suicide attempts in patients with threshold depressive disorders.

(2) *Treatment.* No specific treatments exist for this disorder. One study has found serotonin reuptake inhibitors to be ineffective.

d. *Mixed anxiety-depressive disorder.*

(1) *Description. Mixed anxiety-depressive disorder* is defined as an admixture of at least *four depressive and anxiety symptoms.* The symptoms must be present for at least 1 month, include a dysphoric mood, and cause significant distress or impairment in functioning.

Mixed anxiety-depressive disorder does not pertain to patients who qualify for a threshold depressive disorder and also have symptoms of anxiety. Threshold depressive disorders with concomitant anxiety symptoms are common, but they have different treatment implications. Mixed anxiety depression is a *subthreshold* classification and does not meet the criteria for any DSM depressive or anxiety disorders.

Mixed anxiety-depressive disorder has been the subject of several studies in primary care settings. Patients with mixed anxiety depression have demonstrable reductions in occupational and role functioning. Unfortunately, as in the other subsyndromal disorders, no proven treatment approaches exist.

VIII. Treatment of the "subthreshold depressive syndromes" (DSM-IV: depression not otherwise specified)

Clinicians are advised to return to the "dimensional assessment" of patients for guidance on the treatment of patients with moderate depressive symptoms and functional impairment who meet criteria for subthreshold depressive disorders only.

We suggest that clinicians ask themselves the following questions:

- How severe are this patient's symptoms?
- How many symptoms does this patient have?
- How severe are this patient's functional limitations?
- How long has this patient been symptomatic?
- Does this patient have a family history of depression?
- Does this patient have a personal past history of major depression?
- Does this patient have a coexisting personality disorder?

Patients with depression not otherwise specified who have more severe symptoms, longer duration of symptoms, greater functional impairment, and a personal or family history of depression should be considered for antidepressant treatment and specific psychotherapies. Patients who have lesser symptomatology and shorter durations of symptoms may not need formal treatment interventions and can be managed with the nonspecific measures described in the Initial Management Strategies section. Patients who have coexisting personality disorders as well as subthreshold depressive symptoms may benefit from referral for formal psychotherapy, even if the current episode is of short duration, because they are liable to have recurrent difficulties.

References

1. Katon W, Schulberg H. Epidemiology of depression in primary care. Gen Hosp Psychiatry 1992; 14:237–247.
2. Wells K, Stewart A, Hays R, et al. The functioning and well-being of depressed patients: Results from the medical outcomes study. JAMA 1989; 262:914–919.
3. Simon G, VonKorff M, Barlow W. Health care costs of primary care patients with recognized depression. Arch Gen Psychiatry 1995; 52:850–856.
4. Wilson DR, Wider RB, Cadoret RJ, Judiesch K. Somatic symptoms: A major feature of depression in family practice. J Affect Disord 1983; 5:199–207.
5. Kroenke K, Spitzer R, Williams J, et al. Physical symptoms in primary care: Predictors of psychiatric disorder and functional impairment. Arch Fam Med 1994; 3:774–779.
6. Zich J, Attkisson C, Greenfield T. Screening for depression in primary care clinics: The CES-D and the BDI. Int J Psychiatry Med 1990; 20:259–277.
7. Spitzer RL, Williams JB, Kroenke K, et al. Utility of a new procedure for diagnosing mental disorders in primary care: The PRIME-MD 1000 Study. JAMA 1994; 272:1749–1756.
8. Weissman MM, Olfson M, Leon AC, et al. Brief diagnostic interviews (SDDS-PC) for multiple mental disorders in primary care: A pilot study. Arch Fam Med 1995; 4:220–227.
9. Elkin I, Shea T, Watkins J, et al. National Institute of Mental Health Treatment of Depression Collaborative Research Program. General effectiveness of treatments. Arch Gen Psychiatry 1989; 46:971–982.
10. Wyshak G, Barsky A. Relationship between patient self ratings and physician ratings of general health, depression and anxiety. Arch Fam Med 1994; 3:419–424.
11. Kendler KS, Kessler RC, Walters EE, et al. Stressful life events, genetic liability, and onset of an episode of major depression in women. Am J Psychiatry 1995; 152:833–842.
12. Keller M, Shapiro R. Major depressive disorder: Initial results from a one year prospective naturalistic follow up study. J Nerv Ment Dis 1981; 169:761–768.
13. Cooper-Patrick L, Crum R, Ford D. Identifying suicidal ideation in general medical patients. JAMA 1994; 272:1757–1762.
14. Horwath E, Johnson J, Klerman G, Weissman M. Depressive symptoms as relative and attributable risk factors for first-onset major depression. Arch Gen Psychiatry 1992; 49:817–823.
15. Kessler RC, McGonagle KA, Zhao S, et al. Lifetime and 12-month prevalence of DSM-III-R psychiatric disorders in the United States. Results from the National Comorbidity Survey. Arch Gen Psychiatry 1994; 51:8–19.
16. Wells K, Burham A, Rogers W, et al. The course of depression in adult outpatients. Arch Gen Psychiatry 1992; 49:788–794.
17. Pepper C, Klein D, Anderson R, et al. DSM III R axis II comorbidity in dysthymia and major depression. Am J Psychiatry 1995; 152:239–247.
18. Lapierre Y. Pharmacological therapy of dysthymia. Acta Psychiatr Scand 1994; 89(Suppl 383):42–48.
19. American Psychiatric Association: Diagnostic and Statistical Manual of Mental Disorders. Fourth Edition. Washington, DC: American Psychiatric Association; 1994.
20. Tannock C, Katona C. Minor depression in the aged: Concepts, prevalence and optimal management. Drugs Aging 1995; 6:278–292.

8

JOHN F. GREDEN, MD

THOMAS L. SCHWENK, MD

Major Mood Disorders

I. Evaluation and diagnosis.

A. Introduction and terminology.

Major depressive disorder (MDD), also known as *unipolar depression,* is a serious problem in primary care settings. Depression is the most common psychiatric problem that primary care clinicians encounter, and it may be the most common of all primary care problems. This prevalence is not surprising, because MDD develops in 15% of people (approximately 20% of women, 10% of men), during their lifetime, and an estimated 70% to 80% seek treatment from their primary care physician (PCP). Depressed patients have garnered a reputation for being frustrating and problematic for the PCP because their symptoms tend to become chronic and because depressed patients tend to overuse the health care system. This troublesome reputation is no longer justified. Major mood disorders are eminently treatable, and effective maintenance programs are now available.

Manic-depressive illness, also called *bipolar disorder,* is much less common than MDD in primary care settings. Referral to psychiatric specialists is often required. Symptoms and major treatment strategies are summarized in this chapter.

Major depressive disorder and manic-depressive illness are characterized by *genetic predisposition,* generally *good premorbid functioning, onset* of clinical symptoms occurring most commonly *during adolescence or young adulthood* (occasionally during childhood), and an *episodic, recurrent lifetime course* that tends to worsen with each additional episode.

B. Onset.

Onset of symptoms peaks in late teenage years, earlier than generally believed. During the early stages, depressive symptoms are commonly overlooked because they tend to be mild to moderate in severity and only worsen with repeat episodes. Symptoms are often missed, attributed to stressful lifetime events, or dismissed as events that will pass. Often, these disorders are misdiagnosed as other disorders. For these reasons, MDD and bipolar disorder are often assumed to have their onset in middle age. This is erroneous. Primary care clinicians have an excellent opportunity to identify and treat major mood disorders during earlier stages of life and should strive to do so. They should be especially alert to the presence of mood disorders in anyone with a family history of these problems.

C. Pathophysiology.

1. *Brain dysregulation.*
   Major depressive disorder and manic-depressive illness are brain disorders that are attributable to dysregulation (imbalance) of central nervous system networks that control pleasure, pain, motivation, reward and reinforcement, biologic rhythms, appetite, sexuality, psychomotor function, cognition, and numerous other functions. Although specific abnormalities are not yet characterized, thousands of studies over the past 30 years have confirmed that patients with depression or mania have changes in brain neurotransmitters, neuroendocrine and neuropeptide hormones, second-messenger systems, receptor functions, signal transduction, gene expression, and other important neurobiologic actions. Changes in brain metabolism and regional cerebral blood flow during depression and mania have been demonstrated with positron-emission tomography, single-photon emission computed tomography, and electrophysiologic measures, such as sleep electroencephalography.

2. *Role of stress in mood disorders.*
   Depressive episodes are often precipitated by major stressful life events, such as death in the family, separation, divorce, assault, rape, major accident, or significant financial setback. *The role of stressors in precipitating depression is more evident during earlier episodes of depression, being identifiable in approximately 60% of first episodes, 35% of second episodes, and 25% or fewer of subsequent episodes.* This pattern has prompted some neuroscientists to hypothesize that each new episode of depression or mania sensitizes the brain, producing possible changes in gene expression and increasing the likelihood that milder stressors

might initiate a future episode or that depressive episodes develop in the absence of stressful events. *The presence of stressors should never be the major determinant in the decision of whether pharmacotherapy is used. The decision of whether medication is used should depend on severity, longitudinal course, history of prior episodes, and degree of dysfunction.* However, stressors should always be addressed. Clinicians should assess for recent traumatic life events and should always strive to aid patients and families in preventing future repetitions or in developing strategies to cope with them. In the past, the term *reactive depression* was often used to describe depression coincident with an evident stressor. Unfortunately, this determination frequently led to a treatment with antianxiety agents and sedative hypnotics or to a decision to provide no treatment at all. No substantial support exists for the assumption that the presence of stressors means that antidepressants should not be used. Stressful events *interact* with genetic neurobiologic substrates. Depression is more likely to develop after a major stressful life event in people with greater genetic risk, just as angina or infarct is more likely to develop after a major stressful life event in those with pre-existing cardiovascular ischemia. The PCP should cease struggling with the question of "reactive" versus "biologic" depression because the disorders are always interactive. We recommend that the term reactive depression be discarded from clinical formulations.

Table 8–1
Disorders of Depressed Mood that Commonly Present in Primary Care Settings*

Common
Mood disorder due to a general medical condition
Major depressive disorder
Dysthymic disorder
Bereavement
Seasonal affective disorder
Alcohol-induced mood disorder
Less common
Other substance-induced (including medication-induced) mood disorder
Adjustment disorder with mixed anxiety and depressed mood
Mixed anxiety-depression
Least common
Recurrent bipolar I disorder
Bipolar II disorder

*Organized according to estimated prevalence.

Case Study

Mrs. A. is a 35-year-old mother of three children, aged 7, 4, and 1 year, who consults the PCP about her headaches. She is married, but the marriage is "shaky." She feels considerable stress and little support from her husband since the birth of their last child. She was not overtly depressed after delivery, noting that her husband was temporarily attentive and helpful, but she says that

D. Clinical features, primary care presentation, and initial diagnostic steps.

Clinical features for major mood disorders were recently summarized in the publication *The Diagnostic and Statistical Manual of Mental Disorders, Fourth Edition—Primary Care Version* (DSM-IV-PC). This unique compilation resulted from a collaboration among primary care and psychiatry specialists. It was designed to address the special circumstances encountered by the PCP and to aid them in the prompt recognition and identification of common psychiatric diagnoses. Disorders of depressed mood that commonly present in primary care settings are listed in Table 8–1.

Patients with MDD generally present with combinations of depressed mood, profound decreases in interest or pleasure in usual activities, problems with appetite and weight (loss or gain), sleep dysregulation (too little or too much), loss of energy or fatigue, psychomotor slowing or agitation, problems with thinking or concentration, and feelings of low self-worth or suicidal thoughts. This profile generally persists for at least 2 weeks before a diagnosis of major depressive episode is made. Official DSM-IV-PC criteria are listed in Table 8–2.

A characteristic patient is presented in the case study.

Table 8–2
Criteria for Major Depressive Disorder

I. At least five of the following symptoms have been present during the same 2-week period, nearly every day, and represent a significant deterioration from previous functioning. At least one of the symptoms must be either (1) depressed mood or (2) loss of interest or pleasure:
   A. Depressed mood (alternatively, irritable mood in children and adolescents).
   B. Markedly diminished interest or pleasure in all, or almost all, activities.
   C. Significant weight loss or weight gain when not dieting.
   D. Insomnia or hypersomnia.
   E. Psychomotor agitation or retardation.
   F. Fatigue or loss of energy.
   G. Feelings of worthlessness or excessive or inappropriate guilt.
   H. Diminished ability to think or concentrate.
   I. Recurrent thoughts of death, recurrent suicidal ideation without a specific plan, or suicide attempt or specific plan for committing suicide.

II. Symptoms are not better accounted for by a mood disorder due to a general medical condition, a substance-induced mood disorder, or bereavement (normal reaction to the death of a loved one).

III. Symptoms are not better accounted for by a psychotic disorder (e.g., schizoaffective disorder).

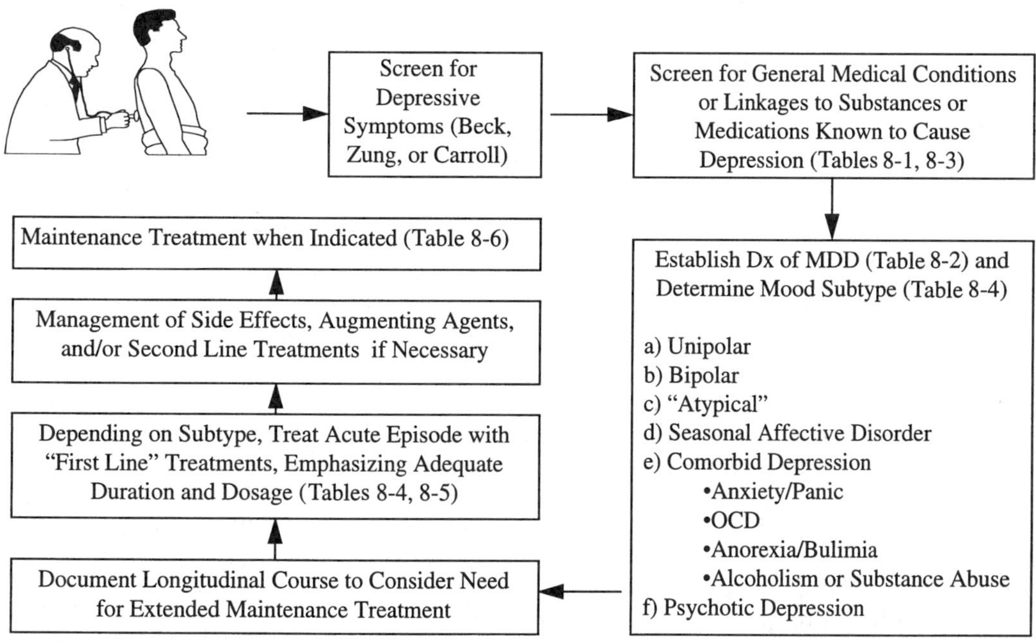

Figure 8–1
Recommended steps for use when primary care physicians encounter patients with clinical profiles suggesting depression. MDD, major depressive disorder; OCD, obsessive-compulsive disorder.

lately he has been consumed by his work and is rarely available to help with the children. Mrs. A. had some type of "breakdown" in college, about which she can say little, but she withdrew from school for one semester. She has no known other psychiatric or medical disease, and she takes no medications. Her mother has a lifelong history of depression, her paternal grandfather was a heavy drinker who committed suicide at the age of 50, and she has a sister who is being treated with some sort of antidepressant. In addition to fatigue, she complains of frequent headaches and back pain, poor sleep, spontaneous tearfulness and emotional lability, inability to carry out her home and parenting responsibilities, and feelings of guilt over her poor performance as a mother. She and her husband have not had sexual intercourse since the baby was born.

When the PCP encounters patients with clinical profiles suggesting depression, we recommend that five steps be followed, summarized in Figure 8–1.

1. *Screen for depressive symptoms.*
Self-rating depression scales (Beck, Carroll, Center for Epidemiologic Studies, and Zung depression mood scales [see appendix]) are recommended for the screening of new or established patients who present with disturbances of sleep or appetite, fatigue, chronic pain, or mood or psychophysiologic dysfunction. Rating scales are one to two pages long. They are simple, inexpensive, well accepted by patients, reliably scored by office staff in 1 to 2 minutes, and, like vital signs, provide an initial indication of whether depressive symptoms are prominent and require further investigation. The scale can be completed after the patient checks in for an appointment. Scores can be quickly tallied and included in the medical record for the physician's use during the initial visit and at subsequent visits. If the total score is greater than a selected cut-off point (e.g., a Beck Depression Scale score $\geq$ 16), the PCP should include specific questions about depression in the medical history. Rating scale items also may assist the PCP in formulating easily asked questions.

2. *Screen for general medical conditions or linkage to substances or medications.*
If the patient's clinical history reveals that symptoms developed during or within a month of significant substance intoxication or withdrawal, or that they followed the use of a medication (including over-the-counter products), a possible association between the two events must be considered. The medications that most commonly cause depression are listed in Table 8–3.
Because no definitive laboratory tests exist to determine when substances or medications might cause depression or mania, a routine strategy should be to eliminate common offending agents whenever they are being used by someone who is also depressed, unless the agents are medically essential. If mood symptoms improve within several weeks of stopping the causal med-

Table 8–3
Pharmacologic Agents that Commonly Cause Depression

Alcohol
Analgesics (e.g., codeine)
Sedative-hypnotics
Anxiolytics
Steroids
Oral contraceptives
Antihistamines (with long-term use)
Chemotherapy medications
Cardiac medications (antihypertensives)
Anticholinergics (antispasmodics)
Amphetamines
Cocaine
Cannabis
Hallucinogens

ication, other interventions may be unnecessary. Patients with an underlying mood disorder diathesis are apparently more susceptible to depression when they are exposed to selected substances or medications; therefore, specific antidepressant interventions may be required if the mood symptoms fail to resolve within 3 to 4 weeks.

3. *Establish diagnosis of major depressive disorder and determine mood subtype.*
   For any patient with a major mood disorder, the clinician should determine the mood subtype before instituting treatment. Subtype determination is based on onset, family history (genetics), premorbid functioning, clinical features, laboratory data, prior response to treatments, and longitudinal course and outcome (Table 8–4). Options include
   a. Unipolar (MDD or dysthymia).
   b. Bipolar (mania or hypomania).
   c. Atypical depression.
   d. Seasonal affective disorder (SAD).
   e. Comorbid depression, especially.
      (1) Anxiety or panic disorder.
      (2) Obsessive-compulsive disorder.
      (3) Anorexia/bulimia.
      (4) Alcoholism or other substance abuse.
   f. Psychotic ("delusional") depression.

   Subtype determinations are important because treatment interventions differ among the subtypes. Key characteristics for each subtype are provided in Table 8–4.

4. *Document longitudinal course (prior episodes).*
   Major mood disorders are commonly episodic, recurrent lifetime disorders, with additional episodes tending to occur closer together, to last longer, and to become more severe. For anyone with three or more significant episodes of depression, the risk of relapse without maintenance treatment within 1 to 2 years is estimated to be greater than 75% and probably becomes greater with each progressive episode. For this reason, after determining the subtype, the PCP should focus on documentation of prior episodes and charting of the longitudinal course. Prior medical records and family input are always helpful. The physician is encouraged to compile a brief sketch illustrating the course of the illness. A sample is shown in Figure 8–2.

   Indefinite maintenance medication treatment should be considered for any patient with three or more significant episodes, especially if there is a family history of depression or mania or if prior episodes have been severe or treatment resistant.

II. Initial treatment and management recommendations.

A. Determine antidepressant medication strategy.

The PCP should ask five questions related to antidepressant medications:

1. Should I prescribe medications?
2. If so, which should I use and in what dosage?
3. What should I do if the patient fails to improve?
4. How long should I continue antidepressant pharmacotherapy?
5. How should I discontinue medication therapy?
   These determinations—arguably the most important in the treatment of patients with MDD—should be based on degree of severity, longitudinal lifetime course, and level of dysfunction, *not* on whether the depressive episode seems to be precipitated by psychological or stressful life events.

   For many patients, medications play a vital role in the resolution of the acute episode of depression. *All antidepressants appear to work approximately equally well in resolving acute episodes ("efficacy") but differ considerably in side effect profiles.* Side effects are most important in determining compliance and "effectiveness." Thus, the initial choice of medication should be heavily weighed by side effects and long-term considerations, with the goal being selection of an acceptable drug. Without compliance, neither resolution of the acute episode nor effective long-term maintenance will occur.

B. Determine whether patient meets specific criteria for antidepressant pharmacotherapy.

1. *Patients with moderate or severe depression that has persisted for 1 month or longer with or without psychotic features should receive full-dose antidepressant medications.* Without pharmacotherapy,

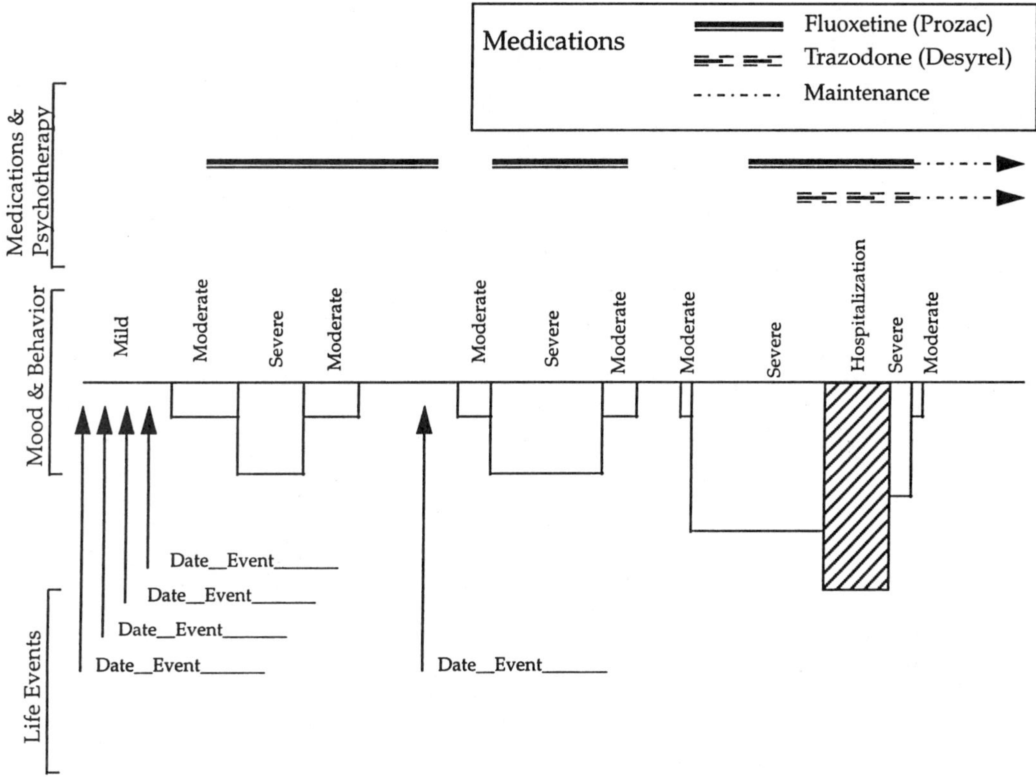

Figure 8–2
Sample brief sketch by primary care physician that illustrates the course of illness of a major mood disorder.

most patients have prolonged episodes or fail to improve.

2. *Patients with mild or mild-to-moderate depression that is chronic and interferes with routine functions of living, social relationships, or occupational performance* should receive a trial of full-dose medication. Mild symptoms do not always have mild consequences. When symptoms become chronic, significant disability may result. Diagnosis may be more difficult because patients with mild depressive symptoms characteristically fail to label the symptoms as "depressive," dismiss them as secondary to recent life events ("I'm just stressed"), or express overt reluctance to a proffered diagnosis of depression ("I'm not depressed doctor, I'm just tired"). If this erroneous formulation is too readily accepted, those with mild chronic depression may receive no treatment, brief or cursory advice ("back off at work a bit"), or nonspecific medication treatment (e.g., benzodiazepines) targeted at anxiety and stress or sleep dysregulation.

   In many primary care settings, prescriptions of antianxiety agents (benzodiazepines) or sedative-hypnotics remain traditional interventions before antidepressant therapy is begun. This tradition warrants reconsideration. *If depressive symptoms, even mild, have lasted ≥ 6 months or are interfering with everyday function, antidepressant therapy should be considered.* Mild symptoms should not equate with mild treatment. If medications are prescribed for patients with mild, prolonged depression (called dysthymia), treatment should be at full dose, the same as for patients with more severe syndromes.

3. *Patients with multiple episodes of major mood disorder* should be treated with full-dose medication and, in all probability, long-term maintenance therapy. When first evaluating depressed individuals with three or more well-documented prior depressive episodes *the PCP should tell the patient at the beginning of treatment about the likely need for continued maintenance treatment indefinitely after the acute episode resolves.*

4. *Depressed patients for whom other appropriate treatments are unavailable* should be considered for a trial of full-dose medication. Psychotherapy or counseling is sometimes considered an alternative to medications for major mood disorders, but a more accurate concept is that psychotherapy and medications support and sometimes augment each other. Two specific psychotherapies, cognitive behavior therapy (CBT) and interpersonal therapy, have been developed for mood disorders. Both have been shown to be

Table 8–4
Characteristics and Treatments for Subtypes of Depression

Clinical Subtype	Clinical Features	First-Line Treatments	Second-Line Treatments	Augmenting Agents	Maintenance Treatments
Unipolar	DSM-IV criteria for major depressive disorder (MDD)	SSRI (fluoxetine, sertraline, paroxetine) Venlafaxine Nefazodone	Bupropion Desipramine Nortriptyline	Lithium T_3/T_4 Pindolol Divalproex	Continue full dose of antidepressant + augmenting agent
Bipolar	DSM-IV criteria for MDD with history of hypomania or mania (e.g., grandiosity, decreased sleep, verbosity, impulsivity)	SSRI (fluoxetine, sertraline, paroxetine) Venlafaxine Lithium Divalproex	Bupropion Desipramine Nortriptyline	Divalproex Carbamazepine T_3/T_4 Pindolol (for SSRIs)	Lithium Divalproex Carbamazepine Combinations
Psychotic	MDD + delusions, hallucinations, other psychotic features (mood congruent or mood incongruent)	Imipramine or desipramine plus Neuroleptic (haloperidol, clozapine)	Electroconvulsive therapy	Lithium T_3/T_4 Pindolol (for SSRIs) Valproate	Continue full dose of antidepressant + neuroleptic + augment (discontinue neuroleptic therapy first)
Atypical	Mood reactivity, hyperphagia, hypersomnia, leaden paralysis, rejection sensitivity, chocolate craving, often with seasonal pattern + MDD criteria	SSRI (fluoxetine, sertraline, paroxetine) MAOI (phenelzine) Venlafaxine Nefazodone	Bupropion	Phototherapy T_3/T_4 Pindolol (for SSRIs) Lithium Combinations	Continue full dose of antidepressant + augmenting agent + seasonal bright light
Seasonal affective disorder	Mood reactivity, hyperphagia, hypersomnia, leaden paralysis, rejection sensitivity, chocolate craving, with regular temporal pattern (usually winter)	Phototherapy SSRI (fluoxetine, sertraline, paroxetine)	Venlafaxine MAOI (phenelzine)	T_3/T_4 Pindolol (for SSRIs) Lithium	Phototherapy Continue antidepressant prn

Dysthymia	Depressed mood and other symptoms ≥ 2 y, but doesn't meet MDD criteria now	SSRI (fluoxetine, sertraline, paroxetine) Venlafaxine Desipramine	Bupropion MAOI (phenelzine) Nortriptyline	Lithium T_3/T_4 Pindolol (for SSRIs)	Continue full dose of antidepressant
Comorbid: anxiety, panic	DSM-IV criteria for MDD + criteria for anxiety, panic, or phobia	SSRI (fluoxetine, sertraline, paroxetine) MAOI (phenelzine) Imipramine	Alprazolam Desipramine	T_3/T_4 Lithium Pindolol (for SSRIs)	Continue full dose of antidepressant
Comorbid: obsessive-compulsive	DSM-IV criteria for MDD + features of OCD (obsessive thoughts, impulses, behaviors)	SSRI (fluoxetine, sertraline, paroxetine)	Clomipramine MAOI (phenelzine)	Pindolol (for SSRIs) Lithium T_3/T_4	Continue full dose of antidepressant + augmenting + CBT
Comorbid: anorexia	DSM-IV criteria for MDD + criteria for anorexia nervosa (e.g., refusal to gain weight, binge eating)	Imipramine SSRI (fluoxetine, sertraline, paroxetine)	Desipramine	? T_3/T_4	Continue full dose of antidepressant + CBT
Comorbid: bulimia	DSM-IV criteria for MDD + criteria for bulimia nervosa (e.g., binging, vomiting, taking laxatives)	SSRI (fluoxetine, sertraline, paroxetine) Venlafaxine	Imipramine Desipramine	T_3/T_4 Lithium Pindolol??	Continue full dose of antidepressant + CBT

Alphabetized list of generic (Brand) names used in Table 8–4: alprazolam (Xanax), bupropion (Wellbutrin), carbamazepine (Tegretol), clomipramine (Anafranil), clozapine (Clozaril), desipramine (Norpramin), divalproex (Depakote), fluoxetine (Prozac), haloperidol (Haldol), imipramine (Tofranil), levothyroxine (T_4) (Synthroid), liothyronine (Cytomel), lithium (Eskalith, Lithobid), nefazodone (Serzone), nortriptyline (Pamelor), paroxetine (Paxil), phenelzine (Nardil), pindolol (Visken), sertraline (Zoloft), valproate (Depakene), venlafaxine (Effexor).

DSM-IV, *Diagnostic and Statistical Manual of Mental Disorders,* 4th ed; MAOI, monoamine oxidase inhibitor; SSRI, selective serotonin reuptake inhibitor; prn, as necessary; OCD, obsessive-compulsive disorder; CBT, cognitive behavior therapy.

considerably better than no treatment for selected patients with mild depression, but neither is as efficacious as pharmacotherapy for those with moderate or severe depression. When symptoms are mild but psychotherapy is not available for geographic, financial, or practical reasons, such as unavailability of trained therapists, medications should be prescribed.

C. Choose medications and dosage.

Many antidepressant medications are available (Table 8–5). In clinical settings, the selection of specific antidepressants should be made on the basis of subtype and other important features, such as

1. *Side effects.*
   This variable is the most important for the maintenance of compliance. If possible, medications with the most favorable side effect profiles should be prescribed so that compliance is enhanced. The patient's age, occupation, and prior experience with a particular medication (or others in its class) should be considered when the PCP is trying to determine the medication's acceptability. The experience of a first-degree biologic family member with a particular medication may be relevant as well.

2. *Comorbid symptoms.*
   Obsessive-compulsive features, eating disorder symptoms (binging, purging, or anorexia), and alcoholism are at least partially linked to serotonin dysregulation. *Medications that predominantly alter serotonin reuptake are preferred for such patients.* Options include selective serotonin reuptake inhibitors (SSRIs), such as fluoxetine (Prozac), sertraline (Zoloft), or paroxetine (Paxil), or newer antidepressants, such as venlafaxine (Effexor), nefazodone (Serzone), or clomipramine (Anafranil). Monoamine oxidase inhibitors (MAOIs), such as phenelzine (Nardil), and tranylcypromine (Parnate) are less effective but are preferable to tricyclic antidepressants.

3. *Presence of atypical features.*
   Some depressed patients are referred to as "atypical" because they have unusual symptoms, such as hyperphagia (excessive eating), hypersomnia (excessive sleeping), or extreme reactivity to disappointing life events. Some report seasonal affective disorder, or "winter depression." *Patients with atypical depressive features should be treated with antidepressants that predominantly alter serotonin reuptake* (medication options are listed earlier for comorbid symptoms). These agents are far more effective than tricyclic antidepressants (TCAs) for patients with the atypical subtype.

4. *History of prior response.*
   Patients should be asked about prior responses to antidepressants because documented prior success to a specific medication may predict similar favorable outcome in the current episode, and past failure *despite an adequate trial* would suggest that alternative approaches should be sought. The doctor should be cautious about concluding that a prior treatment has failed, however, because many patients may have used a medication for only a brief period, stopped taking it because of side effects, and yet concluded that the treatment was not effective. Such a conclusion is unwarranted.

5. *Potential drug-drug or metabolic interactions.*
   Patients receiving multiple medications may have *drug-drug interactions* that alter the expected impact of prescribed antidepressants. Many of the interactions occur because many medications, including most antidepressants, are metabolized via the same enzymatic system in the liver *(cytochrome P_{450})*, and the addition of one medicine often alters the metabolism of another. Antidepressants also have different degrees of protein binding. This characteristic may be of importance for those receiving other medications, such as warfarin (Coumadin); in such cases, an antidepressant with low protein binding (e.g., venlafaxine) should be selected so that the warfarin is not displaced.

6. *Coexisting medical problems.*
   Some antidepressants, especially TCAs, may have adverse effects on coexisting medical problems, such as cardiac disease (e.g., increased risk of arrhythmias, hypertension, dizziness, or orthostatic hypotension), diabetes complications that interfere with cognitive functions, and neurologic diseases. Newer antidepressants generally produce fewer medical interactions than do traditional TCAs (e.g., amitryptyline [Elavil]).

7. *Patient or family preferences.*
   Patient preferences tend to be subjective and often are not based on scientific data. *However, strong preferences provide clues about likely compliance and should not be ignored,* except when the preferred choice is not supported by a prior history of good response and is contraindicated by data (e.g., tricyclics for atypical depression) or when the patient indicates a preference for anxiolytic medications that are not effective in treating the complete depressive syndrome.

8. *Cost.*
   Antidepressant prices vary widely. The first priority is selection of an antidepressant with optimal side effect and safety profiles because such a selection protects the patient and increases long-term compliance; however, cost considera-

Table 8–5
Common Antidepressant Medications

Generic Name	Brand Name	Therapeutic Plasma Levels (ng/mL)	Common Dosage (mg/dy)*	Commonly Used Available Routes and Strengths	Sedation	Cardiac Conduction Effects	Anticholinergic Effects	Orthostatic Hypotension
Tricyclic, Cyclic								
Amitriptyline	Elavil	>120†	150–200	Coated tablets: 10, 25, 50, 75, 100, 150 mg Injection: 10 mg/mL	+ + + + +	+ + + + +	+ + + + +	+ + + + +
Clomipramine	Anafranil	?	150–200	Capsule: 25, 50, 75 mg	+ + + +	+ + + +	+ + + +	+ +
Desipramine	Norpramin	>125‡	50–300	Coated tablets: 10, 25, 50, 75, 100, 150 mg	+ + +	+ + +	+ + +	+ + + +
Doxepin	Adapin, Sinequan	?	150–200	Capsules: 10, 25, 50, 75, 100, 150 mg Concentrate: 10 mg/mL	+ + + + +	+ + + +	+ + +	+ + +
Imipramine	Tofranil	>225	150–200	Coated tablets: 10, 25, 50 mg Capsules: 75, 100, 125, 150 mg Concentrate: 25 mg/2 mL	+ + + +	+ + + + +	+ + + +	+ + + + +
Nortriptyline	Pamelor	50–150	75–100	Capsules: 10, 25, 50, 75 mg Concentrate: 10 mg/5 mL	+ +	+ +	+ +	+ +
Protriptyline	Vivactil	?	15–40	Coated tablets: 5, 10 mg	+ +	+ +	+ +	+ +
Trimipramine	Surmontil	?	150–200	Capsules: 25, 50, 100 mg	+ + + +	+ + + +	+ + + +	+ + +
Selective Serotonin Reuptake Inhibitors§								
Fluoxetine	Prozac	?	20–40	Capsules: 10, 20 mg Concentrate: 20 mg/5 mL	±	±	0	±
Fluvoxamine	Luvox	?	150–200	Scored, coated tablets: 50, 100 mg	±	±	0	±
Paroxetine	Paxil	?	20–40	Scored, coated tablets: 20 mg Coated tablet: 30 mg	+	±	+	0
Sertraline	Zoloft	?	75–150	Scored, coated tablets: 50, 100 mg	±	±	0	0
Other Compounds								
Bupropion	Wellbutrin	?	300–400	Coated tablets: 75, 100 mg	−¶	0	±	±
Bupropion sustained release	Wellbutrin	?	300–400	Coated tablets: 100, 150 mg	−¶	0	±	±
Nefazodone	Serzone	?	300–500	Scored, coated tablets: 100, 150 mg Coated tablets: 200, 250 mg	+ +	±	0	+
Trazodone	Desyrel	?	300–500§§	Coated tablets: 50, 100, 150 mg Scored, coated tablets: 300 mg	+ + + + +	±	0	+ + +
Venlafaxine	Effexor	?	75–225	Coated tablets: 25, 37.5, 75, 50, 100 mg	+	±	0	**
Mirtazapine	Remeron	?	15–45	Coated tablets: 15, 30, 45 mg	+ + +	±	±	±
Monoamine Oxidase Inhibitors (MAOIs)¶								
Phenelzine	Nardil	?	45–60	Coated tablet: 15 mg	+ +	+‡‡	+	+ + + + +
Tranylcypromine	Parnate	?	30–50	Coated tablet: 10 mg	+ +	+‡‡	+	+ + + + +

*Common dosage range produces a therapeutic response in most patients; however, for a maximum therapeutic effect, many patients require doses greater than the upper end of the range.
†Total value is sum of amitriptyline plus nortriptyline values.
‡Total value is sum of imipramine plus desipramine values.
§± means there is a small effect that is variable across patients and the direction of the effect cannot be predicted with certainty.
¶(minus) means bupropion predictably produces stimulation and alertness and mild insomnia, especially at the beginning of treatment.
**Venlafaxine causes dose-dependent and sustained diastolic hypertension in some patients, especially at doses exceeding 200 mg/d.
††MAOIs, as a class, interact with certain foods (e.g., aged cheese) and certain drugs (e.g., ephedrine) to produce a hypertensive crisis that may be countered by administration of 10 mg of nifedipine (Procardia) tablets in an amount proportional to the increase in blood pressure.
‡‡Based on limited data, MAOIs do not significantly affect cardiac conduction. Of course, a drug-induced hypertensive crisis affects cardiovascular and cerebrovascular performance.
§§Trazodone (Desyrel) is commonly combined with SSRI at bedtime for sedative-hypnotic purposes, at doses of 25–50 mg.
0, none; ±, equivocal, sporadic; +, minimal; + +, mild; + + +, moderate; + + + +, strong; + + + + +, severe; ?, not well established.

tions are important. Newer antidepressants generally have more favorable side effect and safety profiles, but they are more expensive than traditional TCAs in the short term. Nevertheless, they appear to be cost-saving in the long term because of increased compliance, which leads to enhanced treatment success.

C. **Psychotherapy and counseling.**

Psychotherapy or verbal counseling with depressed patients in primary care settings should be open, honest, supportive, practical, and directive. Brief, frequent contacts are preferable to lengthier sessions. The PCP needs to move smoothly and comfortably in order to enable time-efficient discussion of symptoms, medications, relationships, and strategies for dealing with grief or recent stressors. Two approaches have been developed, studied, and shown to be effective in patients with depression.

1. *Interpersonal therapy focuses on resolution of problematic interpersonal relationships or stressful events evident in many patients with depression.* The doctor should seek to determine if the patient has abnormal grief, conflicts regarding roles, or interpersonal deficits. When abnormal grief is present, the clinician's objective is to facilitate the mourning process by encouraging discussion about the loss while aiding the patient in re-establishing former interests and developing new relationships. For role disputes, such as in marital conflicts, the doctor should strive to guide the patient to a practical plan of action that modifies the problematic relationship or communication style. A common interpersonal deficit is social isolation. Practical suggestions, such as joining a social, religious, or political group; enrolling in night school; joining a cooking class; and taking a vacation with a tour group, may help such patients. Interpersonal therapy is not a replacement for antidepressant medications, especially for those with moderate or severe symptoms. Scheduled sessions may help the patient deal with symptomatic flare-ups at times of stress or anniversaries, thus avoiding unnecessary changes in medication.
2. *Cognitive behavior therapy stems from the observation that depressed patients have negative views of self, world, and future.* The task in treatment is to provide specific "homework" assignments that enable the patient to accumulate information and experiences that challenge their often erroneous negative cognitive sets; these assignments also enable the patient to gain new skills, enhance confidence, and broaden social circles. Homework assignments that are likely to go well should be emphasized so as to enable the patient to overcome fear of failure.
3. *The clinician chooses from a hierarchy of treatments according to subtype of depression.* Table 8–4 conveys recommendations for first-line treatments, second-line treatments, augmenting agents, and maintenance strategies.

As evident, newer antidepressants, such as fluoxetine (Prozac), sertraline (Zoloft), paroxetine (Paxil), venlafaxine (Effexor), bupropion (Wellbutrin), and nefazodone (Serzone), have become first-line treatments for most mood subtypes for compelling reasons. Newer agents have better side effect profiles, which improve compliance and result in fewer requests for alternative medications (which interfere with adequate therapeutic trials); they are significantly more effective in treating depressive syndromes with comorbidity, such as obsessive-compulsive features, anorexia, bulimia, and alcoholism; they appear to be equally effective in treating patients with concomitant anxiety and panic; and they are effective in treating those with atypical features, whereas TCAs and other traditional antidepressants are not. In the elderly or in patients with psychotic depression, the newer agents have not been studied as extensively as tricyclics. Long-term experience with the newer agents is similarly not as extensive as that with TCAs. Note that MAOIs are not emphasized in this table; although they are effective for selected subtypes, their drug and dietary interactions make their use complex, and they are rarely needed in primary care. Their perceived need may signal the value of consultation or referral to a psychiatrist.

In summary, effective pharmacotherapy usually resolves meaningful depressive episodes; reduces occupational dysfunction; enhances quality of life; reduces risk of marital disharmony, separation, or divorce; prevents unnecessary visits for other medical complaints that are secondary to depression; lowers total costs; makes patients more capable of benefiting from counseling and psychotherapy; enhances coping with stressors; reduces the risk of suicide (which exists for many, even when symptoms are mild); and possibly reduces the risk that neurobiologic sensitization and greater risk of recurrences will develop.

Antidepressants must be used in adequate dosage for appropriate durations if they are to work. An appropriate dosage is usually 4 to 6 weeks, *not* 2 to 3 weeks, as was once believed. Patients who respond to the therapy usually do so by 10 to 12 weeks after its initiation. Although practical constraints in primary care settings usually prevent such lengthy treatment trials, *rarely should major treatment changes be made before 4 to 6 weeks of full-dose treatment has been tried.* Recent studies have shown that if patients do not experience at least a 20% improvement after 4 to 6 weeks of fixed-dose fluoxetine treatment (as monitored by depression rating scales), they are unlikely to respond to longer courses of treatment, and switching to an agent of a different class is recommended.

IV. What to do if the patient fails to improve.

Altering the treatment strategy should be considered after 4 to 6 weeks if patients fail to improve, but it should rarely be considered before then. *We recommend that five steps be followed in sequence:*

A. Amplification of dosage.

When patients who are believed to be compliant to treatment have failed to respond, inadequate dosage and/or duration is most often the cause. A logical first step for treatment refractoriness is increasing the dosage. The exceptions to this are nortriptyline, which has a "therapeutic window" of 50 to 150 ng/mL, and TCAs, when plasma levels are known to be increased.

B. Augmentation with selected agents.

1. *Lithium:* the plasma level should be between 0.7 and 0.9 mEq/L, and the augmentation trial should last at least 6 to 8 weeks.

2. *Pindolol [Visken]:* this agent, which has been used to augment SSRIs or MAOIs, should be initiated slowly (2.5 mg/d), then increased gradually to a dosage not to exceed 5 mg three times a day. Although pindolol is a beta blocker, it appears to augment by enhancing serotonin function rather than by blockading beta receptors. A trial of 6 to 8 weeks is recommended. Cardiovascular status should be monitored.

3. *Liothyronine T_3 [Cytomel]:* this agent is preferred, but some clinicians use levothyroxine (T_4 [Synthroid]. Cytomel dosage should begin with 12.5 μg/d, with an increase to 25 μg/d after 3 to 5 days. The dosage can be adjusted to 50 μg/d over 3 to 4 weeks. A trial of 6 to 8 weeks is recommended before the PCP concludes that the therapy is of no benefit.

4. *Phototherapy ("bright light treatment"):* this agent should be considered as an augmenting agent for patients with seasonal winter onset or accentuation and atypical clinical features, such as excessive sleepiness, increased appetite, lethargy, and physical fatigue. Bright light, which often is used as the sole initial treatment in patients with mild seasonal affective disorder, probably acts by increasing brain serotonin function. Alteration of melatonin function may also occur. Case reports indicate that phototherapy occasionally causes hypomania or mania, so the treatment effects should not be underestimated. The treatment is administered by use of specially designed bright light boxes. The patient generally sits several feet from the light box, reading, using a computer, sewing, or performing some other activity. Staring directly into the light should be avoided. Duration of exposure to the light varies with the intensity (dose-response curve). If the light box provides 2500 LUX (the measure of illumination intensity), approximately 2 hours of daily exposure is necessary. If 5000 LUX is provided, approximately 60 to 75 minutes is necessary, and with 10,000 LUX, 30 to 45 minutes daily is necessary. Morning exposure to light (simulating sunrise) is recommended by many but is probably not essential.

5. *Estrogen (Premarin):* this agent should be considered as an augmenting agent for women who are depressed and have undergone menopause. The recommended dosage is 0.625 mg. An additional benefit is increased bone mineralization. Obviously, several other critical factors and contraindications (e.g., history of breast or uterine cancer) must be considered when estrogen is prescribed.

C. Combination of antidepressants.

For hundreds of thousands of patients receiving SSRIs, it has become commonplace to prescribe trazodone (Desyrel), 25–50 mg at bedtime, to help overcome the insomnia sometimes produced by SSRI medications. Such an approach is favored over nighttime prescription of benzodiazepines. TCAs and SSRIs are sometimes combined, but supporting evidence for such an approach remains scanty, and side effects may occur. MAOIs such as phenelzine (Nardil) and tranylcypromine (Parnate) should not be used in combination with SSRIs, because the patient may develop a severe hypertensive crisis. With the introduction of the SSRIs and venlafaxine, MAOIs are less likely to be used in the future than they are now, even though they are effective agents.

D. Switching to different antidepressants.

This step is usually initiated too early in the course of treatment. Premature switching characteristically delays the favorable treatment response that would be expected if treatment were sustained.

E. Referral to a specialist.

Patients should be considered for referral when they have

1. Failed to respond to initial treatment steps and augmenting strategies.

2. Severe suicidal features.

3. Severity of such a degree that psychiatric hospitalization is indicated, such as an inability to care for oneself or a degree of psychomotor retardation that precludes completion of daily responsibilities.

4. Coexisting comorbidity with obsessive-compulsive syndrome, eating disorders, or substance abuse that fails to respond to routine treatments.
5. Psychosis or manic-depressive patterns that fail to respond to routine treatments.
6. Coexisting medical problems or inability to tolerate antidepressant medications.
7. The need for electroconvulsive treatment.
8. Requested referral.

V. Long-term maintenance treatment.

A. Long-term medication maintenance.

For most patients, depression is a recurrent disorder; an estimated 75% or more of patients have multiple episodes. *Unless maintenance treatment is provided, recurrence appears to be the rule rather than the exception.* Untreated, the median number of recurrences over a lifetime is high, approximately five for patients with unipolar depression and eight for those with manic depression. Many untreated patients have 10 episodes or more. The pattern of recurrences varies greatly from one individual to another. As illustrated in Figure 8–2, for many patients, the depression-free interval tends to shorten after each new episode. Bouts of depression often cluster closer together. Recurrences tend to become more severe, last longer, and become more difficult to treat. For all these reasons, relapse prevention becomes critical.

The number of prior episodes appears to be key in predicting future relapses, with the likelihood of relapse over a 2-year span being 75% or greater for those with three or more episodes. *For patients with three or more prior episodes, especially when there is documented genetic predisposition (a family history), older age, or prior history of suicide attempts, indefinite or extended lifetime treatment is indicated* (Table 8–6).

B. Rating scales.

Rating scales can aid the PCP in monitoring progress and in helping sustain patient cooperation during the early stages of treatment. Scores collected over 3 to 4 weeks that reveal decreases in severity can be compiled on a simple graph and shown to hopeless, frightened, sometimes complaining patients or families. The improvement evident in the graph helps to counteract concerns about "no progress" and to allay requests to change treatments. Rating scales also quantify suicidal ideation and provide some degree of medicolegal protection. Self-rating scales are among the best investments that primary care clinicians can make. Samples of several scales are shown in the appendix at the end of this chapter.

Table 8–6
Clinical Indications Supporting Indefinite Antidepressant Maintenance Medications

Three or more episodes
One or two prior severe episodes with
Suicidal behavior
Treatment refractoriness
Psychosis
Chronic dysthymia followed by major depressive disorder ("double depression")
Prompt relapse following prior treatment discontinuation
Strong family history of recurrent mood disorders
Coexisting medical problems or complication of aging that would make a future episode hazardous
Initial episode occurring after the age of 50 y
Personal or occupational circumstances that make any recurrence unacceptable

Each has a slightly different construction, but all are useful in primary care practice.

C. Patient diaries.

Patients with mood disorders often have characteristic monthly (usually premenstrual) or seasonal accentuations. Such chronobiologic rhythms are difficult to identify or monitor without regular assessments. Patients with major mood disorders should be encouraged to keep a daily diary, plotting the severity of depression on a zero to 4 scale, medication dosages (varying with the medication selected), and administration of other treatments. Women of reproductive age should note their menstrual cycle so that premenstrual accentuations can be identified.

D. Return visits.

During acute stages of depression, weekly contacts of standard office visit length are recommended. These visits provide regular opportunities for assessment of progress, evaluation of suicidality, and more timely adjustment of treatment regimens. Frequent visits also reassure the patient and family. Scheduled telephone appointments can be blended with personal brief appointments. Visits of usual length may not be adequate if the patient is severely depressed or suicidal, although such severe patients are usually referred to psychiatrists after the initial evaluation. After patients have begun to improve, appointments every few weeks are generally adequate until the patient is stable. During the maintenance stage, most patients can be seen quarterly or even twice a year, but they should be instructed to call should symptoms return.

VII. What to tell the patient and family.

The social stigma associated with psychiatric illness, especially depression, is steadily lessening, but many individuals, especially elderly individuals or those with little understanding of mental illnesses or brain function, continue to view depression as a sign of weakness or moral inadequacy. Such viewpoints often lead to poor compliance and outcome. The doctor's initial attitude is important in counteracting this perspective. The most effective approach is to convey the diagnosis with forthrightness, factual verbal and written information, and appropriate optimism because mood disorders have favorable prognoses. Pamphlets, audio tapes, or videocassettes are helpful. The term *depression* is preferred to nebulous terms, such as *exhaustion, fatigue,* or *nervous breakdown.* Such labels often interfere with long-term compliance and may actually induce distrust of the doctor (e.g., the patient may question why he or she should take expensive antidepressants if the problem is "exhaustion").

A. What to tell the patient and family in the beginning.

Initial instructions to the patient and family affect long-term compliance and often determine outcome. After completing the evaluation and formulating the diagnosis, the doctor might state matter-of-factly something like the following:

Mrs. A, you have depression. Depression is a common illness, caused by biologic abnormalities in the brain. The usual symptoms include changes in functions regulated by the brain, such as sad mood, abnormal sleep and appetite, loss of motivation, loss of interest in sexual activities, decrease in energy, difficulty concentrating, a sense that things are no longer enjoyable, and troubling physical symptoms, such as pain, constipation, fatigue, and a feeling of being slowed down. Often, people feel so badly they don't want to go on living. Many even have thoughts of suicide. This list of symptoms probably sounds familiar to you because they are the ones you have been having. You can read a bit more about depression in this pamphlet I am giving you.

You and your family will probably be most interested in knowing that depression is very treatable. We are going to get you better. We have excellent new medications that work well and are safe, nonaddicting, and generally well tolerated. Antidepressants take an average of about 4 to 8 weeks to work, but that time will pass more quickly once you start feeling better. The antidepressants also should help with your sleep problems and your (specific somatic symptoms the patient reports, e.g., headaches, stomach pains, appetite problems), so we will try to avoid other types of medications for these problems. Additional medications don't really treat the underlying problem, and in fact, they sometimes interfere with the antidepressants or even make the depression worse. For this reason, I'm going to discourage you from taking any other medications, including over-the-counter drugs. For our next appointment, I would like for you to bring in each bottle of medicine that you are taking so we can review them.

B. What to tell the patients and family about the role of traumatic life events.

We also need to talk about ways to help you cope with the recent stresses that you have been having. It's a major blow for anyone to go through what you have recently experienced (e.g., your separation, a family member who is seriously ill, a financial setback, the recent death of a family member or friend). We have learned that for people with depression, traumatic life events sometimes set off new episodes. I think that is what happened with you. This, by the way, is no different than stressful events setting off bouts of angina or chest pain for those with heart disease; the only difference is that with angina, the stress affects the heart, and with depression, the stress affects the brain.

Together, we will get through this. In fact, once we start treatment, I am confident that you will get better. People who are depressed usually feel hopeless and pessimistic, however, so I wouldn't be surprised if you were a bit skeptical about what I have just told you about feeling better. That pessimism is caused by your depression; it is part of your illness. But hopelessness is not warranted. Please trust me on this, Mrs. A.; you are going to feel better, but you must follow the treatment guidelines.

C. What to tell the patient and family about the specific treatment.

I am going to give you a prescription for (specific brand of antidepressant). The reasons for selecting this agent are that it is effective, especially for your type of depression, and that it has fewer side effects than some of the older antidepressants. You need to take (dosage) of this medication at (frequency). I will write this down for you, and it will also be written on the bottle from the pharmacist. I am also going to tell you about major side effects and give you a written list.

D. What to tell the patient and family about recurrences (after a first episode).

As I mentioned, Mrs. A., depression tends to recur. In some cases, up to 75% of people can expect to have recurrences unless they continue maintenance treatment. This sounds frightening, but you should know that antidepressant treatments are effective in preventing future recurrences. Unfortunately, we don't yet have any laboratory tests or other ways to identify those few people who might *not* have repeat episodes. However, it is premature to worry about whether you will have a recurrence just now because this is your first real episode, but I want you to know as much as possible about this disorder so that we can work together to overcome it.

E. What to tell patients with multiple episodes who ask, "How long can I expect to remain well between episodes?"

It is impossible to predict for any specific patient who has just gotten over an episode of depression how long the patient might feel well before he or she has another episode, but we do know some information. The average time before a recurrence after the first real episode is about 3 to 4 years, but this figure varies a great deal. A few lucky people never have another, a few go 10 to 20 years or more without recurrences, and some have recurrences within a year or two, but the average recurrence without maintenance treatment is 3 to 4 years in the early stages. Unfortunately, the well time between episodes gets shorter with each new episode. We do know that once someone has had three or more episodes, the time interval between episodes may be as short as 1 to 2 years unless some measure is taken to prevent recurrences. You might recall that this is the fourth time that you have had something like this. That is why we are going to want to continue with your treatment even after you feel better, so that we can try to prevent those recurrences. When you get over this episode, we don't want you to have a fifth episode, so we need to discuss now how we will prevent another one by having you continue to take your antidepressant medications indefinitely. Many studies have shown that maintenance treatment works, but I have learned from experience that most people want to stop taking their medicines once they feel better. I need to tell you that for most who have had prior episodes, stopping treatment makes it very likely that the depression will return. It is important, Mrs. A., that you take the pills regularly and at the doses that we prescribe. Once you feel better, I wouldn't be surprised if you asked me to stop your treatment. Should that happen, I'll remind you of our conversation today and tell you again how important it is to continue maintenance treatment. In the long run, taking a few pills every day is a lot better than having another episode of depression. It is just like taking insulin for diabetes or taking blood pressure medication for hypertension. Most importantly, it works.

F. What to tell the patient and family about other measures that can be taken in order to prevent recurrences.

There are many things you should do, Mrs. A., to help keep this depression under control. The most important is to follow your medication schedule, but other things are also important. You should avoid stressful life events, if possible. I know that this is hard, but if unavoidable bad things do happen, look for help from others to cope with them. Don't be embarrassed to talk about these things with your family, and if you feel the need, call me. More extensive counseling or psychotherapy might be worth considering. Keep your sleep pattern regular. If you are planning to take any long trips that require traveling across three or more time zones, discuss it with me beforehand because travel often changes sleep patterns, and changes in sleep patterns sometimes set off new depressive episodes. Don't take any new medicines without discussing them with me first. Avoid excessive alcohol intake and avoid all other types of drug use unless you consult me first. In fact, don't use any medicines, even over-the-counter kinds, such as cold medicines, without discussing with me. I really mean that. Also, develop a regular exercise routine. I know this sounds a little bit like summer camp, but research has shown these things really do help. You can do a lot to prevent recurrences, Mrs. A. If you can include these things into your everyday life, it *will* be worth it.

A summary of nonpharmacologic treatment interventions is presented in Table 8–7.

Table 8–7
Nonpharmacological Treatment Interventions

Individual psychotherapy (e.g., interpersonal psychotherapy, cognitive-behavioral therapy, marital therapy)
Education (e.g., audiotapes, cassettes, films, videocassettes, Internet sites)
Family involvement
Written diary and graphs of clinical progress
Monitoring for key predictor symptoms of relapse
Participation in support or advocacy groups (e.g., National Depression and Manic-Depressive Association [NDMDA], National Alliance for the Mentally Ill [NAMI])
Special precautions during high-risk times (e.g., deaths, illnesses, seasonal changes, travels, surgeries)

VIII. Management of antidepressant side effects.

Side effects or adverse drug reactions are an inevitable part of treating patients with antidepressant medications. Considering the millions of people who are treated with antidepressants each year, medically serious side effects occur only rarely, but they often are discomforting enough to threaten compliance. The following steps aid the clinician in dealing with side effects.

A. Differentiate side effects from depressive symptoms.

Sleep abnormalities, sexual dysfunction, anxiety, agitation, dizziness, gastrointestinal symptoms, fatigue, impaired cognition, and increases or decreases in appetite are common side effects of antidepressants, but they also are core features of mood disorders. *To avoid the trap of considering a symptom a side effect when it is actually a manifestation of depression, the PCP should document the symptom profile before starting a medication regimen.* Self-rating scales completed before treatment help accomplish this.

B. Prevention of side effects by choice of appropriate antidepressant.

The most troubling side effects are often anticholinergic in origin. Happily, they can usually be prevented by initial selection of antidepressants that have fewer and less troublesome side effects than those of the tricyclics. Traditional TCAs, such as amitryptyline (Elavil), and imipramine (Tofranil), and MAOIs, such as phenelzine (Nardil) and tranylcypromine (Parnate), alter many neurobiologic functions and predictably induce many side effects. Newer antidepressants, such as fluoxetine (Prozac), sertraline (Zoloft), venlafaxine (Effexor), nefazodone (Serzone), and mirtazapine (Remeron), are relatively selective in targeting only serotonin and/or norepinephrine and produce considerably fewer side effects, especially of the anticholinergic and antihistaminic types. Because of these characteristics, compliance is higher with newer agents, and fewer patients request medication changes. Thus, when treating patients who are having new episodes, the doctor should generally strive to avoid products that have high anticholinergic potency, such as amitryptyline and imipramine. In patients who are being successfully treated with these agents and tolerate them well, the therapy should not be changed, however. (See Chapter 2 for additional information about the newer antidepressants.)

C. Educate about side effects.

All antidepressants produce some side effects. The clinician should avoid multiple medication changes while searching for an agent that is "free" of side effects because none exists. *The best approach is to start with a class of antidepressant (e.g., the SSRIs or venlafaxine) with the most favorable profiles,* reassuringly informing the patient about the most common adverse effects associated with the agent selected so that the patient is not frightened when side effects develop, and conveying the expectation that side effects are generally manageable. The doctor might say:

Side effects are not severe with this medicine, but some people encounter the following (specific side effects of the medication the patient is taking). The good news about side effects is that they often go away after a little time, and we can often minimize them by adjusting the time when you take the drug or by changing the dosage. Sometimes, we can give specific treatments to counteract them. By the way, side effects are an indication that the medication is taking effect. You and I may not like them, but they indicate that the treatment is starting to fix the chemical imbalances in the brain. I wish side effects weren't there, but keep reminding yourself that side effects are a lot better than depression. So bear with me as we go through the next month or so, because if we try to get rid of all the side effects, then we'll never be able to give you enough treatment so that your depression will go away.

Medically serious side effects associated with TCAs and MAOIs, such as orthostatic hypotension, warrant special—even written—instructions, especially for elderly patients. Pamphlets may help. For patients starting SSRI therapy, the *prospect of sexual side effects should be mentioned* because their unexpected appearance often leads to discontinuation of the therapy, especially with men.

Patients should be told that several steps can be taken to deal with most side effects. In sequence, we recommend the following.

1. *Allowing time for tolerance.*
   Many patients develop tolerance for common side effects over the span of several weeks. Unless adverse events are dangerous medically or interfere with routine functions, patients should be encouraged to allow time for tolerance to develop.

2. *Changing time of day.*
   Changing the time of day of administration often diminishes the severity of side effects; for instance, the agent may be taken at bedtime if sedation is occurring or in the morning if sleep disruption is occurring. Adjusting the time of day the agent is given should be attempted before the dosage is decreased to ineffective levels.

3. *Adjusting dosage.*
   A *transient* decrease in dosage may be helpful in diminishing severe side effects, but this strategy should be used only if side effects are truly troublesome, and only if patients are simultaneously informed that full dosage is generally essential for good outcome and that dosage will be increased again within 3 to 4 days.

4. *Treating side effects.*
   a. *Anticholinergic effects.*
   Dry mouth, blurry vision, constipation, tachycardia, apathy, impaired cognition, and fatigue are unpleasant and poorly tolerated, and they reduce compliance. The major anticholinergic offenders are TCAs, especially amitryptyline (Elavil) and imipramine (Tofranil), and MAOIs. Elderly individuals are especially vulnerable to, and troubled by, anticholinergic effects. Antidepressants are not the only offending agents, so drug-drug interactions must be considered. *Of the 25 most commonly prescribed drugs for the elderly, 14 produce detectable anticholinergic effects. The most notable examples are ranitidine (Zantac), codeine, dipyridamole (Persantine), warfarin (Coumadin), digoxin (Lanoxin), nifedipine (Procardia), and prednisolone (Prelone).* When antidepressants with anticholinergic effects are prescribed for patients receiving such medications, the cumulative consequences can be significant. *Prevention is the best strategy.* Newer antidepressants, such as SSRIs and venlafaxine, have virtually no anticholinergic effects, one of the strongest justifications for their selection.
   If medicines are prescribed that do produce unpleasant anticholinergic effects, the severity of the side effects can be reduced with specific interventions; for instance, dry eyes may be helped by artificial tears; constipation, by exercise and adequate fluid and fiber intake; and dry mouth, by grapes (sucking, not eating) or sugar-free mints. Bethanechol (Urecholine), 10 mg to 30 mg taken three times a day, can be tried for urinary retention. For emergency cases of anticholinergic toxicity, physostigmine (Antilirium), 1 mg given intravenously, promptly reverses severe symptoms, but this regimen requires careful medical monitoring and is probably best administered in a hospital or emergency department setting, rather than the PCP's office. The toxicity may return several hours later, when the physostigmine is metabolized.
   b. *Cardiovascular effects.*
   Orthostatic hypotension, sinus tachycardia, conduction delays, and arrhythmias may occur

with TCAs; hypertensive crises are a rare but serious risk with MAOIs. As with anticholinergic effects, prevention remains the best antidote. Orthostatic hypotension, which is especially troublesome in the elderly, can be alleviated by dosage adjustment, hydration, Jobst (or comparable) support stockings, and instructions to sit for a few minutes and rise slowly when getting up after lying prone. Caffeine should be reduced or eliminated for patients in whom tachycardia or arrhythmias develop.

c. *Somnolence, sedation and fatigue.*
The PCP should allow time for tolerance; emphasize a regular sleep-wake routine, avoidance of alcohol and benzodiazepines, and prescribe medicines to be taken close to bedtime. Judicious use of daytime caffeine may be encouraged, but caffeine intake is accompanied by an increased risk of anxiety, sleep disruption, and cardiovascular symptoms. For those with severe symptoms of fatigue or somnolence, the PCP may consider adding methylphenidate (Ritalin), 5 mg once, twice, or three times a day (but not after 5:00 p.m. so that the patient does not develop insomnia).

d. *Akathesia, myoclonus, restless legs syndrome.*
This is an uncommon but annoying side effect that can usually be managed by avoiding alcohol, limiting caffeine, and experimenting with a change in time of medication administration. Transient dosage reduction may be necessary. Levodopa (L-dopa) combined with carbidopa (Sinemet) or clonazepam (Klonopin) is often effective in alleviating restless legs syndrome if symptoms become severe, but the original antidepressant therapy needs to be continued. Referral to a psychiatrist specializing in mood disorders may be necessary if restless legs syndrome symptoms fail to resolve.

e. *Insomnia, "jitteriness," or tremor.*
These adverse events are relatively common with SSRIs, venlafaxine (Effexor), or bupropion (Wellbutrin), but they also occur with TCAs and MAOIs. Transiently reducing dosage, developing tolerance, and changing time of administration are preferred initial approaches. Although benzodiazepines are often prescribed, it is preferable to administer trazodone (Desyrel), 25 mg at bedtime. Beta blockers may help but are not a first-line treatment. Alcohol is not an effective antidote. Caffeine reduction should be standard management.

f. *Sexual dysfunction.*
Loss of libido, anorgasmia, and difficulties with erection or ejaculation are reported by 20% to 40% of those receiving SSRIs; these effects are generally attributable to changes in serotonin or norepinephrine brain function. Development of tolerance, adjustments in dosage, alteration in time of administration, and avoidance of benzodiazepines and alcohol may improve the problem. If not, cyproheptadine (Periactin), 2 to 4 mg may be given, although this agent may induce fatigue and apathy and seems to reduce the effectiveness of the antidepressant treatment. Males may benefit from yohimbine (Yocon), 5.4 mg taken several hours before anticipated sexual activity, although this is probably uncommonly used in primary care. Several new antidepressants, such as nefazadone, mirtazapine, and bupropion, were designed and marketed to have fewer negative effects on sexual function.

5. *Changing to different antidepressants.*
If side effects are persistent and severe and have not been successfully alleviated by previous interventions, the doctor and patient should discuss instead using an antidepressant known to be relatively free of the most troubling symptoms, usually a medication from a different class. Such changes should rarely be the first step because it prevents completion of a full course of treatment and inhibits good response in many patients. When a change in medication is planned, isoenzyme interactions in the hepatic cytochrome P_{450} system need to be considered. *The dose of TCA may need to be reduced and plasma TCA concentrations temporarily monitored when therapy with an SSRI agent is begun. Venlafaxine has a lower incidence of isoenzyme alterations and is a logical choice in such circumstances.*

IX. Management of special populations and special problems.

A. Women.

Gender is an important variable in mood disorders; it alters prevalence and influences risk times for symptom presentations and treatment decisions. MDD occurs in women approximately twice as frequently as in men, and this difference appears to be genuine rather than a matter of differences in health care seeking behavior or diagnostic patterns. Rates of depression are similar for boys and girls until puberty, when the risk for females increases. Ten percent to 15% of women develop postpartum depression after they give birth (the incidence of postpartum "blues" is as high as 70%), and oral contraceptives are reported to induce mood disturbance in perhaps 5% to 10% of those taking them. The risk of depression associated with abortion appears to be no higher than that associated with childbirth. Postmenopausal women may have an increased severity or a change in the clinical features of their depression, but they do not have an increased risk of new onset of MDD. Pilot studies suggested that estrogen may improve outcomes in elderly women being treated with antidepressants. For all these reasons, the effects of gonadal hormones on neurotransmitter function have been postulated to play a role in the development of mood symptoms, probably by altering the affinity and numbers of neurotransmitter receptors, changing gene expression, and altering other neuroendocrine systems.

When the diagnosis of depression is considered in women, attention should be paid to other identifiable risk factors for women, including a past history of sexual or physical abuse and a current stressful or unsatisfying marriage. Because premenstrual dysphoric disorder (PDD) is common, it warrants special mention. Approximately 3% to 5% of women develop PDD, and many women with MDD experience mood flare-ups in their premenstrual phase, such that PDD is considered by investigators to be a variant of a cyclical depressive disorder. Women with PDD report that several days before or in the early stages of their menstrual cycle, they experience combinations of depressed mood, anxiety, agitation, diminished interest or pleasure, emotional lability, easy tearfulness, and irritability. Symptoms may be severe, but they generally resolve with onset or within several days of onset of menses. Unless diaries and charting are completed, the patient may fail to make an association with the menstrual cycle. Once diagnosed, PDD has been reported to be responsive to treatment with SSRIs (fluoxetine [Prozac] or sertraline [Zoloft]). If a woman is receiving treatment with TCAs and is generally doing well but has some symptoms during the premenstrual phase, the cause may be a change in pharmacokinetics. A transient increase in TCA dosage (by as much as 25% to 50%) can be helpful for such women.

The use of antidepressants in women who are not pregnant or lactating is basically comparable between men and women, but unique differences may warrant consideration. The weight gain associated with TCAs is perceived as a greater problem by some women. SSRIs may have some value for appetite suppression in these patients or in overweight women. Bupropion (Wellbutrin) may be associated with an increased risk of seizures in patients with bulimia, a disorder that is far more prevalent in women than in men. Loss of sexual interest or anorgasmia occurs in both men and women in 30% to 40% of those receiving SSRIs, but presenting symptoms may differ. In all cases, specific inquiries should be made. The use of antidepressants in pregnancy or lactation is not absolutely contraindicated, but MAOIs are not recommended. *TCAs or SSRIs have no well-recognized teratogenic effects, but caution is justifiable because antidepressants do cross the placental barrier. Unless contraindicated by a severe, repetitive prior recurrent pattern, antidepressant therapy should be avoided in the early stages of pregnancy. The anticholinergic effects of TCAs may cause fetal tachyarrhythmias and a neonatal withdrawal syndrome, manifested by tachypnea, tachycardia, and irritability.* Pregnant women may be more susceptible to the usual side effects of TCAs; agents whose serum levels can be more easily monitored (e.g., desipramine [Norpramin], nortriptyline [Pamelor]) should be used preferentially because of the need for increased doses (sometimes by as much as 50%) in some patients as pregnancy progresses. Most antidepressants are secreted in breast milk; unnecessary exposure for the infant should be avoided, if possible (see Chapter 2).

B. Elderly.

Diagnosis of depression in the elderly can be difficult because many depressed patients present with vague, nonspecific somatic symptoms (e.g., physical pains, lethargy, and fatigue), obsessive preoccupations with the past, hostile and demanding behaviors, or the cognitive lapses associated with pseudodementia of depression. Other stereotypic presentations include the cynical, disagreeable patient who is suspicious and somewhat paranoid and the recluse who is increasingly disconnected from family, routine activities, friends, and relatives.

Depression is highly prevalent in the elderly patient with medical illnesses (estimated at 30% to 35% in some studies). Conditions that correlate most highly include cancer, congestive heart failure, myocardial infarction, cardiac bypass surgery, cerebrovascular disease, endocrine diseases, arthritis, chronic pain, and chronic neurologic disease, such as Parkinson's and Alzheimer's disease (see Chapter 12). Depression in the elderly should always be taken seriously and should not be considered an expected complication of another medical problem. To illustrate, depression in the immediate period after myocardial infarction is associated with a death rate estimated at three to five times greater than that for patients with a myocardial infarction without depression.

The evaluation of depressed elderly patients is not different than for other patients, except that particular attention must be paid to the influence of known chronic disease and medications. Tests such as serum chemistries, blood counts, thyroid function, and vitamin B_{12} and folate levels may provide more information than in younger patients.

The selection and dosage of appropriate antidepressants is more difficult in the elderly depressed patient than in the rest of the population. Elderly patients have different patterns of absorption, distribution, protein binding, hepatic metabolism, and renal clearance, often resulting in longer half-lives, higher blood levels, and more side effects. This has led to the folklore of "start low, go slow," in the treatment of elderly patients. This is good practice, but only if therapeutic doses are achieved. The anticholinergic cardiovascular symptoms of tertiary amine TCAs (e.g., amitryptyline [Elavil], imipramine [Tofranil]), such as cardiac conduction disturbances and orthostatic hypotension, are usually more significant and dangerous in elderly patients. Secondary amines, such as nortriptyline (Pamelor) and desipramine (Norpramin), are less troublesome and somewhat safer but often still produce meaningful and dangerous side effects (a fall in an elderly patient often results in a fracture and a deteriorating course). SSRIs may be particularly advantageous for the elderly because of tolerance, dosage simplicity, and safer side effect profile. Sertraline (Zoloft) has a reasonably short half-life, a quality that may offer an advantage for patients taking other medications or facing surgery. Venlafaxine (Effexor) and nefazodone (Serzone) are two new antidepressants with chemical and pharmacologic properties that are different from those of existing antidepressants, and although they have not been studied extensively in the elderly, they may offer the advantages of low protein binding (venlafaxine) and less sleep disturbance (nefazodone). Bupropion (Wellbutrin) has its primary action on the dopamine and adrenergic systems; thus, it is free from anticholinergic, orthostatic, and serotonergic side effects. Methylphenidate (Ritalin) is occasionally used for elderly patients who experience lethargy when treated with antidepressants. We recommend starting methylphenidate therapy at 2.5 to 5 mg in the morning, then slowly increasing (using divided doses) to 10 to 20 mg/d, which often gives an immediate boost in energy in medical or surgical patients who are acutely depressed. Methylphenidate administration after 4:00 p.m. should be avoided because it may impair sleep. Electroconvulsive therapy is occasionally required in the elderly patient who is severely depressed, has not responded to antidepressant therapy, is unable to tolerate antidepressants, or is psychotic or suicidal. These patients have usually already been referred to a psychiatrist because of lack of response.

C. Bipolar patients with prior hypomania or mania.

Some bipolar patients with depression, when treated with antidepressants, may experience a state of restlessness, overactivity, and irritability, often with a lesser need for sleep, boundless energy, impulsivity, poor judgment, and risk taking in financial, social, sexual, and occupational arenas. These hypomanic episodes, although induced by the antidepressant, usually indicate an underlying bipolar condition. The clinician seeking to identify those at risk for medication-induced cycling can look for several "clues," including a family history of manic depression, an onset of first major episode after the birth of a child, a history of substance abuse, a "diagnosis" during adolescence of attention deficit and hyperactivity, and symptoms of psychomotor retardation (versus agitation) and hypersomnia (versus insomnia) during depressive episodes. Should any of these be present, caution and careful monitoring are important in the initiation of antidepressant therapy. *Full-blown manic episodes can occur, but hypomania is more common.* Sometimes, the hypomanic or manic patient shows concomitant sadness, anhedonia, or tearfulness ("mixed" state). For patients with bipolar disorder, whether medication-induced or occurring spontaneously, treatment with mood stabilizers is indicated. For patients with known bipolar disorder who are depressed, lithium (at plasma levels of 0.7 to 0.9 mEq/L) or divalproex (Depakote) should be started 1 to 2 weeks after the antidepressant therapy is initiated so that potential switches are avoided. The mood stabilizers may also help augment the antidepressant response. We recommend that antidepressants be tapered and discontinued in bipolars once the acute depressive episode has resolved and that maintenance treatment be continued with lithium, valproate (Depakote), carbamazepine (Tegretol), or even combinations of these. Alcohol use and caffeine intake should be eliminated in bipolar patients. Antipsychotics need be administered only if severe mania or psychotic symptoms develop or persist. Clozapine (Clozaril) and risperidone (Risperdal) have been reported to be more effective for hypomanic or manic symptoms than traditional agents, such as haloperidol (Haldol). Newer antipsychotic agents, such as olanzapine (Zyprexa), can also be expected to receive widespread use in bipolar patients. In cases in which a "switch" into hypomania or mania has occurred, referral to a psychiatrist should be considered.

D. Mixed (comorbid) anxiety and depression.

Symptoms of anxiety or panic often precede symptoms of depression. Both clusters are present in perhaps one third or more of patients. The presence of anxiety in the face of significant depressive symptoms should not dissuade the PCP from emphasizing the treatment of the mood disorder. Antidepressant medications characteristically resolve anxiety, panic, and depressive symptoms in patients with comorbidity syndromes, whereas antianxiety agents generally fail to improve mood symptoms, and most patients fail to return to normal functioning. The depressive syndrome should be treated, and the associated anxiety or panic tend to dissolve.

E. Rural and financially disadvantaged patients.

For patients in rural areas and those with financial constraints, the frequency of appointments may need to be changed. In such situations, the doctor, patient, and family should develop a strategy for brief, frequent *telephone contacts* in order to monitor progress and compliance. Home nursing, if available, may help. *Self-rating scales* can be completed by the patient at weekly or biweekly intervals and returned by mail. Family members should be incorporated into the treatment plan. In the future, *telemedicine* communication using video cameras, standard telephone lines, and simple computer equipment may enable video observation of selected patients or consultation with specialists in medical centers for complicated patients.

Costs of office visits, antidepressant medications, or psychotherapy may be concerns for patients with limited resources. Practical compromises need to be sought in such circumstances, including the prescription of less expensive generic medications, such as nortriptyline (Pamelor) and desipramine (Norpramin) (both of which are preferred over amitryptyline), but in such circumstances, clinicians should recognize that safety and side effect profiles are somewhat compromised by selection of agents with more troubling side effects. Should such choices be necessary, the doctor must make special efforts to enhance compliance despite the troubling side effects. Lithium, an inexpensive medication, has been shown to maintain euthymia (stable mood) even in unipolar patients, and although it is probably not as effective as antidepressants, it is an inexpensive alternative for long-term maintenance.

Long-term total cost saving actually occurs with newer agents because they are associated with improved compliance, sustained maintenance therapy, prevention of relapse, decreased repeat hospitalizations, better occupational performance, fewer medical complications or symptoms, fewer visits to the doctor, fewer accidents, fewer suicide attempts, and fewer successful suicides. This long-term advantage, although delayed, has been reported to be substantial.

Suggested Reading

American Psychiatric Association: Diagnostic and Statistical Manual of Mental Disorders, 4th ed. Primary Care Version. Washington, DC: American Psychiatric Association; 1995.

American Psychiatric Association. Practice guideline for major depressive disorder in adults. Am J Psychiatry 1993; 150(suppl 8):1–26.

Depression Guideline Panel. Depression in Primary Care: Volume 1. Detection and Diagnosis. Clinical Practical Guideline, Number 5. Rockville, MD: Public Health Service, Agency for Health Care Policy and Research; April 1993. US Department of Health and Human Services, AHCPR publication 93-0550.

Depression Guideline Panel. Depression in Primary Care: Volume 2. Treatment of Major Depression. Clinical Practice Guideline, Number 5. Rockville, MD: Public Health Service, Agency for Health Care Policy and Research; April 1993. US Department of Health and Human Services, AHCPR publication 0551.

Frank E, Kupfer DJ, Perel JM, et al: Three-year outcomes for maintenance therapies in recurrent depression. Arch Gen Psychiatry 1990; 47:1093–1099.

Goodwin FK, Jamison KR: Course and outcome. In: Goodwin FK, Jamison KR, Editors. Manic-Depressive Illness. New York: Oxford University Press; 1990, pp. 127–156.

Greden JF: Antidepressant maintenance medications: When to discontinue and how to stop. J Clin Psychiatry 1993; 54(Suppl. 8):39–45.

Katon W, Von Korff M, Lin E, Bush T, et al: Adequacy and duration of antidepressant treatment in primary care. Med Care 1992; 30:67–76.

Schatzberg AF, Nemeroff CB. Textbook of Psychopharmacology. Washington, DC: American Psychiatric Press; 1995.

Sturm R, Wells KB: How can care for depression become more cost-effective? JAMA 1995; 273:51–58.

Wells KB, Stewart A, Hays RD, et al: The functioning and well-being of depressed patients: Results from the Medical Outcome Study. JAMA 1989; 262:914–919.

Appendix
Self-Rating Scales for Depression

Four scales are listed in this appendix. The Carroll Self-Rating Scale and the Center for Epidemiologic Studies/Depressed Mood Scale (CES-D) are user friendly, whereas the Beck and Zung Scales have been used extensively in primary care research, and they are presented for those who are interested in a better understanding of this scientific literature or want to compare practice characteristics.

Beck Inventory[1]

Next to each question on the Beck is a number: [0], [1], [2], [3]. A total score is obtained by adding the highest numbers marked for each question. The questions all apply to "the past week, including today."

Question 19 is scored other than [0] if the patient answers "No" to the question following question 19: "I am purposely trying to lose weight by eating less." During a subsequent face-to-face examination, the clinician may want to rescore question 19. For example, some depressed patients say that they are trying to lose weight, but on further inquiry, the clinician finds that the amount lost is well beyond the patient's original goal. In this situation, question 19 should be scored as marked.

Example Statements from the Beck Inventory

The patient receives the following written instructions:

Please read each group of statements carefully. Then pick out the one statement in each group that best describes the way you have been feeling the PAST WEEK, INCLUDING TODAY! Circle the number beside the statement you picked. If several statements in the group seem to apply equally well, circle each one. Be sure to read all the statements in each group before making your choice.

The Beck Inventory contains 21 statements. Example items 17 and 19 are duplicated below:

17. [0] I don't get more tired than usual.
    [1] I get tired more easily than I used to.
    [2] I get tired from doing almost anything.
    [3] I am too tired to do anything.

19. [0] I haven't lost much weight, if any, lately.
    [1] I have lost more than 5 pounds.
    [2] I have lost more than 10 pounds.
    [3] I have lost more than 15 pounds.

I am purposely trying to lose weight by eating less. Yes [ ], No [ ]

All items that duplicate the Beck Inventory are reproduced with permission of The Psychological Corporation. For information about obtaining the Beck Depression Inventory, write to The Psychological Corporation, 555 Academic Court, San Antonio, Texas 78204-2498; Telephone 210-299-1061; Fax 210-270-0327.

Carroll Scale[2]

The Carroll Scale is constructed as a fairly direct adaptation of the 17-category Hamilton Rating Scale for Depression. The disadvantage of the Hamilton scale is that a trained person asks the patient questions; in contrast, the Carroll Scale, which has 52 questions requiring yes or no answers, is self-administered.

Each "yes" or "no" answer is scored either as a 1 or a zero and references "the past few days." The total score is a simple addition. The questions on the scale that follows are numbered 1–52.

Yes. When the following questions receive a "yes" answer, 1 is scored: 2–6, 9–14, 16–24, 26–27, 30–31, 33–35, 37–41, 45–52

No. When the following questions receive a "no" answer, 1 is scored: 1, 7–8, 15, 25, 28–29, 32, 36, 42–44

Scoring is simplified by the making of a template on an 8.5- by 11-inch sheet of transparent plastic. The plastic is marked so that when it is placed on top of the patient's completed Carroll Scale, it is obvious which "yes" and "no" responses should be scored 1.

Scoring the Beck and the Carroll Scales

No one cut-off score identifies a patient as depressed or not depressed. The scale scores provide a means of quantifying the severity of depression; the severity score is used by the clinician as a guide for deciding the need for, and the extent of, a clinical assessment of depression and for recommending treatment. The following scoring system guides these clinical decisions.

Severity	Beck score	Carroll score
None or minimal	0–8	0–11
Mild	9–15	12–18
Moderate	16–22	19–25
Severe	23+	26+

Carroll Depression Self-Rating Scale

Patient's Name ______________________________ Date ______________

Answer the following questions in terms of how you have felt in the *last few days,* circle your answers and please do not leave any questions unanswered. Please do not write any comments on this form.

1. I feel just as energetic as always	Yes	No
2. I am losing weight	Yes	No
3. I have dropped many of my interests and activities	Yes	No
4. Since my illness I have completely lost interest in sex	Yes	No
5. I am especially concerned about how my body is functioning	Yes	No
6. It must be obvious that I am disturbed and agitated	Yes	No
7. I am still able to carry on doing the work I am supposed to do	Yes	No
8. I can concentrate easily when reading the papers	Yes	No
9. Getting to sleep takes me more than half an hour	Yes	No
10. I am restless and fidgety	Yes	No
11. I wake up much earlier than I need to in the morning	Yes	No
12. Dying is the best solution for me	Yes	No
13. I have a lot of trouble with dizzy and faint feelings	Yes	No
14. I am being punished for something bad in my past	Yes	No
15. My sexual interest is the same as before I got sick	Yes	No
16. I am miserable or often feel like crying	Yes	No
17. I often wish I were dead	Yes	No
18. I am having trouble with indigestion	Yes	No
19. I wake up often in the middle of the night	Yes	No
20. I feel worthless and ashamed about myself	Yes	No
21. I am so slowed down that I need help with bathing and dressing	Yes	No
22. I take longer than usual to fall asleep at night	Yes	No
23. Much of the time I am very afraid but don't know the reason	Yes	No
24. Things which I regret about my life are bothering me	Yes	No
25. I get pleasure and satisfaction from what I do	Yes	No
26. All I need is a good rest to be perfectly well again	Yes	No
27. My sleep is restless and disturbed	Yes	No
28. My mind is as fast and alert as always	Yes	No
29. I feel that life is still worth living	Yes	No
30. My voice is dull and lifeless	Yes	No
31. I feel irritable or jittery	Yes	No
32. I feel in good spirits	Yes	No
33. My heart sometimes beats faster than usual	Yes	No
34. I think my case is hopeless	Yes	No
35. I wake up before my usual time in the morning	Yes	No
36. I still enjoy my meals as much as usual	Yes	No
37. I have to keep pacing around most of the time	Yes	No
38. I am terrified and near panic	Yes	No
39. My body is bad and rotten inside	Yes	No
40. I got sick because of the bad weather we have been having	Yes	No
41. My hands shake so much that people can easily notice	Yes	No
42. I still like to go out and meet people	Yes	No
43. I think I appear calm on the outside	Yes	No
44. I think I am as good a person as anybody else	Yes	No
45. My trouble is the result of some serious internal disease	Yes	No
46. I have been thinking about trying to kill myself	Yes	No
47. I get hardly anything done lately	Yes	No
48. There is only misery in the future for me	Yes	No
49. I worry a lot about my bodily symptoms	Yes	No
50. I have to force myself to eat even a little	Yes	No
51. I am exhausted much of the time	Yes	No
52. I can tell that I have lost a lot of weight	Yes	No

Center for Epidemiologic Studies/Depressed Mood Scale (CES-D)[3]

The CES-D is especially useful because it is brief, easily self-administered, and scored, and it has broad applicability. Research has identified the 20 symptom items in the CES-D to be consistently accurate measures.

Each item is scored on a 1 to 4 scale, with each number representing a range of days the patient has had the symptom during the previous week (e.g., 2 = some or a little of the time, 1 to 2 days). Only symptom items 4, 8, 12, and 16 are "reverse scored," meaning that 1 is the most severe and 4 is the least severe. This procedure gives the CES-D a range of zero to 60, with higher scores indicating more severe depression.

No cut-off scores have been established for the CES-D. In our experience, the following cut-off scores best approximate the severity stages of depression: 0–9 = none or minimal, 10–16 = mild, 17–24 = moderate, and >24 = moderate to severe.

Center for Epidemiologic Studies/Depressed Mood Scale (CES-D)

Patient's Name ______________________ Date ____________

Using the scale below, indicate the number which best describes how often you felt or behaved this way DURING THE PAST WEEK.

1 Rarely or none of the time (less than 1 day)

2 Some or a little of the time (1–2 days)

3 Occasionally or a moderate amount of time (3–4 days)

4 Most or all of the time (5–7 days)

DURING THE PAST WEEK:

____ 1. I was bothered by things that usually don't bother me.

____ 2. I did not feel like eating; my appetite was poor.

____ 3. I felt that I could not shake off the blues even with help from my family or friends.

____ 4. I felt that I was just as good as other people.

____ 5. I had trouble keeping my mind on what I was doing.

____ 6. I felt depressed.

____ 7. I felt everything I did was an effort.

____ 8. I felt hopeful about the future.

____ 9. I thought my life had been a failure.

____ 10. I felt fearful.

____ 11. My sleep was restless.

____ 12. I was happy.

____ 13. I talked less than usual.

____ 14. I felt lonely.

____ 15. People were unfriendly.

____ 16. I enjoyed life.

____ 17. I had crying spells.

____ 18. I felt sad.

____ 19. I felt that people disliked me.

____ 20. I could not get "going."

Zung Scale[4]

Twenty self-report statements compose the Zung Scale. Each statement is followed by "None or little of the time"(scored 1), "Some of the time" (scored 2), "Good part of the time" (scored 3), and "Most or all of the time" (scored 4), and the patient marks which of these attributes characterized his or her state "during the past week." The scores are most easily placed in the margin, and the value of each item is added for the raw score. The raw score is then converted to a number score from 20 to 100; the number score may be thought of as a percentage. For example, a score of 80 represents the patient as having 80% of the 100% depression measured by the Zung scale.

Zung suggested that his scale may be used as a "depression thermometer."[5] The detection of some amount of depression is but one clue to the presence of major depressive disorder. The results of a clinical examination determine the actual diagnosis. There is no set rule to determine the percentage cut-off score that indicates the need for a clinical examination. We suggest that any score greater than 33% should stimulate a more extensive clinical examination. Scores greater than 50% are highly suggestive of a major depression, and scores greater than 60% are generally indicative of the diagnosis.

Zung Self-Rating Depression Scale

Name ______________________

Age ________ Sex ________ Date ________

	None OR a Little of the Time	Some of the Time	Good Part of the Time	Most OR All of the Time	
1. I feel down-hearted, blue and sad					
2. Morning is when I feel the best					
3. I have crying spells or feel like it					
4. I have trouble sleeping through the night					
5. I eat as much as I used to					
6. I enjoy looking at, talking to and being with attractive women/men					
7. I notice that I am losing weight					
8. I have trouble with constipation					
9. My heart beats faster than usual					
10. I get tired for no reason					
11. My mind is as clear as it used to be					
12. I find it easy to do the things I used to					
13. I am restless and can't keep still					
14. I feel hopeful about the future					
15. I am more irritable than usual					
16. I find it easy to make decisions					
17. I feel that I am useful and needed					
18. My life is pretty full					
19. I feel that others would be better off if I were dead					
20. I still enjoy the things I used to do					

SDS RAW SCORE ____

SDS INDEX ____

Conversion of Raw Scores to The Zung Index Percentage Score

$$\left(\text{Index} = \frac{\text{Raw Score Total}}{\text{Maximum Score of 80}} \times 100\right)$$

Raw Score	Index	Raw Score	Index	Raw Score	Index
20	**25**	40	**50**	60	**75**
21	**26**	41	**51**	61	**76**
22	**28**	42	**53**	62	**78**
23	**29**	43	**54**	63	**79**
24	**30**	44	**55**	64	**80**
25	**31**	45	**56**	65	**81**
26	**33**	46	**58**	66	**83**
27	**34**	47	**59**	67	**84**
28	**35**	48	**60**	68	**85**
29	**36**	49	**61**	69	**86**
30	**38**	50	**63**	70	**88**
31	**39**	51	**64**	71	**89**
32	**40**	52	**65**	72	**90**
33	**41**	53	**66**	73	**91**
34	**43**	54	**68**	74	**92**
35	**44**	55	**69**	75	**94**
36	**45**	56	**70**	76	**95**
37	**46**	57	**71**	77	**96**
38	**48**	58	**73**	78	**98**
39	**49**	59	**74**	79	**99**
				80	**100**

References

1. Beck AT, Ward C, Mendelson M, et al. An inventory for measuring depression. Arch Gen Psychiatry 1961; 4:561–571.
2. Carroll BJ, Feinberg M, Smouse PE, et al. The Carroll rating scale for depression: I. Development, reliability and validation. Br J Psychiatry 1981; 138:194–200.
3. Fischer J, Corcoran K. Measures for Clinical Practice: A Sourcebook. Vol. 2., Second edition. New York: Maxwell Macmillan International; 1994, pp 114–115.
4. Zung WWK. A self-rating depression scale. Arch Gen Psychiatry 1965; 12:63–70.
5. Zung WWK. The role of rating scales in the identification and management of the depressed patient in the primary care setting. J Clin Psychiatry 1990; 51(Suppl):72–76.

9

RANDOLPH M. NESSE, MD

MARK A. ZAMORSKI, MD

Anxiety Disorders in Primary Care

I. Introduction.

As every primary care clinician knows, anxiety disorders are as common as crabgrass. Patients sometimes directly state that they have "nerves," but more often, they complain of fatigue, muscle tension, sleeplessness, nausea, diarrhea, headache, and myriad other manifestations of anxiety.

However, most people with anxiety do not even have diagnosable anxiety disorders. Most anxiety results from what textbooks call "adjustment disorders," and most clinicians call "excessive but completely understandable anxiety." At times, the stimulus causing the anxiety is obvious to the patient and clinician alike. At other times, it is uncovered only after time and effort. Freudian theory notwithstanding, identification of the cause of the patient's anxiety is, unfortunately, seldom curative. Life changes that result from insight can be, however.

II. Epidemiology.

Several estimates have suggested that the rate of anxiety disorders in the population of patients attending a primary care clinic is more than twice as high as that in the general population. This means that *almost a third of patients seeing a primary care physician have an anxiety disorder.* For about a third of those, a symptom related to anxiety is the main reason for today's visit. In addition to patients with a primary anxiety disorder, *many patients in the primary care setting have anxiety as a result of another disorder.* In these patients, anxiety may be a normal response to everyday stresses, major life difficulties, a medical disorder, substance abuse, or another psychiatric disorder, such as depression.

Because anxiety is so common, and because everyone experiences it, anxiety disorders should, by all rights, be simple to recognize, treat, and understand. In fact, recognition takes practice, treatment is only sometimes straightforward, and an in-depth understanding of these disorders eludes most clinicians most of the time. The foundation for the recognition and treatment of anxiety disorders lies, however, in an understanding of the origins and functions of normal anxiety, so that is where we begin.

III. Pathophysiology.

A. What is anxiety?

Anxiety is a useful defense. Just as cough clears foreign material from the respiratory tract, diarrhea clears toxins from the gastrointestinal tract, and pain enables a prompt escape from and avoidance of tissue damage, anxiety is a coordinated cognitive, emotional, physiologic, and behavioral response pattern that helps us escape from current danger and avoid future danger. In 1930, Walter Cannon coined the term *fight or flight reaction* and documented the utility of many manifestations of anxiety. Increased respiration helps to oxygenate the blood and expel carbon dioxide. Increased cardiac rate and output speed oxygen and glucose to muscles and carbon dioxide and lactic acid away from muscles. Sweating cools the body in anticipation of the heat from exertion and makes the body more slippery as well. The effect of adrenaline on platelets increases blood coagulability, and its effect in the liver regenerates glucose so that it is readily available. Although the utility of these physiologic manifestations of anxiety has long been apparent, the utility of the cognitive, emotional, and behavioral changes has been less so, perhaps because these aspects are harder to study.

1. *Anxiety is not a defect.* The key to understanding anxiety disorders is to first understand that *anxiety is not a disease itself, and very often, it does not arise from any defect whatsoever.* It is merely a useful defense. Just as people who lack the capacity to experience pain are usually dead by their mid-twenties, people who lack the capacity for fear would also be expected to suffer early mortality. These "hypophobic" people do not, however, come to clinicians asking for help in increasing their levels of anxiety. Conversely, just as there are people who experience pain in the absence of tissue damage, there are people who experience anxiety in the absence of danger. These people have anxiety disorders.

2. *Anxiety dysregulation and anxiety disorders.* Anxiety is normal and useful only when the right level of anxiety is aroused for the right duration in response to the right cue. Abnormalities can arise at any stage of this process. When anxiety is aroused by a harmless cue, such as a worm, we call the disorder a *phobia.* Excessive anxiety to a cue that is somewhat dangerous, such as a spider, is also classified as a phobia. Similarly, fear with atypical symptoms (e.g., diarrhea, urinary frequency) or fear that lasts too long can be part of an anxiety disorder.

   Complexities arise when clinicians try to understand anxiety that does not seem connected to a particular cue. Although attributing such anxiety to biochemical abnormalities is tempting, it is not clear that these abnormalities are primary. Instead, it seems more likely that in many cases, the brain changes characteristic of anxiety are secondary to higher-level cognitive and emotional processes. When these processes are conscious, for instance, when someone worries about the health of a child, the connection can be understood, although it may be recognized as excessive. When, however, a person experiences fear at the idea of being at a table on which a sharp knife is lying, there may be a link between the person's impulses to use the knife and the fear. When a person experiences anxiety that is free-floating, that is, separate from all cues and thoughts, the simple notion that such a disorder must arise from primary changes in the brain is even more tempting. This is indeed part of the causation in many circumstances. In others, however, the anxiety arises from unconscious wishes or ideas, as evidenced by the sudden relief that sometimes (although infrequently) attends the experience of understanding that kind of connection. This is one reason why an anxiety disorder that is simple to recognize and treat may nonetheless be very difficult to understand.

3. *Causes of anxiety.*
   Anxiety is caused by activation of an evolved defense mechanism. Thus, the cause can be in the environment, in the form of cues that would arouse this mechanism in almost anyone, or it can be an idiosyncratic characteristic of the individual, either in the psychological processing of these cues or in the physiologic regulation of the anxiety mechanisms. These idiosyncrasies can, of course, arise from genetic causes, or life experiences, or some combination.

   In fact, most anxiety disorders are experienced by approximately 15% of the population, who seem to have an extraordinary sensitivity to anxiety (and depression as well) throughout their entire lives. Others, however, are not much bothered by anxiety until the specific onset of a disorder at a certain time in their lives, either after a traumatic experience or seemingly spontaneously. This is of great importance to the clinician. *Treatment for a person who has life-long anxiety of various sorts should be approached very differently from treatment for a person who has not been excessively bothered by anxiety until the current illness.*

   Patients often ask, "Well, doctor, is the cause physical or psychological?" Too many clinicians give a simple answer to this question. The correct answer, in our opinion, is that everyone has a normal capacity for anxiety, that some people are born with a hair-trigger regulation mechanism, and that events in a person's life are liable to set off that hair trigger much more readily in some people than in others. *Thus, almost every anxiety disorder is best understood as a previous disposition that has intersected with a current precipitant.* In short, anxiety disorders always involve physical changes in the brain, but those changes may be from genetic causes, or from life events, or from both.

4. *Anxiety symptoms and the subtypes of anxiety disorders.*
   Is anxiety fundamentally a single tendency that is manifested in different forms in different people, or is each anxiety disorder a distinct disease? This question, although frequently posed, is, in our opinion, a poor one. Each different kind of danger an organism faces gradually shapes a subtype of defensive arousal. Thus, a challenge by another member of the same species, an attack by a predator, and a fall off a cliff all arouse defensive responses. These responses are different in necessary ways so that they protect against each specific kind of danger, but they are also similar because many aspects of the fear response are adaptive in multiple situations. *Thus, the subtypes of anxiety disorder each correspond to partially differentiated subtypes of normal anxiety.* For instance, panic is an appropriate response to any acute life-threatening danger for which fight or flight is an adaptive response, social anxiety is an appropriate response when one's status or group membership is threatened, specific phobias are appropriate when dangerous small animals must be avoided, and post-traumatic stress reactions may, in some cases, be expected sequelae of experiences that nearly lead to death. Obsessive-compulsive disorder (OCD) appears to be, as we shall see, another matter entirely.

IV. Diagnostic overview.

The challenges of diagnosing and treating patients with anxiety disorders in primary care unfold in a five-step process:

1. Recognize anxiety as a possible cause of the patient's presenting symptoms.

2. Determine if the anxiety symptoms result from a general medical condition.
3. Determine if the anxiety symptoms result from another psychiatric disorder, especially substance abuse or depression.
4. If the anxiety symptoms result from a primary anxiety disorder, determine the specific diagnosis and the factors, psychological and physical, that seem to have precipitated the disorder.
5. Finally, select and apply effective therapies, including education, behavior therapy, psychotherapy, and medical therapy.

Given these challenges, it is not surprising that primary care clinicians have not, as a whole, excelled in their treatment of anxious patients. Each of these steps is described in detail below.

A. Recognize anxiety as the cause of patients' presenting symptoms.

This is no small task. As with depression, physicians are slow to recognize that their patients' symptoms are caused by an anxiety disorder. The symptoms of anxiety are almost always multiple, are often somatoform, and usually raise the possibility of at least one other serious illness. Symptoms and care-seeking patterns that may reflect anxiety are listed in Table 9–1. Patients who volunteer one or more of the symptoms of anxiety should be asked about other symptoms. *The more symptoms a patient has, and in particular, the more somatoform symptoms that are present, the more likely it is that an anxiety disorder is present.*

For some of the anxiety disorders, patients readily volunteer their symptoms, even if they do not recognize anxiety as the cause of the symptoms. For other anxiety disorders—particularly blood, injury, or illness phobias; social phobia; or agoraphobia—patients may avoid all contact with the health care system. Others may fail to reveal their psychiatric symptoms because of shame or fatalism about the treatment; this pattern is seen in those with OCD and certain phobias. We have seen, for example, patients who present with severe, refractory hand eczema who do not volunteer that they compulsively wash their hands for hours at a time.

Finally, some patients with anxiety disorders can function well. For instance, a person with a phobia of cats may see no reason to even discuss it with his or her primary care provider. Patients with panic attacks, however, may be reluctant to divulge their symptoms. Given the hidden nature of some anxiety disorders, careful, sensitive questioning is required.

B. Efficiently recognize the very small number of patients who have anxiety or somatic symptoms of anxiety that result from a general medical condition.

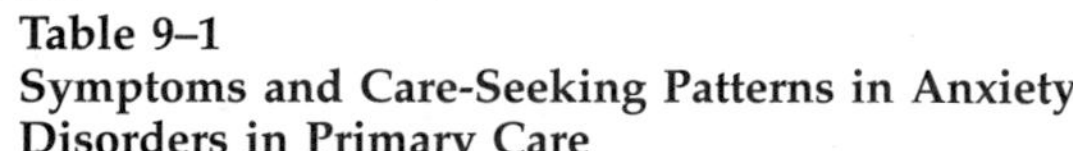

Table 9–1
Symptoms and Care-Seeking Patterns in Anxiety Disorders in Primary Care

Physical symptoms*†
Palpitations
Chest pain
Shortness of breath
Lump in the throat
Dizziness, vertigo, or imbalance
Abdominal pain, nausea, gastrointestinal distress
Pelvic or genital pain
Frequent urination
Sexual dysfunction
Muscular pain
Tremor
Sweating
Paresthesias
Fatigue
Headache
Medical "diagnoses"
Hypoglycemia
Mitral valve prolapse
Care-seeking behavior
Frequent office visits for different complaints
Frequent emergency room visits
Doctor shopping
Psychiatric comorbidities
Substance abuse

*The greater the number of physical symptoms, the more likely it is that an anxiety disorder is present.

†The greater the number of somatoform symptoms (symptoms inconsistent with recognized pathophysiology), the more likely it is that an anxiety disorder is present.

Primary care providers are only too willing to consider a physical cause for a patient's anxiety-related symptoms. Thousands of dollars are often spent on fruitless diagnostic evaluations for symptoms of anxiety. When repeated testing (often of different organ systems) reveals no physiologic cause, patients are sent home with neither a firm diagnosis nor an effective therapy.

Superficially, most symptoms of anxiety can be construed to represent a potentially serious medical illness. The tremor and agitation of the patient with generalized anxiety disorder (GAD) can suggest hyperthyroidism, and the chest pain of panic attacks can mimic ischemic heart disease. At times, a focused medical evaluation is appropriate. More often, the diagnosis of an anxiety disorder is clear from a carefully performed patient history and physical examination. Firm rules about which presentations mandate a medical work-up and which do not are difficult to formulate; we offer several heuristics in their place:

1. *Look for affective content.*
   Simply put, patients with physical symptoms caused by anxiety are anxious. Their anxieties surround not only the concern that their symp-

toms reflect a serious illness but also usually other areas of their life as well. Often, the anxiety strikes the clinician as excessive, and it is often resistant to reassurance. The affective content is usually apparent from body language and the patient's description of his or her symptoms, but several questions and comments are helpful in exploring this area further: "How do you feel when you have symptom X?" "It sounds like these symptoms have been very frightening to you and that you are concerned that they may represent a serious illness." "In addition to your health, what other areas of your life are troubling right now?"

2. *Look for symptom triggers and phobic avoidance.*
   In anxious patients, symptoms are often triggered by certain places or situations. These triggers are usually of diagnostic value. The patient whose chest pain is triggered by exercise may have coronary disease, but the patient whose chest pain is repeatedly triggered by waits in line at the supermarket almost certainly does not. Also characteristic of some of the anxiety disorders is the patient's phobic avoidance of symptom triggers. Patients with stable angina typically continue to engage in activities that trigger it, whereas patients with panic attacks go to great lengths to avoid places and situations in which they occurred. Because some of the triggers may be bizarre and their avoidance shameful for the patient, direct questioning is required: "In what places or situations have your symptoms occurred?" "Have you chosen to avoid those places or situations since the onset of your symptoms?"

3. *Look for multiple symptoms.*
   Patients with anxiety disorders virtually never have just one physical symptom. The more symptoms that are present, the more likely it is that an anxiety disorder is present. In patients who volunteer one symptom of anxiety (see Table 9–1), the clinician should ask about others in an open-ended fashion first, then follow up with a list of other possible symptoms: "What other symptoms do you have when you get symptom X?" "Have you noticed, for example, symptoms Y and Z?"

4. *Look for peculiar symptoms.*
   Patients with physical symptoms of anxiety tend to have somatoform symptoms. These symptoms do not fit into recognized pathophysiologic patterns. For example, intermittent "stocking-glove" numbness and paresthesias are hard to account for pathophysiologically. The symptoms of anxious patients are often hard to describe and characterize. Occasionally, the clinician leaves the examination room unclear as to what precisely the patient was experiencing.

5. *Let epidemiology guide your differential diagnosis.*
   Thankfully for the diagnostician, *anxiety disorders tend to appear in young patients who are at low risk for serious illness.* The young woman with repeated attacks of chest pain is most unlikely to have ischemic heart disease. A positive stress test finding in such a patient is much more likely to reflect a false-positive result than a true positive one, and this fact should be considered before such testing is ordered.

6. *Finally, do not miss the forest for the trees.*
   The reductionism that has proved so powerful for the advancement of medical science may not serve clinicians as well in the diagnosis of anxiety disorders. We see patients who have had negative assessment findings for dizziness, headaches, and chest pain, apparently without the consideration that mental illness could easily account for this particular cluster of symptoms. Anxiety disorders tend to cause symptom clusters and reactions that are virtually unmistakable to the clinician who considers them.

   Diagnostic tests that may be considered in the evaluation of the patient with symptoms of anxiety are listed in Table 9–2.

C. Identify the significant number of patients who have anxiety as a symptom of another psychiatric

Table 9–2
Useful Laboratory and Diagnostic Tests for Patients with Physical Symptoms of Anxiety

Commonly useful tests
Thyroid-stimulating hormone assay
Urine screen for drugs of abuse
Complete blood count and liver enzyme levels (to investigate alcohol abuse)
Follicle-stimulating hormone assay (if menopause is suspected)

Tests that are useful only in selected circumstances
Electrocardiography
Echocardiography
Holter monitoring
Exercise electrocardiography
Coronary angiography
Pulse oximetry
Arterial blood gas determination
Plasma D-dimer level
Imaging studies to exclude venous thromboembolism
24-hour urine sample for levels of catecholamines or indolamines
Abdominal imaging studies
Gastrointestinal endoscopy
Serum chemistry panels
Other thyroid function tests
Computed tomography of the brain
Electroencephalography
Tilt-table testing
Electronystagmography

disorder, especially substance abuse or depression.

Depressed or substance-abusing patients are frequently prescribed benzodiazepines for their anxiety rather than provided with appropriate treatment for their underlying disorder. Both of these disorders are common. Like anxiety disorders, they have distinct therapies; they can be exacerbated by benzodiazepines, and they are potentially fatal. Distinguishing depression from anxiety disorders is indeed difficult, and at times, it defies the skills of the best clinicians (see section XIII of this chapter). Identifying substance abuse can also be challenging; useful strategies are described in detail in Chapter 17. Sadly, substance abuse is often not recognized as the cause of the patient's difficulties, not because of willful deception on the part of the patient (although this does occur), but rather because it was not fully explored by the treating clinician. In a small number of patients with substance abuse, the pattern of abuse may reflect self-medication for symptoms of anxiety. Although this observation is of clinical significance, it should not lead to the conclusion that treatment of the underlying anxiety would eliminate the substance abuse. Instead, appropriate treatment for substance abuse must come first.

D. If the anxiety symptoms result from a primary anxiety disorder, determine the specific diagnosis and the factors, psychological and physical, that seem to have precipitated the disorder.

Once the patient's problem is identified as an anxiety disorder, the differential diagnosis is often not especially challenging. *The Diagnostic and Statistical Manual of the American Psychiatric Association, Fourth Edition*[1] (DSM-IV) identifies the anxiety disorders listed in Table 9–3. The process of differential diagnosis is described in detail in the sections that follow. Significant comorbidity exists among the anxiety disorders, so the identification of a single anxiety disorder should prompt a search for others. For example, 10% to 20% of patients with panic disorder also have a specific phobia. DSM-IV proposes a useful step-wise approach to diagnosis; this approach is adapted as Figure 9–1.

E. Finally, select and apply effective therapies.

Available therapies for anxiety disorders include medical therapy, cognitive and behavioral therapies, and other psychotherapies. Benzodiazepine anxiolytics play a relatively minor role in the management of anxiety disorders. Selection among the different therapies is critical because different disorders mandate the use of very different therapies. For example, behavior therapy is uniquely effective in the treatment of specific phobias, whereas medication is useless. Both behavior therapy and medication help those with social phobia, and patients with panic disorder benefit from these in addition to cognitive therapy. For patients with post-traumatic stress disorder (PTSD), it is not clear that any commonly used interventions offer reliable relief.

V. Overview of cognitive behavior therapy.

A. Overview.

Most clinicians are unfamiliar with cognitive behavior therapy (CBT), the single most effective type of therapy for anxiety disorders. A detailed exposition of the principles and practices of CBT is beyond the scope of this chapter, but the following overview is offered to:

1. Provide practicing clinicians with an understanding of CBT so that they can accurately describe it to their patients.
2. Allow clinicians to select appropriate referral sources for their patients.
3. Permit application of these techniques at their most basic level in the care of patients with anxiety disorders.
4. Stimulate interest in primary care physicians for these powerful techniques.

B. Cognitive therapy.

Cognitive therapy is based on the principle that psychological distress arises, at least in part, from self-defeating, irrational thoughts and beliefs. For example, the terror of a panic attack arises partly out of an inaccurate conclusion that the physical symptoms of the attack reflect a life-threatening illness or that feelings of depersonalization mean that the person is "going crazy." One useful formulation of the cognitive therapy approach has been divided into three phases.

1. *Providing information to the patient on the link between the thoughts and the anxiety response.*
   In the aforementioned example, the patient would be asked to make explicit the implicit conclusions that he or she had reached about the implications of their panic attacks.
2. *Exploring and testing new ways of thinking and "self-talk" that help the patient attenuate the anxiety response to stressors.*
   These can take different forms but consist of a series of self-statements before, during, and after exposure to stresses. In the aforementioned example, these self-statements might take the following forms:
   a. (Before a situation that might trigger a panic attack) "No negative thoughts—worrying won't help. Panic attacks feel dangerous but they are not."

Table 9–3
DSM-IV Anxiety Disorders

DSM-IV Code	Anxiety Disorder	Brief Description
300.01	Panic disorder without agoraphobia	Panic attacks (episode of anxiety and severe autonomic symptoms), at least some of which occur spontaneously, and which are associated with persistent concern about having future attacks, worry about the implications of the attack or its consequences, or a significant change in behavior related to the attacks
300.21	Panic disorder with agoraphobia	As above, but the patient also suffers from agoraphobia, the anxiety about being in places or situations from which escape might be difficult or in which help may not be available in the event of a panic attack
300.22	Agoraphobia without history of panic disorder	Agoraphobia, as described above, which exists in the absence of full-blown panic attacks
300.29	Specific phobia (formerly "simple phobia")	Marked and persistent fear cued by the presence or anticipation of a specific object or situation
300.23	Social phobia	Marked and persistent fear of social or performance situations in which the person is exposed to unfamiliar people or to possible scrutiny by others
300.3	Obsessive-compulsive disorder	Distressing, consuming obsessions (recurrent and persistent intrusive thoughts) and/or compulsions (repetitive behaviors or mental acts that the person feels compelled to perform)
309.81	Post-traumatic stress disorder (PTSD)	Persistent re-experiencing of traumatic events associated with avoidance of stimuli associated with trauma and persistent symptoms of increased arousal
308.3	Acute stress disorder	A reaction to traumatic events similar to PTSD, but limited to 4 weeks' duration
300.02	Generalized anxiety disorder	Six months or more of excessive anxiety and worry about several areas of life associated with several physical or psychological symptoms of anxiety
293.89	Anxiety disorder due to a general medical condition	Prominent anxiety, panic attacks, obsessions, or compulsions due to a general medical condition
291–292*	Substance-induced anxiety disorder	Prominent anxiety, panic attacks, obsessions, or compulsions due to substance intoxication or withdrawal
300.00	Anxiety disorder not otherwise specified	Clinically significant anxiety or phobia avoidance that does not meet the criteria for other anxiety disorders
309.24 (309.28)	Adjustment disorder with anxiety (or with mixed anxiety and depressed mood)	Clinically significant anxiety that occurs in response to an identifiable stressor or stressors

*Code varies according to causal substance.

Adapted from American Psychiatric Association. Diagnostic and Statistical Manual of Mental Disorders, 4th ed. Washington, DC: American Psychiatric Press; 1994, pp. 393–394.

b. (During the attack) "My heart is just beating a little fast—this is unpleasant but not dangerous."
c. (After the attack) "I did it—and I can do it again. I didn't have a heart attack or go crazy and I can remember that the next time I feel panicky."

The patient develops these self-statements in advance with the assistance of a therapist.

3. *Applying the aforementioned responses in stressful situations.*
Obviously, less stressful triggers or situations should be dealt with first so that success can be reinforced. The patient in the earlier example might try imagining being in a place that is currently avoided and trying out the new thought patterns. Gradually, more and more challenging tasks are approached.

Alternatively, panic attacks can be triggered in the office setting—the clinician can help lead the patient through the application of the "script" they have developed together. This strategy is particularly useful with patients who have largely unexpected attacks. A patient whose anxiety is caused by episodes of dizziness could be instructed to spin around frequently in a chair; a patient whose attacks are

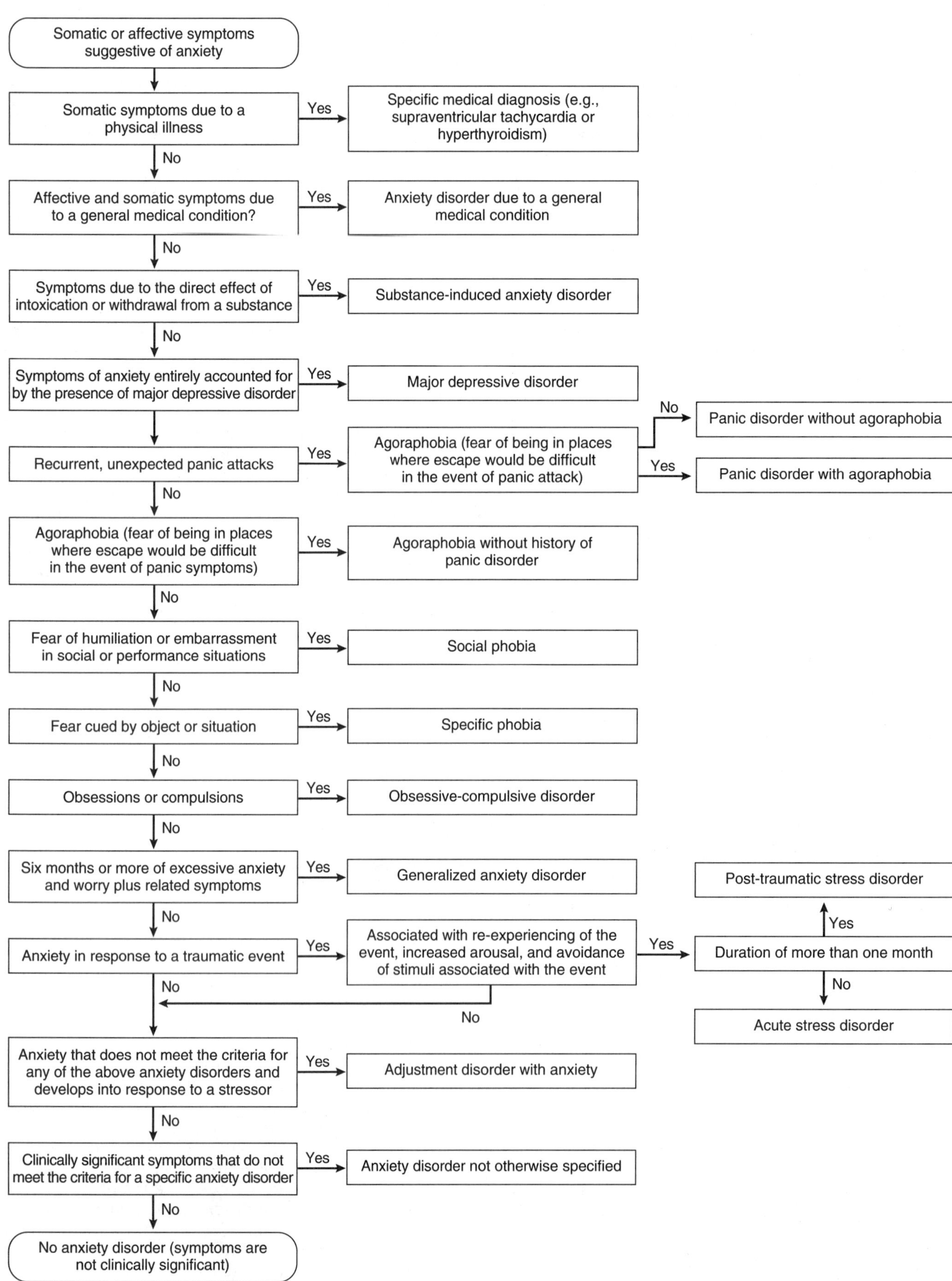

Figure 9–1 *See legend on opposite page*

precipitated by breathlessness or tachycardia could be instructed to climb stairways; a patient whose attacks include prominent symptoms of hyperventilation could be asked to breathe rapidly and deeply. As discussed earlier, the patient can use the new thought patterns before, during, and after the exercise.

These techniques are powerful, and their application to uncomplicated patients is straightforward. As such, the techniques are well suited for use in the primary care setting. In-depth cognitive therapy for patients with more severe or complex anxiety disorders is considerably more involved and is unlikely to be mastered by the generalist.

C. Behavior therapy.

Behavior therapy aims to alter the behavioral response to cues that elicit anxiety. Rather than simply attempting to develop new thought patterns (as in cognitive therapy), behavior therapy helps the patient respond to familiar triggers with different actions. Behavior therapy for anxiety disorders originated with techniques designed to condition a relaxation response to a cue that had elicited anxiety. The expectation was that a person could not be both anxious and relaxed at the same time, and so, with sufficient conditioning, the relaxation response would replace the anxiety response. These treatments involved careful construction of "hierarchies" of anxiety-causing cues, practiced relaxation, and careful attempts to prevent anxiety from arising during the treatment.

Within a few years, however, it was discovered that all the careful attention to the prevention of anxiety was unnecessary. In fact, simple continuous exposure to the anxiety-provoking cue was sufficient to relieve the anxiety, irrespective of whether anxiety occurred. Thus, the principle for most modern behavior therapy of anxiety disorders is *exposure.* Rapid exposure causing high levels of anxiety is called *flooding therapy,* whereas slower treatments are called *graded exposure.*

For example, an agoraphobic patient who has not been in a mall for months would be instructed to go into the mall and wait there until a panic attack occurs, then to stay there for 20 to 40 minutes until the symptoms pass. If the patient leaves the situation during the anxiety, this can make the problem worse—an outcome that is all too common from inexperienced behavior therapists. If the patient is unwilling to get the fear over with quickly, the exercises are changed to whatever the patient will tolerate—perhaps sitting in the car outside the mall for an hour a day. Success depends almost entirely on extended periods of exposure.

Most physicians are uncomfortable with exposure therapy. Although some of this discomfort probably stems from lack of training and experience, much of it seems to come from the idea that these exercises are somehow manipulative, intrusive, or cruel. We offer the following points in response to common misconceptions about behavioral therapy.

1. *"The patient does not really want to change."*
   Although this is true for some patients, the aforementioned approach is predicated on the assumption that the patient has expressed a desire to change. Most people with anxiety disorders want very much to change.
2. *"If the patient wants to change, that's the patient's business—I am not going to tell my patients how to run their lives."*
   Clinicians tell their patients how to run their lives all the time: "Take these medicines." "Go have this test." "Stop smoking." "Don't eat so much fat." "Exercise." Patients rely on clinicians for information on how to live healthful lives and how to alleviate their suffering. Behavior therapy is one way of achieving these goals.
3. *"Exposure therapy is cruel."*
   Although patients can be expected to experience some distress during behavior therapy, administering the therapy is not any more cruel than asking a diabetic to endure daily insulin injections or a depressed patient to experience the side effects of an antidepressant. Patients are willing to accept some discomfort in order to overcome their anxiety and avoidance, and behavior therapy can do just that.
4. *"It makes more sense just to avoid the sources of anxiety."*
   Clinicians see patients who have been told to avoid their phobic objects and situations. This is exactly the wrong approach and is seldom what the patient truly desires. Few patients would willingly choose the shame, humiliation, inconvenience, and anxiety that their phobias occasion—they seek our help precisely so that they may overcome these and lead a less constrained life.

Figure 9–1
A diagnostic algorithm for symptoms of anxiety (somatic symptoms, fear, worry, avoidance, and increased arousal). *Note:* Because of the comorbidity of anxiety disorders with one another, identification of one of these disorders should prompt a search for others. (Adapted from Diagnostic and Statistical Manual-IV, decision trees. Multi-Health System, Inc., Toronto, Ontario, Canada, 1994, pp. 698–699.)

D. Keys to successful cognitive behavior therapy.

Like any therapy, CBT works only if the patient does the exercises as instructed. The following strategies help maximize compliance and effectiveness.

1. *Frame cognitive behavior therapy as a series of "exercises."*
   Ideally, clinicians would be able to briefly instruct their patients in what to do and then have them do it. Although intuitively appealing, this strategy rarely works. It is about as effective as a track coach coming once at the beginning of the season and telling the runners to "run a lot, even when you do not feel like it." Doing those exercises is difficult indeed. Just as patients may feel a bit awkward on initiating a physical exercise program, they may feel similarly about these exercises at first.
2. *Be very specific about assignments.*
   Clinicians' instructions should be as specific as a prescription. They should write the exercises on a prescription form, specifying exactly what the patient has agreed to do, how many times, for how long, and over what time period. The patient should bring the list and documentation progress to the next appointment.
3. *See the patient frequently.*
   Brief, weekly visits to review progress and develop new assignments are ideal.
4. *Contract with the patient for mutually desired behaviors.*
   The clinician should ask the patient to agree to do the exercises as assigned, saying, for example,

   > We've discussed your desire to start driving on your own again and have developed the following exercise, which will move you in that direction. Can I get you to agree to do this exercise as described on this prescription before our meeting next week?

   Written contracting can be used as well.
5. *Refer patients who have intrinsically refractory conditions or those who do not improve during therapy.*
   The minimalist approach to CBT works for many patients in the primary care setting and is especially well suited for patients with panic disorder. *Severely or multiply phobic patients and those with typically refractory disorders, like OCD, should usually be directly referred to a CBT expert* because the minimalist approach is likely to frustrate the clinician and the patient alike.

E. Selecting a referral source.

It comes as no surprise to the practicing clinician that high-quality psychotherapy services can be hard to locate. This is particularly true for behavior therapy. We routinely see patients with anxiety disorders who have received insight-oriented, psychodynamic therapy. These therapies are not reliably effective for anxiety disorders, although they can be useful for other conditions that often accompany anxiety disorders and can clearly be life transforming for certain patients. If the clinician encounters a patient who rejects the clinician's offer of psychotherapy because "it didn't work before," the clinician should inquire as to the nature of the therapy the patient previously received. The clinician can call some therapists in his or her area and ask about their generic approach to such problems as panic disorder and specific phobias. If their treatment skills do not include an approach that the clinician recognizes as CBT, the clinician should keep searching.

VI. Panic disorder and agoraphobia.

Panic disorder is characterized by recurrent panic attacks and their related anxiety and disability. About half of patients with panic disorder also have agoraphobia. These conditions deserve consideration first and in greatest detail for several reasons.

1. Panic attacks are seen in several of the anxiety disorders in addition to panic disorder and are even seen occasionally in many healthy individuals.
2. Panic disorder is common.
3. Panic disorder is frequently not diagnosed promptly in the primary care setting.
4. Patients with panic disorder function poorly, on the average as poorly as depressed patients.
5. Panic disorder is eminently treatable, and the more promptly it is appropriately treated, the easier it is to treat.
6. Patients with panic disorder tend to present to primary care physicians rather than to mental health providers.
7. Many patients with panic disorder receive good care in the primary care setting.
8. The principles of management of panic disorder illustrate well the general approach to the patient with an anxiety disorder.

A. Panic attacks.

1. *Description.*
   Panic attacks are discrete periods of intense fear or somatic discomfort. Attacks begin abruptly and peak rapidly (usually within 10 minutes), then gradually disappear over minutes to an hour. Panic attacks occur in conjunction with several anxiety disorders—these are listed in conjunction with their distinguishing features in Table 9–4.
2. *Signs and symptoms.*
   The signs and symptoms of a panic attack may be nearly identical to those of a myocardial infarction or pulmonary embolus. The patient reports the sudden onset of shortness of breath, palpitations, sweating, chest discomfort, and a feeling of doom. Other common symptoms and the DSM-IV criteria for panic attacks are displayed in Table 9–5.

Table 9–4
Anxiety Disorders in Which Panic Attacks May Occur

Disorder	Distinguishing Features of Panic Attacks
Panic disorder (with and without agoraphobia)	Recurrent panic attacks, at least some of which are unexpected (not triggered by specific places or situations), are associated with persistent anxiety about the attacks or a change in behavior resulting from the attacks.
Specific phobia	Attacks occur in response to exposure to (or thoughts of) a specific feared object, place, or situation.
Social phobia	Attacks occur in only unfamiliar social settings when the patient perceives he or she is subject to scrutiny or criticism.
Obsessive-compulsive disorder	Attacks occur in response to exposure to the content of the obsession (e.g., dirt) or in response to being prevented from carrying out stress-relieving compulsions (e.g., hand washing).
Post-traumatic stress disorder	Attacks occur in the setting of flashbacks of an extremely traumatic event.
Acute stress disorder	Attacks occur in the setting of flashbacks of an extremely traumatic event.
Anxiety due to a general medical condition	Attacks are due to a medical illness, such as coronary artery disease.
Substance-induced anxiety disorder	Attacks are due to intoxication with (or withdrawal from) a mood-altering substance (e.g., cocaine, amphetamine, marijuana, phencyclidine).
None	Up to 30% of the adult population have at least one episode meeting the criteria for a panic attack in a given year. In healthy individuals, such attacks are usually infrequent, are relatively mild, and are not associated with significant anxiety or phobic avoidance.

B. Panic disorder.

Panic attacks do not necessarily mean the patient has panic disorder. In panic disorder, by definition, at least some of the attacks must be unexpected *(uncued),* occurring "out of the blue."

Table 9–5
Criteria for Panic Attack

A discrete period of intense fear or discomfort, in which four or more of the following symptoms developed abruptly and reached a peak within 10 minutes:

1. Palpitations, pounding heart, or accelerated heart rate
2. Sweating
3. Trembling or shaking
4. Sensations of shortness of breath or smothering
5. Feeling of choking
6. Chest pain or discomfort
7. Nausea or abdominal distress
8. Dizzy, unsteady, lightheaded, or faint feeling
9. Derealization (feelings of unreality) or depersonalization (being detached from oneself)
10. Fear of losing control or going crazy
11. Fear of dying
12. Paresthesias (numbness or tingling sensations)
13. Chills or hot flushes

American Psychiatric Association. Diagnostic and Statistical Manual of Mental Disorders, 4th ed. Washington, DC: American Psychiatric Press; 1994, p. 395.

Some of the attacks may be *situationally bound* (always occurring predictably under certain circumstances) or *situationally predisposed* (occurring more frequently in certain circumstances).

In order to merit the diagnosis of panic disorder, patients must have not only recurrent, unexpected panic attacks but also one of the following:

1. Persistent concern about having additional attacks.
2. Worry about the implications of the attack or its consequences.
3. Significant change in behavior related to the attacks.

Two distinct forms of panic disorder are seen, namely panic disorder with agoraphobia and panic disorder without agoraphobia.

C. Agoraphobia.

The formal criteria for agoraphobia—the anxiety or avoidance of places from which escape might be difficult (or help unavailable) in the event of a panic attack or panic symptoms—are shown in Table 9–6.

D. Epidemiology.

Five percent of men and up to 12% of women have panic disorder and/or agoraphobia at some

Table 9–6
Simplified Criteria for Agoraphobia

1. The patient experiences anxiety about being in places or situations from which escape might be difficult or embarrassing or in which help may not be available in the event of panic symptoms.
2. The situations are avoided or else are endured with marked distress or with anxiety about having panic symptoms or require the presence of a companion.
3. The anxiety and phobic avoidance are not better accounted for by another mental disorder.

American Psychiatric Association. Diagnostic and Statistical Manual of Mental Disorders, 4th ed. Washington, DC: American Psychiatric Press; 1994, pp. 396–397.

time during their lifetime. In a 6-month period, panic or agoraphobia is present in 3% of men and 7% of women. Agoraphobia develops in about 50% of people with panic disorder. Good estimates for the lifetime risk of agoraphobia without a history of panic disorder are not available, but experienced clinicians find the presence of panic attacks in more than 90% of people who report having agoraphobia. The age at onset can be in childhood, but the peak is in the early twenties, with first onset rare after the age of 45.

Family and twin studies show that the risk for panic disorder in a first-degree relative of someone with panic disorder is three to five times that of the risk in the general population. Thus, a vulnerability to panic disorder is a strongly inherited trait. It is common for a patient with panic disorder to have first-degree relatives who also have panic or agoraphobia. Of course, just as the patient often has hidden the disorder, parents and siblings may have as well. Quite often, we ask patients who are skeptical about the diagnosis of panic disorder and agoraphobia to question their relatives. On inquiry, they then learn long-hidden family secrets, about, for instance, why mother never drove or father was never willing to go shopping.

No specific gene that causes panic disorder has yet been found, but the search continues. Whether panic disorder results from a discrete genetic abnormality or whether patients with panic disorder are just at one extreme of a continuum of susceptibility to panic attacks remains an unanswered question.

E. Comorbidities.

Panic disorder (with and without agoraphobia) is commonly seen in conjunction with several other psychiatric illnesses. Major depressive disorder is seen in 50% to 65% of patients with panic disorder, with the onset of depression occurring after the onset of panic disorder in most cases. Panic attacks can also be a symptom of major depression, occurring in about a third of patients. *Substance abuse* (particularly *alcohol abuse*) is seen in about 20% of patients with panic disorder. Other anxiety disorders also often coexist; the following comorbidities are commonly seen: *social phobia* (15% to 30%), *OCD* (8% to 10%), *specific phobia* (10% to 20%), and *GAD* (25%). These figures probably overstate the actual comorbidity seen in primary care because they were developed from a clinical sample of severely agoraphobic patients. Nevertheless, the diagnosis of panic disorder (or any anxiety disorder) should prompt questioning about possible comorbidities.

F. Pathophysiology.

The mechanisms that cause panic symptoms are yielding, albeit slowly, to research. At one time, people thought that symptoms resulted from a surge of epinephrine from the adrenal medulla, but some studies have shown no epinephrine increase whatsoever during a spontaneous panic attack. Attention has now turned to the sympathetic nervous system and to peptides like cholecystokinin and corticotropin-releasing factor as possible mediators of panic symptoms.

A large body of literature on substances that provoke panic attacks in susceptible subjects, but not so frequently in control subjects, has looked at lactate, yohimbine, isoproterenol, and many other substances. It is now clear that patients with panic disorder are much more likely (about 80% in many studies) than control subjects (about 20%) to have panic attacks in response to administration of these agents. It remains somewhat unclear whether physiological or psychological mechanisms are more important in precipitating panic attacks. In one recent demonstration, a 2-minute explanation of the expected effects of the drug caused panic symptoms in patients to decrease to almost the same levels as those in control subjects.

Panic symptoms often "spiral" from minimal symptoms only subliminally perceived to a full-blown panic attack. In one especially dramatic experiment, subjects were connected to an electrocardiograph and told that the beeps they heard represented their heart beats. Irrespective of their heart rate, the beeps were increased in frequency. In normal subjects, this slowed the heart rate, whereas in many patients with panic disorder, tachycardia and a full-blown panic attack promptly occurred.

G. Medical differential diagnosis.

1. *Coronary ischemia.*
   Some symptoms of a panic attack that are useful in differentiating it from cardiopulmonary pathology include the patient's feeling that he or she might do something wild and uncontrolled (like jump out of a moving car), the sense of thought racing that makes many patients think they are "going crazy," and the subjective sensation of choking or difficulty swallowing. In fact, however, when a patient

presents with the very first episode of panic, medical evaluation is necessary in order to rule out other pathology. In most cases, a careful history and physical are all that is required.

The most important clues in differentiating a panic attack from cardiopulmonary pathology, however, come from the demographics and the history of the patient. If the patient is a woman younger than 25 years, the chances that the episodes are panic attacks are high. In a person who has a first episode after the age of 50 years, the chances are overwhelming that the cause is something other than a panic attack. Equally valuable is a prior history. Most patients with panic attacks have had similar attacks many times before. Furthermore, the time pattern of a panic attack is characteristic. The symptoms of panic start very suddenly, rise to a peak within 10 seconds to 10 minutes, and then gradually fade over a period of 10 minutes to an hour. An episode that builds gradually over hours, or that lasts for hours, or that goes away suddenly, is not a panic attack.

Important evidence against a medical cause of panic symptoms is the presence of agoraphobia. The clinician should ask if the patient is uncomfortable in grocery store lines, in traffic jams, while riding in a car with someone else driving, or while shopping in large malls or department stores. The patient with cardiopulmonary disease wonders why the clinician is asking these questions, whereas the person with panic disorder with agoraphobia is astonished that the clinician could guess his or her secret.

2. *Pulmonary embolism.*
   Pulmonary embolism can be indistinguishable from a panic attack and, given its potentially life-threatening nature, should be considered in all patients who present with their first panic attack. Obviously, shortness of breath is a prominent feature of the attack. Women taking oral contraceptives are at increased risk for pulmonary embolism, as are pregnant women or those who have just given birth, so these risk factors should be elicited. Most patients with a pulmonary embolism do *not* have signs or symptoms of deep vein thrombosis, so the absence of such cannot be interpreted as being entirely reassuring.

   Pulse oximetry is a good screening test for significant pulmonary embolism. Patients with a panic attack have oxygen saturations of 99% to 100% because of hyperventilation. Values less than this range should prompt determination of arterial blood gases, plasma D-dimer level, or appropriate imaging tests if suspicion of pulmonary embolism persists.

3. *"Hypoglycemia."*
   Most patients with panic disorder are misdiagnosed at first. Some are told that they have hypoglycemia and begin eating very strict diets. When the diet is ineffective, they make the diet still more strict, imagining that some offending food is causing the continuing attacks.

4. *Mitral valve prolapse.*
   Other patients are told they have mitral valve prolapse. Indeed, mitral valve prolapse is a bit more common in patients with panic disorder than in control subjects, but there is no evidence that it causes the disorder. In fact, it seems more likely that the possible sympathetic stimulation associated with panic disorder causes the increased contractility that is the cause of the ballooning mitral valve seen on echocardiography. Excessive attention to mitral valve pathology in patients with panic disorder is often an iatrogenic cause of further anxiety.

5. *Pheochromocytoma.*
   Many patients with panic disorder undergo extensive and frustrating work-ups for possible pheochromocytoma. In a controlled study, however, 32 of 33 patients with true pheochromocytoma did not show manifestations of panic disorder. This is the same prevalence of panic disorder as would be expected in the general population. Patients who have headaches, hypertension, flushing, and tachycardia need a pheochromocytoma work-up. *In patients who have typical symptoms of panic disorder, such a work-up is unnecessary.* If the work-up is pursued, it will likely be found that the urinary levels of catecholamine metabolites are about twice normal levels, as is typical for patients with anxiety disorder. In the presence of panic symptoms, insignificant laboratory abnormalities must not lead to further unnecessary evaluations.

6. *Ménière's syndrome/vestibular neuronitis.*
   Many patients with panic disorder have episodes of dizziness as part of their episode, and sometimes between episodes as well. Sometimes, this is true vertigo and leads to the diagnosis of Ménière's disease, labyrinthitis, or vestibular neuritis. The behavioral treatments for such dizziness, now becoming more common in otorhinolaryngology clinics, are effective, but it is a shame when an underlying panic disorder is not appropriately diagnosed and treated.

7. *Temporal lobe epilepsy.*
   Patients with temporal lobe epilepsy experience unusual mental states, but they are usually distinct from panic attacks. Useful distinguishing factors include the time course of symptoms (more abrupt onset and termination), symptoms that are not typical of panic

attacks (e.g., feelings of déjà vu), and, of course, the lack of prominent anxiety and phobic avoidance.

8. *Cardiac arrhythmias.*
   In the cardiology clinic, patients with panic attacks often undergo Holter monitoring, the results of which sometimes show sinus tachycardia or more ventricular premature complexes than would otherwise be expected. This is rarely of clinical consequence. On very rare occasions, patients present with paroxysmal supraventricular tachycardia. This problem obviously needs to be treated, but in some patients, it recurs much less frequently after appropriate treatment for panic disorder.
9. *Thyroid disease.*
   Hyperthyroidism is commonly considered in patients who present with panic attacks. Although hyperthyroidism can cause some anxiety symptoms (e.g., palpitations, sweating, diarrhea), true panic attacks are not ordinarily seen. Typically, however, patients have enough anxiety symptoms between their panic attacks that hyperthyroidism is worth ruling out with a thyroid-stimulating hormone assay.
10. *Esophageal spasm.*
    Occasionally, a patient presents with a main symptom of esophageal spasm. When treated for panic disorder, many of these patients get good relief from their symptoms.
11. *Bowel and bladder disorders.*
    Some patients have panic attacks manifested primarily by bowel or bladder urgency, rarely with loss of control. These patients typically have other symptoms of panic disorder as well and typical panic disorder treatments are often effective.
12. *Asthma.*
    Asthma is common in young adults, and its presentation may be subtle. Clues to the presence of asthma are initiation by typical triggers and by the presence of cough. Panic disorder often worsens when the patient is treated with beta-adrenergic agonists.
13. *Caffeine.*
    Caffeine is a surprisingly common cause of, or contributor to, anxiety symptoms. Although most patients with panic disorder avoid coffee completely because it causes palpitations and other symptoms of anxiety, other patients may drink three pots of freshly brewed coffee before noon and then continue for the rest of the day, wondering all the while why they keep having attacks of anxiety. Weaning patients from such high doses of caffeine can take months and require supportive treatment and headache relief, but in such cases, this strategy is the key to relieving the anxiety. In our view, one to three caffeinated beverages a day is unwise but acceptable for patients with panic disorder, but any more than three servings daily requires a tapering before treatment for panic disorder is likely to be effective.

In short, the mistake of not recognizing panic attacks and pursuing some other medical cause for the symptoms is common, whereas the mistake of failing to recognize another medical cause when the diagnosis is actually panic disorder is relatively uncommon.

H. Psychiatric differential diagnosis.

The first step is to recognize that the patient is having panic attacks. If the patient is having panic attacks, the clinician should elicit the characteristic reactions of panic disorder, namely worry about having future attacks, worry about the implications of the attacks or their consequences, or significant change in the patient's behavior because of the attacks. If these are present, the patient has panic disorder. If these are absent, the possibility of another psychiatric disorder (particularly *social phobia, specific phobia, PTSD,* or *substance abuse*) should be considered. If patients have had a few panic attacks without evidence of panic disorder or another psychiatric disorder, the clinician should reassure them that uncomplicated panic attacks occasionally occur in healthy individuals.

Panic disorder with agoraphobia can present special diagnostic challenges. In particular, it can be difficult to distinguish from a *specific phobia* when the trigger is a situation (e.g., driving, heights, bridges) that is characteristic of agoraphobia. Patients with panic disorder usually avoid several situations and places. Usually, the phobic avoidance can be traced to a specific panic attack in a particular circumstance. Finally, intercurrent anxiety in patients with panic disorder is often related to fear of having another panic attack. By simply asking, the clinician can determine if the patient feels that the anxiety is mostly fear of panic or if it is also about other matters.

If criteria for both panic disorder and another psychiatric disorder are met, both conditions may be diagnosed. The major pitfall is the failure to distinguish between an occasional panic attack, which may occur in many psychiatric disorders (see Table 9–4), and the recurrent, unexpected panic attacks and associated anxiety and avoidance that characterize panic disorder.

I. Treatment.

1. *Therapeutic overview.*
   The treatment of panic disorder begins with a thorough explanation of the nature of the disorder. For perhaps one of 10 patients, a simple explanation that the symptoms are normal and useful manifestations of a fight or flight response that

is occurring at the wrong time relieves the fears, interrupts the cycle of anxiety, and puts an end to the disorder. For most patients, however, such an explanation is not sufficient.

For patients with more significant symptoms, CBT and medication therapy, alone and in combination, are effective. CBT has the advantage of providing long-lasting benefit after 8 to 15 hours of clinician contact time. The cost (several hundred dollars or more) is balanced against the long-term costs of often expensive medications and their associated side effects, complications, and follow-up visits. If for no other reason, this economic reality makes CBT the superior alternative for patients who accept it.

All patients benefit to some degree from carefully selected patient education materials. In others, bibliotherapy and support groups (Table 9–7) may be helpful. The value of these self-help approaches has not been rigorously evaluated, but we regularly encounter patients who find them useful.

2. *A cognitive behavioral approach to panic disorder.*
The core principle of CBT for panic disorder is simplicity itself. When patients stay for extended periods in a situation that provokes panic attacks, the ability of that situation to provoke panic attacks in the future is decreased. If, however, patients do what comes naturally, namely, running immediately away from a situation that causes panic, the likelihood of panic on subsequent exposure increases. Telling patients to visit a shopping center and stay until they have a panic attack is, as you might guess, not helpful. In fact, it may exacerbate the disorder. Telling patients to avoid situations that cause attacks usually makes the fear worse. Furthermore, helping patients to relax or otherwise trying to ward off attacks is usually counterproductive.

We have found that the CBT approach described in section V can be standardized to a considerable degree, with good results. In one of our settings, we offer a course that meets for 2 hours a week for 6 weeks. During the course, patients learn about the nature of the disorder and the nature of behavior and other therapies, and they commit themselves, each week, to specific behavioral exercises. The next week, they report on compliance and on progress. The other members of the group are often simultaneously more supportive and more firm than the therapist in setting and enforcing expectations, and this leads to vast improvement for many patients. Framing the therapy as a class and not as psychotherapy or counseling appears to help make this valuable intervention acceptable to patients.

Agoraphobia and panic are generally treated together, with exposure being to the very situations the person avoids. In almost all circumstances, the patient avoids the situation because he or she is fearful about having a panic attack there. This can be somewhat awkward when the cue is driving on the expressway, but by increasing exposure gradually, we find that behavioral therapy can be safe and effective even in these circumstances when it is carried out by an experienced clinician.

This treatment is effective indeed. For as many as half of patients, this treatment is entirely sufficient, and 80% to 90% of patients get substantial benefit. Furthermore, relapse is less likely after cognitive behavioral treatment than after medical treatments. Whether performed on an individual basis or as a group, about 8 to 15 hours of contact between the therapist and the patient over several months is usually sufficient.

3. *Medications.*
Medications are appropriate and effective treatments for panic and agoraphobia in many instances. We use them when CBT has proved insufficiently effective, in patients with concurrent depression, in patients who simply do not cooperate with behavioral treatment, and in patients for whom high-quality CBT is not available or accessible. Our impression for primary care patients is that medications usually end up being chosen over CBT, irrespective of what treatment would be best for the individual patient.
   a. *First-line medications.*
   We consider antidepressant medications the drugs of first choice for the pharmacologic treatment of panic disorder. The characteristics of these and other useful antianxiety agents are summarized in Table 9–8. The selection of a particular agent should be guided by considerations of side effect profile, coexisting medical conditions, psychiatric comorbidities, provider familiarity, and cost. The *tricyclic antidepressants* (TCAs) and newer *selective serotonin reuptake inhibitors* (SSRIs) both appear to be effective. Although consistent therapeutic superiority of SSRIs to TCAs has not been established, it is clear that SSRIs are better tolerated and safer, albeit usually more costly. *Monoamine oxidase inhibitors* (MAOIs) are effective in treating panic disorder, but they are not considered first-line therapies (see Alternative Therapies).
      (1) *Tricyclic antidepressants.*
      Which agent is best? *Imipramine* (Tofranil) works well for many patients, but it has anticholinergic and antihistaminic side effects that are bothersome to many people. Its low cost ($5 to $15/mo) makes it appealing to patients who do not have prescription drug coverage. Many clinicians have tried using *desipramine* (Norpramin) as an alternative because it has fewer anticholinergic

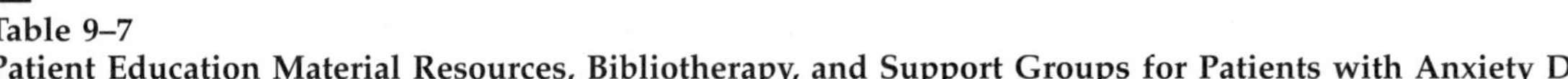

Table 9–7
Patient Education Material Resources, Bibliotherapy, and Support Groups for Patients with Anxiety Disorders

Disorder	Source of Patient Education Resources	Books for Patients and Families	Support Groups
All disorders	National Institute of Mental Health (NIMH) 5600 Fisher's Lane, Room 7C-02 Rockville, MD 20857 (301) 443-4513 Especially useful materials: "Anxiety Disorders" NIH-94-3879 "Medications" DHHS Publication no. [ADM] 92-1509 (on the use of psychiatric medications) NIMH automated fax service: (301) 443-5158	Barlow DH, Craske MG. Mastery of Your Anxiety and Panic. New York: Center for Stress and Anxiety Disorders, University of Albany, State University of New York; 1989 Greist JH, Jefferson JW, Marks IM. Anxiety and Its Treatment. New York: Warner Books; 1986	Anxiety Disorders Association of America (ADAA) 6000 Executive Blvd., Suite 513 Rockville, MD 20852-4004 (301) 231-8368 National Anxiety Foundation 3135 Custer Drive Lexington, KY 40517 (800) 755-1576
Panic Disorder	National Institute of Mental Health Panic Information Line: (800) 64-PANIC Especially useful materials: "Panic Disorder" NIH-93-3508 (available in Spanish [SP-92-1869]) "Understanding Panic Disorder" NIH-93-3509 "Getting Treatment for Panic Disorder: Information for Patients, Families, and Friends" NIH-94-3642	Beckfield DF. Master Your Panic . . . and Take Back Your Life! San Luis Obispo, CA: Impact Publishers; 1994 Handly R, Neff P. Anxiety and Panic Attacks. New York: Fawcett-Crest; 1985	National Alliance for A.I.M. (Agoraphobics in Motion) 1729 Crooks Road Royal Oak, MI
Phobias	Phobia Society of America P.O. Box 2066 Rockville, MD 20852-2066	Peurifoy RZ. Anxiety, Phobias, and Panic. (A Workbook) Citrus Heights, CA: Lifeskills; 1992 Marshal JR. Social Phobia: From Shyness to Stage Fright. New York: Basic Books; 1994	Phobia Society of America P.O. Box 2066 Rockville, MD 20852-2066 Phobics Anonymous P.O. Box 1180 Palm Springs, CA 92263 (619) 322-COPE
Obsessive-compulsive disorder	National Institute of Mental Health Panic Information Line: (800) 64-PANIC (offers information on OCD as well as panic) Especially useful pamphlet: "Obsessive-compulsive disorder" NIH-94-3755	Baer L. Getting Control: Overcoming Your Obsessions and Compulsions. Boston: Little, Brown & Co.; 1991 Livingston B. Learning to Live with Obsessive-Compulsive Disorder. Milford, CT: OCD Foundation, 1989	Obsessive-Compulsive Foundation P.O. Box 70 Milford, CT 06460 (203) 878-5669 Dean Foundation Obsessive-Compulsive Information Center 8000 Excelsior Dr., Suite 302 Madison, WI 53717-1915 (608) 836-8070
Post-traumatic stress disorder	Rape, Incest, and Abuse National Network (RIANN): (800)-656-HOPE (automatically connects the caller to a support agency in his or her community)	Ledray LE. Recovering from Rape, second edition. New York: H. Holt; 1994 (for survivors of sexual assault)	Rape, Incest, and Abuse National Network: (800)-656-HOPE (automatically connects the caller to a support agency in his or her community)

side effects, but it is even more likely than imipramine to cause the single most common and most difficult to manage complication of treatment of panic disorder, namely, intense agitation in the first few days after the medication therapy is started.

After their first dose of an antidepressant, 10% to 40% of patients experience racing thoughts, sweating, pacing, insomnia, and generalized agitation that lead them to call the doctor in a state of high frustration. This outcome can be minimized by (1) choosing an agent that is less likely to cause these effects, (2) starting at very low dosages for the first week (e.g., 10 mg of a tricyclic an-

Table 9–8
Medications Useful in the Treatment of Anxiety Disorders

Medication	Usual Starting Dose	Typical Therapeutic Dose	Typical Cost per Month*	Contraindications	Important Class Side Effects	Advantages	Disadvantages
Tricyclic antidepressants (TCAs)				Glaucoma, Cardiac conduction abnormalities, High suicide risk	Anticholinergic: Dry mouth, Constipation, Blurred vision; Orthostatic hypotension, Weight gain, Somnolence	Some are inexpensive, Long history of use, Treats comorbid depression, Not habit forming	Slow onset of action, May be fatal in overdose, Annoying side effects
Imipramine (Tofranil)	10–25 mg hs	150–300 mg/d	$5				
Desipramine (Norpramin)	10–25 mg hs	150–300 mg/d	$30				
Amitriptyline (Elavil)	10–25 mg hs	150–300 mg/d	$5				
Nortriptyline (Pamelor)	10–25 mg hs	50–125 mg/d	$60				
Clomipramine (Anafranil)	25 mg qhs	100–250 mg/d	$85	As for TCAs	Same as TCAs	As for TCAs, Effective in OCD	As for TCAs, Somewhat expensive
Serotonin-specific reuptake inhibitors (SSRIs)				Use of MAOI within prior 21 days	Somnolence, Agitation, Sweating, Nausea, Anorexia, Sexual dysfunction	Treats comorbid depression, Not habit forming, Well tolerated in most patients	Less published experience compared with use in anxiety disorders, Slow onset of action, Expensive, particularly at higher doses
Fluoxetine (Prozac)	10–20 mg qa.m.	20–80 mg/d	$65				
Paroxetine (Paxil)	20 mg qd	20–60 mg/d	$55				
Sertraline (Zoloft)	50 mg qd	50–200 mg/d	$60				
Fluvoxamine (Luvox)	50 hs	100–300 mg/d	$115				
Nefazedone (Serzone)	100 mg bid	300–600 mg/d	$50				
Venlafaxine (Effexor)	37.5 mg bid	75–375 mg/d	$55		As for SSRIs, Constipation	As for SSRIs, Effective in OCD	As for SSRIs, Can cause hypertension
Monoamine oxidase inhibitors (MAOIs)				Inability to comply with dietary restrictions	Orthostatic hypotension, Insomnia,Agitation, Weight gain, Serious drug-food and drug-drug interactions	Effective in OCD and social phobia, Treats comorbid depression, Not habit forming	Need for dietary and medication restrictions, Slow onset of action, Not inexpensive, Annoying side effects
Phenelzine (Nardil)	15 mg bid	45–90 mg/d	$45				
Tranylcypromine (Parnate)	10 mg bid	10–60 mg/d	$40				
Isocarboxazid (Marplan)	10 mg bid	10–30 mg/d	$50				
Benzodiazepines				History of substance abuse	Sedation, Dizziness, Incoordination, Amnesia, Headache	Rapid onset of action, Safe, Well tolerated, Some are inexpensive, May contribute to depression	Habit forming, Withdrawal symptoms, including seizures
Alprazolam (Xanax)	0.25 mg tid	0.5–6 mg/d	$50				
Clonazepam (Klonopin)	0.5 mg bid	1–4 mg/d	$45				
Chlorazepate (Tranxene)	3.75 mg bid	7.5–60 mg/d	$5				
Chlordiazepoxide (Librium)	5 mg tid	15–100 mg/d	$5				
Diazepam (Valium)	2 mg bid	4–40 mg/d	$5				
Lorazepam (Ativan)	0.5 mg tid	2–6 mg/d	$15				
Buspirone (BuSpar)	5 mg tid	15–60 mg/d	$55		Nervousness, Insomnia, Weakness, Dizziness, Paresthesia, Nausea, Diarrhea	Safe, Well tolerated, Not habit forming, Nonsedating	May not be as effective in GAD as benzodiazepines

*Average wholesale price for least expensive formulation in the middle of the dosage range. Retail prices may be slightly higher and vary from pharmacy to pharmacy.
hs, at bedtime; qa.m., every morning; qd, every day; bid, twice a day; tid, three times a day; OCD, obsessive-compulsive disorder; GAD, generalized anxiety disorder.
Data from Physicians' genRx: The Official Drug Reference of FDA Prescribing Information and Therapeutic Equivalents. Smithtown, NY: Data Pharmaceutica; 1993- (serial).

tidepressant nightly), and (3) explaining this possibility fully to the patient. For approximately half of patients who experience agitation, some kind of adaptation takes place within the first week of treatment, after which it is possible to go up to full doses without further difficulty. For others, continuing agitation persists, and other medications (e.g., *nortriptyline* [Pamelor] or an SSRI) must be tried in sequence until one is found that is tolerable.

A few comments about some other antidepressant agents are in order. *Clomipramine* (Anafranil) is an especially effective agent for panic attacks, often working where other agents do not. Unfortunately, it has an anticholinergic side effect profile very much like that of imipramine, to which it is structurally related.

Amitriptyline (Elavil) is an inappropriate medication for anxiety and depression in almost all cases because of its side effect profile, but some clinicians use it when several other agents have failed because of agitation. The novel antidepressant *bupropion* (Wellbutrin) and the nonbenzodiazepine anxiolytic *buspirone* (BuSpar) are both *ineffective* for panic attacks.

(2) *Serotonin reuptake inhibitors.*
The SSRI agents all seem to be effective for panic disorder and have minimal side effects, except for the usual insomnia, gastrointestinal disturbances, and the agitation discussed earlier. Inhibition of orgasm occurs with many patients and is a common reason for discontinuation of therapy, often without the physician knowing why. Appropriate questioning can reveal the problem and lead to medication or dose changes that may help.

When using *fluoxetine* (Prozac), we often start administration with 10 mg every other day for the first week. Whether any agent is consistently superior in outcome to others seems unlikely, but differences in side effect profiles exist that are, unfortunately, not consistent from patient to patient. *Venlafaxine* (Effexor) seems more likely than other agents to cause agitation, whereas *nefazodone* (Serzone) may be less likely to cause agitation.

b. *Alternate therapies.*
For the very few patients in whom the TCAs and SSRIs are not effective or not tolerated, other medications can be considered. *We advocate trying at least one or two TCAs and one or two SSRIs before pursuing the less desirable therapies discussed later.*

(1) *Monoamine oxidase inhibitors.*
MAOIs are effective antipanic medications and have a therapeutic role, even in the primary care setting. Many clinicians have been reluctant to use these agents because of concern about their potentially serious hypertensive drug-food and drug-drug interactions. Clearly, careful patient education about which foods and medications must be avoided is mandatory—a list of these is available in the drug package insert, which is reproduced in the *Physician's Desk Reference.*[2] Nevertheless, growing evidence indicates that these drugs are much safer than previously believed. One large study of more than 1000 patients taking MAOIs documented only one serious hypertensive reaction. MAOIs also have some unique side effects, especially orthostatic hypotension and insomnia, which should be considered. Still, for patients who are intolerant of other agents or with certain comorbidities (e.g., social phobia and perhaps mixed anxiety and depression), MAOI therapy should be considered. *Phenelzine* (Nardil) is the MAOI for which there is the most experience in anxiety disorders, and it should be selected rather than the other MAOIs for this reason. The typical starting dose is 15 mg twice a day, and typical therapeutic dosages are from 45 to 90 mg/d in divided doses. *MAOIs can interact with other antidepressants. The period for potential drug interaction can be prolonged because of the prolonged half-life of some antidepressants and the irreversible inhibition of MAO by MAOIs.* A medication-free interval of at least 2 weeks should be provided after administration of a MAOI is discontinued and before administration of a TCA or an SSRI is begun. SSRIs with a long half-life (e.g., fluoxetine) should be discontinued at least 6 weeks prior to MAOI therapy; for other antidepressants, a 2-week drug holiday is usually sufficient.

(2) *Benzodiazepines.*
Benzodiazepines are widely advertised and widely prescribed as a primary treatment for panic disorder, but initial treatment with benzodiazepines is, in our opinion, usually a mistake. First of all, the older, less potent, agents, such as *diazepam* (Valium) and *chlordiazepoxide* (Librium), do not relieve panic attacks at conventional doses, although they may be effective at higher doses. They do relieve patients' anticipatory anxiety so that they can leave the house, but patients then have panic attacks just as they did before.

In contrast, *the new high-potency agents, such as alprazolam (Xanax), lorazepam (Ativan), and clonazepam (Klonopin), are effective in stopping panic attacks for most people.* They work faster than the antidepressants and generally have fewer side effects and patients are very appreciative during the first months of treatment. At appropriate doses of these agents, given regularly several times daily, about 70% of patients cease having panic attacks within a few weeks.

Over subsequent weeks, however, problems of one sort or another often arise. Side effects, although not dangerous, are usually annoying. Many patients are sleepy, some notice decreased short-term memory and cognitive dysfunction, and some experience headaches. More likely, however, patients skip a dose or two and immediately notice increased anxiety and perhaps a panic attack. After such experiences, they become much more attuned than ever to their anxiety and begin to check their pocket or purse frequently to ensure that the medication is there. During these weeks, many patients hear from friends, relatives, or other doctors that they are getting "addicted." This is almost never true, because very few patients increase the dose of the medication. The fear, however, leads many patients to suddenly stop taking the medication, whereupon they usually have an enormous increase in anxiety; panic attacks, even if panic attacks have not occurred before; and, occasionally, a seizure. Conversely, the patient's physician may tell the patient to try to decrease the dosage. The patient tries to comply, the anxiety returns, the patient again increases the dosage of the benzodiazepine, and the patient and physician are then locked in a very frustrating conflict.

In fact, as many as half of patients receiving treatment with benzodiazepines for several months can stop taking the agent relatively quickly and experience few withdrawal symptoms. Most patients, however, experience moderate withdrawal symptoms, and some patients, more than 20% in some studies, experience more anxiety and panic attacks than they ever experienced before they were treated.

Is it possible to treat people with long-term benzodiazepine therapy? Certainly. In most cases, the medication continues to be effective for years without the need to increase the dose. Most experienced clinicians have several patients for whom this is an entirely appropriate treatment because other treatments have not worked and the patient and physician have a clear understanding about the nature of the treatment they are pursuing with its risks, side effects, and benefits. Overall, however, in the long run, most patients who are initially treated with medications for panic disorder are better served by antidepressant therapy.

Benzodiazepines are contraindicated in patients with a history of substance abuse and should be used only with hesitation in patients who are at high risk for benzodiazepine abuse. According to an expert panel on this issue, this group includes:

- Patients with current or prior dependence on benzodiazepines and other sedative hypnotics.
- Patients with chronic medical or psychiatric problems.
- Patients with chronic dysphoria or personality disorders.
- Patients with chronic sleep difficulties.

Agents with a long half-life, a slow onset of action, and a high potency are best suited for the treatment of panic disorder. *Clonazepam* has all of these characteristics, and we would consider it the benzodiazepine of first choice for anxiety disorders except that it often causes sedation. *Alprazolam* and *lorazepam* cause less sedation, but their rapid onset and short half-lives may be more likely to result in abuse, dependence, withdrawal reactions, and possibly seizures.

The typical starting dosage of *clonazepam* is 0.5 mg twice a day. This dosage is increased every 3 to 7 days as required and as tolerated up to a maximum of 4 mg/d in divided doses. A common mistake is to underdose benzodiazepines in panic disorder; some patients with panic disorder require doses in the upper range of those listed in Table 9–8; others get good relief from very low doses. The goal is to use the dose that works to control anxiety without causing excess sedation. Patients can expect some sedation, but with time, this effect decreases, even in patients taking the upper end of the dosage range. The main disadvantage of *clonazepam* and *alprazolam* is their high cost—about $30 to $60/mo for the doses required for patients with panic disorder. *Lorazepam* is a less expensive alternative, at about $15/mo for the generic form. High doses of generic low-potency agents, such as *diazepam,* can be considered if an even lower-cost agent ($5/mo) is required, but compared with the more potent agents such as clonazepam or alprazolam, it is not as effective for panic, even at high doses (>30 mg/d).

The most common mistake in using the high-potency, short–half-life agents (those most effective for panic) is irregular administration of the medication. Administering prescriptions on an "as needed" basis seems sensible but is usually counterproductive. Although the physician imagines the dose is being minimized, the patient is constantly checking to see if he or she should take more and often begins taking a pill at times when the anxiety is severe. Taking the medication in this way, when the anxiety level is about to decrease anyway, is an ideal way to cause dependency. The patient should not be constantly monitoring the severity of symptoms to decide, usually with some guilt, about taking another dose.

Alprazolam and *lorazepam* should usually be administered three or four times a day, irrespective of the patient's level of symptoms. Using these agents only at bedtime can cause morning anxiety.

It is tempting to administer a benzodiazepine along with an antidepressant when panic disorder is first diagnosed. This makes pharmacotherapeutic sense because antidepressants take weeks to suppress the panic attacks and associated anxiety, whereas benzodiazepines do so within days. For a small number of patients (e.g., those with frequent, disabling attacks; those with severe anxiety about having more attacks; and especially those with rapidly developing agoraphobia), this approach is appropriate. For the more typical patient, this approach is often not necessary or desirable, given the difficulty of discontinuing benzodiazepine therapy in some patients even after a month or two of therapy. Frequent visits (including urgent, as needed visits in the event of a severe panic attack) often provide adequate symptom management until the antidepressant takes effect.

(3) *Beta-adrenergic blockers.*
Although beta blockers (usually propranolol [Inderal]) have been used in some patients with panic disorder, we cannot endorse their widespread use. In controlled trials, propranolol has performed considerably less well than the agents described earlier and may be no better than placebo. Although it may blunt some of the physiologic (particularly cardiovascular) responses of a panic attack, it does nothing to alter the psychological aspects of the disorder. We would, however, advocate its use:

- In patients who have been successfully maintained on it for long periods of time and in whom weaning from it produces intolerable symptoms.
- In patients in whom all other therapies have failed.
- In patients with annoying but not disabling panic attacks who do not clearly meet the criteria for panic disorder.
- As an adjunctive therapy to help attenuate residual panic attacks or limited-symptom attacks in patients taking other antipanic medications.

4. *Setting reasonable patient expectations.*
The patient should be given the expectations that the panic attacks will become less frequent starting in the second to third week after the initiation of antidepressant medication, and that for most patients, panic attacks are controlled after a month or two of treatment. *Many patients, however, continue to have limited-symptom attacks.* During these episodes, patients feel as if they are about to have a full panic attack and they have some symptoms, but then these symptoms pass without evolving into a full-blown panic attack. It is best to warn patients about this likely outcome and to ask them to simply accept it while waiting for a still better treatment response. Otherwise, patients return demanding more or different treatment because they feel that the limited-symptom attacks are an indication that the medication is not working.

Although antidepressant medications stop the panic attacks, they have no direct effect on the agoraphobia. Many patients who discover on their own that they will not have panic attacks gradually expand their territory and begin to drive on the expressway, go to shopping centers, and even sit in the middle of the row in a movie theater. Others, however, continue their avoidance, and their agoraphobia does not improve until behavior therapy is instituted.

Patients with panic disorder may report having symptoms in response to placebos and may have unrealistic fears about every medication. Very often, they describe themselves as "sensitive" to all medications. Often, they are right. In response to such concerns, we often ask the patient what he or she read about the proposed medication in the *Physician's Desk Reference.*[2] Most patients are surprised that we know they have a *Physician's Desk Reference.*[2] We explain that almost all patients with panic disorder have such fears and that dealing with those fears in a straightforward manner is an ordinary part of the treatment.

5. *Course.*
In general, drug treatment needs to be continued for three or four months after patients have had complete relief from their panic attacks and for at least a couple of months after they are participating in all appropriate activities. Early in this period, brief physician visits every 1 to 2 weeks are typical, with monthly visits being recommended after symptom control is achieved. After several months of adequate symptom control, medication administration is discontinued over a period of 2 months, and a return visit is always scheduled after the complete termina-

tion of medical therapy so that the patient can discuss any anxiety symptoms that have re-emerged and be appropriately reassured. This extra visit seems to decrease the immediate relapse rate. In the longer term, most patients treated with medication alone relapse within a period of a few years.

6. *Relapse and development of comorbidity.* Most patients who present with panic disorder relapse and/or develop a major depressive disorder within five years. Thus, it is unrealistic to expect this disorder to be treated and cured. Instead, we tell patients it is more like peptic ulcer disease in that effective management is almost always available, but in the face of certain provocative events, a return of symptoms is likely at some point and should lead to prompt treatment. Patients need to be specifically told that recurrence is no sign of weakness or failure on their part and that they are welcome to return to treatment at the earliest sign of possible relapse. If the patient returns reporting a single panic attack and no other manifestations of an anxiety disorder, then reassurance is often appropriate. As noted earlier, many people in the general population during the course of a year have an episode that qualifies as a panic attack. When patients with panic disorder know this and the normal functions of panic symptoms, they are less likely to return to the panic cycle.

VII. Specific phobia.

A. Description.

At ages 3 to 6 years, essentially everyone has specific phobias of small animals and insects. Most people lose their phobias with time, but some do not. Some patients report a traumatic onset—a bee sting, a bite from a dog, or some similar event. Others report the concurrence of seeing an object that becomes a phobic object along with some other trauma, such as a family fight on the same day the patient first saw a cat. In most cases, however, simple phobias are merely the persistence into adulthood of fears that are developmentally appropriate in childhood. However, it is not uncommon for situational phobias, such as heights, bridges, and enclosed spaces, to develop later in life.

B. Epidemiology.

The 1-year prevalence of specific phobia is approximately 10%. The sex ratio varies by type of phobia, but in all types, more women than men have them. Specific phobias commonly coexist with other anxiety disorders.

C. Functioning.

Many patients with animal phobias have little or no apparent dysfunction because they can avoid their phobic objects without much effort. Convincing such patients to undergo exposure therapy is usually difficult and may not be necessary. However, because patients may downplay the accommodations they have made for their phobias, these accommodations should be explored in detail. Patients with multiple phobias or those with situational phobias may function less well. Often, patients with long-standing phobias present to the physician for the first time when a change in their life circumstances necessitates increased exposure to their phobic object. For example, a man with an elevator phobia may seek help when a promotion places him in a tall building.

D. Pathophysiology.

Why do some people have simple phobias that persist? Genetic relatives of people with specific phobias have an increased general susceptibility to anxiety but not to panic disorder or depression. When parents have phobias, they often model phobic behavior, and the child learns readily, thus making it hard to differentiate the genetic and environmental contributions. Certainly, in many cases, the phobic object does have unconscious symbolic significance, but understanding that significance is by no means a sure path to a cure of the phobia.

E. Differential diagnosis.

The diagnosis of specific phobia is ordinarily straightforward. As noted earlier, *panic disorder with agoraphobia* can be confused with *specific phobia, situational type* when the agoraphobic fears panic attacks occurring in particular settings. The pervasive anxiety, and phobias of multiple situations, that characterize the agoraphobic patients usually set them apart. *Social phobia* can usually be distinguished by the focus of the fear, namely social interactions in which the patient might come under the scrutiny of unfamiliar people. In *PTSD,* the phobic avoidance is limited to objects and situations that trigger flashbacks of the traumatic event. In *OCD,* the fear surrounds the focus of the obsessions and compulsions, such as contamination from dirt. Patients who have the onset of a specific phobia without a traumatic event later in life are usually found to have more severe psychiatric pathology. The same is true for people with fears of objects that are not usually considered phobic objects. Patients with fears of light sockets, unvarnished wood, and other odd stimuli should receive a comprehensive psychiatric evaluation.

F. Treatment.

1. *Behavior therapy.*
Exposure therapy (see section V.C) offers a reliable method of curing most phobias. If a person stays in close contact with a phobic object for an hour or more, despite the anxiety this proximity entails, the anxiety is reduced on future exposures. A series of such sessions, usually culminating in the patient's handling the phobic object, whether it be a spider or a snake or a dog, usually results in a complete remission of the phobia. This resolution can take anywhere from 2 to 10 hours of treatment, depending on the patient, the therapist, and especially, the expectations of both at the beginning of treatment. Attempts to have the patient relax and/or imagine peaceful scenes while in the presence of the phobic object have proved effective in some cases, but the treatment does not work as reliably or as quickly as exposure therapy.
Exposure therapy should never be forced on anyone and usually requires an experienced guide if it is to be successful with a minimal amount of pain for the patient. Because few primary care clinicians have these skills, their role should be limited to finding appropriate referral sources for their patients with specific phobias.

2. *Medications.*
Medications have essentially no role in the management of an isolated specific phobia. An exception might be the occasional use of a brief course of a benzodiazepine for a patient with a fear of flying who has to take an unexpected trip to attend a funeral out of town.

VIII. Social phobia.

A. Description.

Most people think that they are more shy than other people. In fact, more than half of people in the population report substantial discomfort at having to give a presentation in public. They usually successfully hide this fear, thus letting others imagine that only they have social fears. When is such discomfort a psychiatric disorder? Although the exact cut-off is somewhat arbitrary, the DSM-IV criteria require "marked and persistent fear of one or more social or performance situations in which the person is exposed to unfamiliar people with a possible scrutiny by others." The social phobic recognizes that this fear is excessive but nonetheless avoids situations that arouse this fear (or tolerates the situations with severe distress), and this fear and avoidance interfere significantly with the person's normal life. In short, if the fear is persistent, disturbing, and disabling, it is severe enough to be called social phobia. For many patients, this fear is so overwhelming that it cannot be comprehended by people with ordinary shyness. Some patients leave high school because of fear of being called on in class, take jobs as night watchmen so that they do not need to see anyone, and then live alone, getting most of their supplies by mail order. Treatment for some such patients is a miraculous window to a whole new life, but, of course, most of them fear coming to a clinic.

B. Epidemiology.

The lifetime prevalence of social phobia is between 3% and 13%, with most patients being mildly to moderately affected. The age of onset is usually shortly after puberty. In this anxiety disorder, the sex ratio is relatively equal. As with the other anxiety disorders, a strong genetic predisposition exists.

C. Comorbidity.

As with all anxiety disorders, patients with social phobia are more likely to have other anxiety disorders. Clinically important subtypes of social phobia are those with and those without associated panic disorder. Some people have never been especially concerned about presenting in public until the onset of a spontaneous panic attack while making a presentation causes a conditioned fear of such presentations. For other people, the anticipation of social performance has always been a source of dread, and their symptoms in the situation of social scrutiny are not the sudden unexpected onset of panic symptoms but a steady intense anxiety. This distinction is important clinically because patients with panic-like symptoms often respond well to treatment that stops panic attacks, whereas such medications are less effective for patients who have more typical social phobia.

D. Differential diagnosis.

The overlap with panic disorder is discussed earlier. Confusion with other psychiatric disorders is uncommon.

E. Treatment.

1. *Behavior therapy.*
Behavior therapy (see section V.C) is the initial treatment for most patients with social phobia. This therapy can be conducted in groups in the clinic, or more likely, individually, with exercises to be performed away from the clinic. Exercises involve interacting with people in progressively more and more challenging situations, such as asking a salesclerk for help, asking for a refund, talking

with someone at a coffee shop, and finally, giving a speech. Although it seems paradoxical, we do not recommend that patients practice social presentations more and more until they are perfect. This is, in fact, what has led to the problem for many patients with social phobia. Instead, we instruct them to make embarrassing mistakes in situations in which such actions will not be too harmful. To give an example, we wonder if the managers of the Burger King chain in our area will catch on to the large number of people coming in asking for a "Big Mac." In fact, our patients report that their profound apprehension at such an embarrassing mistake is entirely unjustified. The clerk rarely bats an eye.

2. *Medications.*
It has recently been found that the same group of medications that is effective for panic disorder can also be effective for social phobia. Specifically, the *SSRIs* have been found to be effective in some patients. More patients, however, respond to treatment with *MAOIs. More than 50% of patients, even those with lifelong severe social phobias,* respond well to MAOI therapy. For specific guidelines on the use of MAOIs, see section V.I.

IX. Obsessive-compulsive disorder.

A. Description.

Obsessive-compulsive disorder is fundamentally different from the other anxiety disorders. It seems likely that it will eventually be recognized as the product of damage to the caudate nucleus, and thus its various components will fit together much more like the components of Horner's syndrome, rather than the functional significance that underlies the syndrome of panic or social phobia. Although patients with OCD experience quite a lot of anxiety, anxiety is not the main problem. The main problem is fear that some small oversight will result in unimaginable catastrophe. Thus, one patient retraces her steps for fear that her pill bottle has come open, a pill has fallen out, and a child will ingest it and die. Another patient, a waitress, continually snatches cups of coffee away from customers, concerned that she might have accidentally put a tack in the bottom of the cup and that the person would swallow it and die. Another patient gets up from bed 10 times within an hour in order to check the door locks because of a fear that someone will break in and harm the children.

The mechanisms that people use to try to defend themselves and others against this potential harm are varied. Very often, the patient checks doors, windows, locks, dryers, burners, and so on. The patient may engage in rituals, such as counting things, performing certain tasks in a certain order, walking through a doorway a certain number of times, or touching things a certain number of times. Many patients fear that they will transmit contamination and therefore begin washing their hands or other parts of their body frequently and for long periods, often with strong soaps. On occasion, the washing compulsion arises separate from any fear of harming someone by contamination and even separate from contamination fears at all. Most often, however, the patient fears, not that the patient himself or herself will be hurt by some foreign substance but that he or she will transmit it to others, with harmful effects. The obsessions are intrusive thoughts that enter the patient's mind unbidden and do not make sense to the patient. Many such thoughts are images of harming another person, especially a spouse or a loved child.

Obsessive-compulsive disorder needs to be carefully distinguished from obsessive-compulsive personality disorder. Many patients with OCD are fundamentally normal, with good warm relationships with others and no excessive carefulness until the OCD surfaces. Patients with obsessive-compulsive personality disorder, by contrast, describe what is usually a lifelong history of carefulness, relative intellectuality, coldness, rigidity, and concern with duty and rules. *These two syndromes are distinct.*

B. Epidemiology.

It was previously thought that OCD was exceedingly rare, but it now seems to affect 2% to 3% of the population, with most patients having successfully hidden it from their doctors as well as from their friends and relatives. The mean age of onset is in the twenties, but more patients have the onset in their thirties and forties than occurs in panic disorder. Many patients also report having the onset during childhood. OCD commonly coexists with other anxiety disorders as well as with major depressive disorder.

C. Pathophysiology.

The etiology of OCD is under active investigation, with a particular focus on the neurobiology and genetics of the disorder. The likelihood of an OCD is increased many-fold in patients with first degree relatives with the disorder, and it is also increased in relatives of people who have trichotillomania (hair pulling) or Tourette's syndrome, a disorder that involves ticlike movements of the face and hands and sudden blurted phrases that may include obscenities. Recent positron emission tomography and magnetic resonance imaging studies have shown abnormalities in the basal ganglia, specifically, the caudate nucleus. The most recent research avenue is the possibility that the disorder is an autoimmune complication of streptococcal infection, although this is by no means proved. What is clear is that serotonergic systems are intimately involved in the pathophysiology. Agents that increase serotonin availability at the intrasynaptic cleft relieve OCD symptoms, whereas agents that block serotonin receptors make OCD acutely worse.

D. Treatment.

Treatment of OCD can be frustrating, and incomplete response and relapses are the rule. Nevertheless, patients can show clinically significant improvement with the appropriate therapy. Given the complexity of therapy for OCD and its often incomplete response, most patients with OCD benefit from referral to a specialist.

1. *Behavior therapy.*
As with the other anxiety disorders, behavior treatment (see section V.C) is a mainstay. However, instead of exposure to the cues that cause anxiety, in the case of OCD, the principle of treatment is to either expose the person to the cues that arouse the obsessions and compulsions or to prevent the ritualistic responses that reduce anxiety. The clinician analyzes very carefully, over a period of hours, the exact cues that arouse the concern and the rituals the patient uses to relieve it. For instance, if a patient is obsessing about having hit someone with a car after hitting a pothole and then stops to look and drives around the block to see if anyone has been hurt, the behavioral exercise would likely be to seek out streets that are crowded with people and have many potholes and to keep on driving without looking back, despite the concern that someone might have been hit.

Similarly, if a patient fears accidentally putting a foreign substance into food for the family, the treatment might begin by asking the person to serve meals despite the concern that they might be contaminated. A more advanced exercise might involve keeping an open canister of detergent on the counter while meals are being prepared. For patients who hoard things, some of whom fill their entire houses with newspapers for fear of losing some important item, the treatment is, predictably, to discard the items. However, instead of helping the patient reassure himself or herself that nothing important will be lost, the treatment is very often more effective if the patient semi-intentionally discards several items that are of some consequence, such as a credit card or an important license. Very quickly, such patients learn that the difficulty of replacing such materials is far less than the suffering and impediments they have suffered because of their obsessions and rituals.

Behavior therapy for OCD is not as effective as it is for other anxiety disorders. Although most patients make substantial gains, a relatively small proportion, perhaps 20%, complete treatment and are symptom free. An equal proportion do not get much relief, usually because they are unable to cooperate with the exercises. Overall, behavior therapy alone is about as effective as medication treatment alone, but in most patients, obsessions or compulsions remain.

2. *Medication therapy.*
Drug treatment is indicated for most patients with OCD, ideally as an adjunct to behavior therapy. All of the *SSRIs* are effective, but there are some data that *clomipramine* (Anafranil) may be generally more effective than other antiobsessional agents, despite its anticholinergic and antihistaminic side effect profile. In our clinic, however, we generally start medical therapy with an SSRI; doses at the high end of the range shown in Table 9–8 are typically required for OCD. Although the agitation side effect of these agents is common for panic disorder, patients with OCD are usually much more concerned with the long-term side effects, especially sexual difficulties. Impotence and lack of desire are relatively uncommon effects, but difficulty achieving orgasm is so common and so disturbing to many patients that they stop taking their medications, even when the medication is effective in controlling the OCD. A common mistake in therapy is impatience. Studies have repeatedly shown that patients often do not begin to improve until weeks after treatment has begun and that the improvement is slow and continuous, often over a period of many months. When treatment is stopped, almost all patients experience relapse. If behavior therapy has been instituted, relapse may be less frequent and less severe.

Only about 60% of patients with OCD respond well to pharmacotherapy. When the initial agent does not prove effective, the practice is usually to switch to another agent and subsequently to augment treatment with lithium or antipsychotic agents. *Lithium* has not proved effective in controlled trials, but *dopamine blockers* are effective in a proportion of patients and may be worth a trial, regardless of whether the patient has symptoms of psychosis. Another alternative is the use of antidepressant drug doses that are higher than those usually used. All such complex treatments should be carried out by someone experienced with the treatment of patients with OCD.

X. Post-traumatic stress disorder.

A. Description.

Just as severe physical trauma can leave permanent physical damage, so can mental trauma leave permanent psychological damage. The issue is not quite so simple as that, however, because not all kinds of psychological upset leave a permanent mark. PTSD most often follows exposure to physical violence or situations that could have caused death. It was previously thought that only certain people with predisposing factors would get PTSD after a trauma, but prospective research is showing that the most important variable is the severity of the trauma itself.

Patients often do not mention the traumatic event when they are in a clinic; instead they mention sleep difficulties, especially nightmares; depression; feeling of numbness; outbursts of anger; and hypervigilance. Once the link to the traumatic experience is recognized, the hallmarks of the syndrome are persistent, recurrent, intrusive, vivid thoughts or memories about the event. For instance, a man who tried to rescue his children from a burning trailer said that there was never a minute in the subsequent 5 years when he did not feel the heat on his skin and think about his children dying in the fire. His mental life was literally consumed with these thoughts. Furthermore, he was constantly on edge, could not sleep, had nightmares about the event, and experienced only depression and anxiety, no other emotions. As you might guess, these symptoms often lead to complications. Divorce and job problems are routine. Alcoholism and other attempts to escape the symptoms are equally prevalent.

B. Epidemiology.

Although traumatic, life-threatening events are more common during war time, they are all too common in civilian life. Prevalence studies are limited by difficulties in case ascertainment and sample selection, but the lifetime prevalence of PTSD may be as high as 9%. PTSD develops in about one of four people who experience exposure to a severe traumatic event.

C. Differential diagnosis.

Not all anxiety that follows a stressful event constitutes PTSD. PTSD has several key features that form the foundation for its diagnostic criteria.

1. *A traumatic event.*
   The patient must have experienced or witnessed an event that involved actual or threatened death, bodily injury, or threat to the physical integrity of themselves or others.

2. *Intrusive re-experiencing of the traumatic event.*
   The event is persistently re-experienced through recollections, dreams, flashbacks, and so on.

3. *Avoidance of stimuli associated with the event and numbing of general responsiveness.*
   Patients not only avoid situations, conversations, and activities that they associate with the trauma, they also have a general restriction of affect and responsiveness to the world around them.

4. *Symptoms of increased arousal.*
   These symptoms are similar to those seen in GAD and include insomnia, irritability, angry outbursts, difficulty concentrating, hypervigilance, and exaggerated startle response.

To meet the criteria for the diagnosis of PTSD, the patient must have the symptoms for more than 1 month, and clinically significant dysfunction must be present.

Acute stress disorder has a presentation that is nearly identical to that of PTSD but by definition lasts less than 4 weeks.

Generalized anxiety disorder can include many of the same symptoms of increased arousal, and *confusion can occur when patients do not disclose the traumatic event and its central role in their emotional lives.* For this reason, patients with symptoms of anxiety should be asked about a history of traumatic events. A helpful question might be:

> Sometimes, people who feel the way you do have experienced very traumatic events in the past. Have you ever been in a situation in which you experienced or witnessed a serious threat to life, such as a serious accident, an assault, fire, war, or natural disaster?

Patients should be asked specifically but sensitively about a history of sexual assault or abuse; patients may find this information more difficult to divulge. Patients who acknowledge a history of traumatic events should be asked about the characteristic intrusive re-experiencing, avoidance, and emotional restriction. Patients with GAD have related a lifetime of symptoms of increased arousal, whereas those with PTSD acknowledge onset after the stressor (although not necessarily immediately so). Patients may initially have little insight into the connection between their general dysphoria and the traumatic event.

Adjustment disorder with anxiety is diagnosed when the stressor is less severe (e.g., job loss, divorce) or when the characteristic responses of intrusive re-experiencing, avoidance, and emotional restriction are absent.

Patients can develop a *major depressive disorder* as a result of a traumatic episode, and patients with PTSD usually have depressive symptoms. The characteristic re-experiencing and avoidance should again differentiate these two disorders, although in many patients, both major depressive disorder and PTSD coexist.

D. Comorbidity.

Major depressive disorder is commonly associated with PTSD, and the other anxiety disorders do appear to be more prevalent in patients with PTSD.

Substance abuse is common; it is seen in almost 70% of some samples of PTSD patients. Given its prevalence, contribution to dysfunction, and treatability, its presence should be carefully elicited in patients with PTSD.

E. Treatment.

Patients with PTSD generally benefit less from treatment than do patients with the other anxiety disorders. No particular combination of psychotherapy, behavior therapy, or medication is reliably effective. This having been said, there is little value in fatalism. Many patients do indeed seem to benefit from a long-term, multifaceted treatment program. Although their recovery is seldom complete, their suffering and dysfunction can be lessened.

1. *Psychotherapy.*
   It was previously thought that simple recollection of the trauma would be sufficient to allow symptom relief by catharsis. Although talking about the trauma can be helpful, expressing and reworking the emotions is not a simple or reliable cure, although detailed recollections have been shown to decrease the trauma of rape. In fact, one therapeutic strategy is to train patients to interrupt their traumatic recollections when they occur. Selection of candidates for psychotherapy (and development of a psychotherapeutic plan) usually requires an especially skilled therapist, and for this reason, referral of patients for evaluation is recommended.
2. *Medications.*
   Although extensive research on their use in PTSD is lacking, *antidepressant medications do appear to offer benefit to many patients.* Any of the *TCAs, SSRIs,* or *MAOIs* are certainly indicated in patients with comorbid depression, but some benefit (albeit less dramatic) may be seen in patients without clear-cut major depressive disorder. The symptoms of increased arousal and intrusive re-experiencing tend to respond best to antidepressant therapy. We believe that most patients with PTSD should consider a trial of one or more antidepressant agents at some point in their treatment.

   Benzodiazepines have offered symptomatic relief in some patients, but we cannot advocate their widespread use in patients with PTSD, given the high risk of dependency and abuse in this population. Buspirone has not been systematically studied in PTSD, but occasionally, a patient responds to it. The anticonvulsant *carbamazepine* (Tegretol) has shown some benefit in preliminary trials, but its side effect profile is disappointing, and it is probably best reserved for use by PTSD specialists.
3. *Adjunctive therapies.*
   Treatment for substance abuse often allows improved functioning, and counseling with families can often help them to help the patient manage the disorder as best as possible. Support groups should be encouraged—usually, these are selected on the basis of the nature of the traumatic event. Central referral sources for groups serving veterans and survivors of sexual abuse or assault are shown in Table 9–7.

XI. Acute stress disorder.

A. Description.

Acute stress disorder is a new diagnostic category that was added to DSM-IV. It is a time-limited reaction to an acute severe stressor, such as being involved in a violent crime or a natural disaster. The description and criteria are very similar to those for PTSD, but by definition, acute stress disorder does not last longer than 4 weeks. A major feature of acute stress disorder is the presence of a number of dissociative symptoms, including a subjective sense of numbing or detachment, a reduction of awareness of one's surroundings, depersonalization, derealization, and partial amnesia.

B. Differential diagnosis.

Adjustment disorders also occur in response to traumatic events, but the dissociative symptoms and re-experiencing of the event usually set acute stress disorder apart. PTSD is distinguished by its longer duration.

C. Treatment.

Little has been written about treatment for acute stress disorder. Typically, supportive counseling is offered, and may provide symptomatic improvement. Short-term (< 1 week) use of *benzodiazepines* can be considered. Because the speed with which substance abuse can develop in severely traumatized patients is impressive, close follow-up and firm limits are required.

It is unclear whether any specific steps prevent the development of PTSD in patients with exposure to extreme stressors.

XII. Generalized anxiety disorder.

A. Description.

Generalized anxiety disorder involves excessive anxiety and worry that occur more days than not for at least 6 months about a number of different events or activities. The worry must be difficult to control, and the anxiety and worry cannot simply be related to substance use, depression, panic disorder, OCD, or other major mental disorder. The anxiety (or its symptoms) must cause either significant distress or dysfunction in order to merit the diagnosis of GAD.

B. Symptoms.

In addition to persistent anxiety and worry, the patient must have multiple physiologic symptoms of anxiety, including at least three of the following:

1. Restlessness or feeling keyed up or on edge.
2. Easy fatigue.
3. Difficulty concentrating or mind going blank.
4. Irritability.
5. Muscle tension.
6. Sleep disturbance.

Although these are the symptoms that form the DSM-IV criteria, patients with GAD usually also have many other symptoms of anxiety, as shown in Table 9–1. In primary care settings, patients with GAD tend to present with these symptoms rather than with the worry itself. Patients with GAD usually have little trouble verbalizing their worry if it is directly elicited, but they may have difficulty identifying their anxiety as the cause of their somatic symptoms.

C. Epidemiology.

Epidemiologic surveys demonstrate that about 2% of men and 4% of women meet the criteria for GAD within any given 12-month period. This high reported prevalence conflicts with anxiety experts' impression that GAD is, in fact, uncommon. At least two factors account for this discrepancy: (1) the diagnosis of GAD is among the least reliable of the anxiety disorders, and disagreement frequently exists about the diagnosis in a given patient, and (2) although GAD is usually conceptualized as an intrinsic, lifelong susceptibility to anxiety, most patients in primary care samples no longer meet the criteria for GAD when they are re-examined several years later. It is likely that those whose GAD appears to have resolved never had it in the first place but instead suffered from other conditions described later (see section E below). Comorbidity with other anxiety disorders is said to be common.

D. Etiology.

The etiology is not well understood, but many of these patients have grown up in chaotic homes or suffered specific traumas. Others have a family history of "nerves," or they have a personal history of substance abuse or depression. Genetic studies show that GAD is much more likely to be another manifestation of major depression than of panic disorder, and a high proportion of these patients either have—or will have—associated major depression.

E. Differential diagnosis.

Many clinicians imagine that they see GAD frequently, but usually, they are wrong. GAD is appropriately viewed almost as a diagnosis of exclusion, and its diagnosis should be reserved for patients whose anxiety cannot be better accounted for by another condition.

As mentioned in the introduction, *substance abuse (especially alcohol abuse) often presents with symptoms of generalized anxiety* in the primary care setting. For this reason, patients who are suspected of having GAD should be screened for substance abuse (see Chapter 17). As with other anxiety disorders, a pattern of substance abuse develops in some patients with GAD, at least in part as a result of their attempts at self-medication.

Anxiety is a common symptom of *major depressive disorder* and an even more common symptom of *minor depressive disorders.* Symptomatology more specific to depression, such as anhedonia, sad mood, weight loss, guilt, feelings of worthlessness, suicidality, and thoughts of death, should be specifically sought, and if present, it should suggest the diagnosis of major depressive disorder rather than GAD or another anxiety disorder. Insomnia, difficulty concentrating, and psychomotor agitation can be seen in both anxiety disorders and major depressive disorder, so these symptoms are of no discriminative value. The issue of overlap between anxiety disorder and depression is discussed in a separate section later.

Patients with other anxiety disorders, such as *panic disorder, OCD, PTSD,* and *phobias,* often have some degree of generalized anxiety, but most of their distress surrounds the primary focus of their disorder, such as the panic attacks, the compulsions, the flashbacks, or the phobic objects or situations.

Adjustment reactions of adult life (in which a person who is not otherwise especially prone to anxiety becomes anxious in a particular life circumstance) often present similarly to GAD. The cause of the patient's distress may not be apparent to either the clinician or the patient. Often, the patient describes the difficult circumstances of his or her life but claims to be coping well with them. For example, a patient may fail to see the connection between headaches, fatigue, and insomnia and work as an inner-city police officer. In other cases, hidden psychological conflicts can cause anxiety. Given the importance of distinguishing between GAD and *reactive anxiety* (and the difficulty in doing so), referral to a specialist for diagnostic purposes may be indicated when GAD is a consideration.

A few medical disorders can cause symptoms of generalized anxiety: *hyperthyroidism* is worth ruling out with a thyroid-stimulating hormone assay. *Caffeine* consumption should be assessed and managed as described in section VI.G.13.

F. Treatment.

Far from being easy to treat, GAD is one of the most frustrating and difficult psychiatric disorders to manage.

1. *Psychotherapy.*
   The psychological nature of these symptoms makes it seem as if psychological treatment would be preferred. If specific traumas or psychological issues exist, this is indeed the case, and psychotherapy is recommended. For most patients with true GAD, however, their lifelong worries and physical symptoms do not improve, even through excellent psychotherapy. Behavior techniques can sometimes be effective, but very often, it is hard to find a specific cue to which the person should be exposed. Cognitive techniques involve retraining the person's patterns of thoughts so that the person does not allow entry to the potentially catastrophic expectations that often enter his or her mind as the patient contemplates even an ordinary day. Relaxation training has been tried and seems to be effective in some hands. Even in experienced hands, however, such treatments prove insufficient for most patients. As such, formal psychotherapy cannot be viewed as a principal therapy for true GAD.
2. *Medication.*
   Drug therapy remains the mainstay of therapy for all but the most mildly affected patients with GAD. Thankfully, the number of options available is increasing.
   a. *Antidepressants. Recent studies have shown that antidepressants are effective for most cases of GAD;* they are, of course, particularly appealing in cases with comorbid depression. Perhaps the frequency of this comorbidity is related to the recent finding that the same genes that predispose to GAD also seem to predispose to major depression. The treatment pattern should be the same as described in section VI.I, and the clinician should expect about 70% of patients to get good benefit. Although some agents have been better studied in GAD than others, there is no reason to believe that any agent is reliably superior to any other. For this reason, the clinician is free to select any of the *TCAs, SSRIs,* or *MAOIs,* using the usual considerations of familiarity, cost, side effect profile, safety, and so on. Full antidepressant doses are required for full benefits in most patients.
   b. *Benzodiazepines. These agents are effective for GAD.* Seventy percent or more of patients improve markedly, and although it does not seem to matter which benzodiazepine is used, our pharmacokinetic preferences detailed in the section on panic disorder are relevant here. Low regularly scheduled doses (e.g., 3.75 mg of *clorazepate* (Tranxene) or 10 mg of *chlordiazepoxide* (Librium) are likely to be effective. High-potency agents, including *alprazolam* (Xanax) and *clonazepam* (Klonopin) (which causes more sedation but has a longer half-life), are more expensive but less likely to cause sedation. Taking medication regularly may decrease the psychological dependence that arises when patients are continually monitoring their anxiety levels and postponing taking medication until the level of anxiety is high enough that taking the pill is followed by enormous relief.
      Although the long half-lives of many of the preferred agents would theoretically allow once-daily dosing, most patients seem to have better symptom control and fewer side effects with divided doses. Psychic and somatic symptoms improve in concert. Tolerance develops to the sedative and psychomotor effects, but only rarely to the antianxiety effects. Thus, patients can often be maintained on a stable dose for months to years without difficulty. Escalation of dosage should always raise the possibility of substance abuse. Physiologic dependence does, however, occur, and all of the caveats mentioned earlier with benzodiazepine treatment apply here.
      Overall, it is more appropriate to use benzodiazepines in the long term for GAD than for panic disorder, but alternative treatments often are equally effective. *Given the problems with long-term benzodiazepine therapy, it is our preference to try antidepressants first.*
   c. *Buspirone.* This agent is approved specifically for the treatment of GAD. It is a desirable agent because it causes no withdrawal or dependence and has a mechanism of action and side effect profile that is different from that of other agents. For patients with true GAD, it is a good choice, but the clinician and the patient must realize that side effects (described in Table 9–8) are common and that the patient must take the medication for weeks or even months before it is possible to tell if it will be effective. One report shows that it is not effective in patients who have previously used benzodiazepines, and our clinical experience is largely consistent with this observation.
   d. *Beta blockers.* These agents are sometimes used, but they relieve only the physiologic (not the psychological) symptoms of anxiety. Also, they, too, cause physiologic depen-

dence and withdrawal effects on discontinuation.

G. Course.

True GAD is a chronic condition. Some fluctuation of symptoms may occur in response to acute stressors, but the generalized anxiety persists. Misdiagnosis is common in the best of hands, and many patients may no longer meet the criteria for a diagnosis of GAD at some point after their diagnosis. For this reason, an attempt to taper medication is often indicated after 3 to 6 months of successful therapy. The difficulty in tapering benzodiazepines compared with tapering other effective agents is another reason for using them only when other agents have failed.

During drug titration, physician visits every 2 to 4 weeks are indicated until a stable, effective dose of medication is reached. A follow-up visit after 3 to 6 months of drug therapy allows a discussion about tapering the medication to take place. If the patient continues long-term medication therapy, physician visits every 6 months are acceptable, provided other complicating factors (e.g., prominent somatization) are absent.

XIII. Comorbidity of anxiety and depression.

Although this chapter treats anxiety disorders as if they were distinct from depression, the disorders are intermingled more often than not. More than a third of patients with major depression have panic attacks, and more than half have some kind of substantial anxiety. Conversely, perhaps a third of patients with anxiety disorders have major depression, and most patients with panic disorder develop depression within 5 years. That we lack a satisfactory explanation for this is made clear by the recent publication of an 869-page book on the comorbidity of mood and anxiety disorders. We do know that more than half of the lifetime episodes of anxiety and mood disorders in an epidemiologic survey were accounted for by the 14% of people who had three or more disorders. We also know that the genes that predispose some people to GAD seem to be the same as those that predispose to major depression. Furthermore, we know that panic disorder very often turns into depression, but only very rarely does depression turn into panic disorder. The 2:1 female-to-male ratio for depression may be accounted for by the increased susceptibility of women to anxiety disorders.

Various possibilities may account for the comorbidity. Shared genetic vulnerability may explain much of it, but the genetic evidence points to a possible identity of genes that predispose to depression and GAD, but not to panic disorder or OCD. It may be that panic disorder and depression are a single disorder that progresses from one pattern to the other over time. *We think, however, that it is especially likely that depression is a complication of anxiety.* Anxiety could lead to depression because of brain changes, or because of the social dysfunction caused by anxiety, or just simply because anxiety, like any chronic illness, leads to depression. Consideration of the functions of anxiety raises the possibility that anxiety is caused by threats, and when those threats are realized as losses, depression results. Thus, the comorbidity results from likely correspondences between life events. It is even possible that the comorbidity results from habits of thought that make small threats into big ones and make small losses seem like life is empty and hopeless.

The clinician cannot afford to wait for the research that will clarify these relationships. The important point is that depression and anxiety are profoundly intertwined, and the presence of one should always make the clinician consider the other. Treatments effective for one are generally, but not always, effective for the other. Therefore, more research is necessary.

XIV. Adjustment disorders.

A. Description.

In *adjustment disorders,* the person is anxious for good reason, but the anxiety seems excessive. A relative is sick, a marriage is unraveling, a job is threatened, or the person is worried about the possible outcomes of medical tests or procedures. *This anxiety is normal, but it is not always useful.* In fact, given the low biologic cost of an episode of anxiety, it is not surprising that natural selection has set the regulation mechanism so that anxiety is often more intense than would be useful.

B. Differential diagnosis.

Given the frequency of adjustment disorders, one would think that diagnosis should be as straightforward as that of the common cold. This is, unfortunately, not always the case. The sometimes difficult distinctions between adjustment disorders, PTSD, and GAD are discussed in the relevant sections on those disorders. In addition, of course, some patients may simply be experiencing uncomplicated bereavement. Still, in many cases, patients experience or display evidence of inappropriate anxiety of short duration in response to a stressful event. In such cases, the diagnosis of *adjustment disorder* is clear-cut.

C. Treatment.

1. *Drug treatment.*
   Clinicians can readily block the anxiety of an adjustment disorder with benzodiazepines without subverting the protective role of anxiety and leading patients to engage in foolhardy behavior. We believe the availability of safe and effective treatments for this kind of anxi-

ety should be more widely used than they are for periods of 5 to 7 days. Patients need not undergo a minor surgical procedure having not slept for the previous four nights. On the other hand, *benzodiazepines should be avoided in patients with specific risk factors for their abuse,* as detailed in section VI.I.3.b.(2).

2. *Psychotherapy.*
Supportive counseling (often by primary care clinicians or clergy) seems to help as well. Support groups and patient education materials are also helpful. More in-depth therapy by a mental health specialist is indicated for patients with prolonged or serious symptoms or dysfunction. Some of these more severely affected patients have, or will have, a major depressive episode.

We have emphasized the role of cognitive and behavior therapy for the treatment of anxiety disorders. What about the more traditional forms of counseling and psychotherapy? For one of us, this emphasis comes from the bias of working in a tertiary care setting. The many people who have gotten better with traditional psychotherapy never come to the clinic; we only see those who did not improve. Even aside from this bias, however, cognitive and behavior therapies have proved more effective for serious anxiety disorders. On the other hand, such therapies may be less helpful than insight-oriented psychotherapy for many patients, especially those who experience a lot of anxiety but who do not have a specific anxiety disorder. *In many such patients, early experiences, dysfunctional relationships, trauma, and mental conflicts and fixations are important causes of the symptoms, and psychotherapy may be life changing.*

Deciding what is an anxiety disorder that merits straightforward treatment for symptom relief and what is a manifestation of mental problems that need psychotherapy is a skill born of experience. However, some generalizations can be made. People with a strong family history of anxiety disorders who have suffered from anxiety for their entire lives are unlikely to benefit markedly from psychotherapy, whereas those who have experienced trauma or who have obviously conflicted feelings or difficulty with relationships often benefit more from psychotherapy than any other treatment. Many patients need both. Clinicians must not take the simplistic view that making a diagnosis necessarily indicates the treatment that will be the best for an individual patient.

XV. Considerations for special populations.

A. Disadvantaged populations.

Poverty and its associated problems complicate the management of anxiety disorders. Quality CBT may not be available or accessible. Many medications, particularly the best tolerated ones, may be unaffordable. The chaotic and uncontrollable home lives of disadvantaged patients may undermine the efforts of even the best primary care clinicians. These challenges can be met in several ways.

1. In patients who have medical insurance but lack coverage for CBT, their therapy may be able to be paid for as a "noncontractual benefit." This strategy usually requires calling the insurer and explaining that CBT will decrease their costs overall (e.g., by decreasing unnecessary emergency room visits for a patient with panic disorder).

2. Support groups may need to play a more central role in treatment. Some groups may be able to effectively model CBT techniques for group members.

3. Inexpensive but effective medications, like *imipramine* (Tofranil), are available. Most patients can and do tolerate these if the dose is increased slowly and if time is spent in patient education and support early in the course of therapy. For patients with panic disorder who require them, high doses of generic forms of traditional benzodiazepines can be tried in lieu of the more expensive high-potency agents.

4. Interested primary care physicians can master key techniques of CBT through a self-study program. Examples of learning resources are found in the Suggested Reading.

What should be done for disadvantaged patients who are suffering from a degree of anxiety that seems appropriate for their circumstances? How should the anxiety of the battered woman be treated when her ongoing fear of bodily injury seems realistic and perhaps even protective? Removal of the anxiety in this case might prevent her from taking the steps to free herself from her batterer's control, or it might give her the confidence to leave. What of the anxiety of the homeless man who worries about getting enough to eat, finding a secure place to sleep, and protecting himself from predatory criminals? Treatment of this anxiety might remove his impetus to find a way off of the streets. We offer no simple solution for these all-too-common dilemmas but instead reiterate our opening comments on the adaptive significance of anxiety: *anxiety often serves to protect us from real environmental threats,* and anxiety that serves this purpose should not be medicated away. In fact, some patients actually need to have their anxiety levels increased so that they take self-preserving action.

B. Culture-bound syndromes.

Providers who work with immigrant, refugee, or minority populations benefit from familiarizing themselves with the culture-bound syndromes of their particular patient population. According to the DSM-IV, culture-bound syndromes are "recurrent, locality specific patterns of aberrant behavior and troubling experience that may or may not be linked to a particular DSM-IV diagnostic category."[1] An example relevant to anxiety disorder would be *ataque de nervios,* a culture-bound syndrome common among some Latinos. It is characterized by somatic symptoms (reminiscent in some ways of a panic attack) occurring as a result of a stressful event in the family (e.g., news of the death of a relative, discovery of sexual infidelity) that results in stereotyped behaviors (e.g., shouting, physical violence, fainting, dissociative experiences). As should be clear, a classic *ataque de nervios* does not fit neatly into a single DSM-IV diagnostic category.

The DSM-IV includes a glossary of some of the more common culture-bound syndromes, but its listing is less than encyclopedic. A more useful source of information is likely to be a health professional of the same ethnic origin as the population in question. Patients may also respond to sensitive questioning, such as "Does the problem you are having have a special name back home in ______ ?" *Familiarity with culture-bound syndromes can explain atypical behavioral responses in DSM-IV disorders.* For example, various culture-bound syndromes in which anxiety is prominent are associated with dissociative episodes and behavioral outbursts that would be considered histrionic or even psychotic were they to occur in mainstream culture. This familiarity also helps clinicians understand their patients' explanatory models for their illnesses; these models can have a profound effect on what treatments will be accepted.

Table 9–9
Situations in Which Referral to a Specialist Should be Actively Pursued*

Significant diagnostic uncertainty
Typically refractory anxiety disorders, such as obsessive-compulsive disorder and post-traumatic stress disorder
Anxiety disorders requiring intensive behavior therapy, including specific phobias, social phobias, and moderate-to-severe agoraphobia†
High-grade suicidal ideation
Substance abuse
Before the initiation of long-term benzodiazepine therapy, particularly in patients with an increased risk of dependence and abuse
Psychosis
Failure to respond to initial treatments

*Few patients who meet these criteria are optimally treated in the typical primary care setting.
†Referral in this case should be to a therapist with expertise in behavior therapy.

XVI. Indications for referral.

In some patients, anxiety disorders can be managed as well by a primary care clinician as by a psychiatric specialist. Simple advice and prescription of an SSRI resolve the symptoms for some patients with panic disorder. Prescription of a benzodiazepine for an acute adjustment reaction does not require a specialist. Even simple behavior therapy can be successfully carried out with some patients. Clearly, the publication of this manual is predicated on the assumption that treatment of many mental illnesses in the primary care setting has certain advantages.

Then there are the many patients whom the primary care clinician recognizes would benefit from evaluation and treatment by a specialist. This group includes most patients with OCD and PTSD, some patients with phobias, and many patients with adjustment reactions. These and other guidelines for referral are summarized in Table 9–9.

Referral is unfortunately often impeded by lack of interest or capacity on the part of the patient, lack of resources, lack of adequate referral sources, and so on. For this reason, primary care clinicians find themselves struggling with difficult patients and providing care that they recognize may not be ideal but is the best achievable under the circumstances. For these patients, and for all anxious patients, we hope this chapter helps.

References

1. American Psychiatric Association. Diagnostic and Statistical Manual of Mental Disorders. Fourth Edition. Washington, DC: American Psychiatric Press; 1994. (The chapter on anxiety disorders is well organized and clear and incorporates helpful examples. The sections on differential diagnosis are especially useful and provide more detail than is included in this chapter.)
2. Physicians' Desk Reference, 49th ed, Montvale, NJ: Medical Economics Data Production Company, 1995.

Suggested Reading

Barlow DH. Anxiety and its Disorders. New York: Guilford Press; 1988. (This excellent reference offers special emphasis on psychological aspects of anxiety disorders.)

Blackburn IM, Davidson K. Cognitive Therapy for Anxiety and Depression: A Practitioner's Guide. Boston: Blackwell Scientific Publications; 1990. (A useful guide for practitioners who want to refine or expand their cognitive therapy techniques.)

Coryell W, Winokur G, Editors. The Clinical Management of Anxiety Disorders. Oxford University Press: New York, 1991. (This book offers brief, up-to-date advice on the treatment of anxiety disorders.)

Katon W. Panic Disorder in the Medical Setting. Rockville, MD: U.S. Department of Health and Human Services; 1989. (This slim but richly referenced volume is specifically designed for primary care clinicians by an expert in the field. It is available free of charge by calling the NIMH Panic Disorder Hotline at 1-800-64-PANIC.)

Kleinknecht RA. Mastering Anxiety: The Nature and Treatment of Anxious Conditions. New York: Plenum Publishing Corp.; 1991. (This is a comprehensive but easy to read overview of all of the major anxiety disorders. It gives several useful examples of cognitive behavioral therapy in practice.)

Klerman GL, et al., Editors. Panic Anxiety and its Treatments. Washington, DC: APA Press; 1993. (This text provides a good overview of panic disorder and its treatments.)

Marks IM. Fears, Phobias, and Rituals. New York: Oxford University Press; 1987. (This excellent standard reference covers all aspects of anxiety disorders.)

Turner SM, Editor. Behavioral Theories and Treatment of Anxiety. New York: Plenum Publishing Corp.; 1984. (An advanced guide that describes the theory and practice of behavior therapy for practitioners.)

10

MICHAEL D. JIBSON, MD, PhD

RAJIV TANDON, MD

THOMAS P. O'CONNOR, MD

Psychosis and Schizophrenia

I. Introduction.

Psychosis affects 3% to 5% of the general population at some point in life and thus is sufficiently common that it is likely to be encountered in every primary care practice. Although the long-term treatment of patients with chronic psychotic disorders, such as schizophrenia, should be referred to centers specializing in the treatment of these disorders, *psychosis itself must be viewed as a medical syndrome, and its initial evaluation is well within the purview of primary medical practice.*

Even in the case of schizophrenia, the role of the primary care physician remains extremely important for several reasons:

- In many instances, it is the primary physician who first detects psychotic symptoms, sometimes as the patient's or family's presenting complaint but equally often as an incidental finding.
- Patients with schizophrenia and other psychoses require continued care for unrelated medical conditions, and they may remain in the primary physician's care, even while specific treatment for the psychosis is carried on elsewhere.
- For a small number of very stable patients with psychosis, it may be desirable for the primary care provider to assume responsibility for their long-term management.
- Families of patients with psychosis may seek information or advice regarding the condition and care of their loved ones.
- Finally, some patients may be so resistant to seeking specialized psychiatric treatment that the primary physician must assume responsibility for their care.

It is essential, therefore, that the primary care physician be familiar with psychotic symptoms, their most common causes, and the rationale behind the modes of treatment chosen.

II. Psychosis.

A. Definition and description.

Psychosis is a break with reality, involving hallucinations, delusions, disorganized thinking, bizarre behavior, or catatonia.

1. *Hallucinations* are apparent sensory perceptions, such as hearing voices, seeing things, feeling something crawl on the skin or someone touch the body, or smelling or tasting things others are unable to perceive, in the absence of sensory stimulus.
2. *Delusions* are false beliefs that are firmly held, despite obvious evidence to the contrary and lack of acceptance by others of similar cultural and religious background. Delusions may be divided into common subtypes.
   a. *Persecutory delusions* involve the belief that some person or organization is harassing, spying on, following, stealing from, or plotting against the patient.
   b. *Grandiose delusions* involve a grossly inflated sense of importance, worth, ability, or status.
   c. *Religious delusions* include experiences clearly outside the context of the patient's background and social milieu.
   d. *Erotomanic delusions* involve the belief that another person, generally someone famous or of higher social status, is in love with or has a romantic relationship with the patient.
   e. *Somatic delusions* involve a distorted belief about the appearance or function of the body.
   f. *Delusions (or ideas) of reference* are beliefs that neutral events relate in some special way to the patient. Special messages to the patient from the television, radio, or recorded music are common ideas of reference.
   g. *Delusions of thought control* may take various forms, with the common theme that the patient's thoughts are being influenced in some way from outside the patient. These delusions may include the belief that thoughts are being inserted into, or withdrawn from, the patient's mind; that the patient's thoughts are broadcast aloud to other people; that others read the patient's thoughts or that the patient can read their thoughts; or that the patient's thoughts are controlled by outside forces.
3. *Disorganized thinking* is characterized by a lack of logical connections between thoughts.

Disorganized behavior is chaotic, poorly directed, without a clear goal or purpose, or directed toward some bizarre end.

4. *Catatonia* is a state of immobility, resistance to attempts to be moved, mutism, or stereotyped movements.

B. Diagnostic evaluation.

1. *Patient history* is obtained from both the patient and the family (or others who have observed the patient). In some instances, the patient seeks evaluation specifically because of psychotic symptoms, but on many occasions, these symptoms are not appreciated by the patient. Common scenarios are a family that brings a patient to see a physician because of unusual behavior, or a physician that notes that a patient's thinking is bizarre during evaluation for some other problem. As with any symptom, the onset, duration, and course of symptoms should be elucidated. In addition, other changes in behavior may have occurred and should be sought. These may include loss of interest or motivation, change in social interactions, difficulty with routine tasks, or any uncharacteristic behavior.

   In addition to a history of possible psychotic symptoms, *any history of physical illness that might have a bearing on the current symptoms must be investigated.* Information regarding chronic and acute illness and toxic or infectious exposure is important in this regard. A detailed history of substance use must be obtained.

   A history of illness within the family is also an essential part of the evaluation. Particular attention should be paid to family members with symptoms similar to those of the patient and to illnesses with known genetic predispositions, such as substance abuse, Huntington's disease, schizophrenia, and depression.

   Information from family, friends, colleagues, employers, and others is often more candid and reliable than that obtained directly from the patient. In addition, people in contact with the patient may have observed details of behavior that have escaped the patient's notice or that the patient is reluctant to share. This is especially true for establishing the time course of the illness, which is often of subtle and insidious onset and least obvious to the patient. It is essential to obtain the patient's permission before contact is made with any of these people, including other physicians, except in cases of dire emergency.

2. *Mental status examination* establishes the existence of psychosis and may give additional information that helps characterize the symptoms or their cause. Some mental status abnormalities are typical of patients experiencing psychotic symptoms. Although some areas of inquiry may be awkward for the physician or seem silly to the patient, each should be thoroughly explored in any patient in whom psychosis is suspected. This entire set of questions can be completed in 5 to 10 minutes (Table 10–1).
   a. *Appearance* includes the patient's grooming, hygiene, posture, and motor activity. Patients with bizarre behavior or markedly disorganized thinking may be dressed and groomed in an inappropriate or grossly deficient way, such as wearing heavy clothing on a hot summer day or foregoing bathing and changing of dirty clothes for an extended period. Movements and posture may be strange, awkward, stilted, or stereotypic. Motor activity may be increased or decreased and may include psychomotor agitation. This parameter is assessed by passive observation.
   b. *Speech* is the most direct manifestation of thought. In the psychotic patient, speech may be impoverished (few words) or lacking in content. Connections between one statement and the next may be illogical, hard to follow, nonsensical, or incoherent (loose associations), and there may be rapid, tangential switches from one idea to the next (flight of ideas). Vocal inflection may be reduced, absent, or stilted. The rate of speech may be significantly increased or decreased. The patient may use neologisms (nonwords or words with special meaning for the patient) or word approximations. The patient may show evidence of blocking, in which a thought is terminated in midstream, leaving the patient no memory of it. These qualities are assessed by observation through the course of the interview.
   c. *Mood,* the patient's internal feeling state, may range from very depressed to euthymic to elated, and may include anger, irritability, and anxiety. Mood should be assessed by direct questioning.
   d. *Affect,* the combination of facial expression, tone of voice, eye contact, expressive gesture, and posture that reflects and communicates feelings on a moment-by-moment basis, may be inappropriate, flat, constricted, or labile. This parameter is assessed by observation during the interview.
   e. *Thought process* is reflected mainly in speech and, to a lesser degree, in behavior. Thoughts may be poorly organized, with illogical or bizarre connections. Impoverished thinking shows few spontaneous ideas or logical connections. Racing thoughts move rapidly from one idea to the next, with or without the patient's subjective awareness that the thoughts are moving quickly.
   f. *Thought content* includes hallucinations, delusions, preoccupations, suspiciousness, and other unusual ideas. Thoughts of suicide and

Table 10–1
Mental Status Examination: Detection and Evaluation of Psychosis

Appearance	*Observe for* Poor grooming or hygiene Bizarre or inappropriate grooming or dress Unusual, awakward, stilted, or stereotypic movements or posture
Speech	*Observe for* Poverty of speech Poverty of content of speech Loose associations Tangential associations or flight of ideas Altered rate of speech Neologisms or word approximations Blocking Guarding
Mood	
General	*Ask* How has your mood been? Have you been feeling especially happy or sad?
Depression	*Ask* Do you feel sad, down, or blue? Have you been crying recently? Do you feel that your life is worth living?
Elevation	*Ask* Do you feel unusually high or energetic?
Anger/irritability	*Ask* Are you angry or annoyed with anyone? Have you been irritable or edgy?
Anxiety	*Ask* Are you feeling nervous or tense? Do things bother you more than usual? Are there things that worry you or are on your mind a lot recently?
Suspiciousness	*Ask* Do other people have it in for you? Do you have difficulty trusting people?
Affect	
Range	*Observe for* Blunted or flat affect Constricted affect Labile affect
Content	*Observe for* Inappropriate affect Bizarre affect
Thought and perception	
Organization	*Observe for* Loose associations Tangential associations Circumstantial thinking Poverty of content
Hallucinations	*Ask* Do you hear voices other people can't hear or when no one is around? Do you see things that others don't see? Do you feel people touching you or things on your skin when nothing is there? Do you smell or taste things others don't?
Delusions	*Ask* Is anyone trying to hurt you, following you, spying on you, or stealing from you? Are your thoughts controlled from outside? Is anyone reading your thoughts or putting thoughts into your mind? Do you read other people's thoughts? Do you have any special powers or abilities or a special mission in life? Have you had any unusual religious experiences? Do you have any ideas that you hesitate to share with others because they might think them strange or silly?
Ideas of reference	*Ask* Do you get special messages just to you from the television or radio? When you go into a public place, like a store, do people stare at you or talk about you?
Suicidal ideation	*Ask* Are you having any thoughts of harming yourself?
Homicidal ideation	*Ask* Are you having thoughts of harming anyone else?
Sensorium	
Attention and concentration	*Observe for* Slow or inaccurate calculations Reduced digit span
Orientation	*Observe for* Disorientation to person, place, or time
Memory	*Observe for* Poor immediate, short-term, or long-term memory
Rigidity of thought	*Observe for* Inability to consider other points of view or subject ideas to reality testing
Abstraction	*Observe for* Concrete interpretations of proverbs and similarities Self-referential thinking

homicide may also be present. These ideas may not be readily offered and should be asked about directly in any patient in whom a psychotic process is suspected.

g. *Sensorium* may be assessed with simple tests of memory and attention. Psychotic patients may show evidence of impairment in these areas as a direct result of the psychosis, because of an underlying medical problem or intoxication. Abstract thinking, as reflected in pattern recognition and proverb interpretation, is often deficient in psychotic patients. Concrete thinking is typical of psychosis ("No use crying over spilled milk. Who cares? I never drink milk anyway.") Similarities may include inappropriate categories ("An apple and orange are similar in that they are both carbon-based life forms on earth.")
h. *Insight* may be lacking. The patient may or may not recognize that unusual features of speech, thinking, feeling, and behavior are odd or inappropriate.
i. *Judgment* may be impaired if other aspects of thought and behavior show atypical characteristics.

3. *Medical evaluation* should be performed. *In all cases, psychosis should first be considered a medical problem. A primary psychiatric diagnosis cannot be made until possible medical causes have been ruled out.* Although subtle differences sometimes exist in the presentation of psychosis in medical versus primary psychiatric disorders, these are not sufficiently specific to eliminate the need for a thorough medical evaluation in all psychotic patients. Essential and optional diagnostic tests and procedures are listed in Table 10–2. Optional tests should be used if specific clinical indications, such as exposure to an infectious agent; family history of a disorder; or any unexplained findings in the history, physical examination, or essential laboratory tests, are noted. Practitioners' opinions differ as to whether brain imaging should be considered optional or essential. The current climate of cost containment has driven brain imaging to the optional list, but the procedure should be done in any patient with late-onset psychosis or atypical features.

4. *Psychological tests* may be useful in establishing the existence of psychosis or in elucidating aspects of personality that may predispose the patient to these symptoms. Referral to a qualified psychologist should include a specific request ("Please evaluate for evidence of psychosis."). Procedures that may be helpful include the following:
   a. *Neuropsychological testing* evaluates memory, attention, spatial orientation, constructional ability, language, and calculations and may reveal specific areas of brain dysfunction. This type of testing may be useful in documenting or characterizing loss of cognitive function.
   b. *Projective tests (e.g., Rorschach test) and personality inventories (e.g., Minnesota Multiphasic Personality Inventory)* may detect subtle signs of psychosis or delineate patterns of thought or behavior associated with a psychotic thought process.

Case Study

Evaluation of a possible psychotic disorder:

Mr. B., a 22-year-old single man, comes into the family practice clinic accompanied by his mother. He remains silent as she explains her

Table 10–2
Medical and Psychological Evaluation

Essential Tests		Optional Tests	
Medical	*Psychological*	*Medical*	*Psychological*
Comprehensive physical examination	Mental status examination	CT or MRI scan of the brain	Neuropsychological testing
Serum electrolyte levels, including calcium, phosphate, and magnesium		HIV antibody	Projective testing
Hepatic and renal function tests		Electroencephalography	Personality inventories
Toxicology screen		CSF protein, glucose, cell count, VDRL test	
Complete blood count		Erythrocyte sedimentation rate	
Urinalysis		Lyme antibody	
Thyroid function tests		Antinuclear antibody	
Serum vitamin B_{12} and folate levels		Heavy metals screen	
Fluorescent treponemal antibody (FTA) or rapid plasma reagin (RPR)		Ceruloplasmin, blood copper, and 24-hour urine copper levels	
		Tuberculin skin test	
		24-hour urine porphyrin screen	
		Polysomnography	

CT, computed tomography; MRI, magnetic resonance imaging; HIV, human immunodeficiency virus; CSF, cerebrospinal fluid; VDRL, Venereal Disease Research Laboratory.

concern that her son has become depressed while attending college among the redwoods of northern California. She notes that for 3 weeks, he has made no effort to find a summer job and seems totally unconcerned about the consequences. In addition, he has been largely silent, uninvolved in family activities, uninterested in his usual pastimes of music and tennis, and not socially active—in all regards, a marked contrast to his lifetime pattern.

Although the patient is reticent to give any history, he acknowledges that his mother's description is accurate. He denies, however, that he is depressed or sad. He says that he has made peace with himself and the cosmos and that he has transcended all mundane concerns. He spends his time in meditation about the role he might play in the new world order. He acknowledges that this is a radical departure from his earlier plan to complete a major in biology and attend graduate school. He was sexually active during his first 2 years of college but has lost interest in all social activity over the past several months. He reports frequent drug use at college, particularly marijuana and "ecstasy," and acknowledges occasional marijuana use since returning home.

Physical examination is unremarkable, although he is only marginally cooperative with the eye examination. Mental status examination is noteworthy for psychomotor slowing, poverty of speech, mildly blunted affect, mildly impoverished thoughts, vague peculiarities of thought, and concrete proverb interpretation.

Because of the change in Mr. B.'s demeanor, he receives the essential laboratory tests for psychosis, with toxicology screens repeated over several weeks. Lyme antibody, copper metabolism, and human immunodeficiency virus antibody studies are also performed. He presents no clear delusions, hallucinations, or thought disorganization and is therefore sent for projective psychological testing in order to screen for evidence of possible psychotic symptoms.

Discussion: The primary care physician in this case recognized that there was a major disruption in Mr. B.'s life. As with any illness, the first step was to obtain a thorough history from both the patient and his mother. Next, the patient's condition was investigated by physical and mental status examinations. Because the patient's impoverished and peculiar thinking, blunted affect, and concrete proverb interpretation were suggestive of a psychotic disorder, appropriate laboratory studies and psychological testing were ordered. The initial differential diagnosis included substance abuse, depression, medical illness, and schizophrenia. Results of the laboratory and psychological testing will determine if referral to a psychiatrist is appropriate.

C. Differential diagnosis.

Medical problems always lead the differential diagnoses, irrespective of the pattern of symptoms observed. Although many clinical features may suggest either a psychiatric or a medical cause of the psychosis, these are of limited reliability, and a thorough medical evaluation is required in all cases. A partial list of medical and primary psychiatric causes of psychosis is given in Table 10–3.

Case Study

Substance-induced psychotic disorder:

Mrs. D., a 55-year-old woman, presents to a walk-in clinic indicating that she has heard voices since the previous night. She denies ever experiencing this or any psychiatric symptom before. The voices include several people talking and singing loudly in her room. She appears somewhat unkempt and moves rapidly and frequently. Her speech is poorly focused and disjointed. Her affect is anxious and somewhat agitated. Her thinking is moderately disorganized, and the voices are persistent, but she denies having other hallucinations and any delusions. She is oriented but refuses other cognitive tests.

Physical examination is remarkable for moderately increased heart rate and blood pressure and mild hyperreflexia and clonus but is otherwise within normal limits. Laboratory tests showed mildly elevated liver enzyme levels, including gamma glutamyltransferase, but are otherwise unremarkable. The toxicology findings are negative.

Over the course of the evaluation, she becomes increasingly agitated, while her heart rate and blood pressure continue to rise. With her verbal consent, a telephone call to her family confirms that she has been drinking heavily for the past 2 weeks but stopped abruptly the day before. She is transferred to an emergency facility for treatment of alcohol withdrawal.

Discussion: Medical causes, particularly substance ingestion or withdrawal, must always be considered in the evaluation of psychosis. Clues to this patient's diagnosis included late and rapid onset of psychotic symptoms, unstable vital signs, and elevated liver enzyme levels. Although the diagnosis might have been made without family contact, their additional information facilitated both diagnosis and treatment.

D. What to tell the patient and family.

Although many patients recognize that their fears or unusual sensory experiences represent symptoms of illness, others have no insight into the aberrant nature of their thoughts or experiences. It is important to address this issue with great sensitivity so that rapport with the patient is maintained and enhanced. It is especially important to enlist the patient's cooperation with treatment early in the course of the illness because delusional ideas tend to become more fixed and less amenable to medication when they are left untreated.

Table 10–3
Differential Diagnosis of Psychosis

Substance Induced	Neurologic	Endocrine, Metabolic, and Nutritional	Toxic Reactions and Exposures	Other	Thought Disorders	Mood Disorders	Personality Disorders	Reactive Disorders	Other
Alcohol withdrawal or prolonged use	AIDS- and HIV-related encephalopathy	Acute intermittent porphyria	Anticholinergic agents	Lyme disease	Delusional disorder	Major depressive disorder, severe with psychotic features	Borderline personality disorder	Brief psychotic disorder	Factitious disorder
Amphetamine intoxication	Alzheimer's disease	Cushing's disease	Digitalis	Paraneoplastic syndromes	Schizoaffective disorder	Manic episode, with psychotic features	Paranoid personality disorder	Shared psychotic disorder	Malingering
Cocaine intoxication	Auditory nerve injury or deafness	Hepatic encephalopathy	Dopamine agonists	Systemic lupus erythematosis	Schizophrenia		Schizoid personality disorder		
Inhalant intoxication	Brain abscess	Hypercalcemia or hypocalcemia	Glucocorticoids				Schizotypal personality disorder		
LSD and other hallucinogen intoxication	CNS tumors	Hypercapnea	Heavy metals						
Marijuana or other cannabis derivative intoxication	CVA	Hyperparathyroidism or hypoparathyroidism							
Phencyclidine intoxication	Encephalitis	Hyperthyroidism or hypothyroidism							
Sedative or hypnotic withdrawal	Huntington's chorea	Hypoglycemia							
	Migraine	Hypoxemia							
	Multi-infarct dementia	Korsakoff's psychosis							
	Multiple sclerosis	Pellagra							
	Narcolepsy	Vitamin B_{12} deficiency							
	Neurosyphilis	Wilson's disease							
	Parkinson's disease								
	Seizure disorder								
	Traumatic brain injury								
	Vasculitis								
	Wernicke's encephalopathy								

LSD, lysergic acid diethylamide; CNS, central nervous system; CVA, cerebrovascular accident; AIDS, acquired immunodeficiency syndrome; HIV, human immunodeficiency virus.

1. *What to tell the patient.*
By definition, delusional ideas are not open to correction by evidence to the contrary. In most instances, it is not useful to argue with the patient or to try to prove that delusions are not true, even when this is obviously so. A direct statement acknowledging the patient's belief and the physician's alternative view is preferable, combined with a recommendation for treatment:

> You have been experiencing some very disturbing things in the past few weeks. I know the voices sound very real to you, and the threats seem quite frightening. These experiences are very much like those we see in some types of illness within the brain itself, and I believe that is what is happening to you. These symptoms sometimes occur when there is an infection or injury involving the brain. I have performed tests for these possibilities, and you do not appear to have these problems. Instead, I believe that you have developed a problem in the chemistry of the brain. We don't know very much about why these problems occur, but there are medications that are very helpful in controlling these symptoms, and I recommend that we begin treatment with one of them.

2. *What to tell the family.*
Several issues must be considered when in discussions with family members. As in the case of medical illness, families want accurate, candid information. In the case of psychiatric disorders, it is also useful to reassure the family about the causes of such disorders. An additional consideration is the role the family will play in maintaining the patient's compliance with treatment, a crucial step toward good outcome. The following statement to the parents of a hypothetical young man just diagnosed with schizophrenia addresses these issues:

> The symptoms your son has been experiencing have been very frightening for him and for you. They suggest that his ability to perceive and respond to the world around him has become somewhat impaired. This can be caused by various medical and psychiatric illnesses. I have performed tests for the common medical problems that might cause these symptoms, and everything has turned out to be normal. I checked for evidence of drug abuse, and that did not appear to be the cause, either.
> The diagnosis that most closely fits your son's experience is schizophrenia. This is a disorder of thinking and relating to the world and to other people. We don't know exactly what causes it, but genetic as well as environmental factors appear to be involved. We know that it involves abnormalities in the chemistry and the structure of the brain. We used to believe it was caused by bad parenting, but it is now very clear that parenting style has nothing to do with the development of the illness. What happens in the family from now on is very important, however, because the support that your son receives from you will be critical in keeping him in treatment. Medications are available that will control his symptoms, and you as his family need to be as aware of them as he is.

E. Treatment.

1. *Psychosis secondary to a medical illness.*
Obviously, any underlying medical illness must be treated. Psychotic symptoms may resolve spontaneously with medical intervention alone. In other instances, however, medical illness may be of a chronic or recurrent nature, there may be a substantial delay between onset of treatment and symptom resolution, or the psychosis may present an acutely dangerous situation that requires immediate intervention. In many instances, it is permissible and desirable to begin symptomatic treatment of the psychosis simultaneously with other medical treatments. *In some cases, such as an acutely dangerous patient, antipsychotic treatment may be initiated while the medical evaluation is still in progress.*

2. *Primary psychiatric disorders.*
Treatment of psychotic symptoms should be considered, irrespective of whether they occur in the context of a thought, mood, personality, or reactive disorder. Additional treatments may be appropriate if mood symptoms are also present or if psychosocial factors appear to play a major role in the patient's presentation.

3. *Treatment protocol* (Table 10–4).
   a. *Pharmacotherapy* is the mainstay of antipsychotic treatment, irrespective of the cause of the psychosis. The goal of antipsychotic drug treatment is twofold. Initially, the agitation that may accompany psychotic symptoms should be immediately reduced. Antipsychotic effects are generally seen later, several days to weeks after the medication is started. These include reduction in hallucinations and delusions and better organization of thought. In many instances, these symptoms are significantly reduced, but not completely abolished. Treatment should be considered effective if the residual symptoms do not significantly interfere with the patient's ability to function. *An adequate therapeutic trial of an antipsychotic agent must include 4 to 6 weeks of the full dose of the medication.*

   Conventional antipsychotic medications, also known as typical neuroleptics, operate primarily through blockade of D_2 dopamine receptors. They are divided into high-potency and low-potency compounds (Table 10–5). All are equally efficacious, but their side effects differ somewhat. Major side effects of high-potency, typical neuroleptics include extrapyramidal symptoms (restlessness, muscle rigidity, bradykinesia, dystonic reactions, or tremor), anticholinergic symptoms (dry mouth, constipation, blurred vision, or urinary hesitancy), sexual dysfunction, and sedation (Table 10–6).

Table 10–4
Antipsychotic Treatment Protocol

Option 1	*If*	*Then*
Haloperidol, 5 mg hs	Poor response	Increase dose up to 10 mg b.i.d. Wait 4–6 weeks at full dose Change treatment to risperidone
	Side effects	Decrease dose Add benztropine, 1–2 mg b.i.d.–q.i.d. Add propranolol, 20–40 mg t.i.d.–q.i.d. Add lorazepam, 1 mg t.i.d. Change to risperidone
	Noncompliance	Treat possible side effects Use depot neuroleptic
Option 2	*If*	*Then*
Risperidone, 2 mg bid	Poor response	Increase dose up to 4 mg b.i.d. Wait 4–6 weeks at full dose Change treatment to clozapine
	Side effects	Decrease dose Add benztropine, 1–2 mg b.i.d.–q.i.d. Add propranolol, 20–40 mg t.i.d.–q.i.d. Add lorazepam, 1 mg t.i.d. Change to clozapine
	Noncompliance	Treat possible side effects Use depot neuroleptic

hs, at bedtime; b.i.d., twice a day; t.i.d., three times a day; q.i.d., four times a day.

The side effect profile of low-potency neuroleptics includes more prominent sedation, anticholinergic effects, hypotension, and sexual dysfunction, with less prominent extrapyramidal symptoms. All of these agents may cause tardive dyskinesia and neuroleptic malignant syndrome. Patients must be fully informed of these side effects before they begin treatment.

Atypical antipsychotic drugs include risperidone (Risperdal), clozapine (Clozaril), and olanzapine (Zyprexa). These agents do not operate strictly on the basis of D_2 dopamine receptor blockade and have other pharmacologic actions. They are less likely than typical agents to cause extrapyramidal reactions.

Although a wide variety of protocols for initiation of antipsychotic treatment is available, the following represents one reasonable approach. A brief rationale for each step is presented in order to facilitate understanding and flexibility (see Table 10–4).

(1) *Haloperidol (Haldol), 5 mg orally at bedtime, is given.* This dose is reduced to 1 to 2 mg for the elderly population. If the patient does not respond to this dose, it should be incrementally raised to *10 mg twice daily.* If preferred, the total dose may be given in a single administration, usually at bedtime. Although no general agreement exists on the ideal dose of haloperidol, there is no evidence to suggest that doses higher than 20 mg/d give additional benefit. About 60% to 80% of patients respond to haloperidol therapy. Most treatment failures are related to inadequate dose, patient noncompliance, or insufficient time on the therapy.

Haloperidol is a high-potency, typical neuroleptic. Although it has potentially severe side effects, it also has several compelling advantages. Primary among these is the existence of several available forms of the drug, including pills, liquid concentrate, injectable suspension (to be given intravenously or intramuscularly), and an injectable depot form. This spectrum provides maximum flexibility and assurance of patient compliance. Other advantages of haloperidol include predictable blood levels and therapeutic responses to those levels, ready availability, and low cost. If the patient is unwilling to accept haloperidol or has had an allergic reaction to it, fluphenazine (Prolixin) or thiothixene (Navane) are reasonable alternatives (see Table 10–5).

The major side effects of haloperidol are those of all high-potency, typical neuroleptics: extrapyramidal reactions, anticholinergic symptoms, sexual dysfunction, sedation, and potential for tardive dyskinesia (see Table 10–6).

(2) *Benztropine (Cogentin), 1 mg twice daily,* is commonly administered together with high-potency neuroleptics to reduce extrapyramidal side effects. This agent is often used prophylactically, and it should be given to any patient who experiences restlessness, muscle rigidity, bradykinesia, dystonic reactions, or tremor. *The dose can be adjusted to up to 2 mg four times a day* in order to optimize the response. *Doses greater than 8 mg/d are not recommended.* For the elderly population, 0.5 mg twice daily is a reasonable starting dosage. Alternative medications include diphenhydramine (Benadryl), 25 mg twice a day, which tends to be sedating; trihexyphenidyl (Artane), 2 mg twice daily; and biperiden (Akineton), 2 mg twice daily. These are all anticholinergic agents and as such worsen dry

mouth, constipation, blurred vision, and urinary hesitancy.

(3) *Risperidone, 2 to 4 mg twice daily* (1 mg twice daily for the elderly population), is a reasonable choice if the patient cannot tolerate typical neuroleptics or has not responded to the full dose of conventional antipsychotic administered for 4 to 6 weeks. Risperidone is a newer, "atypical" antipsychotic, with fewer extrapyramidal effects than conventional agents. Its primary side effects include hypotension, restlessness, and sedation. The risks for tardive dyskinesia and neuroleptic malignant syndrome are not fully known but appear comparable to those in typical neuroleptics. Major disadvantages include high cost (about $2000/y) and only one route of administration (pills). Despite these disadvantages, it is rapidly becoming a first-line treatment in some settings and should be considered a favorable alternative choice.

(4) *Depot neuroleptic* should be considered for a patient who responds well to conventional agents but does not take prescribed doses reliably. These agents are injected intramuscularly and are slowly released over about 4 weeks. Although many patients are initially resistant to accepting injections, this mode of administration is extremely useful for a selected group.

A rapid-loading regimen is *haloperidol decanoate, 100 mg intramuscularly on day 1, 150 mg intramuscularly on day 3, and 150 mg intramuscularly on day 5.* This is followed by a maintenance regimen of *150 mg intramuscularly every 4 weeks.* This dosage is equivalent to approximately 10 to 15 mg/d of oral haloperidol. This regimen should be used only in patients who have previously received oral or nondepot injectable haloperidol. Ideally, patients are stabilized on the oral medication before the conversion to the depot form. In that case, the oral dose is halved at the time of the second injection and is discontinued with the third injection.

A depot form of fluphenazine is also available but has a shorter release time (about 2 weeks) and less predictable serum neuroleptic levels. Rapid loading of fluphenazine decanoate is not recommended.

(5) *Other neuroleptics* may be considered if the patient has a history of prior good response, is allergic to the aforementioned recommended agents, or expresses a preference for other reasons. These drugs differ in potency and side effect profile, but are all equally efficacious in the treatment of psychosis.

(6) *Adjunctive agents* should be considered if the patient partially responds to antipsychotics but remains agitated or has persistent decrements in function.

- *Lorazepam (Ativan), 1 mg three times a day,* is especially useful for persistent agitation or restlessness. The dose can be adjusted over a wide range, from 0.5 mg at bedtime to 2 mg four times a day.
- *Propranolol (Inderal), 20 mg three times a day* is recommended for patients with restlessness (akathisia) or marked tremor. The dose can be titrated upward as tolerated by the patient.

(7) *Clozapine (Clozaril)* is reserved for psychotic patients who have failed to respond to at least two other neuroleptics, cannot tolerate other neuroleptics, or have severe tardive dyskinesia. Clozapine is an atypical antipsychotic with greater efficacy against psychotic symptoms than other currently available agents. It does not appear to cause extrapyramidal side effects or tardive dyskinesia. In general, this medication should be started only by practitioners experienced in its use, who have an established monitoring system by which weekly white blood cell counts can be monitored. The major side effects of clozapine include hypotension, sedation, tachycardia, seizures, and anticholinergic effects.

Agranulocytosis occurs in 1% to 2% of cases and is fatal in one case in 10,000. In the United States, clozapine may only be dispensed in 1-week supplies, after the pharmacist has confirmation that the white blood cell count is within an acceptable range that week. In addition, Sandoz Pharmaceuticals, which markets Clozaril, maintains a surveillance system to ensure that any patient who has once developed agranulocytosis is not rechallenged with the drug. Although this level of monitoring has ensured that the rate of fatal complications remains low, it also contributes to the high cost of the drug (about $10,000/y).

b. *Hospital admission* should be considered for these patients and is mandatory for any patient with serious suicidal or homicidal intent, who is physically threatening to others, whose behavior might unintentionally be harmful to himself or someone else, who is too disorganized to provide for basic needs, or who is at risk for grossly irresponsible behavior that might have long-term negative consequences.

c. *Electroconvulsive therapy* is generally reserved for severe depression with psychotic features, mania, or catatonia. In these conditions, it should be considered early if there is an

Table 10–5 Antipsychotic (Neuroleptic) Medications

Generic Name	Brand Name	Relative Potency (mg)	Common Dosage (mg/d)	Available Routes and Strengths	Sedation	Extrapyramidal Effects	Anticholinergic Effects	Orthostatic Hypotension
Typical High Potency								
Droperidol	Inapsine	1		Injection: 2.5 mg/mL	++	+++++	+	+
Fluphenazine	Permitil, Prolixin	1–2	1–20	Tablets: 1, 2.5, 5, 10 mg. Elixir: 0.5 mg/mL Injection: 2.5 mg/mL Depot: 25 mg/mL	++	+++++	+	+
Haloperidol	Haldol	2	5–20	Scored tablet: 0.5, 1, 2, 5, 10, 20 mg Concentrate: 2 mg/mL Injection: 5 mg/mL Depot: 50, 100 mg/mL	++	+++++	+	+
Loxapine	Loxitane	10	60–100	Capsules: 5, 10, 25, 50 mg Concentrate: 25 mg/mL Injection: 50 mg/mL	+++	++++	++	++
Molindone	Moban	10	50–150	Tablets: 5, 10, 25, 50, 100 mg Concentrate: 20 mg/mL	++	+++	+++	++
Perphenazine	Trilafon	8	4–32	Tablets: 2, 4, 8, 16 mg Concentrate: 16 mg/5 mL Injection: 5 mg/mL	++	+++++	+	+
Pimozide	Orap	1	2–10	Tablets: 2 mg	+	+++++	+	+
Thiothixene	Navane	2–5	5–30	Tablets: 1, 2, 5, 10, 20 mg Concentrate: 5 mg/mL Injection: 5 mg/mL	+	++++	+	++
Trifluoperazine	Stelazine	5	4–20	Tablets: 1, 2, 5, 10 mg Concentrate: 10 mg/mL Injection: 2 mg/mL	++	+++++	+	+

Low Potency								
Chlorpromazine	Thorazine	100	100–800	Tablets: 10, 25, 50, 100, 200 mg Sustained-release capsules: 30, 75, 150 mg Syrup: 2 mg/mL Concentrate: 30, 100 mg/mL Suppositories: 30, 100 mg Injection: 25 mg/mL	+ + + + +	+ +	+ + + +	+ + + + +
Mesoridazine	Serentil	50	100–300	Tablets: 10, 25, 50, 100 mg Concentrate: 25 mg/mL Injection: 25 mg/mL	+ + + +	+ +	+ + +	+ +
Prochlorperazine	Compazine	100	50–75	Tablets: 5, 10, 25 mg Sustained-release capsules: 10, 15 mg Suppositories: 2.5, 5, 25 mg Syrup: 1 mg/mL Injection: 5 mg/mL	+ + +	+ + + + +	+	+
Thioridazine	Mellaril	100	100–800	Coated tablets: 10, 15, 25, 50, 100, 150, 200 mg Concentrate: 30, 100 mg/mL	+ + + + +	+	+ + + +	+ + + +
Atypical								
Clozapine	Clozaril	100	300–900	Scored tablets: 25, 100 mg	+ + + + +	+	+ + + +	+ + + + +
Risperidone	Risperdal	1	4–8	Tablets: 1 (scored), 2, 3, 4 mg	+ +	+ +	−/+	+ + +
Olanzapine	Zyprexa	1	10–20	Tablets: 5, 7.5, 10 mg	+ + +	+	+ + +	+ + +

−/+, minimal; +, mild; + +, mild-moderate; + + +, moderate; + + + +, moderate-severe; + + + + +, severe.

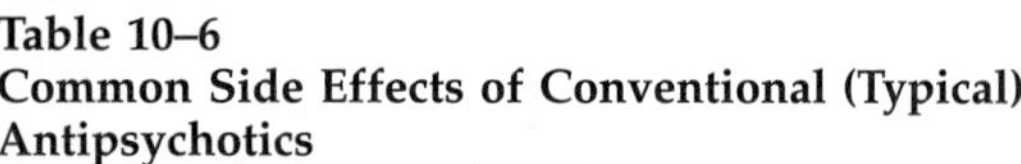

Table 10–6
Common Side Effects of Conventional (Typical) Antipsychotics

Extrapyramidal	Anticholinergic	Other
Restlessness (akathisia)	Dry mouth	Sedation
Bradykinesia	Constipation	Hypotension
Acute dystonia	Urinary hesitancy	Sexual dysfunction
Muscle rigidity	Blurred vision	Neuroleptic malignant syndrome
Tremor		
Tardive dyskinesia		

immediate threat to the patient's safety or well-being, such as refusal to eat or drink.

d. *Psychosocial interventions* should be considered in cases in which readily identifiable stressors exist that may contribute to the patient's difficulties.
   (1) *Patient and family education* regarding diagnosis, prognosis, expected benefits of treatment, and possible medication side effects is essential. Patient compliance, perceived benefits of treatment, family interactions, and maintenance of a family support system are all enhanced by candid, accurate, and timely education.
   (2) *Social skills training* is useful for patients with long-term disorders, such as schizophrenia, so that the deficits in social function that develop during the course of illness can be addressed.
   (3) *Patient and family support groups* are often a valuable resource. Among the most widespread and effective groups is the National Alliance for the Mentally Ill, a support and advocacy group involving many families of severely mentally ill patients.

e. *Discussion with patients about typical neuroleptic medication* occurs in order to explain about, and obtain consent for, the medication. It should motivate the patient to begin and continue with treatment. Usually, the family is involved in helping the patient continue taking the medication and should be given the same information. A frank discussion of side effects is essential both to obtain consent and to ensure compliance.

I recommend that we use a neuroleptic medication to treat your symptoms. The medication is especially effective for treating the voices, unreasonable fears, and disorganization of thinking you have experienced. We can expect the medication to help you distinguish between voices that come from the outside world and those that the brain may be manufacturing itself; it will cause the voices originating in the brain to go away. It will allow you to sort out which ideas and fears you really need to be concerned about and which you don't. It will keep your thinking organized and will help you stay focused on the things in the outside world that are important to you. This may help you get back to doing the things you want to do, without being distracted by these other thoughts and voices.

Like all medicines, this one has some side effects, and I want you to understand them before you take it. The most common side effects are dry mouth, constipation, sleepiness, restlessness, and stiff muscles. If the restlessness and stiffness become uncomfortable, we may want to add another medicine to make that feel better. Somewhat less often, this medicine makes people dizzy, lightheaded, or sleepy. If you take the medicine over a long period of time, you may develop something called tardive dyskinesia. That is a medical term that means "late bad movements," and it refers to a pill-rolling motion of the hands or movements of the jaw or tongue back and forth. About one person in 20 has some of those movements after the first year, and about half of people taking it have them after 10 years. It is usually not a major problem, but in a few cases, it becomes serious, and in rare instances, it even continues after the treatment is stopped. Most people are not terribly bothered by the movements and prefer to continue taking the medication, but the movements can be a problem, and for that reason, I want you to watch for them and tell me if they start to develop.

The medicine takes about 1 to 2 weeks to begin to have an effect and about 6 weeks to have its full effect. The side effects are worst in the first couple of weeks, so it is very important to stay with the treatment through those first few days, when it may be making you uncomfortable and doesn't seem to be doing much. When the medicine starts working, you will be glad you did.

III. Psychiatric disorders.

A. Primary thought disorders.

1. *Schizophrenia* is a heterogeneous disorder consisting of two fundamentally different types of symptoms, classified as *positive* and *negative.* It has no pathognomonic features or specific diagnostic tests, but is identified by a longitudinal pattern of symptoms consistent with the diagnosis, and the systematic elimination of other known medical causes and psychiatric disorders (Tables 10–7 and 10–8).
   a. *Positive symptoms* of schizophrenia refer to active psychosis, including hallucinations, delusions, thought disorganization, bizarre behavior, and catatonia. These need not be present at all times through the course of illness but must be present over a continuous course of at least 4 weeks to meet current diagnostic criteria for the disorder.
   b. *Negative symptoms* refer to aspects of life and social interaction that tend to be deficient in schizophrenia. These symptoms include blunted affect; poverty of speech and thought; loss of interests; loss of pleasure (anhedonia); loss of motivation; psychomotor slowing; diminished capacity for, and interest in, social interaction and intimacy; and poor attention

Table 10–7
Diagnosis and Clinical Course of Schizophrenia

Prodrome (not always present)	Schizoid, schizotypal, or paranoid personality traits Lower-than-expected educational achievement Social withdrawal Unusual behavior or thinking
Active phase (must be present for ≥ 1 mo)	Delusions Hallucinations Disorganized speech Disorganized or catatonic behavior Marked negative symptoms (blunted affect, poverty of speech, lack of motivation, anhedonia)
Deterioration (must be present for ≥ 6 mo)	Marked decline in school or work performance Loss of interest in interpersonal relationships Poor self-care
Residual	Acute phase symptoms are mild or absent Negative or deteriorative symptoms predominate

to social and cognitive tasks. Largely as a result of these symptoms, a deterioration occurs in the quality of life or level of function of schizophrenic patients. This deterioration must continue for at least 6 months for the symptoms to meet criteria for the disorder.

c. *Diagnostic subtypes* of schizophrenia are based on clinical presentation and have some implications for the clinical course and the response to treatment.
   (1) *Paranoid type* is characterized by predominant delusions and hallucinations. Negative symptoms, such as blunted affect, tend to be less severe, and social and occupational function may be less impaired. Medication treatment may dramatically reduce symptoms.
   (2) *Disorganized type* includes prominent disorganization of thought and behavior, accompanied by flat or inappropriate affect. The course tends to be chronic and the symptoms profoundly disabling. Medications tend to be only moderately effective.
   (3) *Catatonic type* is relatively rare and involves immobility or excessive motor activity, mutism, resistance to instructions, and bizarre movements and postures. Catatonic symptoms are more often related to mood disorders than to schizophrenia.
   (4) *Undifferentiated type* refers to symptoms that include elements of more than one of the aforementioned categories or that do not fit any of the aforementioned descriptions.
   (5) *Residual type* may follow an acute episode of another subtype. It is characterized by continued negative symptoms or peculiarities of thought or behavior after the prominent delusions, hallucinations, or thought disorganization have resolved.

d. *The clinical course* of schizophrenia is extremely variable, largely because of the complex interplay of positive and negative symptoms. In general, negative symptoms occur first, in a *prodromal* phase of the illness, often several years before the onset of positive symptoms. The clinician should be alert to the presentation of negative symptoms during this prodromal period. This phase is often mistaken for depression because of the anhedonia, loss of interest, and psychomotor slowing that are common to both disorders. A thorough mental status examination reveals an absence of depressed mood, however, as well as blunted and unresponsive affect.

Table 10–8
Capsule Sketch of Schizophrenia

Positive symptoms	Hallucinations Delusions Thought disorganization Catatonia
Negative symptoms	Blunted affect Poverty of thought and speech Loss of interest and pleasure (anhedonia) Loss of motivation Diminished capacity for social interaction and intimacy Psychomotor slowing Poor attention
Annual incidence	15–20 per 100,000
Prevalence	0.5–1% of adults
Age at onset	Men: 18–30 years Women: 20–40 years
Prognosis	10–15% of patients enter total remission 80% of untreated patients relapse within 1 year 20% of treated patients relapse within 1 year 20–40% of patients do not respond to typical antipsychotics 10–15% of patients respond preferentially to clozapine
Complications	Suicide—10% of patients Depression in 50% of cases Homelessness Commission of crimes incidental to homelessness Frequent victims of both violent and nonviolent crimes Substance abuse in > 50% of cases

In a smaller number of patients, the onset of illness is heralded by a period of florid psychosis (the first psychotic break), after which an incomplete return to the patient's previous level of function may occur. In about half of these patients, a careful history reveals subtle abnormalities of thought or social interaction that predate the psychosis. This may include social isolation or awkwardness (e.g., an adolescent who never dates), scholastic performance below family norms, or peculiar interests and habits (e.g., fascination with extraterrestrials, interest in extrasensory perception).

Once the diagnosis is established, the clinical course of schizophrenia is typically one of intermittent exacerbations of positive symptoms, followed by periods of remission. Negative symptoms, in contrast, tend to be chronic and progressive throughout the course of illness. A small number of patients with schizophrenia (10% to 15%) return to their premorbid levels of function.

e. *Complications* of schizophrenia include depression in up to 50% of patients. At least 10% die by suicide. Substance abuse occurs in more than 50% of cases. Impaired self-care, including deficits in routine activities of daily living, hygiene, and nutrition, often occurs. Social functioning tends to be very poor, and patients have difficulty maintaining family relations, social contacts, and employment. Homelessness is common in this population, in part because of social policy decisions and in part as a direct result of negative symptoms. Petty crime is not unusual, especially violations incidental to life on the streets, such as trespassing, defrauding an innkeeper, or urinating in public. With schizophrenia patients are frequently the victims of robbery and assault for similar reasons. The economic consequences of schizophrenia include not only direct care expenses but also lost productivity, disability payments, and law enforcement costs.

f. *Epidemiology* of schizophrenia is as follows: about 0.5% to 1% of adults worldwide have schizophrenia. The age of onset tends to be in the early twenties for men and the late twenties or early thirties for women. Although it was formerly believed that the illness could not begin after the midforties, this is no longer felt to be true, and a small percentage of cases are diagnosed in the later years.

g. There is a strong *familial pattern* to schizophrenia, although the exact mode of inheritance is unknown. In monozygotic twins, there is a 50% concurrence rate for the illness, whereas in dizygotic twins (and other siblings) the rate is 10%. For the children of one parent with schizophrenia, the frequency of the diagnosis is 10% to 15%, and for those with two parents with schizophrenia, it is 30% to 40%.

h. The *pathophysiology* of schizophrenia is poorly understood. Some evidence implicates dopamine hyperactivity in the limbic system (the "emotional brain"), reduced neuronal activity in the frontal lobes, and structural lesions in the midbrain. The most often replicated finding in biologic studies of schizophrenia is enlargement of the lateral ventricles relative to brain volume, although the lesion responsible for this aberrancy has not been determined. The incidence of schizophrenia is increased in children whose mothers were exposed to influenza in the second trimester of pregnancy. Perinatal anoxia is also associated with the later development of schizophrenia. Other environmental factors are less well characterized.

The former hypothesis that schizophrenia is in some way related to parenting style has been thoroughly discredited. It is true, however, that certain parenting and family communication styles are associated with a less favorable course and outcome of the illness.

Similarly, the belief that substance abuse causes the illness is not supported by the available data. Substance abuse is common in schizophrenic patients, however, and is associated with more frequent acute episodes and hospitalization.

i. The *treatment* of schizophrenia includes biologic and psychological components.
   (1) *Antipsychotic (neuroleptic) medications* are the mainstay of treatment for the positive symptoms of schizophrenia (see section II.E.3). In the acute phase of illness, the medications are intended to induce a remission of psychotic symptoms. In general, once the diagnosis has been established, patients should continue taking these medications indefinitely in order to avoid relapse. In patients in remission who are treated with antipsychotics, the annual recurrence rate is 20%; the rate is 80% for patients who are not treated. Negative symptoms respond poorly to antipsychotic medication.
   (2) The second aspect of schizophrenia treatment is *psychosocial.* Most patients require some degree of intervention in order to maintain an acceptable level of occupational function, social contact, or self-care. In addition, family interactions involving high levels of expressed emotion are especially detrimental to these patients. Psychosocial treatment may include intensive case management, social skills training, family education, and vocational rehabilitation. In many cases, a social worker can ensure that adequate financial and medical resources are

available to the patient. It is largely for this reason that the treatment of schizophrenia should be undertaken in a specialty clinic, where a treatment team may involve each of these disciplines, rather than managed in the primary care setting.

A widespread network of publicly funded community mental health (CMH) clinics is now available throughout most of the United States. These clinics tend to focus on chronic, debilitating psychiatric disorders, such as schizophrenia, and are usually much better equipped to provide the spectrum of services required by these patients. They include interdisciplinary treatment teams consisting of a psychiatrist, a social worker, a case manager, and a psychologist or other therapist, working in close collaboration. Most schizophrenic patients should be referred to their local CMH agencies for long-term management.

2. *Schizoaffective disorder* differs from schizophrenia in that a significant mood component to the illness exists. Under current diagnostic criteria, both a mood disturbance and psychosis must be present, and they must have occurred independently of one another at some point in the illness. Like schizophrenia, schizoaffective disorder is a chronic, debilitating disorder requiring long-term treatment with medications and psychosocial interventions. Patients with schizoaffective disorder often require a combination of antipsychotic and mood-stabilizing medication to induce and maintain remission of acute symptoms.

3. *Delusional disorder* is characterized by the occurrence of delusions without the prominent hallucinations, thought disorganization, blunted affect, catatonia, or functional deterioration that are present in schizophrenia. The delusions typically involve events that might occur in real life but for which there is no basis in fact for the patient involved. For example, a patient may believe that a neighbor is spying on him, that his telephone is tapped, or that his spouse is plotting his murder. Aside from the delusional belief, the patient's appearance and behavior are not abnormal. Hallucinations in all modalities may occur, but they are not prominent. If tactile or olfactory hallucinations occur, they are directly related to the delusional belief. For example, a patient may feel the worms that she believes to be eating her intestines.

   Delusional disorder is uncommon in the general population, occurring with a frequency of less than 0.1%. Symptoms usually begin in the middle or late years of life. The course is variable: there may be spontaneous remissions, followed by recurrence of symptoms, or the symptoms may be chronic and progressive.

4. *Schizophreniform disorder* differs from schizophrenia only in the duration of the illness, which is 1 to 6 months, and in the absence of functional deterioration in some cases. Although most patients with schizophreniform disorder go on to meet the diagnostic criteria for schizophrenia, a significant percentage recover and have no further psychotic episodes.

B. Primary mood disorders.

1. *Major depressive disorder with psychotic features,* the course of a major depressive episode is complicated by the development of psychotic symptoms in about 10% of cases. Delusions, hallucinations, thought disorganization, and catatonia may each occur during the course of the episode. The content of the delusions or hallucinations need not be congruent with the patient's mood.

   Suicide is a major clinical issue in these patients, and suicidality must always be assessed. Such an assessment includes careful questioning regarding the involvement of psychotic symptoms in thoughts of suicide. For example, a patient who says that he does not want to harm himself may be hearing voices ordering him to do so. The presence of command hallucinations to harm oneself is highly correlated with acts of self-harm and must always be taken seriously.

   a. *Treatment* must be directed toward both the depressive and the psychotic symptoms. In general, the use of either an antidepressant or an antipsychotic medication alone is not effective. The two basic treatment options for these patients are medications and electroconvulsive therapy. Hospital admission should be considered for these patients and is essential for any patient with serious suicidal intent.

      (1) *Antipsychotic/antidepressant combinations:* Haloperidol, (Haldol) 5 mg at bedtime and Sertraline (Zoloft), 50 mg daily.

      The two medications may be titrated to an effective dose simultaneously or separately. A selective serotonin reuptake inhibitor is recommended in this case because this class of antidepressants has few side effects in common with neuroleptics. The major drug interaction between neuroleptics and selective serotonin reuptake inhibitors is inhibition of liver microsomal metabolism, with a resulting increase in antipsychotic blood levels. Although sertraline has been reported to have less propensity to increase neuroleptic levels than other selective serotonin reuptake inhibitors, this effect is of minimal clinical significance, and any selective serotonin reuptake inhibitor may reasonably be used.

The combination of a tricyclic antidepressant and a neuroleptic tends to be a less favorable alternative. Although clinically effective, these medications have anticholinergic, hypotensive, and sedating side effects in common and are not very well tolerated. Nevertheless, in patients for whom these side effects have not been a problem, this may be an appropriate combination.

Combination agents, such as Triavil or Etrafon (amitriptyline and perphenazine), lack flexibility, do not include optimal first-line agents, and are not recommended. Similarly, amoxapine (Asendin), which has both antidepressant and antipsychotic efficacy, has an unfavorable side effect profile, lacks flexibility in dosing, and is no longer considered an optimal first-line agent.

(2) *Electroconvulsive therapy.* Depression with psychotic features may be considered an indication for electroconvulsive therapy as a first-line treatment. This is especially true for cases of catatonia, in which the patient's health is immediately threatened by a failure to eat or drink. Electroconvulsive therapy is the surest and most effective treatment of depression with psychotic features and should be considered earlier in the course of this illness than in the treatment of uncomplicated depression.

2. *Manic episode, with psychotic features* includes a distinct period of both mood elevation and psychotic thinking. Elevated mood is indicated by euphoria, expansiveness, or irritability. Accompanying symptoms include grandiose ideas or self-image, decreased need for sleep, increased rate or quantity of speech, racing thoughts, distractible attention, increased purposeful activity, psychomotor agitation, and irresponsible behavior, such as spending sprees and high-risk sexual activity.

   Psychotic features are common in manic episodes and are usually, but not always, consistent with the elevation in mood. These *mood-congruent* symptoms may include voices telling the person to do some great task, such as begin a new movie studio, give advice to the president, or revise the doctrine of an existing church. Delusions may include the belief that the patient is an important historical figure, a religious leader, or a supremely talented artist or entertainer.

   Delusions and hallucinations may cross the entire spectrum of pathology, however, and in some instances are not clearly associated with mood changes. Such *mood incongruent* symptoms may be indistinguishable from those of an acute schizophrenic episode and in some instances may mask the mood symptoms. For example, a manic patient may have such profound persecutory delusions that the mood elevation is no longer obvious. In such cases, the correct diagnosis is determined only after a careful review of the clinical course of the episode.

   Irritability may lead to hostile, sometimes violent, encounters with family, neighbors, or others. Physical assaultiveness is common during these episodes, even among individuals not otherwise disposed to violence. The risk of suicide is also increased, although not to the degree seen during depressive episodes.

   Treatment begins with introduction of an antipsychotic medication. A neuroleptic is the most effective short-term treatment for psychotic symptoms and for mood elevation. It is often advisable to begin a mood-stabilizing medication simultaneously with the antipsychotic agent. In general, a mood stabilizer used alone during the acute phase of illness provides less rapid and less complete resolution of symptoms than the same agent used in combination with an antipsychotic agent. When the acute episode is well controlled, the antipsychotic can be withdrawn, and the patient can be treated with a mood stabilizer alone.

   Hospital admission should be considered for these patients and is essential for any patient with serious suicidal or homicidal intent, who is physically threatening to others, whose behavior might unintentionally be harmful to himself or herself or to someone else, or who is at risk for grossly irresponsible behavior that might have long-term negative consequences.

   For recommendations regarding mood stabilization *as an adjunct to antipsychotics,* see Chapter 8. As with all psychotic patients, these individuals should be referred to a CMH clinic or to a psychiatrist experienced in treatment of the disorder as soon as the symptoms are recognized.

C. Personality disorders.

These disorders are distinguished from major psychiatric disorders in that they represent lifelong, maladaptive patterns of thinking and behaving rather than specific symptoms whose onset represents a deviation in the person's experience. Some personality disorders may include brief episodes of psychotic symptoms. If such symptoms become prominent, are very bizarre, or last longer than a few days, another diagnosis should be considered.

1. *Paranoid personality disorder* is characterized by a pattern of suspiciousness and a fear of hostile intent without any basis for those concerns. People with paranoid personality disor-

der typically suspect that others want to harm or exploit them, distrust those around them, are reluctant to confide in others, bear grudges, see hidden threats to their safety and attacks on their character in innocent situations, and suspect their spouses of infidelity. Their interactions with others tend to be aloof, hostile, and cold.

Although individuals with this disorder are prone to atypical ideas, their beliefs are not bizarre, are not completely foreign to their cultural milieu, and are not formed into well-defined, clearly delusional ideas. Neither do they experience hallucinations or thought disorganization under ordinary circumstances. During times of stress, however, they may develop overt psychotic symptoms for brief periods, rarely more than a few hours. Paranoid personality traits may also be a prodrome to the development of schizophrenia. If psychotic symptoms persist or require medication in order to resolve, a diagnosis of schizophrenia should be considered.

Treatment of paranoid personality disorder is difficult, particularly given the resistance of these individuals to establishing trusting relationships, as is essential for most forms of psychotherapy. *Medication is rarely of benefit in the absence of clear-cut delusional ideas.*

2. *Schizoid personality disorder* is characterized by a lack of interest in social interaction and intimacy and a lack of emotional expression. These individuals have little interest in family or friends; do not confide in other people; tend to engage in solitary work and hobbies; seem cold, aloof, and detached; and seem to derive little enjoyment from most activities.

   Aside from their social indifference, individuals with schizoid personality disorder are not odd in their thinking or behavior. Any psychotic symptoms they develop are limited to very brief periods of severe stress. They do not generally require specific antipsychotic treatment; instead, they rapidly return to their baseline condition once the stressful situation is resolved.

   Schizoid personality disorder may be a prodome to schizophrenia, and that diagnosis should be considered in any patients with schizoid personality disorder who have psychotic symptoms lasting longer than a few days.

3. *Schizotypal personality disorder* includes a lack of social interactions, personal relationships, and intimacy, accompanied by odd behaviors and perceptual distortions. Common characteristics include ideas of reference, eccentric beliefs or habits, unusual patterns of thought or speech, unreasonable suspiciousness, constricted affect, and social anxiety.

   Although these symptoms are similar to those described for schizophrenia, the severity and degree of disability are less with schizotypal personality. The perceptual problems and unusual thinking described here do not meet the definition of psychotic delusions or hallucinations. In some cases, however, the personality disorder is a prodrome to the development of schizophrenia, and individuals with schizotypal personality disorder are at risk for the development of true psychotic symptoms. If psychotic symptoms occur and persist longer than a few hours or days, patients should be given an additional diagnosis (e.g., schizophreniform disorder) and should be treated accordingly.

4. *Borderline personality disorder* is characterized by extreme instability of mood, sense of identity, and personal relationships. Impulsive behavior, suicide attempts, self-mutilation, feelings of emptiness, and extreme sensitivity to rejection and abandonment are common aspects of this disorder.

   During times of stress, individuals with borderline personality disorder may have psychotic symptoms, including hallucinations, delusions, and thought disorganization. These symptoms may last from hours to days and may be indistinguishable from those experienced by patients with schizophrenia or other psychoses. More commonly, however, they are presented in a dramatic and overblown way, and the patient becomes vague and equivocal when examined more carefully.

   Longitudinal history, which is often obtained from family and associates, is essential to the correct diagnosis. Many of the psychotic symptoms disappear when the stressful situation resolves. Some patients with borderline personality disorder benefit, however, from a low maintenance dose of a neuroleptic.

D. Other disorders.

1. *Malingering* is the intentional fabrication or exaggeration of psychotic symptoms to obtain a specific end, such as avoidance of criminal prosecution or qualification for financial compensation. The diagnosis should be considered only if a readily identifiable incentive exists for the patient to falsify symptoms. In some settings, such as where financial compensation is significant for psychotic patients, overemphasis of genuine symptoms may represent a legitimate adaptation by the patient. In general, the societal benefits of feigned psychosis are limited, and malingering should be considered at the end, not at the beginning, of the differential diagnosis list.

2. *Factitious disorders* are a variant on malingering. A factitious disorder is the fabrication of psychotic symptoms for primary, rather than secondary, gain. Assumption of the sick role or placement in the structured environment of

the psychiatric unit are the motivations typically cited in this disorder. Factitious disorders generally occur only in the presence of a severe, coexisting personality disorder. Assumption of a psychiatric diagnosis and placement on a psychiatric unit are not situations to which individuals in modern society typically aspire, and a diagnosis of factitious disorder should be considered only after other diagnostic possibilities have been exhausted.

IV. Practical considerations.

A. Treatment of psychotic patients who have medical illness.

Even in adequately treated psychotic patients, residual symptoms are common. These may include difficulty communicating, inability to distinguish and describe physical symptoms, disinterest, lack of interpersonal skills, and cognitive deficits. In patients who continue to have active psychotic symptoms, treatment of medical illness may be complicated by disorganized thinking, paranoid delusions, somatic delusions, or hallucinations. A further complicating factor may be the presence of medication side effects. Each of these factors must be taken into account when health care is provided for this population.

1. *Symptom presentation.*
In general, psychotic patients tend to underreport physical symptoms. As a consequence, physical illness often goes undiagnosed and untreated. When this characteristic is combined with their often impaired ability to maintain adequate nutrition, hygiene, and physical activity, these patients are at an unusually high risk for both acute and chronic medical conditions but are less likely to recognize and report those conditions. Subtle indications of problems should be actively sought and considered; for example, respiratory or infectious processes should be ruled out in a patient whose behavior or cognition has changed dramatically over a short time.

Patients with psychosis tend to overlap the physical, emotional, and cognitive aspects of the illness. It would not be unusual, for example, for a patient to complain of a "depressed stomach." Likewise, the statement, "There are worms in my legs," may mean that the patient experiences physical discomfort or that the patient has a delusion about the legs. Peculiarities of language further confuse the picture. "I take the pill for my voices; it ills me in the head," may mean that the pill gives the patient a headache, that it causes clouding of consciousness, or that the pill is for mental illness. Each of these possibilities needs to be explored carefully, in clear, concrete terms.

Patients are aware that their medications cause side effects, and they tend to attribute the physical symptoms they experience to those medications. Many patients are ambivalent about the use of psychotropic agents and may express their resistance by attributing symptoms to them. Primary care physicians are often sought as allies by patients seeking to terminate antipsychotic treatment. While investigating physical symptoms, the physician must maintain a balance between an awareness of those side effects, a goal of minimizing them, and a desire to encourage continued compliance with treatment.

Case Study

Presentation of neuroleptic side effects.

Mr. F., a 35-year-old man with a 10-year history of schizophrenia, presents himself to a primary care physician complaining of anxiety. He describes this as a restless feeling that makes it hard for him to sit or lie down, disturbs his sleep, and interferes with his job in a warehouse. It began when he started taking haloperidol, prescribed by a CMH psychiatrist, several weeks ago. He acknowledges that the medication has controlled his hallucinations and that several previous attempts to stop taking the medication resulted in hospital admissions.

Physical examination reveals normal vital signs, mild bradykinesia and cogwheel rigidity at both upper extremities, and moderate hand tremor. Mental status examination is noteworthy for mild inattention to grooming, moderate restlessness, minimal loose associations, blunted affect, and mild thought disorganization.

After discussion with the CMH psychiatrist, it appears most likely that the patient has developed akathisia and parkinsonism in response to haloperidol therapy. Because the haloperidol has effectively stabilized Mr. F.'s psychotic symptoms, it is decided to increase his benztropine from 1 mg twice daily to 2 mg twice daily in an attempt to decrease his side effects.

Discussion: A patient with a long-standing diagnosis who has a recent change in medication is at increased risk for side effects. The physician's awareness of the most common side effects of neuroleptic medication led to a correct determination of the cause of the patient's distress, even though the patient incorrectly labeled it "anxiety."

Case Study

Psychotic presentation of a physical complaint.

Ms. H., a 45-year-old woman with schizophrenia, presents herself to a community physician with stomach pain. She explains that she knows that she is being poisoned by malicious individuals in her neighborhood because she hears them in her house at night and can taste the poison in her food and tap water. She demands that a blood test be performed to identify the poison and prove her suspicions. On physical examination, she has moderate epigastric tenderness and guaiac-positive stool.

The physician explains that there are many reasons why she might have stomach pain and that a series of tests might be necessary to establish the exact cause. Although the patient remains fixed in her belief that she is being poisoned, she responds well to assurance that the physician will work with her to understand and treat the cause of her pain. The physician schedules the appropriate tests, then contacts the patient's CMH psychiatrist to coordinate her care.

Discussion: The physician carefully evaluated the patient's legitimate physical complaint without becoming caught up in, or distracted by, her psychotic symptoms. To the degree that the patient was able to understand and cooperate with the evaluation, the physician involved her in the process.

2. *Doctor/patient relationship.*
   a. *Interpersonal deficits* are characteristic of chronic psychotic disorders and manifest themselves as blunted or bizarre affect, lack of attention to social cues, lack of interest in social relationships, and inability to experience intimacy.
   b. *Regression,* the progressive development of a passive and dependent personality style, is common.
   c. *Ambivalence,* an inability to make a decision or even state with certainty how one feels, is a fundamental characteristic.
   d. *Suspiciousness,* or even overt paranoid delusions, may include virtually anyone in the patient's environment, including the primary care physician.
   e. *Hostility* toward other people in general, and medical professionals in particular, may be present.
   f. *Adaptation to life* with chronic psychotic symptoms and frequent institutional involvement (e.g., with hospitals, social service agencies, or police) may facilitate the development of a defensive or manipulative personality style.
   g. The *bizarre nature* of some psychotic symptoms may strain the credibility of caregivers, leading to erroneous accusations of malingering or factitious symptoms.
   h. The *physician's response* to the patient is affected by each of these factors. A physician who normally is able to establish good rapport and a warm working relationship in the examining room may find doing so difficult or impossible with a chronic psychotic patient. It may be frustrating when a patient is unable to make a decision regarding treatment or expects the physician to take a larger-than-usual role in the decision. Implications or accusations of malevolence may be taken at face value rather than seen as psychotic symptoms, which may place the physician in a defensive posture. Abnormal personality traits may create an impatient, intolerant attitude in precisely the patients for whom patience and tolerance are most essential.

Case Study

Psychosis versus schizotypal personality.

Mr. J., a 50-year-old man, is seen in a family practice clinic for a sore throat, muscle aches, and sinus congestion. In giving a social history, he reports that he has worked happily for many years as a night watchman in an office building, where he makes solo rounds and sits alone watching security monitors. He also shops at night so as to avoid people who might be able to read or influence his thoughts. He maintains a legal collection of handguns and assault weapons because, he says, "You never know who's out there." He has never been interested in friendships, family, and so on. His family history includes schizophrenia in a grandparent, uncle, and brother.

His speech is stilted and odd, although generally well organized. His affect is constricted, and he remains cold and aloof, despite the physician's best efforts to establish rapport. His physical examination is consistent with a viral upper respiratory infection.

The physician offers him a prescription for a decongestant, but he declines, expressing vague suspicions about the reliability of pharmacists. The physician then recommends an over-the-counter decongestant and invites the patient to return if other problems develop. The patient expresses satisfaction with the physician's recommendation and invitation.

Discussion: As important as recognition of psychosis is recognition of what is not psychosis. This patient had many peculiarities of behavior but was happy and functioning well personally and in his job. He had no delusions, hallucinations, or thought disorganization. In the absence of overt psychotic symptoms, personal distress, or deteriorating function, no treatment was appropriate. The physician respected the patient's wishes and worked within his framework.

3. *Competence and informed consent.*
   a. *Medical decisions.* Psychotic symptoms alone are not an indication of legal or medical incompetence. Despite the presence of psychotic symptoms, most patients retain the legal right to determine questions of medical treatment. In the absence of clear evidence that their psychosis impairs their ability to make those decisions, patients should be allowed to do so.

      Typically, patients with psychosis have some cognitive deficits that limit their ability to grasp the full implications of information presented to them and the options available. These deficits may manifest as concrete thinking, poor memory, or difficulty processing new information. In most instances, these deficits require the physician to address the patient in simple, direct terms, often discussing the same material several times.

Psychotic symptoms that may interfere with a patient's competence to handle these issues include disorganized thinking, extreme suspiciousness, and somatic delusions. If these symptoms clearly interfere with reasoned judgments about a specific medical problem and if the failure to deal with that problem may result in significant harm to the patient, a court order for treatment should be sought (see section IV.B). To proceed with treatment in the absence of the patient's consent or a court order is legally and ethically indefensible. The only exception to this rule is a case of *immediate, life-threatening danger,* criteria rarely met in a primary care office.

b. *Psychiatric treatment.* In the treatment of psychiatric symptoms, the legal standard of consent is even more strict. The basis for a separate standard of consent for psychiatric treatment arises from several legal assumptions. First, many psychiatric patients are significantly impaired, and society historically recognizes a duty to provide special protection to these individuals. Second, most current laws were enacted in response to real and imagined past abuses of psychiatric patients in locked facilities. Third, psychiatric treatments, particularly the use of neuroleptic agents, are felt to have unusually high risk-benefit ratios, which require special legal attention.

Informed consent for all psychiatric treatments must be carefully documented. Many venues require that written information be given to the patient and written consent for all psychiatric medications be obtained. This is true even when those medications have other, nonpsychiatric, uses (e.g., use of valproic acid for mood stabilization requires such consent, whereas use of the agent for seizure control does not). For patients who are unable to give this consent and for whom treatment is required in order to avoid danger to themselves or others, or who are so disabled that they cannot provide their own food, clothing, or shelter, a court order for treatment should be sought (see section IV.B). In the absence of such an order, treatment cannot be given, except as a short-term measure in order to avoid an *immediate* threat to the safety of the patient or others.

B. Civil commitment.

Most legal jurisdictions provide for the involuntary hospitalization and treatment of patients who are immediately dangerous to themselves, are dangerous to others, or are so gravely disabled that they cannot provide their own food, clothing, or shelter (Table 10–9). In addition, a guardian or conservator may be appointed by the court for a patient who is not immediately dangerous but is unable to understand and make reasoned decisions about medical or psychiatric care.

Table 10–9
The Three Criteria Commonly Required for Civil Commitment

Criteria	Brief Definition
1. Major psychiatric disorder.	"Major" means a disorder that severely impairs reality testing and/or judgment (e.g., major depression). Adjustment disorder is *usually* unacceptable.
2a. Dangerousness to self or others, and/or	"Dangerousness" means suicidal and/or homicidal ideation, intent, and/or behavior. Serious inattention to personal safety or neglect of essential medical needs are acceptable.
2b. Grave inability to care for self.	"Grave" means a life threatening inability to obtain food, clothing, or shelter.
3. Unwillingness or inability to accept needed treatment.	"Needed" means that if treatment is withheld, criteria 1, 2a, and 2b become more severe and/or more life threatening.

The mechanism by which a court order for treatment is obtained is different within each venue. If the question arises, ready sources of information include the local CMH agency, hospital psychiatric emergency facilities, and the probate court.

Case Study

Suicide risk in a depression patient with psychotic features.

Ms. L., a 45-year-old woman with bipolar disorder, is seen by her community physician for a routine gynecologic examination. She appears very preoccupied, and the physician asks if something is bothering her. She responds that she is increasingly troubled by feelings of worthlessness and hopelessness and that she feels that God has decreed that she be punished for her many sins. On questioning, she acknowledges that she hears voices telling her that she deserves to die and must kill herself. She states that she does not want to die but is not sure she can resist the voices.

Her physical examination is deferred.

Her mental status examination shows her to be mildly agitated. Her speech is slightly slowed and fixed on themes of hopelessness and punishment. Her mood is depressed, and her affect is constricted and tearful. Her thoughts include auditory command hallucinations, delusions of guilt, and thoughts of suicide.

She adamantly refuses to consider hospitalization because she does not want to be labeled as "crazy." The physician has a nurse stay with the patient, contacts a CMH clinician for advice and assistance with involuntary hospitalization, calls an ambulance, and returns to explain to the patient what steps have been taken and why. The nurse remains with the patient until she is safely transported to a psychiatric emergency facility.

Discussion: The physician recognized Ms. L.'s distress and made appropriate inquiries regarding her mood and thoughts, with particular reference to suicide. The peculiar nature of her guilt feelings led to specific questions about psychotic symptoms. The physician recognized that depression and command hallucinations are two major risk factors for suicide and took the appropriate steps to ensure the patient's safety, despite her objections.

C. Confidentiality.

As with informed consent, special consideration is given in the law for confidentiality of psychiatric patients. As a result, many medical centers have historically maintained separate medical and psychiatric charts. With the integration of psychiatric care into the larger framework of medical practice, separation of charts is becoming less common. It is not necessary (and may be unwise) in a primary care setting to exclude psychiatric information from a patient's medical chart, but special care should be taken with regard to discussions with family members, other physicians, and so forth. It is advisable to obtain written consent from the patient before discussing any such information, although in the case of close family members, documentation in the chart of verbal consent may be adequate.

D. Agitated, threatening, or violent behavior (see Chapter 3).

Numerous studies have shown that psychotic patients are no more dangerous than the general population and in fact are more likely to be the victims, rather than the perpetrators, of violent crime. The potential for violence by a patient who is severely agitated, paranoid, or disorganized is, however, real and must be taken seriously.

1. *Goals of treatment* of an acutely agitated, psychotic patient are threefold:
   a. Assurance of safety of *all* concerned (e.g., patients, staff, and family members).
   b. Reduction of acute agitation.
   c. Long-term alleviation of psychotic symptoms.
2. *Physical intervention* by individual treatment providers is not recommended. A "show of force" involving a sufficient number of staff, clinic security personnel, and police is often useful to prevent violent outbursts in even the most psychotic patient. Involvement of law enforcement personnel is essential if the patient is armed.
3. *Medication* treatment is most successful when antipsychotic therapy is begun as for any psychotic patient and when agitation is reduced in the short term with a benzodiazepine. A typical medication protocol is
   a. Haloperidol, 5 mg twice daily orally or intramuscularly (1 to 2 mg twice daily for the elderly).
   b. Lorazepam, 1 to 2 mg orally or intramuscularly every 2 to 4 hours as needed for agitation (0.5 to 1 mg for the elderly).

The use of larger doses of neuroleptics has not been found to be helpful and may lead to severe side effects, such as extrapyramidal reactions, akathisia, and anticholinergic effects. Benzodiazepines have been found to be safe and effective for the treatment of acute agitation and are the preferred short-term agents.

The issue of informed consent for these medications may be deferred only when there is an *immediate threat of significant harm, and other measures are not adequate to ensure the safety of the patient and others.*

V. Referral for psychiatric treatment.

Optimal treatment for patients with long-term psychotic disorders, such as schizophrenia, includes not only a physician but also an interdisciplinary team of psychologists, nurses, social workers, case managers, and activity therapists with expertise in the treatment of the disorder. Most areas of the United States now have publicly funded CMH agencies that offer some or most of these services. In some areas, appropriately staffed private treatment programs are also available. In general, individual psychiatrists are less well equipped to provide the broad-based treatment these patients require, and referral to a specialty program is preferred.

The stigma still attached to some psychiatric disorders often discourages patients and families from seeking out specialized care. Although many people are comfortable accepting a referral to a psychiatrist, others react negatively, particularly if the referring physician is also uncomfortable. The best approach is to be clear about why the referral is being made. Most mental health agencies expect the patient or family to contact them directly, but the additional contact from a referring physician is very helpful.

It was good that you decided to come in and get this problem sorted out, and I think we have made a good start. With difficulties like this one, it is usually a good idea to work with someone who specializes in this type of illness. I want to give you the name of one of my colleagues who has a lot of experience in this area. She is a psychiatrist in community mental health. She works with the kind of difficulties you have experienced, and she has access to specialized treatments that you might not otherwise be able to find. With your permission, I will also give her a call and bring her up to date on what we have done here.

Selected Reading

Carpenter WT, Jr, Buchanan RW. Schizophrenia. N Engl J Med 1994; 330:681–690.

Kane JM. Drug therapy: Schizophrenia. N Engl J Med 1996; 334:34–41.

Wyatt RJ, Alexander RC, Egan MF, Kirch DG. Schizophrenia, just the facts. Schizophr Res 1988; 1:3–18.

11

NORMAN E. ALESSI, MD

PAUL E. QUINLAN, DO

JAMES E. DILLON, MD

Common Emotional and Behavioral Problems of Children and Adolescents

I. Introduction.

The identification and treatment of psychiatric disorders in children and adolescents is among the most difficult tasks facing primary care physicians. *Of children visiting a primary care physician, 20 to 25% have psychiatric disorders, with depression, anxiety, and conduct disorders being the most frequently identified.* The physician therefore must attend to the role of behavioral and emotional factors, irrespective of the presenting complaint.

When should the primary care physician suspect the presence of a psychiatric disorder? What information is needed for the evaluation of a potential psychiatric problem, and where can it be obtained? How are disorders of childhood and adolescence different from their counterparts in adults? What should a physician tell a family, and what impact does diagnosing a child have? Which interventions are likely to be effective? How safe are medications? What myths and misconceptions may deter necessary treatments or promote ineffective ones? When should the physician seek assistance?

This chapter answers these and related questions. Several tables have been designed for easy reference in order to facilitate recognition of psychiatric disorders in young patients and to suggest useful probes in eliciting history.

II. When to suspect an emotional, behavioral, or developmental abnormality.

Two distinct yet complementary approaches help in identifying emotional, behavioral, or developmental abnormality. The *developmental approach* gauges behavior and skill acquisition against statistically established age norms, and the *medical approach* uses symptoms and signs as indicators of disorder.

A. Developmental approach.

Childhood and adolescence encompass the period from birth to age 18, during which new skills and behaviors are rapidly acquired while older ones are either transformed or discarded. Normative development reflects the accomplishment of these complex emotional, behavioral, cognitive, interpersonal, and social skill sets. When a child's development deviates from expectation by virtue of either the rate or quality of development, it is appropriate to ask whether the deviation is significant with respect to current functioning and future development.

Table 11–1 gives approximate milestones for expected progress in several domains of functioning. This milestone approach is particularly helpful when developmental delays exist. *Failure to meet milestones raises the possibility of retarded development or a psychiatric disorder and should be noted for further evaluation.* Significant *regression* in development, especially with respect to major cognitive, linguistic, and motor skills, may signify the presence of major disorders, including dementing processes and autism.

B. Symptom and sign approach.

Psychiatric disorders may also present as signs or symptoms. *Signs and symptoms may include alterations in mood and affect, such as depression or prolonged sadness associated with a depressive disorder; in cognition, such as difficulties in concentration seen in attention deficit disorders; perception, as in psychotic disorders characterized by hallucinations; or in behavior, such as school avoidance associated with separation anxiety disorder or tantrums seen in oppositional defiant disorders.* They may also include alterations in physiologic functions, such as eating and sleeping.

Disturbed physiology should always prompt consideration of medical illness. *The absence of an obvious medical disorder does not imply that the patient is feigning symptoms or somatizing psychological distress.* Psychiatric diagnosis needs to be founded on affirmative behavioral data, not merely upon the absence of medical findings. Therefore, when a psychiatric disorder is suspected as the basis for unexplained somatic complaints, further assessment is indicated.

III. Myths and misconceptions about child and adolescent emotional and behavioral disorders.

Addressing these problems requires an appreciation of one's own values and one's beliefs regarding emotional

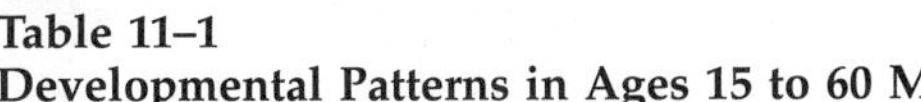

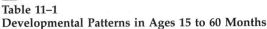

Table 11–1
Developmental Patterns in Ages 15 to 60 Months

Age	Motor	Fine Motor/Adaptive	Language	Social
15 months	Stands, then walks alone.	Builds tower of 3 cubes, can scribble	Says "da da", speaks first words, responds to names	Can indicate needs by pointing, hugs parents
18 months	Starts to run, climbs up stairs with one hand held	Makes tower of 4 cubes, imitates scribbling, imitates vertical stroke	Knows 10 meaningful words	Feeds self, calls for help when needed
24 months	Runs well, goes up and down stairs one step at a time, can open doors, can jump	Builds tower of 7 cubes, imitates horizontal stroke, imitates folding paper in half	Can create 3-word sentences (subject, verb, noun)	Handles spoon well, refers to self by name, listens to stories and follows pictures
36 months	Alternates feet while climbing stairs, can ride tricycle, stands briefly on one foot	Builds tower of 10 cubes, copies a circle	Knows age and sex, can count 3 objects, has large vocabulary	Understands taking turns, engages in parallel play
48 months	Can hop on one foot, can cut with scissors, climbs well	Copies a cross	Understands several prepositional directives, e.g., under, in front of	Plays cooperatively with other children
60 months	Skipping, has anal sphincter control	Copies a square, can draw a man, can count 10 objects	Names primary colors, can identify coins	Dresses self, prints a few letters

and behavioral disorders in children and adolescents. Based on the sum total of one's experience, these values and beliefs become one's personal myths about development, childhood, and psychopathology.

A. "These aren't disorders, they're just problems."

A broad range of psychiatric disorders can occur in young people. The thrust of organized child and adolescent psychiatry and psychology for the past 25 years has been to identify and differentiate disorders from variants of normal development. This work has demonstrated that the diagnosis and presentation of psychiatric disorders are relatively uniform across geographic, economic, social, and age groups. This consistency has been documented in infants, children, and adolescents with disorders of affect and mood, aggression, cognition and concentration, motor activity and coordination, thought, and social behavior.

B. "This child is too young to have a mental or psychiatric disorder."

Emotional and behavioral disorders in children and adolescents respect no age limits. Major developmental disorders, such as autism and mental retardation, usually begin in infancy. Severe behavioral difficulties and excessive anxieties are common in toddlers and preschool-aged children, and even depressive syndromes have been documented in children younger than 5 years. The belief that children cannot have psychiatric disorders reflects the limitations of physicians' conceptual systems and observational abilities. Table 11–2 lists the average age of onset for major disorders.

C. "Children and adolescents are reacting to something in their lives."

The development of criterion-based diagnoses has helped physicians appreciate both their prevalence and, increasingly, their etiology. Emotional problems once thought to be reactive to environment or to be manifestations of the vicissitudes of development are now often recognized as early presentations of well-established adult psychiatric disorders. Family studies have strongly implicated genetic contributions to the majority of psychiatric disorders across the life span.

Reactive responses do exist, yet even these are now viewed differently than before. After exposure to "trauma," whether from abuse, cataclysmic events, or exposure to such events, children and adolescents may suffer post-traumatic stress disorders that become an enduring part of the child's psychobiology, much as an athlete recovering from torn cartilage remains vulnerable to reinjury.

D. "The child will outgrow this problem."

Of all the myths, this may be the most pernicious. All parents want to hear it. Offering false hope to a parent with overwhelming fear may give immediate relief, but its long-term effects can be immensely destructive. Family conflict often ensues. In the public school setting, teachers are told that the child or adolescent is "normal" or that problems are transient. Unrealistic expectations lead to the forfeiture of essential services, academic failure, and behavioral disturbances. What could be a site for growth

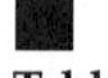

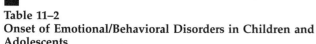

Table 11–2
Onset of Emotional/Behavioral Disorders in Children and Adolescents

Disorder	Comments
Major depressive disorder	The peak age of onset is 14–15 y and 16–17 y. Depression can occur in children as young as 3–4 y of age. Bipolar disorders rarely seen before puberty (ages 12–14 y)
Anxiety disorder	Seen as early as age 4–5 y, especially separation anxiety disorder and school phobia. Adults have noted the onset of their panic attacks as early as age 6–8 y.
Attention-deficit hyperactivity disorder	Symptoms present before the age of 7 y. Adults with this diagnosis must have impairment due to symptoms before the age of 7 y.
Disruptive disorders	Oppositional disorders can begin as early as 4 to 5 y. Conduct disorders are usually not thought of beginning before the age of 7 to 8 y because of the heavy emphasis on antisocial behavior.
Learning disorders	Given that learning disorders require that a level of functioning not be obtained, the earliest most disorders can be identified would be ages 6–8 y.
Mental retardation	Identification can occur as early as 18–24 mo, when a delay in reaching significant milestones occurs.
Enuresis	Functional enuresis cannot be diagnosed before the age of 5 y.
Encopresis	Cannot be identified before the age of 4 y.

becomes the battle ground for disagreement, confusion, and hostility.

Unfortunately, the development of symptoms, signs, or a full-blown disorder during childhood or adolescence may foreshadow a lifelong disorder and the need for indefinite care from parents. Disorders causing impairment throughout the life cycle include mental retardation, autism, major depressive disorders, bipolar disorder, schizophrenia, panic disorders, and attention-deficit hyperactivity disorder (ADHD).

E. "It is better not to identify the problem."

Not identifying the problem is better for whom, the parents, the patient, or the physician?

Physicians identify disorders for many reasons: to identify a cause, to focus therapeutic interventions, to determine prognosis, or to help patients plan the future.

Emotional and behavioral disorder should be identified unless there is either no disorder or uncertainty about the diagnosis. In the latter case, consultation, which may be informal, is advisable. Child and adolescent psychiatrists and empirically oriented clinical child psychologists are usually the best resources, and general psychiatrists, behaviorally oriented pediatricians, developmental psychologists, and social workers often possess relevant expertise as well. The clinician should not allow lingering doubts to go unaddressed—any doubt should be pursued to its resolution, either by the physician or by a specialist.

Can a stigma result from the identification of the problem? Of course it can, but it is better to identify and deal with the existence of the problem than assume that ignoring it will make the situation better. Stigma, like any other side effect of medical practice, can be managed, sometimes to the patient's advantage. *Fear of stigma should never deter the physician from making the diagnosis.*

IV. Using psychotropic medications in children and adolescents.

Nothing in child psychiatry elicits more concern, doubt, skepticism, pessimism, and hopefulness than a recommendation for a psychotropic medication. A basis for these complex responses exists. Advances in neurobiology, neuropharmacology, and psychopharmacology during the past 25 years have been remarkable. Knowledge of the relationship between neurotransmission and specific psychological phenomena has led to increasingly specific remedies for well-defined disorders. Families are often aware of these developments and come to the physician's office with high hopes.

Despite these advances, however, the clinical indications for psychotropic medication and the severity of disorder necessitating treatment in children and adolescents can be vague. Although some question exists about whether science has proved the efficacy of medication in children and adolescents, the growing literature supports a wide range of psychotropic uses in this population.

Medication is not a panacea in the treatment of emotional or behavioral disorders in children or adolescents. Occasionally, medications are all that are needed. In some cases, involving depression or ADHD for example, medication may be the central intervention, leaving issues that require parental support. Other patients, however, may require a broad range of services. Some require several medication trials, involving careful introduction and discontinuation of each medication and monitoring of symptoms from multiple observers in different settings. Some cases require many medications. Comorbidity of disorders in children and adolescents is so common that polypharmacy is not just a consideration but often a necessity and is considered the standard practice. With the growing number of medications and the increasing complexity of treatable disorders, the number of possible drug regimens has increased geometrically.

V. Mood disorders.

A. Introduction.

No psychiatric syndrome in children and adolescents is more insidious than a mood disorder. A long prodromal phase may be marked by social withdrawal, often mistaken for taciturnity; disorganization and lack of concentration resembling ADHD; or behavioral difficulties attributed to oppositional behavior or conduct disorder.

Sadness is a normal reaction to life events, such as loss or disappointment, and can be seen in children and adolescents of all ages, but it is not the same as a depressive disorder. A depressive disorder is a serious condition entailing emotional suffering and impaired academic and social functioning. The child or adolescent may be ostracized by his or her peers because of irritability, unreliability, or avoidant behavior. Suicidal ideation is common, and completed suicide is an important complication, especially in older teens. In white American teenagers, suicide is the second leading cause of death.

B. Epidemiology.

The prevalence of major depressive disorder in prepubertal children ranges from 1% to 2.7%. Children as young as 4 years of age have been determined to have depressive disorders. Adolescent depression rates range from 3.7% to 8.3%, in the later teen years approaching the rates observed in adults. Children and adolescents with somatic complaints, such as stomach aches and headaches, are especially likely to be depressed. *Depressive disorders are the most common emotional disorder in pediatric primary care populations.* Therefore, in patients with chronic unexplained headaches, stomach aches, and other vague complaints, depression needs to be considered in the differential diagnosis.

C. Evaluation and diagnostic overview.

In the medical evaluation of children and adolescents, the physician should vigilantly watch for depression and suicidality.

1. *Mood disorders need not present with sadness.* Instead, they may present with pain, low energy, irritability, or aggression. *A major mood disorder is more likely if there have been prior episodes, a family history of mood disorder, a family history of suicide, concurrent chronic illness, concurrent substance abuse, or recent stressful events.*
2. *An interview of the child or adolescent and a family member should be conducted.*

   Interviewing a depressed teenager can be taxing. If the adolescent patient attributes his or her internal distress to external sources (e.g., parents) or if the patient regards himself or herself as so unlikable that the patient cannot imagine anyone wanting to help him or her; then the patient may appear hostile, treating the doctor's inquiries as intrusive and insincere. Sensitivity and persistence, which require more time than is usually allotted to a primary care visit, are needed in order to establish a relationship with such adolescents before meaningful diagnostic data can be obtained.

   In children, a similar clinical presentation can occur. For the child with limited communication skills, aggression and other displays of hostility may replace speech. If these behaviors are interpreted without recognition of the underlying mood state, behavior may be labeled oppositional and may be managed, usually unsuccessfully, as a primary behavior problem.
3. *Somatic complaints and illness should be addressed medically, if possible, before treatment of depression is undertaken.* This is especially true when the medical problem may be the cause of mood symptoms.
4. *If a mood disorder is present, it may not be the primary or sole disorder.* Comorbidity can include substance abuse, eating disorders, obsessive-compulsive disorder (OCD), or panic disorders.
5. *Grief responses typically last 2 to 8 months and, during the acute phase, may resemble major depression.* For some children and adolescents, however, grief reactions evolve into mood disorders requiring treatment, including medications. This is more likely in the context of a personal or family history of affective disorders.

D. Specific diagnosis or problem.

1. *Major depressive disorder.*

   Major depressive disorder exhibits signs and syndromes that can be distinguished from normal reactions to life events. Depressed mood may be inferred from the presence of marked irritability, loss of interest in usual activities, or inability to experience pleasure (anhedonia). It is accompanied by several core symptoms, including
   - Changes in eating and sleeping patterns.
   - Fatigue or loss of energy.
   - Poor concentration and indecisiveness.
   - Feelings of worthlessness or excessive guilt.
   - Suicidal behavior, recurrent suicidal ideation, or morbid preoccupation with death.
   - Psychomotor retardation or agitation.

   In children and adolescents, many additional behaviors can be indicative of depression, including
   - Withdrawal from friends.
   - Violent or rebellious behavior.
   - Drug and alcohol use.
   - Change in habits of personal hygiene and dress.
   - Marked personality change.
   - Violent, delinquent, or rebellious behavior.

- Persistent boredom, difficulty concentrating, or decline in the quality of schoolwork.
- Somatic complaints, such as stomach aches, headaches, or fatigue.
- Intolerance of praise and reward.
- Withdrawal from friends and activities.

If core symptoms persist for 2 weeks, then the diagnosis of major depressive disorder is made. Table 11–3 lists signs and symptoms of depression and how they may present in children and adolescents.

The evaluation of depression requires information from both the child and the parents. Although parents can describe the external manifestation of their child's difficulties, the child or adolescent is much more attuned to his or her internal state. Table 11–3 presents a series of questions that can be used during interviews with children, adolescents, and parents.

Major depressive disorder in children and adolescents often relapses, sometimes becoming chronic and refractory to medications. After successful treatment of a single episode, therefore, close follow-up is important.

2. *Dysthymic disorder.*
Dysthymic disorder is a mood disorder in which depressed mood or irritability is experienced on most days, along with poor appetite, poor sleep, low energy, low self-esteem, poor concentration, and feelings of hopelessness, for 1 year. This disorder is sometimes thought to be a "minor" form of major depressive disorder because individual symptoms may be less severe and less conspicuous than in "major" depression. *There is nothing minor, however, about the degree of impairment imposed by chronic mood symptoms, which may insinuate themselves into every aspect of a child's academic, social, and personal life.* Furthermore, major depressive disorder subsequently develops in more than 60% of children and adolescents who have dysthymic disorders.

3. *Bipolar disorder.*
Bipolar disorder, also called manic-depressive illness, is an uncommon yet extremely serious form of mood disorder that can be accompanied by hallucinations and delusions. Onset in childhood or adolescence is usually associated with a family history of the disorder. *In childhood, bipolar disorder mimics attention deficit disorders, whereas in adolescence, it may be confused with conduct disorder, substance abuse, or schizophrenia.* Key symptoms of mania include grandiosity, reduced need for sleep, pressured speech, racing thoughts, distractibility, agitation, and excessive involvement in pleasurable activities. Depression in bipolar disorder is similar to that of major depressive disorder, but it is more likely to be accompanied by hypersomnia, psychomotor retardation, and psychotic features. Antidepressants frequently catapult children and adolescents with bipolar depression into manic episodes.

E. General management guidelines.

The first priority in the management of this disorder is safety: when a patient poses a danger to himself or herself or others, immediate intervention, which may entail sedation or hospitalization, is required. If a psychiatric hospital is unavailable, the patient may need one-to-one supervision in a pediatric unit. If hospitalization is not an option, better functioning families may be able to provide round-the-clock observation.

1. *Suicide assessment and prevention.*
The patient with a mood disorder is presumed to be at high risk until suicidal potential has been thoroughly assessed.
   a. *Assessment of ideation and intent.* The patient must be asked directly about suicidal ideation, although the question is better posed and the answer more reliable once rapport has been achieved and the adolescent has displayed a willingness to reveal other confidences. If suicidal ideation is acknowledged, further questioning should establish the potential for action. The patient should be asked for details concerning a suicidal plan—how, where, and when would it be accomplished? Where would the patient get the proposed implement of suicide (e.g., pills or a gun)? What would it take to prompt the patient to carry out the plan? What already has been done in preparation? Has the patient prepared a will or a suicide note, or purchased rope, a weapon, or pills? Has the patient given valuable things away?
   It is inadequate to rely solely on the patient's history of suicidal ideation. Adolescents can appear stable emerging from a crisis, but if the source of the crisis is not identified and treated, the suicidal risk remains high. The parent's report of the crisis and their concerns must be elicited as well, in order to substantiate or refute what the patient has said.
   b. *Risk assessment.* Risk assessment must determine the possibility of the child or adolescent's possibly wanting to hurt himself or herself. Factors that would further heighten concern include the following:
      (1) *Suicide threats.* These should never be seen merely as attempts to get attention. Most patients who successfully commit suicide have told others of their inclination, often within a day of the event. Suicide threats are sometimes characterized as "pseudocide"; the physician should not be lulled into this simplistic analysis.
      (2) *Previous suicide attempts.* A person who has previously attempted suicide and failed should not be seen as a "failure,"

but as someone in need of serious attention and help. Fifty percent of female adolescents and 25% of male adolescents who successfully complete suicide have made previous attempts.

(3) *Statements revealing a desire to die.* Suicidal statements may be direct or indirect. The physician should listen for both. Statements such as "I won't be a problem for you much longer," "Nothing matters," "It's no use," "I won't see you again," may reveal a suicidal motivation.

(4) *Preoccupation with death.* Adolescents may develop fascinations with popular cultural heroes who represent themes of death and suicide or with occult activities glorifying death in movies, books, graphic comics, music, music videos, or role-playing games. Depressed adolescents contemplating suicide may begin asking questions about death.

(5) *Behavior related to getting affairs in order.* The patient may give away favorite possessions, clean his or her room (for the first time), or throw away important belongings.

(6) *Contagion effect.* Adolescent suicide risk is especially high after the suicide of a friend, classmate, or acquaintance; after suicide has been reported in the media; and after a popular television or movie production glamorizes suicide.

(7) *Personality changes or odd behavior.*

(8) *Apathy, moodiness, anger, crying, sleeplessness, or lack of appetite.*

(9) *Loss of interest in usual activities.*

(10) *Isolative behavior.*

(11) *Statements about hopelessness, helplessness, or worthlessness; complaints of being "rotten inside."*

(12) *Sudden appearance of happiness and calm* after a period of some of the aforementioned characteristics.

c. *Professional responsibility for the suicidal patient.* Even when the family and patient refuse psychiatric evaluation for suicidal ideation, the primary care physician must act to protect the patient. Adolescents whose parents refuse emergency care may be referred to child protective services (or a comparable organization in the physician's state) for medical neglect. The primary responsibility of the health professional assessing the patient is the maintenance of patient safety.

2. *Psychosis.*
Acute psychosis, as a manifestation of psychotic depression, mania, or thought disorder (schizophrenia), should also be considered a psychiatric emergency because psychotic patients unpredictably engage in violence, suicide, or other seriously harmful behaviors. Obtaining a *substance abuse history* and *toxicology screen* is critical in evaluating psychotic, depressed, and suicidal patients.

F. Treatment.

The treatment of mood disorders usually requires a mixture of therapeutic interventions, including medications, counseling or psychotherapy of the patient, and sometimes family therapy. Interventions in the school and other settings are sometimes needed.

1. *Medical treatment for major depression and dysthymic disorder.*
Antidepressants are the drugs of choice in treating major depressive disorder and are often used in the treatment of dysthymia. Despite limited evidence from double-blind placebo-controlled studies, the use of antidepressants has grown in the past several years with the advent of the selective serotonin reuptake inhibitors (SSRIs), such as fluoxetine (Prozac). Care should be taken to assess for the history of bipolar disorder before antidepressants are prescribed because these agents may induce mania.

Table 11–4 contains a list of the most frequently used antidepressants in children and adolescents. It also lists the starting and maximum doses of the medications, frequent side effects, and serious adverse events.

a. *Selective serotonin reuptake inhibitors.* The SSRIs include fluoxetine, sertraline (Zoloft), paroxetine (Paxil), and fluvoxamine (Luvox).

(1) *Clinical effects. SSRIs are usually the drugs of choice for children and adolescents with unipolar depressive disorders.* Clinical effects in this population are similar to those in adults with mood disorders, and they typically require several weeks to fully develop. The first sign of improvement may be the parent's observations that the child is more affable and less irritable. Acute vegetative symptoms, often less prominent in the clinical presentations of young persons than in adults, may improve less dramatically.

Among the SSRIs, only fluoxetine has been subjected to controlled trials in the younger population with depression; presumably, sertraline and paroxetine are equally effective, distinguished mainly by their metabolism and pharmacokinetics. Fluvoxamine has achieved less use in depression than in OCD, but it is more likely to be sedating than the other SSRIs.

(2) *Administration.* Before administering antidepressants, the physician should establish that there is *no history of bipolar disorder* because antidepressants often induce mania in susceptible children. If bipolar disorder is present in first- or second-degree relatives, antidepressants should be adminis-

Text continued on page 197

Table 11–3
Presentation of Depressive Disorders in Children and Adolescents (Questions That Can Be Asked of Children, Their Parents or Adolescents)

	Children			Adolescents	
		Questions(s) to Ask			
Symptom/Sign	*Presentation*	**Child**	**Parent**	*Presentation (assume same presentation as child, unless otherwise noted)*	*Question(s) to ask (assume same questions as child, unless otherwise noted)*
Depressed mood	Looks sad. Quieter than usual. Smiling less. Not laughing as much.	Are you feeling down, sad, blue? Do you feel unhappy? You don't look as if you're happy today, is there something wrong?	Is your child feeling sad, down or depressed? How would you describe your child's mood? Is this a change? Do you talk with your child about his or her feelings? Has there been anything that may have happened that would have made your child unhappy or depressed? How long has your child been feeling sad or depressed? How bad is it?	More reclusive. Spending more time alone in room. Possibly listens to culturally acceptable yet morbid music.	Same *plus* How long has he or she been feeling sad or depressed? How bad has it been? Can you describe the feeling? Does anything make it better? For how long?
Impaired concentration	Unable to follow directions in class or home. Taking longer to complete work/homework. Bringing more work home. More incorrect answers on seemingly the same work. Spending less time watching television or playing video games.	Are you having problems in school? Can you do what your teacher is asking? Is your work harder in school? Can you do your work? Is it harder? Do you watch television or play video games? What are your favorites? Are you watching more or less? Is it more difficult to follow?	Is your child having difficulties in class? Is he or she taking longer to do their work in class or their homework? Is your child bringing more homework home now? Is your child enjoying the classroom work less? Does he or she watch television? How much? Is he or she paying attention or just sitting there?	Grades drop for no apparent reason. Work becomes increasingly difficult. Becomes more forgetful.	Is it more difficult to concentrate in class? Are you having trouble in your classes? Has there been a change in your academic performance? Have your grades gotten worse?

Insomnia/hypersomnia	Altered bedtime routine. Not falling asleep at usual bedtime. Waking up at all times of the night. Waking up earlier than expected. Sleeps all the time. Increased number of naps. Comes home looking tired, wanting more naps than usual.	Are you sleeping well? What time do you go to bed? Are you having a lot of bad dreams? Have you been waking up mommy and daddy? Do you take a lot of naps? How many? How often?	What is your child's bedtime? How long does it take for your child to fall asleep? Does he or she wake up during the night? Is he or she sleeping longer or about the same? Does he or she take naps? How often and are they increasing?	Increased sleep more common than insomnia. Sleeps for prolonged periods without restfulness.	
Fatigue (loss of energy)	Tired. Not rested after adequate sleep. Taking longer to fall asleep. Getting up in the night and awakening parents due to "bad dreams" or being frightened in the night. Sleeping all the time. Taking more frequent naps, but not apparently due to increased physical exertion.	Are you tired a lot? Do you take naps after school? Are you tired after school? Do you get tired during school? Do you ever put your head on the desk and just fall asleep?	Does your child seem more tired? How do you know? Does your child tell you? Is your child taking more naps after school? Does that help him or her when tired? Does your child fall asleep watching television more often than usual?		
Weight loss/gain	Poor appetite. Eating fewer things and eating less. Weight loss greater than 5–10% of body weight. Not eating packed lunch at school. Not eating snacks at home.	What do like to eat? (Offer what you like best?) Are you eating okay? Do you take your lunch to school? What do you take? Do you eat it all?	Is your child eating okay? What's his or her favorite food? Is your child eating that as well? Does your child take a lunch to school? Does your child eat it? Is this a change in behavior? Has your child gained or lost any weight? When was the last time you weighed him or her?	Loss of appetite, not just weight loss as part of a diet. Body image would not be disturbed as might be seen in anorexia nervosa or bulimia.	Are you eating? Have you noticed a weight loss? How much over what period of time? Are you trying to lose weight? Do you think that you're fat? Do you think that you need to lose weight?

Table continued on following page

Table 11–3
Presentation of Depressive Disorders in Children and Adolescents (Questions That Can Be Asked of Children, Their Parents or Adolescents) *Continued*

	Children			Adolescents	
		Questions(s) to Ask			
Symptom/Sign	*Presentation*	**Child**	**Parent**	*Presentation (assume same* presentation *as child, unless otherwise noted)*	*Question(s) to ask (assume same* questions *as child, unless otherwise noted)*
Psychomotor agitation/ retardation	More active than usual. Restless. Unable to sit in seat. Getting up often and roaming the room. Wringing hands. Getting into more fights with peers, siblings, and parents/authority figures. Losing temper more frequently, yelling and even hitting. Moving more slowly. Gets tired relatively rapidly in games and sports. Complaining of feeling sick, e.g., muscle aches and pains, joint discomfort.	Are you able to sit still in class? Do you have to get up a lot? Does your teacher ask you to sit down? Do you bother other students (kids) in your class? Do you lose your temper a lot with your friends, kids in class, brothers and sisters, parents, or teachers? Have you been getting into more fights? Does it feel like more kids are picking on you? Do you feel slowed down? Does your body feel like it's not able to move as fast? Does your body feel like it hurts a lot? Where?	Has your child become more active recently? Not able to settle down? Appears more disobedient? Has he or she been arguing more than usual? Fighting with siblings and friends? Has your child been more tired than usual? Appear to drag himself or herself around. Doesn't appear to enjoy himself or herself as before?	Restlessness noted in all settings including home, school, and with friends. Can be an annoyance to others, especially if not present before. Body will feel different, heavy, bloated. Physically uncomfortable.	Are you feeling restless? Does it bother you or others? Do you feel tired? Does your body feel different, heavy, slowed down.
Feelings of worthlessness (guilt)	Feels bad about himself or herself. Refers to self as stupid. Says that no one likes him or her. Can be seen hitting self in the head when discussing these issues.	Do you like yourself? What do you like the most about yourself? Is there anything that you don't like about yourself? Are there things that you would change about yourself? When you grow up what would you like to be?	Does your child talk about not liking himself or herself or that people don't like your child? Does your child hurt himself or herself more than you would expect? Falls, injuries, and so on?		

Somatic symptoms	Increase in the frequency of headaches, stomach aches, general aches and pains?	Does your tummy hurt? All the time? When? Does your head hurt? Where? When?	Has your child been getting sick lately? Headaches? Stomach aches? Has he or she missed more school because he or she has been sick?		
Recurrent thoughts of death and suicide	*Ideas of death:* thinks about dead relatives, pets, or famous people. Wonders about what it would be like to be dead. *Ideas of suicide:* thinks about what it would be like to be dead. It might be better for him or her, family, and others. Questions whether he or she is a burden to others and if his or her death would be a relief. Thinks about how he or she would die (when, where, possibly how). *Plan of suicide:* makes plans for his or her death (when, where, how).	Do you ever think about an animal or relative that's passed away? How do you think they are doing? Do you know what suicide means? Could you tell me? Do you ever think about suicide? What do you think it would be like? If yes, have you ever thought about how?	Do you ever hear your child talking about not liking himself or herself? Wishing he or she were dead? Have you seen anything from school (pictures, stories) that would suggest that he or she is feeling bad toward himself or herself?	May become "obsessed" with someone who writes about death and dying.	Have you been thinking about death a lot? What kind of things are you thinking about? Are there books, music or movies that you've seen that are about death that you keep seeing over and over? What are they and what makes them interesting?

Table 11–4
Medical Treatment of Depressive Disorders in Children and Adolescents

Medications	Dosage			
Antidepressants	*Child*	*Adolescent*	Side Effects	Psychopharmacologic Considerations
Selective serotonin reuptake inhibitors (SSRIs)				
Fluoxetine (Prozac)	Age, 5–8 y Liquid, 5-mg starting dose Dose range, 5–20 mg Age, 8–12 y Capsule, 10 mg starting dose Dose range, 10–40 mg	Age, >12 y Capsule, 10-mg starting dose Dose range, 10–60 mg	Nausea, weight loss or gain, anxiety, insomnia, excessive sweating, headache, agitation, diarrhea, sedation, decreased sexual drive or ability, tiredness, tremor, blurred vision, and constipation. Induction of mania. Death if interacting with MAOI.	Prozac can often produce feelings of hyperactivity, especially at bedtime. If this occurs then diphenhydramine 10–25 mg, or trazadone, 10–50 mg, approximately 30 minutes before sleep will assist sleep. May need to give in the p.m. if sedation is noted during the day. The principle difficulty is the long half-life (about 2 wk) if the patient does not respond. If another antidepressant will be used, can do immediately, as long as it is not an MAOI; then must wait at least 4–6 weeks.
Sertraline (Zoloft)	Age, 5–8 y Tablet, 25-mg starting dose Dose range, 25–75 mg Age, 8–12 y Tablet, 25-mg starting dose Dose range, 25–125 mg	Age, >12 y Tablet, 50-mg starting dose Dose range, 100–200 mg	Same as with fluoxetine.	Sometimes preferred due to its shorter half-life, as compared with fluoxetine. Dosage needs to be raised slowly until therapeutic effects reached.
Paroxetine (Paxil)	Age, 5–8 y Tablet, 10-mg starting dose Dose range, 10–30 mg Age, 8–12 y Tablet, 10- to 20-mg starting dose Dose range, 20–30 mg	Age, >12 y Tablet, 20-mg starting dose Dose range, 20–50 mg	Same as with fluoxetine.	
Tricyclic antidepressants*				
Imipramine (Tofranil)	Age, 5–8 y Tablet, 10-mg starting dose Dose range, 25–75 mg Age, 8–12 y Tablet, 25-mg starting dose Dose range, 175–150 mg	Age, >12 y Tablet, 25-mg starting dose Dose range, 100–250 mg	Dry mouth and sinuses, constipation, urinary hesitancy, esophageal reflux, orthostatic hypotension, palpitations, intracardiac conduction slowing, sweating, elevated blood pressure, tremor, skin rashes, stimulation, sedation, delirium, myoclonic twitches (high dose), nausea, speech blockage, extrapyramidal symptoms, weight gain and impotence, and sudden death. High suicidal potential if taken as an overdose. Parents as well as children should be instructed to keep medications away from children.	Plasma drug concentration of imipramine + desipramine level must be followed if this is used in the treatment of depression. Plasma levels of 125–250 ng/mL should be sought, but the dosing can be increased to 4.5 mg/kg. ECGs should also be monitored during the medication trial to look for prolongation of the Q-R interval. All tricyclics have been described as causing an "irritability" that can be misidentified as a part of the disorder. Observe carefully for irritability and agitated behavior.

Desipramine (Norpramin)	Age, 5–8 y Tablet, 25-mg starting dose Dose range, 25–75 mg Age, 8–12 y Tablet, 25-mg starting dose Dose range, 50–125 mg	Age, >12 y Tablet, 25-mg starting dose Dose range, 75–150 mg	Same as imipramine.	Same as imipramine. Sudden death reported in children and adolescents who took the medication for ADHD; unclear if there is a proven association. Blood levels appear to help less in the monitoring of the medication. Given reported sudden death, a baseline ECG and screening for cardiac disease should be obtained before starting the medication.
Amitriptyline (Elavil)	Age, 5–8 y Tablet, 10- to 25-mg starting dose Dose range, 10–75 mg Age, 8–12 y Tablet, 25-mg starting dose Dose range, 25–75 mg	Age, >12 y Tablet, 25-mg starting dose Dose range, 30–60 mg	Same as imipramine except extremely anticholinergic. Symptoms noted below are usually worse than with the other tricyclics. Dryness of mouth, sleepiness, dizziness due to orthostatic alterations in blood pressures. *Note*: most frequently prescribed at bedtime due to sedating effect. Also, most helpful in cases in which there might be more severe symptoms of aggression.	Same as imipramine. Blood levels appear to help less in the monitoring of the medication. Therapeutic window is often described. Would obtain blood levels at higher levels as well as serial ECG.
Nortriptyline (Pamelor)	Age, 5–8 y Tablet, 10-mg starting dose Dose range, 25–50 mg Age, 8–12 y Tablet, 25-mg starting dose Dose range, 50–75 mg	Age, >12 y Tablet, 25-mg starting dose Dose range, 125–150 mg	Extremely anticholinergic. Symptoms noted below are usually worse than with the other tricyclics: dryness of mouth, sleepiness, dizziness due to orthostatic alterations in blood pressures. *Note*: Most frequently prescribed at bedtime due to sedating effect. Also, most helpful in cases in which there might be more severe symptoms of aggression.	High suicidal potential if taken as an overdose. Sudden death reported in children and adolescents who took the medication for ADHD.

Table continued on following page

Table 11–4
Medical Treatment of Depressive Disorders in Children and Adolescents *Continued*

Medications	Dosage			
Antidepressants	*Child*	*Adolescent*	Side Effects	Psychopharmacologic Considerations
Other antidepressants				
Buproprion (Wellbutrin)	Age, 5–8 y Half tablet, 37.5-mg starting dose Dose range, 37.5–75 mg/d Age, 8–12 y Tablet, 37.5- to 75-mg starting dose Dose range, 75–100 mg/d	Age >12 y Tablet, 75-mg starting dose Dose range, 75–150 mg/d, may require up to 450 mg/d divided b.i.d. to t.i.d.	Headache, insomnia, nausea, restlessness, agitation, irritability.	An alternative to tricyclics after treatment failure with SSRIs.
Mood Stabilizers				
Lithium†	Age, 5–8 y 75- to 150-mg starting dose Dose range (see below) Age, 8–12 y 150- to 300-mg starting dose Dose range, q.d. to t.i.d. and adjusted by monitoring the level of lithium to an optimal range of 1.0 mEq/L ± 0.2 mEq/L. Side effects may limit reaching this blood level.	Age, >12 y Tablet, 300-mg starting dose Dose range, q.d. to t.i.d. and adjusted by monitoring the level of lithium to an optimal range of 1.0 mEq/L ± 0.2 mEq/L. Side effects may limit reaching this blood level.	GI complaints, including nausea and vomiting, diarrhea (improves when given with food), weight gain, mild cognitive impairment, exacerbate seizure disorders, ataxia, tremor, dysarthria, polyuria, hypothyroidism, dermatologic changes, avoid in sick sinus syndrome.	Used primarily in bipolar disorder but can augment treatment with antidepressants (augmentation doses typically 300 mg/d), avoid combination with fluoxetine and haloperidol, which results in parkinsonian syndrome, severe ataxia.

q.d., every day; b.i.d., twice a day; t.i.d., three times a day; GI, gastrointestinal; ADHD, attention-deficit hyperactivity disorder; MAOI, monoamine oxidase inhibitor.

*Obtain electrocardiogram (ECG), complete blood count. Perform liver function tests.

†Obtain baseline ECG; electrolyte levels, including blood urea nitrogen, creatinine, thyroid-stimulating hormone, and monitor. If patient is female of child-bearing years, obtain pregnancy test before start of treatment; do not use if patient is pregnant.

tered cautiously, and lower initial doses and more gradual titration should be used.

For otherwise healthy children receiving monotherapy, *baseline laboratory examinations are unnecessary* before treatment with SSRIs is begun. Because drug interactions are common, however, other medications metabolized through the hepatic cytochrome P_{450} system should be monitored with extra care when SSRIs are added to any regimen. Monoamine oxidase inhibitors, including isoniazid, are contraindicated in patients receiving SSRIs. Drugs with quinidine-like effects at higher serum levels, such as tricyclic antidepressants (TCAs) and terfenadine (Seldane), should be administered with utmost caution.

Sertraline therapy is usually started at a dose of 25 mg and titrated upward as tolerated to 50 to 100 mg daily, usually in a single morning dose. If no response occurs after about 3 weeks, the dose may be advanced in adolescents and larger children to a maximum 200 mg/d, often in divided doses. A steady state level of sertraline and its active metabolite may not be achieved for about 2 weeks after the initiation of therapy. Sertraline probably has a somewhat more favorable profile of drug-drug interactions than do fluoxetine and paroxetine.

Treatment with *fluoxetine,* which is available both as 10- and 20-mg capsules and as a liquid, can be initiated in younger children at doses of 4 mg or less daily, and the dosage usually needs to be raised to 10 to 20 mg daily for therapeutic effects to be obtained. Higher doses, when needed, are often well tolerated, but dosing should not be advanced rapidly, because steady state levels of the parent drug and an active metabolite are not reached for several weeks after the therapy is initiated.

Paroxetine is administered like fluoxetine, except that therapeutic doses are commonly somewhat higher (≥ 50 mg daily).

(3) *Common side effects.* Common side effects of these agents are listed in Table 11–4.

(4) *Maintenance treatment.* Maintenance treatment should continue for at least 6 to 12 months unless a placebo response is strongly suspected. The dosage may then be tapered slowly over a period of 1 to 3 months and discontinued if symptoms to do not re-emerge.

b. *Tricyclic antidepressants.* TCAs, such as imipramine (Tofranil), desipramine (Norpramin), and nortriptyline (Pamelor), have been used in children with enuresis and attention deficit disorder for more than 2 decades. Although most clinicians believe that these drugs can be dramatically effective for children with depression as well, several controlled trials have failed to demonstrate their efficacy.

The side effect profile of TCAs is much less favorable than that of SSRIs. TCAs are thus second-line drugs unless another condition requiring tricyclic therapy coexists with the affective disorder.

(1) *Clinical effects.* When effective, response to TCAs resembles that to SSRIs.

(2) *Administration.* Family history of early sudden death is a relative contraindication to use of TCAs in children. A baseline complete blood count, liver function results, and electrocardiogram (ECG) should be obtained before treatment is begun. If the ECG shows a conduction defect, another medication should be considered. The complete blood count and liver function tests should repeated about 4 to 6 weeks after therapy is initiated and thereafter at intervals of 6 to 12 months. The ECG should be obtained two to three times during titration of medication to therapeutic levels.

A low starting dose of 10 to 25 mg/d of imipramine may be titrated up to 2 to 3 mg/kg/d in the first week of therapy. The timing and frequency of dosing depends mainly on side effects; most patients prefer to take medication at bedtime. In the interpretation of the ECG, the clinician should pay special attention to changes in PR, QRS, and QTC intervals. Doses producing primary block or QTC intervals in excess of 0.45 second should be avoided. If the ECG is normal, the dose may be raised to 3.5 to 4 mg/kg/d (but not more than 300 mg/d), at which point, a second ECG and a serum tricyclic level should be obtained. Therapeutic levels of imipramine and desipramine (imipramine's active metabolite) are usually about 150 to 250 ng/mL; levels greater than 300 ng/mL should alert the physician to potential toxicity.

When a therapeutic level has been achieved, the dose should be maintained for at least 4 weeks before therapy is changed or augmented. If a therapeutic level has not been achieved, the dose may be raised to a maximum of 5 mg/kg/d (not to exceed 300 mg/d) and the ECG and blood levels should be periodically monitored.

(3) *Side effects.* Side effects include anticholinergic effects, sedation, sweating, tachycardia, postural hypotension, and ECG changes consistent with a quinidine-like effect. Several children receiving desipramine have died unexpectedly.

c. *Other or atypical antidepressants.* The novel antidepressants, including bupropion (Wellbutrin), venlafaxine (Effexor), nefazodone (Serzone), and trazodone (Desyrel), have not been studied for the treatment of depression in children. Bupropion and trazodone have been used for ADHD and aggression, however, and appear to have acceptable safety profiles.

d. *Augmentation.* Several strategies have been used to augment the effects of antidepressants in children and adolescents with disorders that are resistant to maximal doses of single drugs, although none have undergone formal trials.
   (1) *Lithium,* usually in doses from 300 to 900 mg/d, may be added to an antidepressant regimen and may trigger rapid alleviation of symptoms. The *dose and serum levels used in lithium augmentation of antidepressants are usually lower* than those needed for bipolar disorder.
   (2) *Stimulant medications* can augment antidepressant effects in adults and are especially appropriate in children with comorbid attention deficit disorders. Augmentation of TCAs should be performed with caution because TCA levels may increase with stimulants. Therefore, TCA levels and electrocardiograms should be monitored closely, considering the side effect profiles of both medications. The SSRI augmentation with stimulants is less of a risk; however, side effect profiles of both medications also need to be monitored because augmentation is likely to increase side effects, regardless of whether treatment response improves. The stimulant should be started at a dose equivalent of 5 mg of methylphenidate and adjusted according to the degree of symptom improvement versus tolerated side effects.
   (3) Low doses of *thyroid hormone* (liothyronine [Cytomel]) can be added to an antidepressant regimen at dosages beginning at 5 μg/d. The dose can be adjusted to 20 to 25 μg for adolescents.

e. *Innovative treatments: treatment-refractory cases.* Two situations may arise in which multiple medications may be necessary.
   (1) *Depression does not respond adequately to a single agent.* The augmentation strategies described earlier may be used (i.e., lithium, liothyronine or levothyroxine [Synthroid], or stimulants.) Alternatively, two antidepressants can be used simultaneously. Many combinations, unfortunately, produce serious drug interactions. SSRIs can usually be safely combined with bupropion and trazodone. *Monoamine oxidase inhibitors should not be combined with other antidepressants in children and adolescents under most circumstances. Their combination with SSRIs, in particular, may produce a fatal serotonin syndrome.* TCA levels can rise dramatically in the presence of SSRIs and must be monitored closely if this combination is used.
   (2) *At least one other disorder is present.* For comorbid disorders, a single medication addressing all symptoms is optimal. A TCA, for example, can be used for depression in a child with enuresis and ADHD, although it is not the best treatment for any of these conditions individually. Many psychiatrists, however, would use three different medications (e.g., an SSRI, a stimulant, and desmopressin acetate) because these may be more effective than antidepressants and, even collectively, have a superior side effect profile to that of the TCAs.

   Sometimes, many medications are needed for the treatment of a single disorder. *Psychotic depression,* for example, usually requires both antidepressant and, during the acute phase, antipsychotic medications. Long-term use of antipsychotic medications should be avoided because the risk of tardive dyskinesia is increased in patients with affective disorder.

f. *Frequently asked questions.*
   (1) *Does Prozac increase the likelihood of suicide?* Patients receiving any antidepressant are less likely to commit suicide. Prozac is similar to other antidepressants in this respect.
   (2) *How long will improvement take during medication?* Somatic symptoms, such as difficulties with sleep and concentration, improve within days to weeks; depressed mood often lifts within 2 to 5 weeks; and chronic feelings of inadequacy improve more slowly.
   (3) *How long will my child or adolescent need to be taking this medication?* Duration of treatment varies. After 6 to 8 months of remission, it is reasonable to attempt a gradual tapering of medication. If relapse occurs, medical therapy needs to be resumed. Patients with multiple episodes of depression and strong family histories may require indefinite treatment.
   (4) *What happens if the medication does not work?* Many alternative medications and combinations exist.

2. *Medical treatment for bipolar disorder.*
   a. *Lithium.* Lithium, which has been widely used in children with aggression and in adolescents with bipolar disorder, is usually well tolerated. The drug appears to be relatively safe when it is properly monitored, although long-term effects have not been adequately studied. It is not known whether lithium is as effective in children and adolescents as it is in adults.
      (1) *Clinical effects.* Lithium stabilizes mood in cyclical disorders. It has a more pronounced effect on mania than on depression.
      (2) *Administration.* Children requiring lithium therapy should usually be treated in consul-

tation with a psychiatrist, because of both the severity of the underlying problem and the peculiarities of this drug. Treatment is usually started with 300 mg once or twice daily, with subsequent dosage increments based on trough lithium blood levels obtained at least three days after a dosage change. The target blood level is 1.0 ± 0.2 mEq/L. Blood levels are approximately linearly related to dosage. Blood levels need to be obtained frequently early in treatment, but levels in children receiving stable maintenance regimens need be checked only every few months.

(3) *Common side effects.* Lithium has many side effects, both annoying short-term effects and potentially serious long-term effects. Short-term effects include a metallic taste, nausea and vomiting, diarrhea, polyuria, tremor, and aggravation of acne. Lithium toxicity, which is uncommon in children, usually emerges insidiously later in treatment, often when a change in metabolism of the drug has gone undetected. This effect can occur in the summer months, when sweating and sodium depletion reduce lithium clearance. The effects of lithium on developing human kidneys have not been studied.

b. *Anticonvulsants.* In adults, carbamazepine (Tegretol) and valproate (Depakene) are as effective in stabilizing mood as lithium, although they are not necessarily effective in the same patients. Administration of anticonvulsants for mania in children and adolescents is handled in a manner analogous to that used in seizure control.

3. *Psychosocial treatment.*
Supportive and educational interventions involving both the patient and the family can be administered by the primary care physician. When these fail, psychiatrists, psychologists, or social workers can offer more specialized techniques.

a. *Individual interventions with the child or adolescent.* Interventions should be specific and supportive. The primary care physician should assure the patient of the reality of what he or she is feeling, explain what a mood disorder is, and help the patient understand that the problem is treatable. Although the trust of a depressed youngster who feels hopeless and undeserving of help may be difficult to achieve, it is important that the physician be perceived as understanding and willing to help.

The approach to the patient should be direct and concrete, focusing on immediate concerns with simple, straightforward solutions. This is especially important during the early phase of recovery, when concentration and abstract thinking are impaired.

The *cognitive behavior approach* to therapy calls for helping the youngster challenge negative beliefs about himself or herself. The child who says that he or she cannot do anything should be helped to make a list of things that he or she *can* do. The adolescent who believes that he or she is stupid should be helped to make a realistic appraisal of his or her achievements, especially intellectual ones. The physician should not offer *false consolation;* self-criticism is always colored by depression and often promotes it.

Behavioral management consists of quickly returning the patient to his or her usual lifestyle. If he or she is experiencing overwhelming stress at school or is unable to minimally function there, a brief respite is acceptable. Longer interruptions of school promote school avoidance, which becomes more difficult to treat than the depression that gave rise to it. Although complete restoration of function, including the capacities to concentrate and socialize in a school setting, may require weeks, the child should sustain friendships and keep up with schoolwork to the extent possible during the recovery period. If the youngster's inability to attend school lasts for more than a few days, he or she should minimally attend school for an hour, say "hello" to his or her friends, and pick up his or her homework assignments.

The cognitive distortion commonly found in depression can severely limit the person's functional capability and is best treated by removal of barriers to a normal routine.

b. *Family interventions.* Family interventions include educating the family about the illness and addressing guilt in parents who hold themselves responsible for the child's distress. In some instances, unfortunately, a certain amount of guilt may be warranted; in that case, the physician should encourage the parent to constructively resolve family or personal problems that may have triggered or maintained the depressive process. Treatment plans should not be formulated around unrealistic expectations for parent behavior.

G. What to tell the patient and family.

1. Depression is an illness, not a character flaw.
2. *The disorder will take time to resolve.* Typically, physical manifestations resolve first, followed by cognitive symptoms. Insight about the illness and a balanced appraisal of one's own personality and attributes are the last to occur. Depressive episodes typically last 2 to 6 months.
3. *The course of treatment needs to be continued beyond the resolution of symptoms.* Because insight is late in returning, the patient is likely to express confusion or dismay when family members insist that the child is better.

4. The natural history of affective disorders needs to be discussed with the parents, although not necessarily at the outset of treatment. If the child has bipolar disorder or a strong family history of recurrent mood disorders, multiple episodes across the life span can be expected. Some mood disorders respond incompletely to multiple treatments; rarely, treatment is without benefit. However, even in a seemingly hopeless situation, there is reason for optimism. Dozens of medications are now available, new remedies are in production all the time and in countless combinations. In addition to medications, somatic treatments such as phototherapy and electroconvulsive therapy are currently available and others are being studied.

H. When to refer.

A comorbid conditions such as an eating disorder or thought disorder may require the involvement of a child psychiatrist. If the disorder proves to be refractory to antidepressants alone and alternative interventions prove necessary, a consultation with someone with expertise in the use of medication combinations may be beneficial.

VI. Anxiety disorders.

Life is replete with fear and worry. Infants may experience intense anxiety when removed from a primary caretaker, and toddlers may panic if the parent leaves the room or may hide behind a parent when confronted by a stranger.

All children have fears. Many fears are age-appropriate and characteristic of normal development, including the following:

- *Birth to 6 months*—Loss of physical support; loud noises; large, rapidly approaching objects.
- *7 to 12 months*—Strangers.
- *1 to 5 years*—Loud noises, storms, animals, the dark, separation from parents.
- *3 to 5 years*—Monsters, ghosts.
- *6 to 12 years*—Experiencing bodily injury, being victimized by burglars, being sent to the principal, being punished, failing.
- *12 to 18 years*—Tests in school, social embarrassment.

Fears and worries that are developmentally appropriate and predictable in response to specific cues may be pathologic when they occur at a later age, with excessive intensity or persistence, or in response to atypical triggers. *Separation anxiety disorder, overanxious disorder, panic disorder, phobias, and OCD* are conditions in which pathologic anxiety is the critical defining feature.

These disorders can be debilitating, as in the child who refuses to attend school or the adolescent whose compulsive hand cleaning prevents him or her from working and having a social life.

A. Epidemiology.

Separation anxiety disorder occurs in approximately 3% of school-aged children and commonly coexists with depression. Ten percent of children and 3% of adolescents have phobias that may require treatment. Panic disorder occurs much less frequently in children and adolescents than in adults, and in younger people, it is usually associated with comorbid depressive illnesses and a family history of panic or depression. In OCD, obsessive thoughts and compulsive rituals become a dominant part of a person's life. One percent of the population has OCD, which has a very strong pattern of inheritance.

B. Evaluation and diagnostic overview.

Anxiety disorder should be suspected in children or adolescents with multiple fears and worries, avoidance behavior, preoccupation with potential disasters, excessive social reserve, multiple or chronic unexplained somatic complaints, ritualistic behavior, or nervous habits, such as nail biting and hair pulling.

1. *Children or adolescents with an anxiety disorder may not present with specific complaints of anxiety.* They may present with social awkwardness, headaches, or stomach aches. Physical manifestations of acute anxiety, such as tremor, sweating, clammy skin, and pupillary dilation, may not be present. *The likelihood of a major mood disorder being present is increased if there have been prior episodes or a family history of an anxiety disorder and recent "stressful events."* Hyperactivity may be present, especially in acute stress reactions, although most anxious children tend to be reserved and quiet rather than active and rambunctious.
2. *If you suspect an anxiety disorder, an interview of the child or adolescent and a family member should be conducted.* Communication by phone or questionnaire with teachers and others with whom the patient has daily contact is often useful. The interview is apt to be difficult because the fearful youngster feels awkward and apprehensive offering confidences to a relative stranger. If the child is silent or speaks little, this should not be interpreted as oppositional or resistant behavior until the diagnoses of anxiety, depression, and language problems can be excluded.
3. *If the patient presents with somatic complaints or a chronic illness, this must be taken care of first to make certain that the patient is medically stable.*
4. *Comorbidity is common.* Substance abuse, eating disorders, and depressive disorders frequently coexist with anxiety disorders and with anxiety as a symptom.

C. Specific diagnosis or problem.

Five anxiety disorders are reviewed in this section: separation anxiety disorder, overanxious disorder, panic disorder, phobias, and OCD.

1. *Separation anxiety disorder.*
   The primary symptom of this disorder is exces-

sive anxiety, relative to development, in the face of separation from a significant person. The anxiety may prevent the separation from occurring or may persist well beyond the separation, despite the presence of an adequate substitute caretaker, such as a teacher or a babysitter. A considerable degree of apprehension is normal in a younger child. By the age of 5 years, however, the youngster should be able to overcome the mild anxiety attendant on going to kindergarten or having a first sleep over. Anxiety that prevents a child from engaging in activities common among his or her peers is suspect.

Separation anxiety displays several of the following characteristics:

a. Unrealistic and persistent worry about possible harm befalling major attachment figures or fear that they will leave and not return.
b. Unrealistic and persistent worry that an untoward calamitous event will separate the child from a major attachment figure, such as that the child will be lost, kidnapped, killed, or the victim of an accident.
c. Persistent reluctance or refusal to go to school in order to stay with major attachment figures or at home.
d. Persistent reluctance or refusal to go to sleep without being near a major attachment figure or to go to sleep away from home.
e. Persistent avoidance of being alone, including clinging to and "shadowing" major attachment figures.
f. Repeated nightmares involving the theme of separation.
g. Complaints of physical symptoms, such as headaches, stomach aches, nausea, and vomiting, on many school days or on other occasions when separation from major attachment figures is anticipated.
h. Recurrent indications of excessive distress in anticipation of separation from home or major attachment figures, such as temper tantrums, crying, or pleads with parents not to leave.
i. Recurrent signs or complaints of excessive distress when separated from home or major attachment.

Somatic complaints such as headaches, stomachaches, nausea, or vomiting, sometimes mistaken for physical illness, are especially characteristic of separation anxiety disorder and typically play a role in school refusal. In separation anxiety, the symptoms disappear on weekends and when the child is reassured that the separation will not occur.

2. *Simple phobias.*

Simple phobias are diagnosed when excessive anxiety relates to a specific stimulus other than separation (*separation anxiety disorder*) and social activities (*social phobia*). *In a medical setting, especially in chronically ill children, phobias often include blood, needles, and medical personnel.* Most phobias remit spontaneously, but occasionally they persist to seriously restrict a youngster's activities. Phobic avoidance may also occur as a feature of other anxiety syndromes. In post-traumatic stress disorder, for example, the patient fears stimuli associated with the trauma. In such cases, the diagnosis of simple phobia is usually not made.

Some fears appear to be innate, such as the fear of snakes and the fear of heights, and serve an obvious adaptive purpose. Others result from association of the stimulus with a specific fear-provoking event, as in a dog phobia that develops after a child has been bitten by a dog. This distinction can be helpful in setting realistic treatment goals and in conceptualizing interventions.

3. *Panic disorder.*

Panic disorder can occur in children and adolescents but is uncommon, especially in children. It usually presents as chest pain or, in children, as a feeling of overwhelming terror with no obvious precipitant. In some respects, panic attacks mimic separation anxiety: the child may avoid separation and other situations perceived as evoking an attack. Adults with panic disorder may restrict their activities to home (*agoraphobia*), whereas children and adolescents are more likely to avoid separation from their parents.

It is important to ask the child or adolescent directly about symptoms of panic disorder because the parent may be unaware of the child's suffering. Although the physician knows that anxiety produces somatic distress, the patient may believe that a serious illness has caused the anxiety. If the patient does not think of it as panic attack, he or she will deny having had one. Therefore, it is better to ask about the specific symptoms, namely, intense fear or fear of dying accompanied by manifestations of sympathetic arousal, including tachycardia, chest pain, palpitations, dizziness, sensation of choking or shortness of breath, sweating, tremor, numbness and paresthesias, and nausea and vomiting. Even though the fear is psychogenic, it should be addressed as (and, in fact, it *is*) a powerful biologic process with very real effects on well-being and development. The child who regards these feelings as strange or whose parents convey the view that such complaints are insubstantial may be reluctant to disclose the extent of the problem.

4. *Overanxious disorder.*

Overanxious disorder of childhood is synonymous with generalized anxiety disorder in adults. In this condition, excessive and unrealistic worries are wide ranging, with no specific focus, in contrast to simple phobia or separation anxiety disorder. The clinical picture is dominated by apprehension rather than by panic. In children and adolescents, common symptoms include the following:

- Excessive or unrealistic worry about future events.
- Excessive or unrealistic concern about the appropriateness of past behavior.
- Excessive or unrealistic concern about competence in one or more areas, such as athletic, academic, and social.
- Somatic complaints, such as headaches and stomach aches, for which no physical basis can be established.
- Marked self-consciousness.
- Excessive need for reassurance about a variety of concerns.
- Manifestations of physiologic anxiety, such as restlessness, easy fatigability, poor concentration, irritability, muscle tension, and sleep problems.

In the evaluation, it is important to recognize similar symptoms in the parents, especially with respect to fears, worries, and perfectionism. The primary care physician should also note the presence of habits such as nail biting, hair pulling, and, in children, thumb sucking.

Table 11–5 describes the presentation of several of these symptoms and offers specific questions designed to elicit history from children, adolescents, and parents.

5. *Obsessive compulsive disorder.*
Obsessive-compulsive disorder consists of persistent thoughts and rituals that dominate the patient's life. Rituals often involve counting, cleaning, and checking, and obsessions frequently implicate violence, such as the fear that the patient may kill another or the fear of sex. Early in the course of the illness, rituals can be suppressed outside the home, but later, rituals may increase in number and severity, interfering with daily activities, school attendance, and friendships.

People with OCD are usually secretive about their symptoms. Recognition that symptoms are illogical is a defining feature of the disorder. Because obsessions may occur in the absence of overt behavior, a careful interview may elicit the child's first description of the problem. The questioning should be designed to place the child at ease and to minimize embarrassment in the disclosure. The interviewer may say, "Some kids have thoughts over and over. Sometimes, they can't get the thoughts out of their heads, even though the thoughts seem silly or unpleasant. Do you have thoughts like that? What thoughts do you have?" With respect to compulsions, which are usually observable if they are not practiced in complete secrecy, parents may give a more reliable account of the frequency and the severity of the problem.

D. General management guidelines.

The first step in managing anxiety disorders is distinguishing normal from abnormal fears and worries. Just as medications would be inappropriate for a 6-year-old child who fears spiders, failure to medicate an adolescent with severe obsessions and compulsions could prolong misery and render future treatments less effective.

1. *Normal variant.* When anxiety is developmentally appropriate in kind and degree or arises from simple phobias, reassurance and simple behavioral interventions, such as relaxation and desensitization, are indicated. *Relaxation* typically involves progressive relaxation of muscle groups in a cephalocaudal direction, accompanied by visualization of calming scenes. Many variants of this approach, including meditation and mild hypnotic states, are also acceptable. Once practiced, relaxation techniques can be used in anticipation of a frightening situation. *Desensitization* involves gradually increased exposure to the feared stimulus. Exposure may be increased in intensity, proximity, or duration and may be carried out initially as a pure mental exercise if the actual stimulus is intolerable or unavailable. The child should use relaxation techniques to cope with the anxiety and can be *rewarded* for successfully achieving each level of exposure.
2. *Anxiety disorder.* For generalized anxiety, panic, and separation anxiety disorders and OCD that do not respond to behavioral interventions, medication is indicated.

E. Treatment.

Treatment of severe anxiety disorder requires both medications and behavioral therapy. In some cases, especially where desensitization is required, treatment may require the cooperation of a teacher or school psychologist.

1. *Medical treatment.*
   a. *Selective serotonin reuptake inhibitors.* Fluoxetine (Prozac) and fluvoxamine (Luvox) have been used extensively in the treatment of OCD and are supported by data in both adults and children. Separation anxiety disorder and panic disorder may benefit from SSRIs as well. These drugs are better tolerated than alternatives such as clomipramine (Anafranil) for OCD and imipramine (Tofranil) for separation anxiety disorder.
      (1) *Clinical effects.* In children with OCD, measurable and clinically significant reductions in habitual behaviors can usually be discerned after several weeks of treatment.
      (2) *Administration.* In the treatment of panic disorder and separation anxiety disorder, SSRIs are used in the same manner as they are used in the treatment of depression. Treatment of OCD, however, often requires higher doses ($\leq$ 80 mg/d of fluoxetine in an adult-sized adolescent) and longer periods of treatment for maximal effects to be achieved. Fluvoxamine, which is more likely to be sedating than the other SSRIs, can be

given at night, beginning with doses of 25 to 50 mg and increasing to a daily maximum of 200 mg.

(3) *Common side effects.* Common side effects of SSRIs are presented in Table 11–4.

b. *Tricyclic antidepressants.*

(1) *Clinical effects. Clomipramine* is at least as effective, and possibly more effective, than SSRIs in the treatment of childhood OCD. *Imipramine* has been used for separation anxiety disorder in a fashion analogous to its use for depression.

(2) *Administration. Clomipramine* daily doses should not exceed 3 mg/kg or 200 mg/d. The dosage usually needs to be advanced slowly because of sedative and anticholinergic effects.

(3) *Common side effects.* Clomipramine is highly sedating and often poorly tolerated because of its anticholinergic side effects. It is more apt to induce seizures than other TCAs, and its use should therefore be avoided in epileptic patients.

c. *Benzodiazepines.* Benzodiazepines have generally been not been used in child psychiatry, presumably with the rationale that reliance on a habit-forming drug should be avoided during youth. "Paradoxic" excitement from benzodiazepines has also been a rationale for their avoidance in children, although it is not clear that this characteristic represents a major problem. Benzodiazepines originally marketed for nonpsychiatric purposes, mainly clonazepam (Klonopin), have been much better received.

Benzodiazepines and benzodiazepine derivatives, such as alprazolam (Xanax), may be helpful in treating acute, disabling anxiety in children, especially in combination with behavioral interventions, such as relaxation techniques and systematic desensitization, and antipanic drugs, such as the SSRIs. A benzodiazepine could be used, for example, to reduce anxiety about a specific phobic stimulus (e.g., flying) or to assist a child with separation anxiety disorder in returning to school.

(1) *Clinical effects.* Benzodiazepines reduce anticipatory anxiety at low doses. In the doses ordinarily administered to children, these agents do not have useful antipanic properties.

(2) *Administration.* Alprazolam is available as 0.25-, 0.5-, 1-, and 2-mg scored tablets, and clonazepam is available as 0.5-, 1-, and 2-mg scored tablets. Low doses (0.125 mg of alprazolam or 0.25 mg of clonazepam) may be administered once or twice for acute anxiety or in a three times daily regimen for up to 1 or 2 weeks.

(3) *Common side effects.* Side effects include sedation, ataxia, and paradoxic excitement.

d. *Buspirone (Buspar).*

(1) *Clinical effects.* Buspirone reduces chronic, generalized anxiety but is ineffective in blocking panic. It has occasionally been useful in augmenting SSRIs in treatment-resistant cases of depression and OCD. Responses in children are rarely dramatic, but the drug is well tolerated.

(2) *Administration.* In children or adolescents with chronic anxiety, buspirone may be given in doses ranging from 2.5 mg twice a day to 10 mg three times a day. Effects appear gradually over a period of several weeks. Since the effects may not be obvious, it can be helpful to have a parent supply regular ratings of target symptoms.

(3) *Common side effects.* Buspirone rarely produces side-effects of consequence. It is not habit forming or addictive, posing little risk of abuse.

e. *Innovative treatments: treatment insensitive patients.* Of significance are two possible situations that may necessitate use of two or more medications.

(1) *The anxiety is only partially responding to the antidepressant.* In the first case, several strategies can be used to deal with depression that partially responds or does not respond (refractory). These can include the use of more than one antidepressant or the addition of other medications (augmentation) to the antidepressant regimen.

(2) *There is at least one other disorder present.* In the case of two comorbid disorders, it is usually advisable to chose a medication that will most parsimoniously treat both of them. Examples include the use of a TCA in patients with both an anxiety disorder and ADHD. If this does not seem to remedy the situation, then adding a second medication, such as a stimulant, may prove necessary for a maximum benefit. In some cases, medications are absolutely necessary for the patient to be adequately treated.

2. *Psychosocial treatment.*
In almost all cases of anxiety disorder in children or adolescents, a form of psychological therapy is necessary. In cases of normal developmental anxiety or phobia, separation anxiety, and, in some cases, panic disorder, the most useful therapeutic interventions are behavioral. This requires the setting of specific goals with the parents and sometimes with the child, indicating the need to help the child overcome the fear or anxiety. This step is followed by specific recommendations regarding desensitization or other methods to help the child diminish his or her fears.

F. What to tell the patient and family.

1. Anxiety and fears can be normal for a child; they do not characterize a child or adolescent as being weak.

Table 11–5
Presentation of Anxiety Disorders in Children and Adolescents (Questions That Can Be Asked of Children, Their Parents, or Adolescents)

	Children			Adolescents	
		Question(s) to Ask			
Symptom/Sign	*Presentation*	**Child**	**Parent**	*Presentation (Assume same* presentation *as child, unless otherwise noted)*	*Question(s) to ask (Assume same* questions *as child, unless otherwise noted)*
Excessive anxiety or worry	Has something on his or her mind. Worried about something almost all the time. Looks preoccupied. Often seems self-absorbed and difficult to get attention from. Increased fears of going to school, leaving or being away from his or her parents. Onset of increased fears about specific things or situations, such as darkness, being alone, animals, heights.	Is there anything that you are worried about? Can you tell me about it? Does it scare you? Are you worried about going to school? Are you worried about going to school or being away from your parents? Are there things that you are afraid of? (name them for the child or adolescent)	Does your child report feeling worried about anything? Does he or she act as if worried? Does your child talk as if something bad may happen to someone he or she knows or cares about?		Is there anything that's bothering you? A great deal? Can you talk about it? Are there things that you can't get off your mind? Do they frighten you?
Restlessness	Feels as if he or she cannot relax. Moves around without purpose. Fidgety. More active than usual. Restless. Unable to sit in seat. Getting up often and roaming the room. Wringing hands.	Do you feel that it's difficult to sit still? Can you sit still? Are you able to sit still in class? Do you have to get up a lot? Does your teacher ask you to sit down? Do you bother other students (kids) in your class?	Does your child seem restless? Unable to relax? Moves around a lot?		Do you feel that it's difficult to sit still? Can you sit still? Are you able to sit still in class? Do you have to get up a lot? Does your teacher ask you to sit down? Do you bother other students (kids) in your class?
Difficulty with concentration	Unable to follow direction in class or home. Taking longer to complete work/homework. Bringing more work home. More incorrect answers on the same work. Spending less time watching television or playing video games.	Are you having problems in school? Can you do what your teacher is asking? Is your work harder in school? Can you do your work? Do you watch television or play video games? What are your favorites? Are you watching more or less? Is it more difficult to follow?	Is your child having difficulties in class? Is he or she taking longer to do work in class or homework? Is he or she bringing more homework home now? Is your child enjoying the classroom work less? Does he or she watch television? How much? Is he or she paying attention or just sitting there?		Are you having problems in school? Can you do what your teacher is asking? Is your work harder in school? Can you do your work? Is it harder? Do you watch television or play video games? What are your favorites? Are you watching more or less? Is it more difficult to follow?

Insomnia	Bedtime routine becomes altered. Not falling asleep at usual bedtime. Waking up at all times of the night. Waking up earlier than expected. Taking longer to fall asleep. Getting up in the night and awakening parents due to "bad dreams" or being frightened in the night.	Are you sleeping well? What time do you go to bed? Are you having a lot of bad dreams? Have you been waking up mommy and daddy? Do you take a lot of naps? How many? How often?	What is your child's bedtime? How long does it take for your child to fall asleep? Does your child wake up during the night? Is your child sleeping longer or about the same? Does your child take naps? How often and are they increasing?		Are you sleeping well? What time do you go to bed? Are you having a lot of bad dreams? Have you been waking up your mother and father? Do you take a lot of naps? How many? How often?
Fatigue (loss of energy)	Tired. Not rested after adequate sleep. Sleeping all the time. Taking more frequent naps, but not apparently due to increased physical exertion.	Are you tired a lot? Do you take naps after school? Are you tired after school? Do you get tired during school? Do you ever put your head on the desk and just fall asleep?	Does your child seem more tired? How do you know? Does your child tell you? Is your child taking more naps after school? Does that help him or her being tired? Does your child fall asleep watching television more often than usual?		Are you tired a lot? Do you take naps after school? Are you tired after school? Do you get tired during school? Do you ever put your head on the desk and just fall asleep?
Muscle tension	Feels tense. Complains of headaches that are tension in origin. May also complain of sore muscles in arms and legs. This tension may also make it difficult to sleep.	Do your arms or legs hurt a lot? Do they feel like you have been running and were hurt or just ache? Can you make the ache go away or is it always there?	Is your child complaining of aches and pains? Are you giving him or her aspirin or other pain relievers because of too many aches and pains? Where are they? What makes them better?		Do your arms or legs hurt a lot? Do they feel like you have been running and were hurt or just ache? Can you make the ache go away or is it always there?
Irritability	Getting into more fights with peers, siblings, and parents/authority figures. Losing temper more frequently, yelling and even hitting.	Do you lose your temper a lot with your friends, kids in class, brothers and sisters, parents, or teachers? Have you been getting into more fights? Does it feel like more kids are picking on you?	Has your child become more active recently?		Do you lose your temper a lot with your friends, kids in class, brothers and sisters, parents or teachers? Have you been getting into more fights? Does it feel like more kids are picking on you?

2. *If their child or adolescent has a disorder, it is important for the parent to understand the difference between fears that are a normal part of development and those that represent manifestations of a disorder.* If a disorder is present, then the family needs to understand that these are illnesses and are not present either because the child or adolescent is bad or because he or she has a character flaw.
3. *The disorder will take time to resolve.*
4. It is important that the family understand the steps necessary to help the child or adolescent. Because treatment requires the implementation of a behavioral plan, the parents must be adequately educated as to the steps necessary and must be supported in their efforts.
5. *The course of treatment needs to be continued beyond the resolution of symptoms.*
6. Parents need to be informed that some anxiety disorders do not resolve and may be lifelong disorders. Some individuals may not respond to treatment. These rather negative outcomes should not be broached in the earlier stages of the disorder unless a family history of such illnesses exists. Rather, it is important to provide hope to the child or adolescent and family in what often seems to be a hopeless situation.

G. When to refer.

Most disorders usually respond to a combination of medical and behavioral therapy. In cases in which there appears to be little to no response, a second opinion is recommended, either from a child psychiatrist, especially for younger patients, or an adult psychiatrist in adolescents.

VII. Disruptive behavior disorders.

Disruptive behavior disorders, including ADHD, conduct disorder (CD), and oppositional defiant disorder (ODD) make up most cases seen in child psychiatry clinics in the United States.

Attention-deficit hyperactivity disorder is probably the most prevalent and important of these syndromes from the family practitioner's perspective, because parents, schools, and nonmedical mental health specialists often rely on the primary care physician for definitive somatic intervention. The ADHD concept has become increasingly controversial because the label is applied to, and sometimes offered as an "excuse" for, a widening range of behaviors in children and adults. It has justified the prescription of stimulants for large numbers of school children, sometimes on slender indications.

Ambiguities in the attention-deficit disorder concept arise from two false but implicit assumptions: (1) ADHD is an etiologically distinct disorder rather than a heterogeneous group of problems with common symptomatic manifestations, and (2) the border demarcating "normal" from "pathologic" attention span and activity level is both qualitatively distinct and nonarbitrary. The result of these false assumptions is reification of the syndrome of inattention and overactivity as if it were a unique and distinct disorder, like a fracture, that a patient either has or does not have. It may well turn out that subgroups of ADHD conform well to such a model, but it is far less likely that the heterogeneous group of problems satisfying current behavioral definitions of ADHD represents a single entity that can be sharply distinguished from normal.

The terms *attention-deficit disorder, hyperactive child syndrome, hyperkinesis,* and *minimal brain damage* refer to similar problems but reflect older hypotheses about the nature and causes of the disorder.

Conduct disorder is a behavioral syndrome of multifactorial etiology that overlaps with the legal classification of "delinquency." *ODD* first appeared in the *Diagnostic and Statistical Manual of Mental Disorders,* Third Edition (DSM-III) in 1980, in an effort to classify relatively mild antisocial behaviors characterized by defiance. It is uncertain whether ODD is best viewed as a distinct disorder or as part of a continuum with CD.

A. Epidemiology.

Rates of ADHD in the general population of children and adolescents ranges from 0.1% to 20%. The best available data, using DSM-III criteria for attention-deficit disorder with hyperactivity, give a *prevalence of 8% in children aged 6 to 9 years,* with lower rates in preschool and adolescent populations.[1] *All studies show considerably higher prevalence in boys than in girls, the sex ratio ranging from about 2:1 to 9:1.*

Oppositional defiant disorder is thought to have a prevalence roughly similar to that of conduct disorder, with estimates ranging from *2% to 16% of the population.* In prepubertal children, ODD is more common in boys than in girls, but by adolescence, the gender gap disappears. Estimates of the prevalence of CD range from *6% to 16% in boys and 2% to 9% in girls.* University clinics and family practices may see fewer adolescents with severe conduct disorders because such adolescents are often detoured into the juvenile justice system.

B. Evaluation and diagnostic overview.

A referral may arise out of a specific crisis, such as suspension from school. Alternatively, it may appear to represent the culmination of years of frustration in managing difficult behavior. In the latter case, some trigger usually impels referral at a particular time; an important unstated agenda may need to be addressed. A single mother, for example, may present a child for treatment because his or her behavior jeopardizes a new romance, or the child may have been assigned to a classroom whose teacher has a zero-tolerance policy on disruptive behavior.

1. *History.*
   a. *Sources. The history, much of which can be collected from teachers and parents from question-*

naires before an office visit, should come from multiple sources. Correlations among parent, teacher, and child ratings are usually low. The elementary school classroom teacher can sometimes offer the most objective appraisal of a child's behavior, whereas the school-aged child's version of the history should usually receive little weight. Often, a *teacher's brief written narrative,* specifically requested in some questionnaires, provides the most useful and specific information. The parent can deliver an envelope to the teacher that contains relevant rating scales and is addressed for return to the physician's office. The consistency of behavioral problems over time and across raters can be assessed by review of the comments teachers have made on *report cards* over the years.

Mothers and fathers may give contrasting perspectives on a child's behavior, although a mother's complaints should never be discounted simply because the child is better behaved in a father's presence.

Disparities among witnesses often reflect actual differences in behavior across social contexts rather than inconsistent reporting. Some apparent differences resolve when specific behaviors are described in detail.

b. *Obtaining a detailed history of present illness.* The history of present illness should include descriptions of behavior that reflect temperamental predispositions, such as short attention span and high energy level, as well as recurring behavior problems that may be context-specific or situation-specific, such as defiance and aggression.

(1) *Obtain specific examples of behaviors. The primary care physician should not accept generalizations or conclusory statements.* For example, if the parent says the child is inattentive, *the parent should be asked to describe specific situations* in which this occurs and *the specific behavior* being characterized as inattentive. This precision allows the clinician to establish whether the physician and parent are using a common language. Some parents, for instance, describe a *disobedient* child as inattentive, because "He doesn't pay attention to what I tell him!" From the behavioral description, the physician can also ascertain whether the parent has unrealistic developmental expectations. A preschool-aged child, for example, should not be expected to spend an hour doing chores.

(2) *Have the parent identify a specific situation occurring in the past week* that is characteristic of the presenting complaint, and ask the parent to describe the event in minute detail. General characterizations of typical behaviors are much less useful than detailed descriptions of specific events that are fresh in the parent's memory.

(3) Follow the **ABC rule** in assessing specific problem behaviors:

Antecedent conditions and behaviors:

- What was happening *immediately before* the index behavior?
- What was the child doing before the problem occurred?
- What were other people doing?
- What time was it?
- Where did the events occur?
- Who else was there? What seemed to trigger the problem behavior?

Often, a recurring behavior problem can be minimized by alterations in the conditions that triggered it. If a child always disagrees with his or her little sister's choice of television program, for example, the conflict might be resolved simply by having the children watch different televisions in different rooms. If the child repeatedly steals things from his or her sister's bedroom, then locking the bedroom door may remedy the problem.

Behavior itself: a detailed description containing quantitative estimates should be obtained. "She was mean to her little brother" is much too vague.

- What did he or she say?
- What did he or she do?
- How many times did he or she do it?
- How long did it go on?

These rough measures provide a gauge of the baseline severity of a problem and also help in prioritizing problems for behavioral therapy.

Consequences of the behavior: if the behavior is recurring, then obviously the consequence was not entirely adequate.

- Was the child scolded?
- Was he or she spanked or sent to his or her room?
- Did he or she get what he or she wanted?
- Did the parent threaten punishment but fail to carry it out?
- Were punishments timely and proportionate to the misbehavior?
- Do the same negative consequences occur whether the child behaves appropriately or not?

When a child gets what he or she wants, the effective behavior is reinforced. Parents who yield to tantrums make future tantrums more likely. On the other hand, punishments that are dispensed randomly or inconsistently have little effect on behavior other than to make a child fearful, defensive, and avoidant.

(4) *To assess attention span, persistence, and activity level, inquire about behavior in specific situations, including:*

- *Watching television.* How long does the child remain at the television set? Does he or she rush off during commercials?

Does he or she usually do something else, like playing with a toy, while watching television? Does he or she shift position or move around in his or her seat, even during his or her favorite shows? (Children with ADHD often have good sustained attention exclusively in the contexts of watching television and playing video games.)

- *Reading a book or being read to.* How long does the child stay with the activity? Does he or she stop before completing a relevant section? Does he or she skip pages and push ahead to the end of the book?
- *Doing homework.* Does he or she do homework? Does he or she avoid it? Once started, can he or she continue to do it? Is it messy or carelessly completed? Does he or she forget to turn it in?
- *At a family meal.* How long can he or she remain at the dinner table? How many times is he or she up and down during a meal? Does he or she rush through a meal, or, owing to distractibility and talkativeness, does he or she take forever to finish?
- *At a restaurant.* Does the family avoid restaurants because of the child's behavior? Does the child intrude on other families? Does he or she insist on leaving his or her seat and wandering about?
- *Doing chores.* Does the child refuse to do chores? Does he or she initiate chores cooperatively but become distracted by more entertaining pursuits?

(5) *Establish whether the behavior is a marked departure from the child's usual behavior.* Usually, children with ADHD have had similar problems in the past, although perhaps never as troublesome as the events leading to the medical referral. An abrupt change in behavior suggests the occurrence of an unusual stressor, the onset of a new psychiatric disorder, or, less commonly, the advent of a serious medical condition.

2. *Interview of the child.*
Interviews are helpful in excluding other causes of disruptive behavior, such as depression, psychosis, and pervasive developmental disorder, and in identifying obvious learning or communication deficits. No interview findings are specific to the disruptive behavior disorders, although some children display obvious hyperactivity in the course of an interview. Contrary to popular belief, anxiety tends to *reduce* locomotor activity in children. Thus, *even decidedly hyperactive children may appear subdued during an interview by a relatively strange adult,* especially one known to administer shots. This may give the false impression of *depression,* a possibility that can be checked against the child's demeanor in the waiting room.
   a. The *interview may be arranged topically* around themes such as home, school, family, friends, moods (anger, fear, sadness), specific worries, scary experiences, nice people, not-so-nice people, sleeping, and dreaming.
   b. *Several simple rules,* summarized in Table 11–6, *can facilitate interviews with prepubertal children.*
   c. *Conduct interviews away from parents. It is not always essential to interview prepubertal children apart from their parents* if the clinician knows the family well enough to exclude suspicion of child abuse and has a good sense of the quality of

Table 11–6
Interviewing Prepubertal Children

Do	Minimize distractions, e.g., toys.
	Establish your authority in a friendly way.
	Sit close to the child and lean toward him or her while exuding a friendly and receptive attitude. *The distance between you and the child should be inversely proportional to the age and activity level of the child.*
	Inquire about simple matters, e.g., school, family, place of residence, to establish rapport and determine whether the child understands questions and can give simple, factual responses.
	Inquire about sadness, worries and fears, anger, boredom, and habits.
	Use simple vocabulary and short sentences.
	Standardize your interviews enough that you can make valid comparisons among different children interviewed under similar conditions.
Do not	Play with the child or offer him or her fascinating toys if you wish to have a seated, face-to-face conversation. Play interviews are specialized techniques of limited value in diagnosing disruptive behavior disorders.
	Offer the child a chair that rolls or rotates.
	Open the interview by discussing a disciplinary problem, which could cause the child to cower in shame and silence. Instead, discuss a neutral topic (e.g., How old are you? What grade are you in? How do you like school? What do you like to do in your free time?). It is not always necessary to discuss the problem behavior at all.
	Routinely offer the child gratuitous advice on reforming chronic behavior problems.

family interactions. Some children, however, reveal animosities, especially toward step-parents, only in private interviews.

Adolescents often have important secrets that they will not reveal in the presence of their parents. These secrets may include substance abuse, sexual behavior, truancy, serious antisocial behavior, suicidal thoughts, and gang activity.

d. *Social behavior can be sampled* through brief observations in the waiting area, especially if other similarly aged children are attending the clinic. It is useful to conduct the parent interview at least partly in the child's presence, especially when time is limited. This allows the physician to observe symptomatic behaviors directly (e.g., frequent interruptions, inability to sit still) and to assess the quality of family interactions, including a parent's approach to obtaining compliance from a reluctant or bored child. The physician needs to be sensitive, however, to family secrets or embarrassing information that parents may not wish to disclose to the child (e.g., that he or she is adopted or that a relative committed suicide).

e. *Adolescents often inquire about or need reassurance that their communications will be kept confidential.* The adolescent should be told that the primary care physician will protect his or her confidentiality unless the physician feels that the information must be disclosed in order to ensure his or her safety and health or that of others. This implicitly covers reporting requirements relating to infectious disease, child abuse, or anticipated violence.

3. *Rating scales and detailed history forms.*
The *Conners rating scales* have been popular because of their long established use in children with ADHD and because of their simplicity of administration and scoring. The "hyperactivity index," derived from items on these scales, is useful for measuring response to medication.

Other scales, such as the *ADD Comprehensive Teacher's Rating Scale* (ACTERS), have been designed specifically for the diagnosis of ADHD and are easy to administer and score. Both the Conners rating scales and the ACTERS can be obtained from Psychological Assessment Resources, Inc., P.O. Box 998, Odessa FL 33556 (1-800-331-8378). The Stony Brook Child Symptom Inventory—4 is a checklist covering the gamut of child psychiatric disorders. This instrument can be obtained from Checkmate Plus, Ltd., P.O. Box 696, Stony Brook, NY 11790-0696.

4. *Physical examination.*
Although the results of the physical examination are usually negative, they can suggest a broad range of medical problems associated with inattention or hyperactivity. Minor physical anomalies and neurologic soft signs are frequently present but facilitate diagnosis only if they point to a specific inherited syndrome, such as fragile X syndrome, or if they are markedly asymmetric, suggesting a localized lesion.

Vision and hearing screening should be obtained if these have not been performed recently.

5. *Psychological, educational, and language testing.* When learning disabilities are suspected, a psychoeducational testing battery should be performed by the school, at the parents' request, or by a psychologist familiar with ADHD and learning disabilities.

C. Specific diagnosis or problem.

1. *Attention-deficit hyperactivity disorder.*
(ADHD) Attention-deficit hyperactivity disorder is characterized by two core symptom clusters: *inattention*, especially lack of *sustained* attention; and *hyperactivity-impulsivity.* The classic presentation involving both symptom clusters is called *ADHD, combined type*; children with prominent symptoms from only one cluster may be diagnosed with *ADHD, predominantly inattentive type* or *ADHD, predominantly hyperactive type.* The disorder must begin before the age of 7 years and in most cases is first noticed in the preschool years. The specific behaviors by which the DSM-IV defines inattention and hyperactivity are summarized in Table 11–7.

Generally, activity level decreases and attention span increases from infancy to adulthood, both in normal people and in hyperactive people. Thus, *adolescents with ADHD are usually more active than other adolescents, but they are not as active as they may have been at school age.* A subset of hyperactive children become *underactive* in adolescence, but attentional problems typically persist.

Comorbidity with other disruptive behavior disorders and other psychiatric disorders is common. *Poor peer relationships and school underachievement, with or without learning disabilities, are common complications.* Older children, adolescents, and adults often display *dysphoria* and *demoralization* in the absence of frank affective disorder. *Low self-esteem* associated with social rejection and academic failure becomes more apparent as the child matures.

a. *Identification and course of ADHD during childhood and adolescence.*
   (1) *Infants and preschool–aged children. The classic presentation of ADHD begins in the preschool years.* The traits of hyperactivity, impulsivity, and inattentiveness can be noted in infants, but they rarely constitute a problem before a child begins to walk. Normal children who are frustrated or upset may transiently appear to be strikingly hyperactive. The physician who happens to observe a major tantrum in his or her office should guard against too hastily diagnosing ADHD. Generally, however, *children who consistently meet the criteria for ADHD over a period of 6 to 12*

months as preschoolers continue to warrant the diagnosis by the age of 6 years. Thus, the persistence of the problem is probably the best indicator of an accurate diagnosis in very young children.

(2) *School-aged children. The classic picture of ADHD usually emerges by the early elementary years.* The child may be seen as a troublemaker—or may fit the job description for "class clown." Even with high intelli-

Table 11–7
Symptom Clusters in Attention-Deficit Hyperactivity Disorder

Signs and Symptom	Presentation	Questions to Ask
Inattention	Often fails to give close attention to details or makes careless mistakes Often has difficulty sustaining attention to tasks or play activities Often does not seem to listen when spoken to directly Often does not follow through on instructions; fails to finish schoolwork or chores Often has difficulty organizing tasks Often avoids, dislikes, or is reluctant to engage in tasks requiring sustained mental effort Often loses things necessary for tasks Is often easily distracted Is often forgetful in daily activities	How does your child behave during a family meal? Is he (or she) up and down several times, even when he's (or she's) on his (or her) best behavior? How does your child behave in a restaurant? Describe a time you took your child to a restaurant. Does your child like to have you read stories to him (or her)? If not, why not? Does your child sit patiently for the duration of the story, or does he (or she) start turning the pages or moving about? Describe a recent time when you read a story to your child. Does your child watch television? If not, why not? Does your child sit patiently, mesmerized for hours on end, or is television watching a fairly active process, with commercials being opportunities to run into the next room? Have you stopped taking your child places because of his (or her) behavior? What happens when your child goes to visit friends? What happens when you take your child to visit your friends? Tell me about a specific time. Is your child a "daredevil" engaging in activities heedless of danger? Give an example.
Hyperactivity and impulsivity	Often fidgets with hands or feet, squirms in seat. Often leaves seat in classroom or in situations in which remaining seated is expected Often runs about or climbs excessively Often has difficulty playing or engaging in leisure activities quietly Is often "on the go," or acts like "driven by a motor" Often talks excessively Often blurts out answers before questions are completed Often has difficulty waiting turns Often interrupts or intrudes on others	*To parent of prepubertal child:* Is your child the class clown? Does the teacher complain that your child cannot sit still or that your child frequently leaves his (or her) seat much more often than other kids? Does your child always need to be first in line or first to answer a question? Does your child talk too much? When your child's legs aren't in motion, does his (or her) mouth usually take over? Does your child rush through homework, do sloppy and careless work, or forget to turn in assignments? *To parent of an adolescent:* What was your child like when he (or she) was younger (refer to above questions). Does your child tap his (or her) foot continuously when compelled to remain seated? Does your child have special difficulty with longer assignments, planning his (or her) time poorly or waiting to the last minute? Describe the process of getting homework completed. *To the adolescent:* Do you have trouble sitting through an entire class? Does your mind start wandering early in a lecture, so that you are completely lost when the teacher calls on you? Do you feel restless when you have to sit still for a long time? Do you just want to get up and DO something?

Table 11–7
Symptom Clusters in Attention-Deficit Hyperactivity Disorder *Continued*

Signs and Symptom	Presentation	Questions to Ask
Defiance and anger	Often loses temper Often argues with adults Often actively defies adult requests Often deliberately annoys people Often blames others for mistakes or misbehavior Is often touchy or easily annoyed Is often angry or resentful Is often spiteful or vindictive	*To the parent:* Is your child touchy, irritable, and intolerant? Does he (or she) anger easily or argue without cause? What happens when your child does something wrong? Does your child admit it? Does he (or she) blame his (or her) little sister or friend? Give an example. Does your child flatly refuse to obey? Does your child hear an instruction and march off with no intention of complying? Does your child behave this way with everyone, or just with you? What is different about the people your child is "good" for? Does your child do mean things to get back at people?
Aggression	Often bullies, threatens, or intimidates others Often initiates physical fights Has used a weapon that can cause serious physical harm Has been physically cruel to people Has been physically cruel to animals Has stolen while confronting a victim Has forced someone into sexual activity	*To the parent:* How frequently does your child get in fights? Describe one. Does your child start the fights? What motivates the fights? Does your child like to fight, or does he (or she) just have a quick temper? Is your (child's) fighting mainly in self-defense? Is your child a bully? Does your child pick on other kids? Does he (or she) do mean things just for the fun of it? Has your child ever been arrested? For what? If not, has your child done things he (or she) could have been arrested for (burglary, mugging, vandalism, shoplifting, and so on)? Describe. Have you seen stolen property at home, or unaccounted for valuables? Do you have any reason to suspect gang activity or substance abuse? *To the adolescent:* If you knew you wouldn't get caught, would you kill someone? Rape someone? What would you do? Do you ever feel sorry for people you have hurt?
Destruction of property	Has set a fire with the intent of causing serious damage Has deliberately destroyed other people's property	*To the parent of an adolescent:* Has your child ever broken windows at school, in stores, or in residence, other than by accident? Has your child ever set fires that did or could have caused significant damage to persons or property? Were other children involved, or did your child act alone? *To the adolescent:* Have you engaged in or been arrested for vandalism or firesetting? Have you ever broken windows at school, in stores, or in residences, other than by accident? Have you ever set fires that did or could have caused significant damage to persons or property? Were other children involved, or were you acting alone? What motivated these acts (e.g., revenge, alcohol abuse, received payment)?
Deceit, theft	Has broken into someone else's house, building, or car Often lies to obtain things or to avoid obligations ("cons" others) Has stolen valuable items without confrontation of victim	*To the adolescent:* Do you belong to a gang? How often do you drink alcohol, smoke marijuana? How many different drugs have you used? Did you ever sell drugs? Are you sexually active? Since what age? How many partners have you had?
Violations of rules without harm to others	Often stays out late at night, beginning before age 13, despite parental prohibition Has run away from home overnight at least twice (or once for a lengthy period) Has been a frequent truant, beginning before age 13	*To the adolescent:* (If you ran away from home) where did you go? What did you do? Are there some people you would like to punish if you could? Who? How would you do it? Do you plan to do it?

gence and normal academic capacities, the child may fall behind in school or earn grades that poorly reflect the knowledge he or she has acquired and his or her potential for above-average performance. Peer problems, aggression, defiance, and antisocial behavior emerge in the school years.

(3) *Adolescents. In teenagers, the core symptoms of ADHD may be less apparent than secondary problems, such as conduct disorder, ODD, substance abuse, legal conflicts, and school failure.* Adolescents typically present themselves to adults as if they were fully in control of their own behavior, reflecting the striving for independence emblematic of teenage development. They may deny that they have a problem with inattention, externalizing blame for incomplete homework assignments to their teacher or to the quality of the assignment itself. They would rather be deliberately defiant and affirmatively neglectful than be perceived as unable to meet their responsibilities. *ADHD symptoms may therefore be hard to detect, and diagnosis may hinge on tracing the continuity with ADHD symptoms that began in childhood.*

2. *Oppositional defiant disorder.*
Oppositional defiant disorder is defined on the basis of two major symptom clusters, defiance and hostility lasting at least 6 months. To constitute psychopathology, the pattern of oppositional behavior should be characteristic of the child's relationships with authority figures generally rather than symptomatic of one or two distressed relationships. Because of the prominence of irritability and anger, an important differential diagnostic consideration in children meeting criteria for ODD is affective disorder or emerging affective disorder. Specific behaviors defining the symptom clusters are shown in Table 11–7. *Major breaches of social norms, such as overt aggression and acts that would constitute felonies if committed by an adult, suggest the diagnosis of CD.* Because ODD was conceived as a mild form of CD, the diagnosis of CD pre-empts that of ODD.

In some children with ODD, but certainly not all, more serious antisocial behavior develops in later childhood and adolescence.

3. *Conduct disorder.*
Conduct disorder has four major groups of symptoms:
   - Aggression and cruelty, such as bullying, frequent fighting, cruelty to people or animals, and rape.
   - Arson and other forms of vandalism.
   - Deceit, stealth, or theft, as in burglary, "running cons," and larceny.
   - Violations of major rules and so-called "status" offenses, that is, behaviors for which juveniles but not adults can be arrested, including truancy, running away from home, and curfew violations.

A diagnosis of conduct disorder implies that at least three symptoms from any of these clusters are present and that the behavior represents a pattern of at least 6 months' duration.

Conduct disorder appearing de novo in adolescence carries a much more favorable prognosis than that beginning in childhood and persisting into adolescence. Multiple, severe, and chronic symptoms carry the worst prognosis.

4. The differential diagnosis of disruptive behavior disorders is extremely broad because inattention, hyperactivity, and aggression are among the most ubiquitous symptoms of child psychopathology. Attention, which has evolved to an extraordinary degree in the human brain, is one of the first functions compromised by even mild cerebral insults. Closed head injuries, for example, may produce significant attentional incapacity in the absence of any focal signs of damage on physical or radiologic examination.
   a. Normal children may seem hyperactive during ordinary play, during states of excitement, and during group activities with boisterous and provocative peers. Indeed, hyperactive children and normal children are often indistinguishable from one another on the playground.
   b. *Substance abuse* should be suspected when a child or adolescent undergoes a change in personality, has symptoms that are uncharacteristic of previous behavior, or becomes unusually secretive in his or her activities.
   c. *Acute, severe stress* and *post-traumatic stress disorder* produce a state of autonomic hyperarousal with increased locomotion and extreme hypervigilance that resembles distractibility.
   d. *Sleep deprivation,* whether caused by sleep disorders, such as apnea and narcolepsy, or caused by an erratic sleep/wake schedule, impairs attention and may produce paradoxic excitement.
   e. Children with frank mental illnesses, such as *major depression, bipolar disorder,* and *schizophrenia,* typically display inattention and varying degrees of locomotor excess.
   f. *Pervasive developmental disorders* (e.g., autism and autistiform conditions) are typically associated with disruptive and hyperactive behavior. Prominent disruptiveness can obscure the core symptoms of pervasive developmental disorder, especially in higher-functioning children.
   g. *Tourette's syndrome* and other tic disorders can be associated with ADHD; about half of children with Tourette's syndrome also meet criteria for ADHD. Children with undiagnosed Tourette's disorder frequently present with complaints related to ADHD.
   h. Children with *mental retardation, communication disorders,* and *learning disabilities* often have difficulty in comprehending a teacher's lecture or instructions and so may appear to be restless and inattentive.

i. *Sensory-perceptual impairment,* especially deafness, can resemble ADHD.

j. Most medical conditions producing inattention and hyperactivity are fairly distinctive and present trivial differential diagnostic problems, mainly because behavior problems are the least salient treatment issue. However, virtually any medical condition that affects brain structure can also produce behavioral manifestations that outlive the primary medical complaint.

k. A broad array of prescribed and over-the-counter medications can mimic or aggravate hyperactivity. Commonly implicated medications include phenobarbital, antihistamines and over-the-counter cold preparations, and theophylline derivatives. Hyperactivity induced by an antidepressant should raise the question of bipolar disorder.

5. No routine laboratory investigations need to be conducted on most children with behavior problems. More extensive work-ups may be helpful in cases with atypical presentations, treatment-refractory cases, and in cases in which physical symptoms have been identified.

D. General management guidelines.

1. *Limits and efficacy of treatment.*
Abundant evidence indicates that specific treatments, including medications and behaviorally oriented psychotherapies, have robust short-term effects, although long-term effects have yet to be conclusively demonstrated. *Traditional psychotherapies, including play therapy and loosely structured "talk" therapies, have no demonstrable effect on the core symptoms of ADHD or conduct disorder.* These may be useful in selected cases for secondary symptoms such as low self-esteem, especially in older children and adolescents.

2. *General measures.*
Regular, frequent, and vigorous exercise, a healthy diet that is low in simple carbohydrates, good sleep hygiene, and involvement in organized activities that promote self-discipline, self-esteem, and wholesome moral values are good general measures to treat hyperactivity. Martial arts training can be particularly valuable. Parents fear they may generate a "black belt with an attitude," but most children outgrow their "attitude" long before developing lethal skills.

3. *Role of diet.*
Most diets used for ADHD have not proved beneficial when subjected to controlled study.

E. Treatment.

1. *Medical treatments for inattention and hyperactivity.*

a. *Stimulants.* Stimulants such as methylphenidate (Ritalin), dextroamphetamine (Dexedrine and Adderall), methamphetamine (Desoxyn), and pemoline (Cylert) can be used to treat ADHD.

(1) *Clinical effects.* The stimulants are the drugs of choice for inattentive children. Most children with typical presentations of ADHD respond favorably to either methylphenidate or dextroamphetamine. Those who do not respond to one drug usually respond to the other.

Both methylphenidate and dextroamphetamine are available in short-acting forms, lasting 3 to 4 hours, and in long-acting forms, lasting 6 to 8 hours. Administration of pemoline, with clinical effects persisting for 6 to 8 hours, requires liver function testing early in therapy and every 6 months during maintenance treatment.

(2) *Administration.* Before treatment, blood pressure, pulse, height, and weight should be assessed. *Liver function tests should be performed before and periodically during therapy with pemoline, but otherwise routine laboratory examinations are unnecessary during stimulant treatment.*

These medications have almost immediate effects when the correct dose is given. Usual doses range from 0.3 to 0.7 mg/kg/dose of methylphenidate or 0.15 to 0.3 mg/kg/dose of dextroamphetamine, given twice or three times daily, typically at 8 a.m., noon, and, if the drug is needed at home, 4 p.m. It is wise to begin at a low dose followed by rapid upward titration, because great variation exists in the responses of individual children, and adverse effects from the first dose could jeopardize compliance. If the drug will be given during school hours only, the parents, who are most apt to detect adverse effects, should be invited to administer test doses at home.

For documentation of drug effects, rating scales (as discussed earlier) should be completed by observers in the settings in which the treatment is being given, usually school. Late afternoon ratings from a parent are not helpful in establishing whether a noon dose of medication affects classroom behavior.

(3) *Common side effects.* Common side effects include anorexia, insomnia, abdominal pain, headaches, and behavioral activation.

- Most children lose weight when treatment is initiated, but this rarely jeopardizes health.
- Reduced growth velocity is common, especially in children who are treated on a daily basis throughout the calendar year rather than during school sessions only. Stimulant effects

on ultimate growth are thought to be minimal; most decelerations are compensated for during the adolescent growth spurt.

- The advent of tics should prompt a closer investigation of the possibility of Tourette's disorder.
- Psychosis is rare at the doses ordinarily given and may reflect underlying psychopathology in some cases.

Limited data suggest that children having inattention without hyperactivity are somewhat less likely to respond to a single stimulant and that the dose required by those who respond is somewhat lower than that usually needed in hyperactive children. Stimulants can aggravate anxiety, a common feature in the predominantly inattentive type of ADHD, and should be used cautiously.

b. *Nonstimulants.*

Tricyclic antidepressants.

(1) *Clinical effects. TCAs are the best studied and possibly the most effective alternatives to stimulants in children with ADHD, but they also are the most toxic.*

(2) *Administration and side effects.* Administration and side effects of TCAs for ADHD are generally similar to their use in depression, with differences as noted in Table 11–8. Following reports of several deaths in children undergoing treatment with desipramine, many clinicians have been reluctant to prescribe this and other TCAs.

Alpha$_2$ agonists. These agents include clonidine (Catapres) and guanfacine (Tenex).

(1) *Clinical effects.* Alpha$_2$ agonists are sympatholytics whose major central effect is inhibition of arousal, blood pressure, and other aspects of sympathetic tone. They reduce activity level, impulsiveness, and aggression but enhance attention only indirectly. Although it is marketed as an antihypertensive drug, clonidine rarely produces significant decrements in blood pressure in normotensive children at the doses typically required for behavioral effects. *Clonidine is commonly used as an alternative or an adjunctive treatment to stimulants.* Guanfacine, a longer-acting drug with similar therapeutic properties, has recently won some popularity, despite an absence of controlled trials. Advantages of alpha$_2$ agonists include safety and, when given at night, hastened sleep onset. In many children with Tourette-spectrum disorders, clonidine benefits both tics and behavior. Disadvantages of clonidine include sedation, possible impairment in attention, need for frequent dos-

Table 11–8
Tricyclic Antidepressants for Attention-Deficit Hyperactive Disorder (ADHD), Depression, and Enuresis

Conditions	ADHD	Depression	Enuresis
Evidence for efficacy	Strong	Weak (children and adolescents)	Strong
Therapeutic levels	Probably irrelevant	Presumably similar to those for adults	Irrelevant due to low dosage
Effective dose	Highly variable; some children respond to as little as 20 mg of imipramine daily, so starting dose should be low	Usually 3.5–5 mg/kg/d	Maximum dose is 2.5 mg/kg/d; typical upper dose in children is 50 mg at bedtime; preadolescents may require 75 mg at bedtime
Dosing schedule	Can be given once daily, at night or in the morning; but may be most effective when given in divided doses, like stimulants	Based on convenience and tolerance of the patient	Given at bedtime
Maintenance treatment	Higher doses often required	Same as effective dose	Same as effective dose
Advantages over first-line treatment	Effects are much more consistent than with stimulants, with minimal rebound effects; sleep and appetite typically improve	Few advantages over SSRI antidepressants	Less risk of electrolyte abnormalities than desmopressin, rapid onset compared with behavioral interventions
Onset of effects	Rapid	Weeks	Rapid

SSRI, selective serotonin reuptake inhibitor.

ing, and inconsistency of effects over the course of a day. Evidence for the efficacy of clonidine is rather limited considering its widespread use.

Alpha$_2$ agonists should be avoided in children with pure inattention. Although virtually no published clinical experience exists, one would expect this class of drugs to impair neuropsychological performance in inattentive children.

(2) *Administration.*

Clonidine (Catapres) Pulse and blood pressure should be obtained before therapy is initiated, on changing of a dose, and regularly thereafter. Most children experience sedation when oral treatment with clonidine is initiated. Treatment should begin with a low dose of 0.025 mg twice daily, increasing in increments of 0.025 mg every few days as tolerated. Daily doses ranging from 0.1 to 0.3 mg/d in two to four doses are usually helpful, although higher doses may be given if needed.

The clonidine transdermal patch overcomes problems with sedation, frequent dosing, and rebound phenomena, but it often produces a local dermatitis that is annoying and disfiguring. When severe, this dermatitis may alter the absorption characteristics of the patch, with unpredictable effects. For these reasons, the patch has achieved only limited use.

For patch administration, a 0.1 mg patch is affixed to a clean area of the back that is not readily accessible to roaming hands. The patch usually needs to be changed about every 5 days, rather than weekly, as suggested in the packaging instruction. The full effect is not experienced for about 3 days, and a similar period of time is needed for clearance of the medication after discontinuation of therapy. For discontinuation of clonidine therapy, the dose should be tapered over 1 to 2 weeks, depending on the initial dose and duration of treatment.

Guanfacine (Tenex) The chief advantage of guanfacine is that it can be given in a single bedtime dose with minimal daytime sedation. Many parents report the waning of effects by late afternoon, presumably reflecting the more vigorous metabolism of children. The major disadvantage of guanfacine is the absence of controlled trials demonstrating its efficacy in behavior disorders.

Therapy should be initiated at 0.5 mg at bedtime, raising the dose in weekly 0.5 mg increments, as needed and tolerated, to a maximum of 3 mg at bedtime.

Bupropion (Wellbutrin).

(1) *Clinical effects.* Bupropion is a promising alternative to stimulants for ADHD. Its mild dopaminergic properties give it stimulant-like effects and enhance attention, as measured on neuropsychological tests. Side effects are generally mild and resemble those caused by stimulants. Bupropion therapy is contraindicated in patients with epilepsy and eating disorders.

(2) *Administration.* Bupropion is available in 75-mg and 100-mg tablets. The initial dose should be low (e.g., 37.5 mg twice a day). For avoidance of seizure induction, the dose should be advanced in 37.5-mg increments every 3 to 4 days. Doses should be at least 4 hours apart, and no single dose should exceed 3 mg/kg. The highest published doses in children are 6 mg/kg/d, in two to three divided doses. We have treated individual patients with higher doses without ill effects. Onset of effects, although usually more subtle than for stimulants, should be fairly rapid once an adequate dose has been achieved.

Other drugs for inattention/hyperactivity. Many other medications have been used for ADHD and represent reasonable alternatives in special situations or situations in which conventional treatments have failed. Monoamine oxidase inhibitors, such as selegiline (Eldepryl) and tranylcypromine (Parnate), are effective but require dietary restrictions that few children can follow. Diphenhydramine (Benadryl) in high doses ($\leq$ 10 mg/kg/d in two to three doses) showed promise for younger children (< 10 years of age) in early trials in the 1960s, but these were never followed up with properly designed studies. Carbamazepine (Tegretol) may be useful in some cases.

2. *Medical treatments for aggression.*
   a. *Types of aggression that respond to medication.* Aggression may be *impulsive* and thoughtless, driven by powerful and unanticipated emotions, such as anger or fear; or it may be *predatory,* executed with a purpose in mind, such as intimidation or elimination of an obstacle. Impulsive aggression may respond to drug therapy; predatory aggression does not respond to drug therapy, except to the extent that the therapy produces sleep and apathy.
   b. *Treating the primary disorder.* In cases in which aggression arises in the context of another disorder, treatment should first be directed at the primary disorder. Thus, aggressive patients with ADHD should first receive stimulants, those with depression should receive antidepressants, and so on.
   c. *Choosing a drug.* Conventional wisdom has it that the preferred drug should have the support of controlled, double-blind studies. Un-

fortunately, the drugs with this advantage are also the most hazardous and difficult to administer, such as neuroleptics and lithium. Medications like trazodone and clonidine, the effects of which in aggression are supported mainly by anecdotal reports, are far easier to use and are better tolerated. A medication such as lithium, however, might be preferred in cases of ADHD with aggression in which there is a family history of bipolar disorder or in which the aggressive behavior is precipitated by dramatic changes in mood.

d. *Trazodone (Desyrel).* Trazodone has been extremely effective in treating aggressive patients in our clinical experience. It is safe, generally well tolerated, and can be given in extremely high doses (> 1 g/d). It is also inexpensive.

(1) *Clinical effects.* The calming effect of trazodone is presumably mediated by a serotonergic mechanism, including a direct receptor effect.

(2) *Administration.* Administration should begin with 25 mg (1/2 tablet) at night and advanced as tolerated. Parents should be instructed to watch for sustained erections and to contact the physician or an emergency room if an erection persists for longer than 30 minutes. The dose may be advanced in 25 to 50-mg increments every day or two as tolerated. Daytime doses should be added as tolerated, the limiting factor being excessive sedation. Children may respond to doses ranging from 12.5 mg to 1200 mg daily, usually in two to four divided doses. Daily doses of 200 to 300 mg/d are usually well tolerated without intolerable side effects.

(3) *Common side effects.* Trazodone is highly sedating, but patients requiring higher doses usually become tolerant of the sedating effect. Clinical efficacy for aggression does not depend on sedation.

Orthostatic hypotension is also fairly common. Several cases of priapism have been reported in adults; this phenomenon probably occurs in children as well, but is rare. No cases of permanent sexual dysfunction in children have been reported in association with trazodone use.

At higher doses, trazodone may induce electrocardiographic changes. At lower doses, however, routine electrocardiographic monitoring is unnecessary.

e. *Clonidine.* Clonidine may be used to treat aggressive behavior, particularly when the behavior is associated with extreme sympathetic arousal. The drug is handled the same as it would be for target symptoms of hyperactivity and impulsivity.

f. *Lithium.* The value of lithium in reducing aggression has been demonstrated in studies in prepubertal children, as well as in several less rigorous studies in adult populations. After neuroleptics, it is the best studied drug for aggression in children. Unfortunately, statistical differences between lithium and placebo have not been matched by robust clinical effects. Use of lithium requires regular blood monitoring, and side effects are common.

(1) *Clinical effects.* Aggression arising in association with rapid mood fluctuations, even in children without frank affective disorder, may improve as the result of lithium therapy. The drug has been effective in developmentally disabled adults and in incarcerated prisoners as well as in children with conduct disorder. Lithium has no direct effect on symptoms of ADHD, although children with both ADHD and aggression can benefit.

(2) *Administration.* Treatment of children receiving lithium should generally be conducted in collaboration with a psychiatric consultant. Treatment is usually started with 300 mg once or twice daily, with subsequent dosage increments based on trough lithium blood levels obtained at least 3 days after a dosage change. The target blood level is 1.0 ± 0.2 mEq/L. Blood levels are approximately linearly related to dosage. Blood levels need to be obtained frequently early in treatment, but blood levels of children receiving stable maintenance regimens need to be checked only every few months.

(3) *Common side effects.* Lithium has many side effects, both annoying short-term effects and serious long-term effects. Short-term effects include a metallic taste, nausea and vomiting, diarrhea, polyuria, tremor, and aggravation of acne. Lithium toxicity is uncommon in children and usually emerges insidiously later in treatment, often when a change in metabolism of the drug has gone undetected. This phenomenon can occur in the summer months, when sweating and sodium depletion reduce lithium clearance. The effects of lithium on developing human kidneys has not been studied.

g. *Neuroleptics.*

(1) *Clinical effects.* The classic neuroleptics most commonly used in children and adolescents are haloperidol (Haldol) and thioridazine (Mellaril). These agents are indisputably effective in curbing aggression, but they have the least desirable side effect profile of any class of psychotropic medication and generally tend to blunt behavior. Risperidone (Risperdal), an atypical neuroleptic that has only recently been used in children, produces many of the benefits of classic neuroleptics with-

out a high rate of extrapyramidal side effects. Most clinicians resort to neuroleptics in nonpsychotic, nonautistic children only when other treatments have failed. The classic neuroleptics are effective antipsychotic agents and can reduce agitation in acutely excited patients.

(2) *Administration.* Neuroleptics should be given at the lowest possible dose and titrated slowly because some of the effects (including antipsychotic effects) may be delayed. The daily dose may be given entirely at night, but best effects are usually achieved by dividing the doses. Close evaluation for extrapyramidal effects, including akathisia masquerading as hyperactivity, needs to be conducted regularly. Children with withdrawal dyskinesias may be at risk for tardive dyskinesia.

Risperidone may pose a lower risk for tardive dyskinesia than other neuroleptics, but data on its long-term use in adults are limited, and none exist concerning its long-term use in children. It is usually given in two doses, beginning with 0.5 mg at bedtime. Until further data in children are available, daily doses in excess of 6 mg should be avoided.

(3) *Common side effects.* Neuroleptics produce *extrapyramidal symptoms, anticholinergic effects, postural hypotension, and sedation.* Neuroleptic malignant syndrome, a rare but potentially lethal complication, has been reported in adolescents. *Tardive dyskinesia* can occur in children, and *withdrawal dyskinesias* are common.

The popularity of thioridazine rests mainly on a low incidence of acute extrapyramidal effects and postural hypotension. The cost is relatively marked sedation, anticholinergic effects (which may compromise cognition), and potential *quinidine-like effects* on the electrocardiogram, especially when combined with other anticholinergic drugs, such as imipramine. For these reasons, low doses of haloperidol are preferred if the agent can be administered without producing akathisia or parkinsonism.

Risperidone has very mild extrapyramidal effects in most patients at the doses ordinarily used, and it has minor anticholinergic effects. It is highly sedating.

h. *Other medications.* Various other medications have been used in aggressive children, but data are limited. SSRI antidepressants have antiaggressive effects in animals and sometimes reduce human aggression. Carbamazepine (Tegretol) and other anticonvulsants may be used much as they would be used in the treatment of epilepsy, but effects are typically modest. Beta-adrenergic blocking agents, such as propranolol (Inderal), have been used in some centers, but efficacy, dosing, and course of response are uncertain, thereby limiting their appeal.

3. *Psychosocial treatments.*

a. *Parent management training.* Parent management training (or parent training) programs teach parents communication skills and effective application of rewards and punishments. Topics such as tangible rewards (stickers, tokens), time out, and spanking are usually addressed. These programs are well supported by empiric studies and are often appropriate for clinical populations. Russell Barkley's program is geared to defiant children with ADHD.[2, 3] It is available from Guilford Press, complete with parent handouts and rating scales. An enterprising nurse with some mental health experience can easily learn to administer this treatment in an office setting.

Parent training is most effective for intact families without major interpersonal conflicts or adult psychopathology. Single, depressed parents with many children, poor social networks, and limited economic resources are poor candidates for parent training.

b. *Other behaviorally oriented treatments.* Social skills training and anger management training, often offered in a group therapy format, may be useful for some children. These programs require some degree of motivation on the part of the child, however, and are less consistently useful than parent training.

c. *Individual cognitive behavior therapy.* Cognitive behavior therapies for impulsive children, although heralded by several learned books, have been disappointing in clinical practice. These approaches are probably more helpful in highly motivated adolescents than in prepubertal children.

d. *Family therapy.* A broad range of family-oriented treatments have been advocated, but few have been empirically validated. When troubled families are unable to consistently implement parent training programs or specific behavioral techniques, family conflicts must be addressed directly.

e. *Parent therapy.* Parents with psychiatric disability, character disorders, or chronic stress often can best help their children by helping themselves with appropriate psychiatric treatment. Chronically low-functioning parents often benefit from having a therapist—who may be the primary care physician—to offer moral and common sense support during recurrent crises. In such cases, the physician should try to resist feelings of resentment that may be provoked by the parent's unwillingness to follow through with *real* therapy. The physician's accessibility and thoughtful advice sometimes is the real therapy.

4. *School-based interventions.*
   a. *Individualized educational planning committee.* Children with emotional, learning, or physical disabilities that interfere with academic achievement are entitled to special services under federal law. The formal mechanism by which a parent obtains these services is the individualized educational planning committee, which can be sought either at the child's school or, in the case of preschool children, at the intermediate school district. The parent's request triggers an assessment that typically includes intellectual and psychoeducational testing and assessment by a social worker or school psychologist. Children with ADHD often qualify for services as learning disabled, emotionally disturbed, or "physically or otherwise health impaired." Obtaining an appropriate classification and services can be a taxing process that challenges the parent's capacity to advocate in behalf of her child, especially in school districts with limited resources.
   b. *Special classrooms.* The child may qualify for a classroom with a favorable teacher-student ratio and individualized instruction. The desirability of such classrooms varies greatly from school to school and can be assessed only on a case-by-case basis.
   c. *Classroom modifications.* Children with ADHD benefit from a large array of classroom modifications and teaching devices. These include placing the child close to the teacher; giving the child frequent reinforcement (praise) for sticking to his or her work; using multisensory teaching approaches that integrate seeing, hearing, and touching; varying the subject matter frequently; and allowing extra time for tests and assignments.
   d. *Daily home/school report.* Satisfactory school performance in children with ADHD requires regular communication and consistency between teachers and parents. Daily reports should document the child's success in meeting target goals and summarize homework assignments. A grid showing achievement of four or five goals during each classroom period is especially effective when linked to a point or token reward system implemented at home.

5. *Parent support groups.*
   Children with Attention Deficit Disorder is a national support group with hundreds of local chapters through which parents can locate competent therapists, educate themselves about treatment alternatives, obtain readings, seek advice about handling specific problems, and find dozens of sympathetic listeners. Because many of the parents also have ADD, the meetings can be animated and entertaining.

F. What to tell the patient and family.

1. Attention-deficit hyperactivity disorder is usually chronic, reflecting a temperamental style as much as a disorder. The good news is that even in hyperactive children, activity level diminishes and attention span improves with maturation.
2. Many positive characteristics are associated with ADHD. If the child's energy, friendliness, and gusto can be channeled effectively, it can form the basis for high achievement later in life.
3. The child can take medication for as long as it proves helpful. Although only a small number of children completely outgrow ADHD, adults with persisting symptoms do not necessarily require treatment.
4. Stimulants are not habit forming in children and adolescents. Addiction is exceedingly rare. Although many adolescents and adults with ADHD abuse alcohol and drugs, those who have been treated with methylphenidate (Ritalin) as children tend to avoid stimulants later in life.
5. Growth decrements relating to stimulant use are usually made up during the adolescent growth spurt. Long-term effects of stimulants on growth are minimal in most patients.
6. Attention-deficit hyperactivity disorder, predominately inattentive type, is more like a learning disability than a behavior problem.
7. Parents who are persistent in advocating for their children, consistent in their love and discipline, and clear in their moral convictions usually succeed in producing children with similar qualities, with or without ADHD.
8. Distressed families and parents need to address their marital and personal problems directly to the extent that this is possible. On the other hand, the physician should recognize and empathize with the problems individual children can pose for parents. Family mental health is a reciprocal phenomenon.
9. Not all behavior problems are amenable to psychiatric treatment. The prognosis for children with severe, persistent conduct disorders and psychopathic dispositions is poor.
10. Behavior problems occurring de novo in adolescence usually do not persist into adulthood.

G. When to refer.

1. *Role of the primary care physician.*
   a. *Typical presentations of ADHD.* Most children with ADHD respond favorably to either methylphenidate or dextroamphetamine (Dexedrine) with results that can be quite dramatic.

b. *Mild behavior problems.* Many children display mild behavior problems from time to time, and in more persistent cases, these may warrant a specific diagnosis. Forty percent or more of preschool-aged children display behaviors that their parents view as problematic, including defiance, tantrums, conflicts with siblings, and episodically overactive behavior. Common disruptive behaviors in school-aged children include arguing, refusing to do chores or homework, and lying to escape punishment. Adolescents seeking an identity separate from that of their parents may join peer groups in which temptations to engage in mild or serious antisocial acts may be overwhelming. Adolescents often argue with and defy adults to establish their independence as much as to achieve any stated goal. They may test limits through staying out late, cutting classes, or experimenting with drugs. For otherwise well-functioning families, the primary care practitioner can sometimes offer straightforward advice to parents that helps them decide where to draw limits and how to manage misbehavior.

c. *Severe conduct disorders.* Children whose violations of social norms are multiple, persistent, and extremely damaging to the victim respond poorly to treatment of any kind. Children who seem cruel by nature, lacking empathy or concern for the distress of other living beings, are especially resilient to intervention. The role of the family practitioner in managing such cases is generally to exclude treatable medical or psychiatric causes, to address symptoms amenable to pharmacologic treatment (e.g., inattention and overactivity), and to offer parents guidance in seeking other services.

2. *Problems warranting psychiatric referral.*
   a. Atypical presentations of ADHD symptoms, including late onset, autistic-like presentations, and complicated comorbid symptoms, may benefit from psychiatric consultation.
   b. Atypical responses to stimulants and other medications, especially psychoses and marked behavioral activation, may indicate more serious psychopathologic processes.
   c. The patient may fail to respond to ordinary treatments.
   d. Chronic and serious parent or family problems may exist. These may not be amenable to treatment, but the possibility should be considered.
   e. Serious antisocial behavior of recent onset or escalating intensity may indicate the advent of new psychopathology.
   f. Children and adolescents exhibiting aggressive behavior that endangers the physical welfare of others, and those with recurrent or persistent homicidal behavior, should be referred for possible hospitalization. Antisocial adolescents are also at increased risk for suicide.

VIII. Enuresis and encopresis.

Many children with elimination disorders feel embarrassed and guilty about the problem, and their parents are frustrated by repeated failures to help their children master bowel and bladder control. Regrettably, the role of psychological factors in causing and curing elimination problems has been exaggerated, leading parents and many clinicians to expect simplistic behavioral programs that use reward and punishment to solve longstanding problems. The clinician should reassure the family that elimination disorders can be effectively managed in the home with behavioral and medical treatments supervised by the primary care physician. Reassurance that treatment usually succeeds helps families persevere for the several months of treatment often required.

A. Epidemiology.

1. *Enuresis.*
   By the age of 5 years, 7% of boys and 3% of girls display clinically significant enuresis, and a larger proportion have occasional accidents. About 2% of teenagers and 1% of young adults continue to have accidents. Seventy-five percent of children with enuresis have a first-degree relative with a current or past history of the disorder. Enuresis is more common in children with psychiatric and developmental disorders and in those with medical conditions that increase urine flow or compromise bladder innervation.

2. *Encopresis.*
   About 1% of 5-year-old children are encopretic, with a predominance in boys. About 15% of their fathers were also encopretic. The incidence drops off rapidly after the age of 7 years. *Factors that increase the risk for developing encopresis include birth of a sibling, family conflict or separation, beginning of school attendance, pre-existing psychiatric or developmental disorder, and abnormal rectosphincteric reflex.*

B. Evaluation and diagnostic overview.

1. *Enuresis.*
   Children should be reassured that they are not to blame for wetting. This is almost always true, and cases of "voluntary" enuresis are rare in primary practice settings.

   Whereas occasional episodes of nighttime wetting in response to stress are expectable, chronic nocturnal enuresis is usually functional (developmental), having neither a specific psychiatric nor a medical cause. *Diurnal enuresis occurring after the age of 5 years and secondary enuresis occurring after a period of several months of continence are more likely to have underlying behavioral or medical causes.*

2. *Encopresis.*
Encopretic children may appear either ashamed or indifferent about soiling. *Involuntary encopresis is more likely than voluntary soiling to be associated with shame and embarrassment. Some involuntary soilers, however, appear untroubled by their problem.*

C. Specific diagnosis or problem.

1. *Enuresis.*
Usually, the history of enuresis is straightforward, and the parent can offer an account of the frequency of wetting in terms of nights per week. Older children occasionally present when parents realize that the supply of underpants has been exhausted, the child having sequestered them somewhere to conceal his or her wetting.
To introduce the subject with a reluctant child, the interviewer might say, "Boys and girls feel sad or worried when they lose a favorite toy, wet their bed, or get mad at their mommy. Do any of those things make you feel sad?" A more direct approach with a teenager can be followed: "I see a lot of teenagers who sometimes wet their beds. Does that ever happen to you?"
   a. *Types of enuresis.* In *functional enuresis* a medical explanation for wetting cannot be identified; it may be either *primary,* if bladder control has never been achieved, or *secondary,* when existing bladder control is lost.
   b. *Criteria for the diagnosis of enuresis.* Diagnosis should be reserved to cases in which children have repeated episodes over a period of months. The minimum age for the diagnosis is arbitrary, but most authorities select age 4 or 5 years.
   c. *Differential diagnosis of enuresis.* Specific medical causes for enuresis can be identified in 2% to 4% of case, and in many instances, the physician is already aware of these. The differential diagnosis includes problems in the urinary tract, such as *infection, malformation, obstruction,* and *injury,* including sexual abuse; seizures; *neurogenic bladder,* as in manifest spinal disease or occult myelodysplasia; endocrinopathies, such as diabetes mellitus causing *increased urine volume;* medication, substance, or diet-induced diuresis, such as that caused by lithium, alcohol; bladder compression due to constipation; and hyperhydrophagia.
   d. *Examination and laboratory tests.* A thorough history and physical examination with attention to the neurologic examination should be conducted. Urinalysis is an adequate laboratory screen unless other aspects of the evaluation point to a specific disease or defect. Invasive urologic procedures are unnecessary in most cases.

2. *Encopresis.*
Encopresis is a problem precisely because the diagnosis is usually so obvious, although many children conceal individual episodes of soiling and, if extremely resourceful, a series of episodes. Families often try different techniques to manage encopresis before they consult their primary care doctor or may have adapted to soiling by preparing "soiling kits" consisting of clean underwear, a change of clothing, or a can of air freshener. Sometimes, parents resort to diapers, which usually indicates that parents and child have given up the effort to restore normal continence. The history should explore bowel habits, including the place, the frequency, and the time of day that defecation usually occurs; the size and consistency of the stool; the need for straining when fecal material is passed; and retentive posturing. Diet may contribute to painfully hard stools and fecal retention. Anal fissures may cause or result from retention. Although specific psychological stresses, such as starting school or arguing with parents, may contribute to early retention of stool, by the time incontinence has developed, these are often forgotten or insignificant. Younger children occasionally have conditioned fears or imaginative fantasies about toileting that lead to avoidance of the toilet seat altogether.
   a. *Types of encopresis. The term functional encopresis* implies the absence of a specific disease process and may be either primary or secondary, the latter having followed an extended period of continence.
   Retention of stool followed by constipation and overflow incontinence is the most common and treatable pattern of functional encopresis. Expansion of the rectum from retained and hardened stool compromises sensory afferents and the reflex relaxation of the internal anal sphincter that makes normal defecation possible. Smudges on the underpants, rather than large, completely formed stools, result from seepage of stool around the hardened rectal mass.
   b. *Criteria for the diagnosis of encopresis.* Diagnosis of encopresis should be reserved for cases in which children have repetitive episodes over a period of months. The minimum age for the diagnosis is arbitrary, but most authorities select the age of 4 years.
   c. *Differential diagnosis of encopresis.* Medical conditions presenting with fecal incontinence or constipation include diarrheal disease; cathartic agents, including sorbitol-based and mannitol-based candy; Hirschsprung's disease; rectal stenosis; anal trauma; and metabolic diseases, such as hypothyroidism, lactase deficiency, and myelodysplasia.

D. General management guidelines.

1. *Treatment of enuresis.*
   Medication and behavior management are often combined in the treatment of enuresis. The child's support must be enlisted in order for any behavioral plan to succeed. If this is not possible, medications may be preferred over elaborate, conflictual, and failed behavioral remedies.
   a. *Behavioral treatment.* Simple changes, such as limiting fluids before sleep and eliminating caffeine (a diuretic) from the diet, are often attempted by the parents even before the child presents to the physician's office.
      - A *toileting schedule* is very helpful for *diurnal* enuresis. The child should urinate on a schedule, typically every 2 hours, and be rewarded for going to the toilet, for actually urinating, and for *reducing* the frequency of incontinence.
      - *Bladder stretching exercises* are also useful for *diurnal enuresis,* but not for nocturnal enuresis. The child is asked to hold his or her urine for as long as possible and, when the child does urinate, to interrupt the process several times. This process "expands" the bladder, strengthens urethral muscles, and encourages conscious mastery of the process (bladder urgency containment). Rewards for complying with the treatment plan and for reducing the frequency of diurnal wetting help sustain the child's motivation over the several months often required for completion of the process.
      - *Labeling underpants* prevents corruption of the reward process in children who secretly substitute clean for wet pants to present to parents.
      - *Moisture or urine alarms (bell and pad)* are the treatments of choice for enuresis occurring only at night. The alarm works by pairing the stimulus of urinary urgency with the behavior of awakening. *The alarm thus conditions the child over time to respond to a full bladder by waking.* The child should then go to the bathroom, if necessary, with a parental escort. It is irrelevant whether the child awakens quickly enough to interrupt urination. Conditioning requires several months and most often fails when the child sleeps through the alarm. In such cases, the parent must himself awaken the child on hearing the alarm until the child begins to do so without assistance.
      - *Maintaining cleanliness* should be delegated to the child. The child should be taught to go to the toilet before bedtime. If the child awakens after wetting, he or she should go to the toilet, clean himself or herself, put on clean clothing, and change the sheets. *Punishment is not helpful. The cleaning activities should not be rewarded, either, because this may inadvertently encourage the wetting as well.*
      - *Dry nights should be rewarded* as part of a routine of checking sheets in the morning.
      - *Awakening the child frequently at night* reduces the laundry burden, but at the expense of lowered quality and amount of sleep. It is not nearly as effective as an alarm in bringing about lasting change.

      Reinforcement of the desired behavior of using the schedule and eventually maintaining dryness is the means to success. This is particularly helpful for children who become so involved in activities that they fail to recognize the sensation of a full bladder.
      - *Combining techniques* into a program provides the best results.

   b. *Medical treatment.*
      (1) *Imipramine (Tofranil).*
      Imipramine can be given in doses titrated from 10 mg to 75 mg at bedtime, not to exceed 2.5 mg/kg. At least half of children respond to this drug, although enuresis remits as soon as the therapy is discontinued. Onset is immediate once the right dose has been achieved. Serious side effects are rare at this dosage, and annoying side effects are mitigated by sleep. Abrupt withdrawal of higher doses can produce a transient flu-like syndrome, so withdrawal over about 1 week is preferred.
      (2) *Desmopressin.*
      Desmopressin, a synthetic analogue of arginine vasopressin, is a nasal spray administered in doses from 10 to 40 μg (one to four sprays) at bedtime. Onset of action occurs within a few days. Side effects, including headache, drying of mucous membranes, nosebleed, nausea, cough, nasal congestion, abdominal cramps, and irritation of the nasal mucosa, are uncommon. *It should not be prescribed in children with known or potential electrolyte abnormalities.*

2. *Treatment of encopresis.*
   Treatment involves cleansing the bowel, maintaining soft stools, and establishing regular toileting habits while strengthening rectal musculature.
   - *Cleansing the bowel* may be achieved by more vigorous means, including hypophosphate enemas twice daily for one to three days; by using bisacodyl (Dulcolax) suppositories twice daily until the bowel is clear; or by using relatively large quantities of mineral oil, 15 to 30 mL/year of age each day, up to 240 mL/d for 3 to 4 days. Small quantities of mineral oil may not help to clear hardened stool from the rectum. A creative alternative is to offer the child a meal of sugar-free chocolate sweetened

with sorbitol or mannitol. In one young child, however, this regimen proved more effective in curing the child of his craving for chocolate than in resolving his constipation.

- *Stool softeners,* but *not* cathartic agents, need to be given for the next several months, as healing of the rectal neuromuscular apparatus proceeds. *Mineral oil* given in doses of 15 mL/year of age each day, up to 90 mL/d, or *lactulose* can be used to accomplish this. When the child has achieved good control, stool softeners should be discontinued gradually. Supplements to replace fat-soluble vitamins are sometimes recommended in children receiving mineral oil but are probably unnecessary in most cases. Diet should be adjusted to maximize dietary fiber.
- *A toileting schedule should be established* in which the child sits on the toilet for 5 to 10 minutes after each meal and before bedtime. The child should practice pushing at stool during these periods in order to strengthen rectal musculature whether or not stool is forthcoming.
- *The parent should assume a matter-of-fact attitude to episodes of soiling* while systematically rewarding successful toileting with praise and concrete rewards. Punishment is not helpful.

Much has been said about the invasiveness of enemas and suppositories, as though ordinary pediatric treatments were relatively unobjectionable and encouraged the child's sense of mastery and self-esteem. Mastery and self-esteem are best enhanced by decisively fixing the problem.

E. What to tell families.

Discussion of the genetics of enuresis and the physiology of encopresis destigmatizes the problems and discourages moralizing. The family needs to be warned in advance that treatment will require much time and perseverance but will probably achieve the desired result. The National Enuresis Society can be contacted at 1-800-NES-8080 and provides literature and support for families.

F. When to refer.

Cases failing to respond to behavior interventions with medication management after complete medical evaluation should be referred for psychiatric evaluation. "Voluntary" encopresis, characterized by fully formed stools of normal consistency and an attitude of apparent indifference, may be indicative of more serious psychiatric or developmental problems that warrant psychiatric assessment. Families that scapegoat the child and resist the possibility that the child's problem represents anything other than moral turpitude, on the other hand, may benefit from intervention by a mental health specialist.

Summary

Primary practitioners develop varying levels of interest and competence in treating psychiatric disorders in children and adolescents. All such clinicians need to recognize important psychiatric problems when they arise, however, and many want to implement first-line treatments, seeking consultation after an initial treatment trial fails. Even when psychiatric consultants are needed for diagnosis and treatment recommendations, however, family practitioners and pediatricians can usually conduct maintenance treatment at greatly reduced cost to the family (or to the capitated practice, as the case may be), often in a setting more congenial and accessible to the family.

On the other hand, the primary provider should not hesitate to seek assistance. Only a few important examples of the wide range of psychiatric disturbances seen in children and adolescents could be addressed here; often, these bear superficial but misleading similarities to the more common conditions. Psychosis may thus present as depression, Tourette's syndrome as ADHD, high-level autism as psychosis, and narcolepsy as mood disturbance. The physician must therefore remain alert for atypical features and be prepared to reconsider diagnoses in patients who fail to respond to well-established treatments.

References

1. Szatmari, Offord DR, Boyle MN. Ontario Child Health Study: Prevalence of attention deficit disorder with hyperactivity. J Child Psychol Psychiatry 1989; 30:205–218.
2. Barkley RA. Defiant Children: A Clinician's Manual for Parent Training. New York: Guilford; 1987a.
3. Barkley RA. Defiant Children: Parent-Teacher Assignments. New York: Guilford; 1987b.

Suggested Reading

Introduction

American Psychiatric Association. Diagnostic and Statistical Manual of Mental Disorders. Fourth Edition—Primary Care Version. Washington, DC: American Psychiatric Association; 1995.

Costello EJ, Costello AJ, Edelbrock C, et al. Psychiatric disorders in pediatric primary care: Prevalence and risk factors. Arch Gen Psychiatry 1988; 45;1107–1116.

Gureje O, Omigbodun OO, Gater R, et al. Psychiatric disorders in a paediatric primary care clinic. Br J Psychiatry 1994; 165:527–530.

Giaconia RM, Reinherz HZ, Silverman AB, et al. Age of onset of psychiatric disorders in a community population of older adolescents. J Am Acad Child Adolesc Psychiatry 1994; 33:706–717.

Wilens TE, Spencer T, Biederman J, et al. Combined pharmacotherapy: An emerging trend in pediatric psychopharmacology. J Am Acad Child Adolesc Psychiatry 1995; 34:110–112.

Depression and suicide

Alessi NE. Refractory childhood depressive disorders from a pharmacotherapeutic perspective. Adv Neuropsychiatry Psychopharmacol 1991; 2:53–63.

Alessi N, Naylor MW, Ghaziuddin M, Zubieta JK. Update on lithium carbonate therapy in children and adolescents. J Am Acad Child Adolesc Psychiatry 1994; 33:291–304.

Ambrosini PJ, Bianchi MD, Rabinovich H, et al. Antidepressant treatment in children and adolescents: I. Affective disorders. J Am Acad Child Adolesc Psychiatry 1993; 32:1–6.

Ambrosini PJ, Bianchi MD, Rabinovich H, et al. Antidepressant treatment in children and adolescents: II. Anxiety, physical, and behavioral disorders. J Am Acad Child Adolesc Psychiatry 1993; 32:483–493.

Beasley CM Jr, Dornseif BE, Bosomworth JC, et al. Fluoxetine and suicide: A meta-analysis of controlled trials of treatment for depression. BMJ 1991; 303:685–692.

Kovacs M, Goldston D, Gatsonis C. Suicidal behaviors and childhood-onset depressive disorders: A longitudinal investigation. J Am Acad Child Adolesc Psychiatry 1993; 32:8–20.

Rao U, Weissman MM, Martin JA, et al. Childhood depression and risk of suicide: A preliminary report of a longitudinal study. J Am Acad Child Adolesc Psychiatry 1993; 32:21–27.

Ryan ND. The pharmacologic treatment of child and adolescent depression. Psychiatr Clin North Am 1992; 15:29–40.

Anxiety disorders

Bernstein GA, Perwien AR. Anxiety disorders. Child Adolesc Psychiatr Clin North Am 1995; 4:305–322.

Birmaher B, Waterman GS, Ryan N, et al. Fluoxetine for childhood anxiety disorders. Am Acad Child Adolesc Psychiatry 1994; 33:993–999.

DeVeaugh-Geiss J, Moroz G, Biederman J, et al. Clomipramine hydrochloride in childhood and adolescent obsessive-compulsive disorder: A multicenter trial. J Am Acad Child Adolesc Psychiatry 1992; 31:45–49.

Kutcher SP, Reiter S, Gardner DM, et al. The pharmacotherapy of anxiety disorders in children and adolescents. Psychiatr Clin North Am 1992; 15:41–67.

Leonard HL, Swedo SE, Rapoport JL, et al. Treatment of obsessive-compulsive disorder with clomipramine and desipramine in children and adolescents: A double-blind crossover comparison. Arch Gen Psychiatry 1989; 46:1088–1092.

Riddle MA, Scahill L, King RA, et al. Double-blind, crossover trial of fluoxetine and placebo in children and adolescents with obsessive-compulsive disorder. J Am Acad Child Adolesc Psychiatry 1992; 31:1062–1069.

Attention-deficit hyperactivity disorder

Barkley RA. Attention Deficit Hyperactivity Disorder: A Handbook for Diagnosis and Treatment. New York: Guilford; 1990.

Dulcan MK, Bregman JD, Weller EB, Weller RA. Special issues in the treatment of childhood and adolescent disorders. In: Schatzberg AF, Nemeroff CB (eds): Textbook of Psychopharmacology. Washington, DC: American Psychiatric Press; 1995.

Egger J, Carter CM, Wilson J, et al. Is migraine food allergy? A double-blind controlled trial of oligoantigenic diet treatment. Lancet 1983; 2:865–868.

Egger J, Carter CM, Graham PJ, et al. Controlled trial of oligoantigenic treatment in the hyperkinetic syndrome. Lancet 1985; 1:540–545.

Hunt RD, Arnsten AFT, Asbell MD. An open trial of guanfacine in the treatment of attention-deficit hyperactivity disorder. J Am Acad Child Adolesc Psychiatry 1995; 34:50–54.

Offord DR, Boyle MIH, Szatmari MD, et al. Ontario child health study: II. Six-month prevalence of disorder and rates of service utilization. Arch Gen Psychiatry 1987; 44:832–836.

Safer DJ, Krager JM. A survey of medication treatment for hyperactive/inattentive students. JAMA 1988; 260:2256–2258.

Enuresis/encopresis

Dulcan MK, Bregman JD, Weller EB, Weller RA. Special issues in the treatment of childhood and adolescent disorders. In: Textbook of Psychopharmacology. American Psychiatric Press; 1995.

Fournier JP, Garfinkel BD, Bond A, et al. Pharmacology and behavioral management of enuresis. J Am Acad Child Adolesc Psychiatry 1987; 26:849–852.

Fritz GK, Anders TF. Enuresis and encopresis. Psychiatr Clin North Am 1982; 5:283–296.

Kaplan SL, Breit M, Gautheir B, Busner J. A comparison of three nocturnal enuresis treatment methods. J Am Acad Child Adolesc Psychiatry 1988; 28:282–286.

12

DAVID J. KNESPER, MD

A. E. EYLER, MD, MPH

Common Neurologic Disorders: Alzheimer's Disease, Parkinson's Disease Dementia, HIV/AIDS, Stroke, Multiple Sclerosis, and Epilepsy

I. General Management Guidelines Across Disorders.

A. General clinical considerations.

All of the disorders considered in this chapter have neurobehavioral complications that occur at rates significantly higher than those of physical illnesses of comparable severity but without central nervous system (CNS) involvement. Consultation is recommended whenever psychiatric illness appears to coexist with unexplained neurologic symptoms or whenever patients with a neurologic disorder experience significant social or behavioral complications or cognitive decline.

B. Prevention.

Like any other medical problem, in neurologic disorders, treatment is more effective when the problem is identified early. Patients and families should be warned about the signs and symptoms of each neurobehavioral complication and asked to seek medical help at an early stage. A false alarm and an opportunity for further education is far better than, for example, a severely depressed and suicidal patient needing emergency services.

C. Medication management.

Neuropsychiatric patients are often sensitive to medications and may respond to them in idiosyncratic ways. Accordingly, it is often best to disregard the drug manufacturer's recommendations for a starting dose by beginning with a fraction of the recommended initial dose and to proceed with a slow increase of the dosage. For example, the patient may start with one quarter of the recommended dose and increase the dose every 3 days until a known effective therapeutic dose is reached. Applying this rule of thumb to the antidepressant sertraline (Zoloft), the patient may start therapy at 12.5 mg by cutting the tablet and adding 12.5 mg every third morning until taking 50 mg every morning. Regardless of the drug class, because of unexpected drug responses, a test dose should be given in the morning in order to provide an opportunity for easy physician contact in the event of unanticipated problems. Thus, whenever possible, avoid starting new drug therapy during a weekend or after 5 p.m.

D. What to tell the patient and family.

The family should be told to expect delays and slow improvement. The physician can make a statement like

> This will require your patience. The treatment of your depression (for example) is more complicated because of your neurologic disease. Our drugs often take 3 or more weeks to work, and the first drug we try may not even work. Sometimes, patients with a neurologic disease are unusually sensitive to medications, so we need to start at a low dose and work our way up to a higher therapeutic dose and, at the same time, watch for unusual side effects.

Then, the physician explains the usual side effects and ends with cautious optimism.

E. Return visits and general follow-up care.

If, for example, an antidepressant is prescribed on a "go slow, stay low" basis to a patient with Alzheimer's disease (AD), the first follow-up visit can be 3 or 4 weeks after the patient has reached a therapeutic dose. The aforementioned explanation and slow increase allow for a smooth onset of action and avoid side effects and associated unnecessary telephone calls. The patient returns when some response should be observable. Sometimes, if the patient or family is anxious, they should be asked to call an identified person working with the doctor and give a descriptive report. The contact person should have criteria for contacting the doctor. Unless an obvious focus for family and/or patient counseling exists, our preference is to give the medication time to work before a specific counseling intervention is added.

F. Relapse prevention.

Relapses are to be avoided because they usually are more severe and treatment resistant than the original episode. *A therapeutic response is sustained by maintaining the therapeutic dose until a persuasive reason to change exists.* The sometimes used rule that an antidepressant therapy can be discontinued after the patient is asymptomatic for 6 to 12 months does not apply to mixed neurologic-psychiatric states, because the neurologic illness is ongoing and likely has a causal link to the depression. If some persuasive reason exists for discontinuing a therapeutic agent, decreasing the dosage slowly over several weeks to months is reasonable because early symptoms of relapse can be identified and the medication can usually be more rapidly increased and a relapse avoided.

II. Alzheimer's Disease.

A. Evaluation and diagnostic overview.

1. *Differential diagnosis.*
Dementia is determined by comparison with a previously known estimated baseline of cognitive function; dementia is an acquired and slowly progressive impairment of memory (always impaired in AD) and a subset of such other cognitive functions as language, visuospatial skills, and calculations. Dementia must be distinguished from an acute confusional state (delirium), the dementia of depression (pseudodementia), and such focal neurologic syndromes as aphasia and amnesia. The diagnosis of AD usually can be made on the basis of a characteristic onset; in AD, memory and learning impairment are early symptoms, usually followed by word-finding and naming difficulties.

   Frontal lobe disease is characterized by relative preservation of memory and cognitive functions. Office testing finds impaired verbal fluency (e.g., "Name as many vegetables as you can in a minute."), disabled sequential hand movements, and deficient executive functions (e.g., goal-directed and motivated behavior and decision making). One of many alternatives to testing sequential hand movements has the examiner demonstrating with his or her hand a "fist, slap, chop" sequence and then asking the patient for a duplication. Word and conversational theme perseveration and apathy are common symptoms. *Parkinson-like extrapyramidal features are common, and the associated frontal lobe symptoms are frequently and mistakenly attributed to depression.*

2. *Laboratory and neuropsychology tests.*
No one standard work-up exists for the dementias. Tests should be selected that best investigate a particular patient's problems; however, all patients should receive, at the very least, a full battery of routine tests such as complete blood count, erythrocyte sedimentation rate, electrolyte levels, blood chemistries, vitamin B_{12} and folate levels, thyroid function, and Venereal Disease Research Laboratories (VDRL) tests. There is a growing consensus that an imaging study is mandatory. If clinical features suggest a delirium or a seizure disorder, results from an electroencephalogram reduce uncertainty. Blood tests for AD-related chemicals, such as apolipoprotein E, are available, but their predictive value is limited.

   The most widely used office neuropsychological screening test is Folstein's Mini-Mental State Exam (see chapter appendix). This assessment should be extended with supplements that are tailored to the baseline skills of the patient. Example supplements are similarities and differences (e.g., picture frame versus window), abstraction (proverbs), and current events and world landmarks (e.g., name the Great Lakes and world capitals for a geography teacher). The patient's response behavior is helpful for identifying the dementia of depression, in which attention and concentration are the most prominent features of cognitive impairment. The depressed, not demented, patient must be severely depressed (e.g., unmotivated for personal hygiene) to score poorly on the Mini-Mental State Examination. Moreover, a depressed person learns three words with repeated effort; a patient with severe AD does not learn. When the results of office examinations are inconclusive, expert neuropsychological testing is indicated. Personality testing is of little value.

B. Epidemiology and pathophysiology.

Most dementias occur in people older than 65 years. Dementia is an epidemic in part because of the rapid increase in the size (absolute number and percentage) of the elderly population. Persons aged 65 to 69 years have a 0.2% prevalence rate, and this rate doubles every 5 years, giving those aged 85 years an 18% prevalence rate. AD accounts for 40% to 60% of all dementias. AD most severely affects the temporal and parietal cortices. Neuronal alterations include neurofibrillary tangles and amyloid plaques; cholinergic neurons are most affected. Inherited susceptibility is conferred by at least three different genetic loci. Genes for β-amyloid precursor protein and apolipoprotein E have received most attention.

C. The depressions of Alzheimer's disease.

Several varieties of depression exist in AD, ranging from reactive sadness and subsyndromal depressions to major depressive disorder; each of these may be partners with anxiety symptoms. *Depression and more severe AD do not generally commingle.* Depression is less and less likely as AD progresses. In patients with less severe AD, no more than 10% have the classic neurovegetative symptoms of major depressive disorder (e.g., loss of appetite, sleep disturbance), and these patients improve with antidepressant therapy. Another 10% to 15% have less severe and atypical forms of depression. *An antidepressant trial is indicated when behavior and emotions include any one or more of the following: frequent episodes of crying: frequent references to death, suicide (even if tangential), and futility, and more or less continuous failure to experience pleasure and enjoyment.* Such nonverbal manifestations of depression as irritability, complaining, demandingness, dependency, and clinging may be improved by antidepressant therapy. Selective serotonin reuptake inhibitors (SSRIs) may increase emotional stability (e.g., less frequent and shorter episodes of dysphoric mood states, easier distractibility from depressive themes, more calm and fewer angry periods). Classic frontal lobe symptoms do not usually respond to antidepressant therapy.

1. *Risk factors.*
   A personal and family history of depression and an early onset of dementia have been found to predict the coexistence of depression with dementia.
2. *Medication management.*
   a. *Recommended treatments.* With the possible exception of paroxetine (Paxil), *any of the SSRIs are reasonable choices.* At the initial 20 mg dose, paroxetine has minimal anticholinergic properties, but if the dose needs to be increased, anticholinergic properties are more of a concern.
   b. *Possible treatments. Because they have significant anticholinergic effects, the tricyclic antidepressants are of limited value in AD.* A history of a low-dose previous response favors their use. If used, the least anticholinergic tricyclic antidepressants (nortriptyline [Pamelor], desipramine [Norpramin]) are recommended, and blood level determinations are needed to ensure the lowest possible effective dose (for nortriptyline, 50 to 150 ng/mL; for desipramine, >150 ng/mL).
   c. *Innovative treatments.* Little information is available about AD and the newer agents fluvoxamine (Luvox), venlafaxine (Effexor), and nefazodone (Serzone); they all lack significant anticholinergic activity. Because fluvoxamine is an SSRI, a patient with AD who is intolerant to an older SSRI would likely have trouble with fluvoxamine. Venlafaxine is a mixed norepinephrine-serotonin reuptake inhibitor, and it is asserted to be effective when other agents are not. Moreover, venlafaxine has been well tolerated by elderly patients without AD.

   Mirtazapine (Remeron) is largely untried in AD. Mirtazapine is excreted mainly in urine and use has been associated with significant increases in serum glutamic-pyruvic transaminase. Consequently, elderly patients with impaired renal or kidney function will require close monitoring. Mirtazapine-caused neutropenia is a rare adverse event (see Chapter 2).

D. Psychosis in Alzheimer's disease.

Psychotic symptoms develop in 50% of patients with AD; psychosis may be associated with more severe dementia. Hallucinations are common. False beliefs that can be easily attributed to memory impairment (e.g., "someone stole my watch") may not represent psychosis if an explanation (e.g., "you misplaced it") easily diminishes concern. False beliefs are considered psychotic and delusional when the patient with AD clings to the false beliefs, uses aggression and/or hostility against suspected villains, and is verbally abusive, irritable, and aggressive. However, agitation is not considered a psychotic syndrome. Psychosis is often mistaken for delirium.

1. *Risk factors.*
   A past personal history of psychosis and a low premorbid intelligence are thought to predispose patients with AD to psychosis. Psychosis is associated with more severe AD and behavioral dysfunction.
2. *Medication management.*
   a. *Recommended treatments. Low-dose haloperidol (Haldol) remains the treatment of choice* in patients without significant extrapyramidal findings. Sometimes, very low doses (e.g., 1.25 mg, in the liquid preparation measured with a tuberculin syringe) are effective, but usually 1 to 2 mg either at bedtime or in divided doses are necessary.
   b. *Possible treatments.* Thioridazine (Mellaril) 12.5 to 50 mg/d, may be helpful, most likely because of its sedative properties; 100 to 200 mg/d is its maximum dose in the AD population; anticholinergic properties limit its use.
   c. *Innovative treatments.* Risperidone (Risperdal), 0.25 to 0.5 mg twice daily, has been used with success; hypotension and headache may occur and are more likely to occur at higher doses. Risperidone has low anticholinergic side effects. Olanzapine (Zyprexa) is now available, but its anticholinergic effects will limit use for AD psychosis.

E. Agitation in Alzheimer's disease.

In AD, agitation is a poorly defined syndrome characterized by generalized behavioral perturbation and arousal and by one or more of the following symptoms: motor restlessness, pacing, repetitious vocalizations and/or acts, self-abusiveness and/or aggressiveness toward others, anger and hostility, irritability with minor stimulation, belligerence, fearfulness, and sleeplessness, often with day-night reversal.

Agitation is not the same as psychosis. Agitation may accompany any primary psychiatric illness, and treating the primary psychiatric illness simultaneously treats concurrent agitation.

When a primary psychiatric illness is superimposed on dementia, distinguishing the psychiatric problem may be hard. It is useful to consider a description of depression (for example) that would be concurrent with a dementia. Pacing, easy tearfulness, and reduced motivation and eating could describe mixed dementia-depression syndrome. *The diagnosis of AD-associated agitation should be made when agitation cannot be attributed to a superimposed delirium or acute (e.g., urinary tract infection) or chronic (e.g., congestive heart failure) medical illness or new neurologic illness (e.g., stroke) and when CNS side effects from medications have been ruled out.* If the patient has a known concurrent medical condition, optimizing treatment often diminishes the severity of agitated behavior. A decrease in environmental stimulation or a reversal of recent environmental changes is almost always helpful.

1. *Risk factors and precipitants.*
   Cognitive dilapidation, pain, hypoxia, CNS medication effects, sensory loss, and innumerable acute medical illnesses are risk factors and precipitants for agitation in patients with AD. Sometimes, the precipitant is an environmental change (e.g., new room, unexpected visitors).

2. *Medication management.*
   a. *Recommended treatments. Trazodone (Desyrel) is often effective because of its sedating and calming properties.* Treatment begins with 25 to 50 mg at bedtime, and the dose is gradually increased to 150 mg or more. Postural hypotension is a potential side effect. Trazodone in divided doses may be used during the daytime. Another choice is a slow increase of buspirone (BuSpar) to 5 to 10 mg three times a day used either alone or to augment trazodone. If the patient is experiencing psychosis, increasing the dosage of haloperidol (Haldol) from 0.25 mg (or less) to 1 to 2 mg at bedtime or given as divided doses may be tried.
   b. *Possible treatments.* Lorazepam (Ativan), 0.25 to 2.0 mg, is reserved for acute agitation. *Because benzodiazepines impair memory, they should be used only until other agents become effective.* Benzodiazepines, in general, may worsen the situation because of their potential for disinhibition. Thioridazine (Mellaril) at 12.5 to 50 mg may be helpful, most likely because of its sedative properties; its anticholinergic properties limit its use.
   c. *Innovative treatments.* Zolpidem (Ambien), a nonbenzodiazepine hypnotic, may be given, starting at 2.5 to 5 mg at bedtime and at 1.25 to 5 mg as needed during the day; zolpidem is especially useful for later-stage AD. Risperidone (Risperdal), 0.25 to 0.5 mg twice daily, has been used with success; hypotension and headache may occur and are more likely to occur at higher doses. If angry and aggressive outbursts are frequent, carbamazepine (Tegretol) or divalproex sodium (Depakote) may be tried in dosages appropriate for seizure control.

F. Behavioral management.

The patient with AD may need tools to change the behavior of caregivers, and caregivers need tools to minimize the objectionable behaviors associated with AD.

1. *Patients with AD may change the behaviors of others by using cognitive aids.* Counseling is possible for demented patients who retain some memory functions and are capable of (limited) meaningful interactions with others. In this situation, it is often the AD patient who has the need to change the behavior of others. Well-intentioned caregivers may make unrealistic demands on the patient with AD or may react in inadvertently punitive ways. Persons with AD may be unable to tell others about their needs and wants.

   Unfortunately, counseling requires repetition, and repetition is unproductive in many demented patients. In this situation, it is useful to provide a small index card on which is written the key concept from a counseling session. For example, an always timid patient gets AD. At a relatively early stage, the patient is at a loss for words when the spouse makes task demands that are beyond the patient. The patient might be given a card on which the phrase "I CAN'T DO THAT" is written (see Case Study). In another situation, a card might read "I AM SCARED." The patient is told to refer to the card whenever trouble comes and a caregiver's behavior needs to be changed. Some patients with AD can manage as many as a half dozen cards of this sort. Others are only able to give the caretaker the pile of cards, and the caretaker must seek out the intended response. For this strategy to work, the caregiver must be sensitive to his or her own limitations and must be willing to "listen" to someone with AD. All too often, the problem is a resentful caregiver who is unwilling to acknowledge personal anger and is unable to change.

2. *Patients with AD may have objectionable behaviors.* Some AD behaviors are insensitive to treatment with medications. Because patients with AD respond to cues and are sensitive to their environments, manipulation of environmental contingencies is a means of modifying objectionable behaviors. The following elements must be present if objectionable behaviors are to be modified. The doctor's main goal is to determine if these elements are suffi-

ciently available to support the use of behavior modification.

a. *Identify problems early.* Objectionable behaviors are best modified when they first appear. Behaviors that are practiced and ingrained for many months are difficult to modify.
b. *Set realistic goals. Success is achieved if the behavior's frequency, duration, intensity, or location is reduced by 50%.* Caregivers should be prepared for such a realistic goal and must be told that any additional success is a bonus.
c. *Measure target behaviors.* The behavior must be sensitive to behavior management. Behaviors that stem mainly from brain dysfunction are unlikely targets. For example, any cognitive improvement (e.g., relearning the names of objects), self-stimulating behavior (e.g., head banging), general restlessness and arousal, and severe depressive symptoms are inappropriate targets for behavior modification. Appropriate target behaviors can be well described and are measurable, such as yelling obscenities, wandering, remaining in a room for 18 h/d, being awake but inactive for 10 hours, and hitting a caregiver during personal care.
d. *Exclude sensory and medical impairment.* Poor hearing and vision can contribute to objectionable behavior, as can pain from any source (e.g., constipation) or discomfort from a medical illness (e.g., urinary tract infection) or treatment (e.g., drug side effects). Moreover, patients must be able to hear and see the cues that may be used in a behavior management program.
e. *Sustained effort required.* Many caregivers express frustration but far fewer are able to make the sustained time commitment required for success. If time is available, caregivers may be reluctant to use reinforcers such as food when more congenial reinforcers like attention and praise prove ineffective. For example, small food rewards are powerful motivators of behavior, but a reinforcement schedule requires the caregiver to go to a behavioral specialist and learn the appropriate skills.
f. *Practical suggestions.* During the evaluation for behavior management, potential home dangers that are identified need to be removed or altered so that they no longer work. If the patient wanders at night, secure door locks need to be installed (with keys quickly available to the caregiver). Stoves need to be disabled if the patient is to be left alone for even a short time. Dangerous chemicals need to be removed. Car keys must be unavailable and/or useless because the car is disabled so that the patient cannot start it.
g. *Implementation.* A primary care doctor rarely has the skills or the time to develop, implement, and monitor a behavior management plan. When the aforementioned foundation is present, referral to a specialist in behavior management may be indicated for complicated situations.

Case Study

Mrs. A. is 74 years of age and is brought to medical attention by her daughter and husband. Mrs. A. is agitated. She does not keep still and moans "nothing is right"; she is able to say in a private meeting, among other things, that "I cannot talk to my husband." Mr. A. has very poor vision, is hard of hearing, has mild short-term memory impairment, and says that he makes every effort to keep his wife occupied. During the evaluation, the daughter reveals that Mr. A. expects more of his wife than she can really do and that Mrs. A. has always had trouble standing up to her husband. For example, he insists that she help him find his hearing aid when it falls from his night stand; Mrs. A. tries, but she usually cannot locate the hearing aid and starts to cry. With the help of her daughter, data are collected that list many tasks that Mr. A. expects his wife to do. Mr. A. is counseled about the inappropriateness of his requests, but he seems to be unable to change because his short-term memory impairment may reduce his desire and motivation for change; he tends to "forget" his desire to change. After some counseling and help from her daughter, Mrs. A. agrees to wear a 3 x 5 card around her neck; the card says in big letters "I CANNOT DO THAT." Progress is monitored according to how many times Mrs. A. shows the card for appropriate reasons. The daughter visits daily to perform the data collection and monitoring and praises Mrs. A. for using her card and praises Mr. A. for "getting the message." Mrs. A.'s agitation is diminished by all accounts.

III. Parkinson's disease.

A. Evaluation and diagnostic overview.

1. *Differential diagnosis.*
Parkinson's disease (PD) is primarily a movement disorder. The distinction between Parkinson's disease with dementia and AD with extrapyramidal features is difficult, but the time course and relative severity help separate these two problems. Either way, the neurobehavioral problem is similar, and a slowly progressive dementia is integral to PD. The major features of PD dementia are initially those of frontal lobe disease followed by increased memory impairment. *Mild cognitive dilapidation is more common than is a rapidly progressive cognitive and behavioral deterioration.*

Numerous conditions and diseases produce a parkinsonian syndrome; perhaps the most common of these is drug-induced parkinsonism (e.g., induced by neuroleptics like haloperidol [Haldol] and thioridazine [Mellaril], antihypertensives like methyldopa [Aldomet], antinausea agents like metoclopramide [Reglan], and other drugs).

2. *Laboratory and neuropsychology.*
The diagnosis of PD is made based on the results of the neurologic motor examination. Neuropsychological assessment is complicated because of slowed motor and speech performance that affects tests that require manual dexterity or are timed. Assertions of depression with psychomotor retardation often fail to recognize the degree of motor impairment due to PD. When the office examination for dementia or depression is inconclusive, the patient should be referred for expert neuropsychological testing.

B. Epidemiology and pathophysiology.

For office populations, PD is comorbid with dementia in 35% to 55% of PD cases. Drug-induced parkinsonism appears within a month in most patients, and within 3 months, 90% of patients are symptomatic. PD affects the basal ganglia and the frontal lobe via neural connections between the two. Autopsy studies of PD dementia have found the pathology characteristic of both PD and AD.

C. Depression in Parkinson's disease.

Depression is comorbid with idiopathic PD in 40% to 60% of cases. Depression in PD may significantly impair cognition but otherwise has many of the clinical features seen in primary major depressions. Because the clinical features of PD (e.g., fatigue, psychomotor retardation, speech without facial expression) have all the appearances of depression, *such psychological symptoms as helplessness, hopelessness, and wishes for death are used to support the diagnosis.* Suicide is rare in Parkinson's patients.

1. *Risk factors.*
Serious depression does not correlate well with the amount of disability and, therefore, should not be considered to be reactive to the disease. Risk factors include a personal and family history of depression and an early age of onset.

2. *Medication management.*
When antidepressant treatment is started, it is logical to match the antidepressant to the severity and the stage of PD.
    a. *Recommended treatments.* For mild depression and minimal-to-mild PD, the dosage of levodopa-carbidopa (Sinemet), which is associated with depressed mood, may be reduced, and bromocriptine (Parlodel), amantadine (Symmetrel), or selegiline (Eldepryl), any of which have beneficial effects on mood, may be added or substituted. Given that anticholinergic agents benefit patients with PD, patients unresponsive to treatment may be given one of the less anticholinergic tricyclic antidepressants, such as nortriptyline (Pamelor) or any of the SSRIs; however, an argument can be made that favors the use of the slightly anticholinergic SSRI paroxetine (Paxil). About 10% of patients with PD have increased motor impairment when they take an SSRI; if this occurs, the therapy must be discontinued. Bupropion (Wellbutrin) is mildly dopaminergic and has been used with success in mild-to-moderate PD. However, bupropion-enhanced dopaminergic effects may account for the few reports of psychosis as an adverse event.
    For later-stage PD with probable dementia, antidepressants with negligible anticholinergic effects are best. Trazodone (Desyrel) is a reasonable choice when agitation and anxiety are emotionally experienced; agitation in PD is often unaccompanied by motor expression. The use of trazodones may be limited by its capacity to cause postural hypotension. Electroconvulsive therapy is effective and temporarily improves PD.
    b. *Possible treatments.* Patients with PD are sensitive to medication, and any medication treatment may produce a negative drug experience, especially combinations of psychiatric drugs with substantial doses of antiparkinsonian drugs. *Combining an SSRI with selegiline is contraindicated.* Amoxapine (Asendin) has neuroleptic properties and should not be used.
    c. *Innovative treatments.* Based on preliminary data, venlafaxine (Effexor) may prove useful in PD; blood pressure must be monitored after a dosage of 225 mg/d is reached and until blood pressure is unaffected at a higher, stable dose. Nefazodone (Serzone) may prove to be useful as well.

D. Psychosis in Parkinson's disease.

Medications used to treat Parkinson's disease, particularly carbidopa-levodopa (Sinemet) and bromocriptine (Parlodel) are usually the cause of psychosis in PD, but every antiparkinson agent has been implicated. Three forms of psychosis may occur alone or together:

- *Benign psychosis:* visual hallucinations are described with an otherwise clear mind. Known or unknown small children or older people are commonly seen. These hallucinations are benign because the patient responds to them only with verbal comment; they are nonthreatening.
- *Disruptive psychosis:* paranoid delusions, visual and/or auditory hallucinations, and distortions of reality are typical. These are disruptive because the patient changes his or her behavior in

response to the misperceptions. For example, the patient may become tearful and upset because dead people are seen in the living room.

- *Psychiatric psychosis:* patients with concurrent psychiatric conditions, such as schizophrenia, exhibit the standard symptoms, often in some admixture with the benign and/or disruptive psychosis previously described.

1. *Risk factors.*
   Dementia and medications are risk factors for psychosis in patients with Parkinson's disease.

2. *Medication management.*
   a. *Recommended treatments.* To the extent possible, administration of the potentially causative adjunctive agents, like bromocriptine, amantadine (Symmetrel), and selegiline (Eldepryl) should be reduced or discontinued. Then, any anticholinergic antidepressant therapy should be discontinued.

   For further treatment, *clozapine (Clozaril) is the drug of choice;* clozapine's efficacy is so compelling that its use in primary care is recommended. (See below for potential alternative drugs.) The therapy should start with 6.25 mg (1/4 of a 25-mg tablet) before bedtime, and the dosage should be slowly increased as tolerated until symptoms resolve or a maximum of 50 to 75 mg at night is reached. Many patients respond within 7 to 14 days to nightly doses of 6.25 to 25 mg. A successful outcome is best measured by improvements in sleep and mental status. The majority of responders are free of psychosis, have a somewhat improved mood, and may have a lessening of PD.

   If the patient has a concurrent psychiatric psychosis (1% chance), a more standard dose of clozapine is necessary. Although uncommon, dystonic and extrapyramidal reactions are possible with clozapine. A small risk of clozapine-induced agranulocytosis exists, and weekly complete blood counts and related weekly reports of white blood cell counts are required before the pharmacy dispenses clozapine. These paperwork chores are minimized with the help of the clozapine sales representative.

   Several "clozaril-like" antipsychotics will soon be available. Olanzapine (Zyprexa) is now available; there are a few favorable reports about its use for PD-related psychosis.

   b. *Possible treatments.* A low-dose neuroleptic, like thioridazine (Mellaril), 1 to 12 mg or more in the liquid form (25 mg/5 mL), is sometimes effective; however, neuroleptics are usually effective only at a dose that increases the severity of PD symptoms.

   Risperidone (Risperdal) may be successful in about 10% to 15% of cases; its dosage is increased every 3 to 5 (or more) days, starting from 0.25 mg daily and increasing to a low-maximum of 0.5 to 1 mg twice daily. *In our experience, risperidone often makes both the PD and the mental status worse, and postural hypotension limits use.*

   c. *Innovative treatments.* If clozapine or olanzapine therapy proves unsuccessful, an innovative choice is oral ondansetron (Zofran), a serotonin antagonist without known effects on motor systems; the initial dose is 4 to 8 mg/day, divided between morning and evening (twice daily), with subsequent increases of 4 to 8 mg/w, and stopping at a total daily maintenance dose of 12 to 24 mg. In preliminary studies of ondansetron alone, patients have been maintained on optimal antiparkinsonian therapy; there are no published reports of combined clozapine-ondansetron therapy. Ondansetron is currently extremely expensive (16 mg/d costs, $1150/mo wholesale).

E. Behavioral management.

The depressive symptoms of Parkinson's disease can be addressed with behaviorally oriented psychological interventions. For patients with PD with major depressive disorder, standard cognitive behavior treatment is used. Patients with PD with minor symptoms often benefit from a more behavioral approach. Minor symptoms are usually related to awareness of decreased personal effectiveness (e.g., patients need more help with tasks, have limitations on activities, and fear that these and similar problems will get worse) and of increased anxiety and tension (e.g., the patient cannot relax yet has limited motivation, feels under pressure to get things done but just gets angry and frustrated).

The goal of the doctor is to dignify these problems as being common to all patients with PD, to suggest strongly that psychological skill building is the solution, and to dismiss any idea that deep psychological problems are the cause. PD support groups for patients and relatives can often provide these skills. Specific self-help groups are sometimes available. Behavioral counseling is another option.

Essentially, counseling sessions consist of seminars in which the topic is whatever is bothering the patient with PD. Being in public places like restaurants, using public transportation, asking for help, and experiencing dissatisfaction with friends and relatives, are common themes. Besides social skills and stress management training, cognitive restructuring, role playing, and role modeling are among the techniques taught.

IV. Human immunodeficiency virus and acquired immunodeficiency syndrome.

A. Evaluation and diagnostic overview.

Acquired immunodeficiency syndrome (AIDS) is

caused by the human immunodeficiency virus (HIV). AIDS is a chronic and eventually fatal illness that is associated with various neurologic and neurobehavioral disturbances. In addition, individuals with HIV and AIDS often experience difficult and stressful social circumstances (e.g., bereavement, homelessness) that negatively affect physical and mental health. In order to successfully diagnose and treat HIV-related neuropsychiatric illnesses, the clinician must understand the physical manifestations of HIV disease and the social context of patients with HIV and AIDS. With this (and all illnesses), it is important to interact with patients in a nonjudgmental manner; reassurances about confidentiality must be provided. Description of the nonpsychiatric aspects of HIV disease and their treatment is beyond the scope of this chapter. General references are provided in the recommended reading list at the end of the chapter.

1. *Differential diagnosis and delirium.*
Neurobehavioral disturbances are often found in association with deterioration caused by an HIV-associated medical or neurologic problem (or by medications used to treat these concurrent problems). Accordingly, the premature diagnosis of a psychiatric syndrome is unwise.

   Altered mental status in an HIV-positive patient is a medical emergency, and infectious and noninfectious causes must be included in the differential diagnosis. HIV-positive patients with altered mental status must be approached in the same way as those who are HIV negative: *the origin of the disturbance should be identified and reversible causes corrected.* The usual causes of delirium and dementia in persons with HIV and AIDS are listed in Table 12–1.

   A thorough history (including an interview of the patient's significant other or caretaker), physical examination, and laboratory evaluation should be performed for each patient who presents with altered mental status. An electroencephalogram (EEG) may be useful in differentiating between delirium and AIDS dementia (Table 12–2). (Background slowing is usually present in the former.) An investigation for infectious causes is mandatory, but other causes should not be neglected, especially medication and substance ingestion and metabolic abnormalities.

   Treatment for delirium in patients with HIV consists of maintaining a safe, medically supportive environment, rapidly determining the cause of the disturbance, and applying corrective treatment.

2. *Laboratory and neuropsychology tests.*
Obvious medical symptoms often occur when the absolute number of CD4 helper cells is less than 500/mm^3, although many patients remain asymptomatic at much lower CD4 levels. One criterion for the diagnosis of AIDS is fewer than 200 CD4 cells (i.e., an indication of active disease).

   Cognitive impairment is positively correlated with disease severity. Infrequently, the results of tests in medically asymptomatic patients are in the impaired range; cognitive and motor deficits are usually minor in these cases. Significant CNS involvement occurs in at least 90% of patients at some time during the course of the illness, especially in the terminal stages. The pattern of deficits is similar to those found in subcortical dementias (e.g., impaired memory, attention and judgment, slowed information processing, and decreased verbal fluency).

Table 12–1
Central Nervous System Causes of Altered Mental Status in Human Immunodeficiency Virus Infection

Dementia

Human immunodeficiency virus (HIV)–associated dementia (especially AIDS dementia complex)
Dementia associated with opportunistic infections
- Bacterial
- Viral
- Fungal
- Protozoal

Dementia associated with central nervous system malignancies
- Cerebral lymphoma
- Disseminated Kaposi's sarcoma

Delirium

Intoxication
- Prescription medications, e.g., narcotics, antibiotics, antineoplastics
- Substance abuse, e.g., alcohol, other drugs

Withdrawal
- Alcohol, sedatives, opiates

Metabolic encephalopathy
- Hypoxia
- Hypoglycemia
- Hepatic, renal, pulmonary, pancreatic insufficiency
- Acid-base disturbances
- Fluid and electrolyte disorders
- Endocrinopathies

Infections
- Systemic, e.g., septicemia, subacute bacterial endocarditis, pneumonia, *Mycobacterium-avium* complex (MAC)
- Intracranial, e.g., cryptococcal meningitis, HIV encephalitis, tubercular meningitis, toxoplasmosis

Seizures
Head trauma
Strokes
Mass lesions, e.g., central nervous system malignancies, abscesses
Hematologic, e.g., severe anemia

B. Epidemiology and the psychosocial context of HIV/AIDS

Human immunodeficiency virus is transmitted through exposure to the body fluids of infected

Table 12–2
Symptoms and Signs of Human Immunodeficiency Virus Dementia

Symptoms
- Early
  - Word-finding difficulty
  - Forgetfulness
  - Poor concentration
  - Confusion
  - Slowed thinking
  - Difficulty performing complex learned tasks
  - Poor handwriting
  - Loss of balance
  - Dropping of things
  - Depression
  - Lower-extremity weakness
- Late
  - Disorientation
  - Severe confusion
  - Delusions
  - Psychosis

Signs
- Early
  - Cognitive impairment
  - Apathy
  - Regression
  - Psychosis
  - Psychomotor retardation
  - Difficulty with abstract thinking
  - Ataxia
  - Tremor
  - Paresis
  - Perseveration
- Late
  - Mutism
  - Incontinence
  - Seizures
  - Perseveration
  - Severe regression
  - Carphologia (picking)

Adapted from Cohen MAA, Alfonso CA. Psychiatric manifestations of the HIV epidemic. AIDS Reader 1994; 4(3): 97–106.

individuals. HIV is the leading cause of death in the United States for persons 25 to 44 years of age. Although HIV infection has been reported among members of all ethnic groups, social classes, and sexual orientations, patients with HIV and AIDS in the United States disproportionately represent men who have sex with men, injectable drug users, and low-income residents of predominantly nonwhite urban areas. Thus, many social stressors and psychiatric comorbidities are more common among people with HIV than among the population at large (Table 12–3).

C. Depression and suicide in HIV/AIDS.

Depression is the most frequently diagnosed psychiatric disorder among people with HIV; prevalence estimates are 4% to 14% among

Table 12–3
The Psychosocial Context of HIV and AIDS

Gay and bisexual men
- Discrimination based on sexual orientation, AIDS diagnosis
- Antihomosexual prejudice and violence
- Bereavement (often multiple)
- Recent separation or loss
- Alienation from family, culture, religion
- Illness-related unemployment, eviction, financial distress

Low-income women and minorities
- Discrimination based on gender, ethnicity, AIDS diagnosis
- Violence
- Sexual assault
- Post-traumatic stress disorder (PTSD)
- Insufficient family or child support
- Multiple losses
- Illness-related or pre-existing unemployment, financial distress, homelessness
- Legal difficulties (especially related to sex industry work and drug use)

homosexual men and non–drug-abusing women, and are higher (≥ 32%) in sociodemographically diverse populations. Rates of depression are thought to be similar among HIV-positive and HIV-negative adults with similar risk behavior profiles. *Even in cases of substantial physical disability, depression should not be considered to be part of the normal disease progression but should instead be evaluated and treated.*

Depression in persons with HIV or AIDS may be diagnosed according to standard criteria, but allowances must be made for symptoms that can be attributed to either depressive illness or HIV infection (e.g., fatigue, decreased libido, anorexia, weight loss). No infallible guidelines exist for distinguishing between these conditions; depression remains a clinical diagnosis that must be made in the context of the patient's total presentation.

1. *Suicide.*
   Several studies have found that *suicide rates in persons with AIDS are 7 to 37 times higher* than those of matched control subjects. Furthermore, as many as one in five HIV-seropositive patients may demonstrate suicidal behavior. Suicide may represent a way to re-establish control of personal destiny or to escape further pain or disability. However, suicidality is often caused by depressive illness (rather than being a "natural" effect of HIV on the CNS) and must be taken seriously and treated aggressively. Persons experiencing bereavement, substance abuse disorders, or lack of social support are at especially increased risk.
   Epidemiologic data regarding the relationship between HIV positivity and suicide must be in-

terpreted with caution because many people with HIV have histories of pre-existing depression and severely challenging social circumstances. Furthermore, mortality resulting from suicide in people with AIDS is dwarfed by mortality attributable to opportunistic infections and malignancies.

Suicide prevention depends on accurate assessment of risk and timely intervention. *Any patient who is experiencing an additional loss, or who appears depressed, should be asked about the possibility of suicide.* Preventive measures are the same as for HIV-negative persons: crisis intervention, treatment for depression, mobilization of interpersonal support, and direct supervision in acute cases.

2. *Risk factors.*
Depression is more common in individuals with a history of this illness before the diagnosis of HIV seropositivity, personality disorders, and poor social support.

3. *Medication management.*
Treatment of depression in people with HIV or AIDS is generally similar to that for HIV-negative patients.
   a. *Recommended treatments.* Patients with HIV or AIDS benefit from SSRI therapy. Among the cyclic antidepressants, desipramine (Norpramin) is energizing in patients with HIV but without AIDS. Nortriptyline (Pamelor) is another cyclic antidepressant with low anticholinergic affinity that has been found to be highly useful. *In general, the same antidepressant dosing guidelines apply for HIV-positive and HIV-negative patients.* Antidepressants do not adversely affect the immune system, and complications from the treatment of depression are rare. However, the adage "start low and go slow" should be followed in cases in which substantial physical wasting or disability is present. Furthermore, patients who are receiving multiple medications for the treatment of AIDS-defining illnesses are more likely to experience dose-limiting side effects or drug interactions.
   b. *Possible treatments.* When HIV illness progresses to AIDS, patients often become physically intolerant of cyclic antidepressants. Bupropion (Wellbutrin), even at low doses, may produce confusion and seizures. Benzodiazepines should not be used for the treatment of depression.
   c. *Innovative treatments.* Venlafaxine (Effexor) has been reported to treat depression and enhance cognition effectively. Psychostimulants, such as dextroamphetamine (Dexedrine) and methylphenidate (Ritalin), may bring prompt relief of depressive psychomotor retardation, low energy, and apathy, but they must be used with caution in patients who are at risk for substance-abusing behavior. Small doses (e.g., 5 to 15 mg daily of methylphenidate) may be used when the response to other agents (e.g., fluoxetine [Prozac]) is inadequate. In this population, psychostimulants do not generally produce weight loss. Psychosis may be produced in a setting of advanced AIDS. Finally, electroconvulsive therapy has been used to treat severe, refractory depressions, such as delusional affective disorders.

D. Mania in HIV/AIDS.

Mania caused by HIV or AIDS is uncommon; however, mania can occur secondary to a concurrent medical or neurologic problem. Intolerance to lithium and standard neuroleptics is the norm in these cases. Risperidone (Risperdal), clonazepam (Klonopin), or divalproex sodium (Depakote) should be used in the lowest effective doses.

E. HIV-associated dementia and psychosis.

Human immunodeficiency virus has an affinity for the brain and can produce dementia, even in the absence of opportunistic infections or CNS malignancies. Minor cognitive and motor deficits can be detected in some asymptomatic HIV-positive individuals by means of expert neuropsychological testing. However, HIV-associated dementia (HAD) is rare in the absence of immunosuppression. Because of subcortical involvement, early-stage HAD may mimic depression, but in HAD, psychomotor slowing and attentional deficits are usually well out of proportion to the affective component. Later-stage HAD is found in the presence of personality changes, psychosis, and progressive neurologic dilapidation. Although HAD is the most common cause of dementia in patients with HIV, a thorough search for reversible causes must be performed for any HIV-positive patient who presents with altered mental status. The aforementioned commentary on differential diagnosis and delirium applies to HAD (see Table 12–2).

Supervision is essential in cases in which the patient retains motor functioning but is severely cognitively impaired; accidental (or perhaps antisocial) behaviors, such as fire setting and public elimination, have been reported. Management of true AIDS dementia (HIV encephalopathy) requires an increase in the level of caretaking and environmental support.

In general, zidovudine (AZT) or other antiviral agents may partially reverse HAD. The side effects are limiting, and the zidovudine dose should be increased as much as tolerated (not to exceed 2000 mg/d).

1. *Early-stage HIV-associated dementia.*
Methylphenidate (Ritalin) is the agent of choice; the dosage should be slowly increased to as

much as 60 mg/d divided at 7 a.m., 10 a.m., and 1 p.m. Dextroamphetamine (Dexedrine) and pemoline (Cylert) are alternatives. In seizure-prone patients (e.g., those with CNS infection), psychostimulants increase the likelihood of seizures, and they may exacerbate any movement disorder.

2. *Late-stage HIV-associated dementia.*
Although little used in primary care, *the antipsychotic molindone (Moban) is a first-line agent;* treatment starts at 5 mg three times daily, and the dosage may be slowly increased to 100 mg/d or higher. Risperidone (Risperdal) may prove to be an important alternative. Because of its potential for causing hypotension, a low dose (e.g., 0.5 mg) should be given an adequate trial; a slow dosage increase may need to follow. All the higher-potency neuroleptics (e.g., haloperidol [Haldol]) are less useful because of their tendency to produce neuroleptic malignant syndrome or unusually severe extrapyramidal side effects in this population. Haloperidol may be tried at a dose of 0.5 mg/d or twice a day.

F. Anxiety states in HIV/AIDS.

High levels of stress and anxiety are common in HIV and AIDS. These states are often associated with severe social circumstances or may be a physiologic response to other aspects of HIV disease. The diagnosis may be complicated because of the many possible origins of the symptoms: hypoxemia in patients with active lung disease, recreational drug use, HIV/AIDS-related medications, and metabolic dysfunction may all be causal. It is wise to ask about the patient's use of investigational and unconventional therapies, herbal agents, and over-the-counter medications.

When an idiopathic anxiety syndrome is diagnosed, such non-pharmacologic therapies as meditation, deep muscle relaxation, and biofeedback are recommended first. Among the benzodiazepines, only the short- and intermediate-acting agents can be recommended. These include lorazepam (Ativan), oxazepam (Serax), and alprazolam (Xanax). Longer-acting agents (e.g., diazepam [Valium]) and ultra–short-acting agents (e.g., midazolam [Versed]) too often cause paradoxic agitation, confusion, and apathy. When relief can be postponed for several weeks or more, buspirone (BuSpar) may be helpful. Slow increase to 15 mg three times a day. Doses well beyond 45 mg/d have been reported to be useful. Trazodone (Desyrel), 25 to 50 mg at bedtime, is useful as a sedative and may be helpful in low doses as a daytime antianxiety agent.

G. Other HIV/AIDS-related disorders.

Substance abuse, pain syndromes, sleep disorders, and adjustment disorders with or without personality disorders have been described in people with HIV and AIDS. In general, treatment is similar for persons with and for those without HIV disease; however, support groups and community-based interventions may play a more significant role in the treatment of HIV-positive individuals with these disorders.

V. Stroke.

A. Overview.

1. *Differential diagnosis.*
The sudden onset of focal neurologic symptoms, with a maximum deficit occurring at onset and persistence for longer than 24 hours, indicates a completed stroke unless standard evaluative procedures prove otherwise.

2. *Laboratory and neuropsychology.*
Unilateral infarctions tend to produce well-described focal syndromes, whereas dementia is usually a complication of stroke when cortical infarctions and ischemic changes are multiple and bilateral.

B. Epidemiology and pathophysiology.

Stroke and related cerebrovascular disease is the third leading cause of death in the United States (10% of all deaths). Neurobehavioral syndromes are common.

C. Poststroke apathy, depression and catastrophic reactions.

Serious depression occurs in both acute and established chronic stroke. *About 20% to 40% of all stroke patients have a depression that benefits from medical management.* The symptoms of depression are generally the same as for elderly patients with major or minor depression. Antidepressant treatment has a positive effect on early rehabilitation and long-term outcome. Apathy (e.g., absent desire for improvement, disinterest in self-care or rehabilitation, lack of motivation) usually precedes depression, and these characteristics are frequently found together. Aphasic patients are prone to *catastrophic reactions* (apprehension, fearfulness and tearfulness, excessive anxiety, anger); this state may be linked to depression, and if it persists, antidepressants may be helpful.

Before medical management begins, the medical and neurologic circumstances should be continuously stable for at least a week. Providing antidepressants sooner may simply complicate overall treatment. For example, if a new symptom develops, it may be incorrectly attributed to the use of antidepressants. Many clinicians believe that many less severe, and some more severe, forms of depression may self-resolve within 6 weeks and therefore recommend that antidepressant therapy be withheld if at all possible during this time. Any significant mood disturbance that persists for 2 weeks or more should be treated.

1. *Risk factors.*
   Anterior left-sided brain stroke lesions, subcortical atrophy, and ischemic changes that predate the stroke predispose to depression after the stroke. Larger left- or right-sided anterior lesions are more predictive than are smaller lesions. Heavy prior use of alcohol is also associated with poststroke depression.
2. *Medication management.*
   a. *Recommended treatments. For rapid improvement in apathy and increased motivation for rehabilitation, methylphenidate (Ritalin)* should be used and slowly increased from 2.5 mg to as much as 30 mg daily (usually given in divided doses with breakfast and lunch). Pemoline (Cylert) is an alternative option; the regimen begins with 18.75 mg with breakfast, and the dosage is increased at weekly intervals to as much as 37.5 mg at breakfast and lunch. Psychostimulants infrequently cause serious complications; anxiety and restlessness are often limiting side effects.

   For patients who become depressed after a completed rehabilitation program or who are intolerant to psychostimulants, any of the SSRIs are reasonable choices. Among the SSRIs, sertraline (Zoloft) may have a slight advantage over fluoxetine (Prozac), which has a long half-life, so side effects may linger, or over paroxetine (Paxil), which has minor anticholinergic effects.

   b. *Possible treatments.* Nortriptyline (Pamelor) treatment is widely recommended on the basis of results from a 1984 double-blind study; however, subsequent experience has found a 20% or higher incidence of delirium, which is most likely the result of excessive doses and/or anticholinergic side effects. *Caution is recommended with the use of tricyclic antidepressants in patients who have had a stroke.*

D. Poststroke emotional lability, agitation, and anxiety-like states.

Any of these symptoms may stem from dementia, or atypical forms of depression, or both. Emotional lability or emotional incontinence (e.g., easily provoked crying or, less often, undue delight) is a common complication of stroke. This behavior is usually appropriate to the circumstances. Episodes of crying or laughing that appear spontaneously, are inappropriate to the circumstances, and are incongruent with cognitive emotional perception may be a severe pathologic variant.

1. *Risk factors.*
   Dementia occurring before stroke predicts agitated and anxiety-like states. Pathologic crying and laughing is related to bilateral cortical lesions and related disrupted innervation of bulbar motor nuclei and subcortex.
2. *Medication management.*
   Trazodone (Desyrel) given in divided doses may improve agitation and anxiety-like states. Postural hypotension is sometimes a problem, especially at higher doses. All of the SSRIs have been used with some success for poststroke emotional lability; success may be the result of the treatment of depression. Pathologic crying and laughing have been improved with nortriptyline at doses that are therapeutic for depression. Neuropsychiatric or geriatric consultation may be of considerable help in determining the differential diagnosis and related treatment.

E. Poststroke psychosis and mania.

Psychosis (e.g., hallucinations and delusions) and mania (e.g., excited disinhibited behavior) are uncommon poststroke problems unless they predate the stroke. Delirium is much more common. Nonstroke causes for delirium should be considered, and *delirium must be ruled out before a diagnosis of psychosis or mania or a treatment is considered.*

1. *Risk factors.*
   Right cortical and subcortical lesions, poststroke seizures, and significant cortical or subcortical atrophy seem to be predictive of psychosis and mania.
2. *Medication management.*
   One to 2 mg of haloperidol (Haldol) at bedtime or twice a day may be helpful. Neuropsychiatric consultation may be indicated when other medication strategies are considered.

F. Behavioral management.

In order to begin a comprehensive treatment approach as soon as possible after the stroke, behavioral management should be initiated concurrently with other rehabilitation work and with the use of medications (e.g., stimulants).

1. *Modest measurable changes.*
   It is important to define a set of skills that are necessary for activities of daily living; these skills should be attainable from physical rehabilitation. The physician should focus on one skill at a time and find a method for measuring progress toward an improved quality of life. For example, changes in ambulation for a stroke patient may be measured by distance walked per unit of time. The patient and/or caregiver should be asked to chart progress. The physician should avoid focusing on large changes that are out of reach in the near term, such as walking around the block; instead, the physician should convey the message that progress is made one step at a time.

2. *Biofeedback.*
The combination of electromyographic biofeedback and physical therapy can be used for neuromuscular re-education. Biofeedback instrumentation is applied to muscles targeted for active recruitment or inhibition. Information in the form of sounds or lights guides the patient's skill development. Each session has only one or two attainable goals and is followed by home practice. Progress is monitored and charted. Biofeedback has been used in the successful treatment of poststroke urinary incontinence and swallowing difficulties. These methods remain controversial and are not widely available.

VI. Multiple Sclerosis

A. Evaluation and diagnostic overview.

Exacerbating and remitting, acute and progressive, and *chronic and slowly progressive (the most common)* describe the three different clinical courses of multiple sclerosis (MS).

1. *Differential diagnosis.*
Diagnostic accuracy is crucial in cases of MS. A remarkable array of neurologic signs and symptoms may characterize MS (e.g., some combination of visual, speech, gait, muscle strength, and sensory and bladder disturbances). Neurobehavioral disturbances may precede the diagnosis of MS by a period of months to years, resulting in inappropriate treatment for hysteria, somatization, or antisocial personality disorder. Conversely, patients with confirmed MS and depression are less likely to receive antidepressant pharmacotherapy than are persons with similar symptomatology but without MS. A thorough history should be obtained, with special attention being paid to medication use, substance abuse, and concurrent illnesses. Coexisting psychiatric dysfunctions, especially depression, should be evaluated, and signs of delirium or dementia should be thoroughly investigated. Magnetic resonance imaging may reveal new or progressive lesions.

2. *Laboratory and neuropsychological tests.*
Early in the course of MS, the results of bedside or informal cognitive testing, such as screening with the Mini-Mental State Exam (see Appendix, this chapter), are often unremarkable. Similarly, intelligence testing (e.g., the Wechsler's Adult Intelligence Scale—Revised [WAIS-R]) may be unrevealing, particularly if the patient's premorbid intelligence was greater than average. Eventually, about 20% of patients have cognitive dysfunction. The degrees of cognitive and motor impairments are usually independent; many patients with significant physical disability are cognitively intact. Basic speech, written communication, and mathematical reasoning generally remain reasonably intact, with short-term memory, conceptual reasoning, and concentration most often affected. People with MS are commonly particularly vulnerable to the effects of distractions and nonrelevant stimuli, and they may perform poorly at tasks in which rapid information processing or intellectual flexibility is needed. However, the spectrum of cognitive functioning among patients with MS is broad, and many individuals exhibit no demonstrable impairment. Functional constellations involving substantial deficits in certain areas and sparing of others are also common. *Patients in whom cognitive changes are suspected should be referred for comprehensive neuropsychological evaluation.*

B. Epidemiology and pathophysiology.

The most common of the demyelinating disorders of the CNS, MS tends to occur in early adulthood; 1% of patients with MS have their first symptoms after the age of 60 years. Perhaps 20% of persons with MS experience a detectable degree of cognitive impairment during the course of the disease (estimates range from 2% to 72%), although global intellectual breakdown, such as is seen in Alzheimer's dementia, is rare.

C. General management guidelines.

Treatment for MS *is multidisciplinary.* Most patients with MS require ongoing assessment and therapy from a neurologist, preventive and routine care from a primary care physician, and, frequently, psychiatric consultation as well. Further research regarding psychiatric disorders among persons with MS is strongly needed, and definitive knowledge concerning optimum treatment is lacking.

1. *Medication management.*
No proven treatment for MS-related cognitive changes currently exists. Pharmacotherapy aimed at improving memory and other cognitive functions has been attempted, and this is an area for further research. Programs involving amantadine (Symmetrel) therapy, immunosuppression, and plasmaphoresis may be helpful. Information regarding current trials can be obtained from the National Multiple Sclerosis Society (1-800-624-8236).

2. *Rehabilitative services.*
Training in personal organization (e.g., using an electronic notebook or lists) may prove helpful. Persons who are experiencing employment-related difficulties can be referred to locally available vocational rehabilitation services and to the National Multiple Sclerosis Society Job Raising Program (1-212-986-3240).

3. *What to tell the patient and family.*

Patients and families generally benefit from a straightforward discussion of the known impairments and remaining strengths. If the patient's personality has been significantly altered, counseling that this phenomenon is caused by the disease process (rather than by the interpersonal relationship) may be reassuring. Referral to support groups, family therapy, and other services is often of crucial importance.

D. Major depression in multiple sclerosis.

Approximately 30% to 40% of individuals with MS experience depression (current estimates of prevalence range from 14% to 57%). Before the onset of neurologic symptoms, rates of depression do not differ significantly from those of young to middle-aged adults without MS. Later in the disease, depressive symptoms are often severe. Several possible causes for depression in MS have been proposed: reaction to a serious illness, direct neurologic degenerative change, common genetic or immunologic factors, and coincidence (especially among young adults). It is likely that many patients experience some combination of these factors.

As with patients without MS, diagnosis of depression is made by diagnostic interview. However, certain cautions must be observed: *fatigue is a prominent feature of MS, and it is not useful in the diagnosis of depression among patients with MS.* Similarly, emotional lability and inappropriate weeping or laughter are more likely to represent the effects of the underlying disease process than a depressive episode. However, feelings of hopelessness, worthlessness, or despair must be taken seriously as representing potential signs of depression and should not be simply accepted as an appropriate reaction to the physical limitations that MS can impose. Excessive anger, worry, and irritability may also indicate a need for treatment. The prevalence of suicide among persons with MS is not definitively known (estimates range from 3% to 12%), but suicidal ideation or plans must be appropriately investigated.

1. *Risk factors.*
   The severity and type of physical disability do not necessarily predict depression, but depressive episodes are more common after an exacerbation of MS that requires steroid therapy and when history of depression prior to MS is present. Patients with lesions of the brain, rather than the spinal cord, are more likely to become depressed. Furthermore, poor social and family support also correlate with clinical depression in people with MS.
2. *Medication management.*
   Experience with newer antidepressants is limited. Clinicians who prescribe serotonergic agents should be alert for symptoms of mania and hypomania, which occur more often in patients with MS than in those with other neurobehavioral disorders.
   a. *Recommended treatments.* Sertraline (Zoloft) is a reasonable treatment for depression in MS, based on a recent report. Fluoxetine (Prozac) has been used with success for MS-related emotional incontinence and, in our experience, fluoxetine is also an effective antidepressant in MS.
   b. *Possible treatments.* Pharmacotherapy with cyclic antidepressants (principally desipramine [Norpramin] and amitriptyline [Elavil]) has been effective, although side effects become prominent at lower dosages than in patients without MS (e.g., at doses of desipramine >125 mg). Anticholinergic effects may improve bladder symptoms but may cause cognitive impairment.
3. *Counseling.*
   Depression in people with MS has been treated successfully with short-term cognitive therapy. Couples or family therapy and partner/caregiver support can also be helpful.

E. Manic-depressive states in multiple sclerosis.

The prevalence of bipolar (manic-depressive) disorder among persons with MS has been estimated at 2% to 13%, compared with 1% in the general population. Generally, the diagnosis of MS predates the development of bipolarity, although mania may also be steroid induced. *Diagnostic criteria for bipolar disorder are unchanged by the presence of MS, and lithium remains the treatment of choice,* including in cases involving steroid therapy. Antiepileptic drugs are largely untried on MS-related mood disorders.

F. Inappropriate responses in multiple sclerosis.

Outbursts of weeping and laughter are characteristic of MS and do not indicate psychopathology. However, this phenomenon can be socially disabling and may require treatment. Amitriptyline (Elavil), 50 to 75 mg daily, or fluoxetine (Prozac), 20 to 40 mg daily, have been shown to reduce this symptomatology, although these treatments have not been widely tested. Levo-dopa, at doses of no more than 1.5 g/d, and amantadine (Symmetrel), at 100 mg/d, have been used for similar symptoms in patients without MS. Patients may experience substantial relief simply by providing their families and associates with information about this aspect of the disease.

Euphoria is also a prominent clinical feature in a small percentage (10% to 20%) of persons with MS. This can manifest as either a profound optimism that appears inappropriate to others or as a jolly or upbeat manner that does not represent the individual's true emotional state. Euphoria does not require treatment; however, the clinician must remain alert for the development of mania.

G. Psychosis in multiple sclerosis.

Psychotic symptomatology may arise in response to treatment with steroids or adrenocorticotropic hormone (ACTH). Paranoid ideation, hallucinations, and schizophreniform thought disorders are found in 2% of patients. Extensive cerebral pathology may also result in psychotic presentations. Research in this area of MS management is lacking. At present, psychosis in patients with MS should be treated in the same fashion as in patients without MS.

H. Sexual dysfunctions in multiple sclerosis.

Approximately 75% of women and men with MS experience some form of sexual dysfunction, and about half of heterosexual patients with MS eventually discontinue having intercourse. (Specific data regarding MS in lesbians and gay men is lacking.) Difficulties arising from fatigue, weakness, spasticity, paralysis, muscle cramps, urologic dysfunction (including catheter dependence), and partnership stresses are experienced by members of both genders. Men also present with erectile dysfunction, decreased orgasm, and diminished libido, whereas women experience reduced genital sensation, orgasmic dysfunction, decreased libido, vaginal dryness, and dyspareunia.

A complete neurologic evaluation should be undertaken for patients with MS and sexual dysfunction. Consultation with a urologist or physiatrist should be obtained when needed (e.g., for catheter management or treatment of spasticity). The treatment of common sexual dysfunctions is discussed in Chapter 20.

VII. Epilepsy.

A. Evaluation and diagnostic overview.

1. *Overview.*

Seizures may be classified into one of two groups: (1) *partial or focal seizures,* which have an onset in a portion of one cerebral hemisphere and (2) *generalized seizures,* which involve the entire brain at their onset. Within the group of partial seizures are *simple partial seizures* (focal seizures) and *complex partial seizures* (CPSs) (temporal lobe epilepsy, psychomotor seizures). Partial seizures can secondarily generalize to grand mal seizures. Within the generalized group are *nonconvulsive absence seizures* (petit mal) and *tonic-clonic seizures* (grand mal seizures), all of which are frequently seen in psychiatric and primary care practices. The treatment of these specific subtypes is described in this section.

An aura precedes 60% of complex partial or secondarily generalized seizures; the phenomenology varies, depending on the seizure's focal origins. For example, visual distortion of size, shape, and arrangement arise from disturbances in the posterior temporal lobe, whereas foul smells or tastes arise from the medial temporal lobe. The aura's manifestations can be almost any symptom or experiential phenomenon.

Absence seizures occur almost exclusively in children, although absence status can infrequently occur in adults. Adults present with an episode of extended confusional behavior or an ictal psychosis. Absence seizures may stop during adolescence, but, in certain epilepsies, they may continue, with grand mal seizures.

During CPSs, the patient has a detached appearance, cannot perform obviously purposeful goal-directed tasks, and may, rarely, become nondirectionally violent, especially if restrained. Behaviors and experiences represent snippets of the person's entire behavioral and experiential profile. By definition, CPSs involve impaired consciousness; automatisms, such as clumsy perseverative motor tasks (groping, "searching"), lip smacking, and repetitive swallowing, occur frequently. The same sequence of CPS events usually occurs with each seizure. In the current world literature, only a few persuasive case reports of extended periods of semipurposeful and goal-directed activity have been published.

An epileptic prodrome may precede any type of seizure by minutes or hours. The prodrome is characterized, for example, by uncomfortable feelings of apprehension, irritability, and distractibility.

Generalized grand mal seizures start with abrupt loss of consciousness and loss of postural tone, immediately followed by bilateral extension of the trunk and limbs (tonic phase); during this time the mouth is open, emitting an "epileptic cry" (guttural noise); and the head may be turned to one side. Thereafter, the mouth clenches shut, and synchronous muscle jerking begins (clonic phase). Excessive salivation causes "frothing at the mouth"; tongue biting is common, urination is less common, and bowel incontinence is least common.

Termination of either a generalized or a partial seizure consists of a confusional state that may last for minutes (mostly in CPSs) to hours. Given the complex behavioral profile of CPSs and confusional states, it is often impossible to separate the ictal from the postictal state. After a generalized seizure, the patient is briefly unarousable, then lethargic and confused, and sleep is the preferred activity.

2. *Interictal behavioral disturbances.*

Psychiatric behavioral phenomena usually appear in a patient with a known history of epilepsy rather than with the onset of the first seizures. Patients with simple partial seizures have psychiatric conditions at a rate similar to that in the general population, whereas those with a lengthy history of severe generalized or complex partial seizures have a high rate of psychiatric conditions. These *interictal alterations* are of four types: (1) *personality changes,* (2) *dementia,* (3) *depression,* and (4) *psychosis.* Interictal manic-depressive disorder is rare in epileptics. Long-term exposure to antiseizure medicines is thought to influence the various behavioral attributes.

3. *The epilepsy personality.*
The epileptic personality and CPSs are often partners because of the peculiar features of the temporal lobe, perhaps because the association is a product of patient selection bias. Although 50% to 75% of seizure patients have personalities well within the normal range, personality disorders are more common among seizure patients, in general, than in the population at large. Regardless, the epileptic personality has been best characterized concurrent with CPSs in cases in which extremes of behavior, values, emotions, and attitudes exist. The most common features are obsessionalism, circumstantiality, humorlessness, irritability, dysthymia, altered sexual interest, hypergraphia, and hypermoralism. Interpersonal contacts are "viscous" or "sticky" (i.e., a discussion while "walking through oatmeal"). The experience is of a labored, slow conversation that is oversubscribed with details and excessively concrete and from which there is no ready escape. Knowledge of these characteristics is helpful in establishing a behavioral baseline against which new complaints that are suggestive of depression or dementia can be contrasted. Often, these "new" complaints are simply progressive extensions of existing personality traits, now recognized in the context of a psychosocial stressor; treatment consists of problem clarification and problem solving that needs several repetitions and avoids abstractions. Dementia and depression are diagnosed when the typical but inordinate deviations from baseline are found.

4. *Epilepsy with dementia.*
The slowly progressive dementias of epilepsy stem from the cerebral insults preceding, precipitating, and/or following epilepsy, coupled with frequent seizure-associated hypoxia and toxic antiseizure medication levels. This profile describes medically refractory seizures, and, indeed, *patients with medically refractory seizures are at high risk for eventual dementia.* In general, left-hemisphere foci impair verbal functions, and right-hemisphere foci impair visuospatial performance. Memory and learning disorders are inevitable after years of poorly controlled seizures. Treatment is similar to that considered in the dementia section of this chapter and takes into account the effects of antiepilepsy medications.

B. Differential diagnosis.

Nonepileptic seizures (pseudogenic or psychogenic seizures) develop from opposing ideas, feelings, and emotions; are under some voluntary control; and occur in 20% of patients with actual epilepsy. Although a few minutes of arrhythmic, asynchronous pelvic thrusting, arm flailing, and general thrashing about describe the classic nonepileptic patient, frontal lobe epilepsy, a relatively uncommon epilepsy, can have similar bizarre manifestations that usually have a brief duration. For many patients, the diagnosis of non-epileptic seizures is made by a combination of in-patient video-EEG monitoring and a compelling psychiatric formulation (e.g., the student who is about to start college who expresses a desire to leave home but has overwhelming dependency needs).

The differential diagnosis of seizures includes transient ischemic attacks (which do not usually lead to loss of consciousness), syncope (subsequent extended confusion or sleepiness is uncommon, as is preceding nausea, weakness, sweating, or dizziness), migraine (concurrent visual field defects and photophobia), and various toxic-metabolic conditions, such as hypoglycemia. Parasomnias occur in children and in adults. In children, they predictably occur in the early part of the sleep cycle, and motor behavior is slow and trancelike. In adults, the automatic behavior syndrome is accompanied by excessive daytime sleepiness.

C. Epidemiology and pathophysiology.

About 1 million Americans are receiving treatment for a seizure disorder, and CPSs are the most common of newly diagnosed adult cases across age groups. The incidence of epilepsy is stable through adult life (15/100,000/y) and slowly increases after age 50 to 130/100,000/y at age 75. The increasing numbers are due, in part, to concurrent increases in occlusive vascular disease, Alzheimer's disease (AD), and alcoholism; however, 50% of newly identified cases have no clear etiology.

CPSs arise from hypersynchronous electrical discharges from neurons in the temporal, frontal, occipital, or parietal brain regions. Foci in the temporal lobe account for 70% of CPSs and provide the basis for the near-equivalent name *temporal lobe epilepsy.* The abnormal brain activity produces complex behaviors characterized by changes in subjective experience, mood and emotion, memory, consciousness, and cognition and usually by bizarre observed behaviors. These seizure-related symptoms make for behaviors that suggest psychiatric conditions. Most CPSs resolve within 2 minutes; prolonged CPSs occur infrequently but can result in mental status changes that may continue for hours or weeks.

D. Laboratory and neuropsychology.

New major psychiatric syndromes with a history of episodic, paroxysmal behavior require careful neurologic examination, and any new findings necessitate further studies. These may include an EEG, imaging, and a spinal tap. *Results of a routine EEG are unremarkable for 40% of patients diagnosed clinically.* Sleep deprivation, photic stimulation, and special electrode placement for two subsequent EEGs increase the yield, but in 10% to 25% of patients, results are still unremarkable. In contrast, epileptiform discharges occur in 1% to 4% of normal healthy children and in 3% of ill adults, all of whom have no epileptic behavior. Therefore, the interictal or routine EEG does not unequivocally make the diagnosis, which must always be made in the context of the entire clinical situation.

Neuropsychological testing must be ordered for the purpose of sorting out the relative contributions from (1) personality and emotional disturbances versus brain disease, (2) psychological versus cognitive impairment, and (3) epileptic versus pseudoepileptic or nonepileptic seizures. Testing results are usually unsatisfying when the differential diagnosis is the most perplexing. Quantification of the relative contributions from the aforementioned attributes must often wait for the appearance of definite neurologic signs or of a typical illness course identified over time. Nevertheless, a baseline of test results enables the comparison of subsequent results *from the same test battery;* with this method, progressive changes or their absence is usually diagnostically helpful. Both because nonepileptic and epileptic seizures often coexist in the same patient and because patients with nonepileptic seizures are heterogeneous, neuropsychological testing finds few if any distinguishing features between these two states, unless functional cognitive complaints, psychosis, or depression are present.

E. General management guidelines.

Psychopharmacologic treatment must take into account the medications used for seizure control and drug-drug interactions that affect antiepileptic blood levels (see Chapter 2). Moreover, paradoxical responses to antidepressants are likely, and *all antidepressants have the potential for lowering the seizure threshold.* In this regard, the antidepressants recommended later carry an acceptable level of risk, provided that the "go slow, stay low" dictum is followed. *Psychoactive agents are most proconvulsant when they are introduced rapidly and at high doses.*

Psychiatric drugs are highly protein bound and may displace anticonvulsants from binding sites, and both compete for liver metabolism. These mechanisms may lead to either increases or decreases in blood levels of free drug for both the anticonvulsant and the neuroleptic. For example, carbamazepine (Tegretol) may lower haloperidol (Haldol) levels by as much as 60%, thereby increasing the risk for recurrent psychosis.

The new antiepileptics lamotrigine (Lamictal) and gabapentin (Neurontin), like their predecessors, will surely be associated with various potential emotional effects. Gabapentin was associated with hypomania in one report. Interactions with psychiatric drugs are likely with any new CNS agent, and careful monitoring is recommended.

Vigabatrin (Sabril) remains investigational in the United States; it may become available in the near future. Mood problems are a major reason for vigabatrin discontinuation, and vigabatrin psychosis has been reported.

F. Depression and epilepsy affective syndrome.

The recognition of interictal depression in patients with epilepsy is important because suicide risk is 7%, five times higher than in the general population (1.4%), and 30% of depressed patients with epilepsy attempt suicide. Unfortunately, depression in epilepsy lacks definitional criteria because most patients have so many atypical features that there is often too little resemblance to typical depression; thus, depression in epilepsy may be a unique affective syndrome. *Epilepsy affective syndrome* is characterized by *any combination* of mood-congruent hallucinations or delusions, paranoia, irritability, and rapid shifting moods with predominant dysphoria or frank depression, superimposed on a personality baseline of chronic dysthymia. Nevertheless, about 10% to 20% of all depressions in epilepsy have the typical depressive symptoms (e.g., sleep, appetite, and interest disturbances) admixed with epilepsy affective syndrome.

1. *Risk factors.*
   The elderly patient with epilepsy is particularly prone to depression. Depression is associated with complex partial seizures from left-sided temporal lobe foci.

2. *Medication management.*
   a. *Recommended treatments. Two new antidepressants are equally effective and may be less epileptogenic than others: fluvoxamine (Luvox) and nefazodone (Serzone); these are reasonable first*

choices. Fluvoxamine is an SSRI that is an effective antidepressant but has been approved only for use in obsessive-compulsive disorders. One recent report claims that fluoxetine (Prozac) acts as an anticonvulsant in some patients.

If possible, carbamazepine (Tegretol) or divalproex sodium (Depakote) should be substituted for antiepilepsy drugs that promote depression (especially phenobarbital; less so, phenytoin); carbamazepine may help control recurrent dysphoria and irritability.

b. *Possible treatments.* Any one of the following is equally effective in the treatment of depression: fluoxetine (Prozac), sertraline (Zoloft), desipramine (Norpramin). The lowest effective dose should be used. These drugs lower the seizure threshold, but the effect is usually of little clinical significance unless the drugs are rapidly introduced.

Antidepressants with marked anticholinergic and/or proconvulsant properties (e.g., maprotiline [Ludiomil], amoxapine [Asendin], bupropion [Wellbutrin], amitriptyline [Elavil], imipramine [Tofranil], clomipramine [Anafranil], and nortriptyline [Pamelor]) should be avoided.

c. *Innovative protocols.* Gabapentin (Neurontin) and lamotrigine (Lamictal) are new and somewhat atypical antiepileptics. Interestingly, gabapentin may improve cognitive, affective, and social behaviors in some patients. Some patients receiving lamotrigine report an elevation in mood; however, recent reports suggest that lamotrigine has antimanic properties. Although these effects remain to be clarified (and they may simply represent a response to improved seizure control or a reduction in adverse affects) when other antiepileptic drugs are withdrawn, a patient with epilepsy who has a severe form of epilepsy affective syndrome might benefit from the use of one of these agents.

G. Psychosis.

The chronic interictal psychotic disorder associated with epilepsy is an active aroused behavioral state that is schizophrenic-like; "quiet" behaviors, such as blunted emotions and social withdrawal, are uncharacteristic, and the premorbid personality is not schizoid. This chronic psychosis is largely unmodified by the use of psychotropic agents.

Alternating psychosis or *forced normalization* is an acute state of epilepsy-related psychosis that appears with a temporary period (e.g., several days) of total or near-total disappearance of seizures. This acute psychosis is often treated with antipsychotic agents. The immediate postictal psychosis or delirium that sometimes follows a single seizure or a prolonged seizure almost always self-resolves.

1. *Risk factors.*
   Episodes of acute psychosis are concurrent with an absence of seizures or a significantly reduced seizure frequency compared with a previous baseline. Periods of frequent seizure activity are generally unaccompanied by psychosis; however, flurries of seizures may result in psychosis and subsequent reduced seizure activity. Patients with CPSs are at the highest risk; left-sided, temporal lobe foci also place patients at risk.

2. *Medication management.*
   a. *Recommended treatments. All antipsychotics lower the seizure threshold;* any of the following antipsychotics is least epileptogenic, and all are equally effective: fluphenazine (Prolixin), haloperidol (Haldol), molindone (Moban), and thioridazine (Mellaril). Anticonvulsant levels must be monitored because they usually are altered during antipsychotic administration.
   b. *Possible treatments.* Neuroleptics with anticholinergic or proconvulsant properties (chlorpromazine [Thorazine], risperidone [Risperdal]) should be avoided because they lower seizure threshold. Clozapine (Clozaril) infrequently induces seizures in patients without epilepsy, so it should be avoided as well.

H. Behavior management of epileptic seizures.

Because psychic life and a neuropsychiatric illness are as closely linked as the mind is to brain and behavior, changes in thought content, feeling states, and daily activities can alter epileptic seizure frequency. *Although the patient who has seizures is not responsible for his or her seizures, behavior management provides tools that may reduce seizure frequency.*

Seizures may be triggered by specific circumstances and situations. This is a type of learning, conditioning, and activation against which countermeasures can be used with some success in about 25% to 35% of patients. The term *reflex seizures* has been used to describe this phenomenon: visual cues, fatigue, interpersonal stress, particular activities, thoughts, and feelings may trigger seizure activity for these patients. Some patients know of mental strategies they can use to suppress their seizures. Knowledge about triggers comes from a two-column log of "possible triggers" and "likely consequences" that patients should be asked to keep. Data collection and hypothesis generation are the main goals. The patient should be asked to record those emotional and behavioral events that happen in the hours or minutes just before the seizure onset (i.e., possible triggers) and to also record what happens in the minutes and hours immediately after a seizure (i.e., possible consequences). Consequences of particular interest are any changes in the behavior or actions of people who in any way might be affected by the seizure. For example, the patient's feeling of anger may provide the trigger for a seizure that, in turn, keeps the parent or spouse at home.

The data collection and log keeping should be a project for everyone who is immediately involved with the patient; participants might include parents and teenager or husband and wife, for example. Separate logs need to be kept, and participants should be asked not to discuss their observations until the doctor is present. This method is introduced by a statement such as

> Seizures may sometimes have triggers that are unknown to both the patient and the family. It is important that we not prejudge these triggers. (Many physicians make this explicit.) Mom and Dad, please don't share information in any way. Some parents want to prove their suspicions, and this is not helpful. What is helpful is the collection of unbiased data.

When, for example, parents report very similar data, the doctor needs to investigate the reason for such similarity.

Sometimes, no triggers are found. The physician may state

> It is all too easy to think of seizures as a means to get attention, and this simple explanation is hardly ever the answer. We all need to keep an open mind and just collect data independently; we are only generating hypotheses at this point.

It is important to insulate the patient and family from theories, such as that the behavior is "attention getting," that only serve to stir up animosity. If a theory like this pre-exists the data collection, it is often better to have the patient alone collect data, assuming that the patient is willing to consider that some triggers may be associated with some unmet need.

The goal for the primary care doctor is to identify triggers or, at least, to gather enough data to suggest that triggers exist. Once this is accomplished, referral to a behavioral psychologist or psychiatrist is appropriate for the development and prescription of specific countermeasures. Contingency management, relaxation, biofeedback, and desensitization are possible prescriptions. When used by itself, counseling or psychotherapy has not been found to be a very successful strategy.

I. Nonepileptic seizures, pseudoseizures, psychogenic seizures, and other names.

1. *Differential diagnosis.*
Nonepileptic seizures is the term we prefer to describe a set of behaviors that in many ways mimic epilepsy but that are produced by emotional events. These phenomena are sudden paroxysmal experiences that are interpreted as being epileptic-like. Moreover, the patient's belief is that the event is quite real and beyond the usual means of voluntary control.

Nonepileptic seizures mimic all types of epilepsy. The pattern of behavior may include just about every symptom associated with epilepsy: 55% of patients have premonitory sensations or auras, and 15% have urinary incontinence and minor self-injuries, such as tongue biting. Coughing, gagging, and foaming can occur. Falls may be frequent, but major, severe injuries are rare, as is fecal incontinence. Nonepileptic seizures occur in public places or places with several witnesses. The most common behaviors include asynchronous, inconstant motor activity with back arching, kicking, slapping, striking out, side-to-side movements of the head and trunk, and pelvic thrusting; long episodes of unresponsiveness; and recall for some features and for surrounding events. *One third of patients with epilepsy have a mixture of epileptic and nonepileptic seizures;* however, with isolated nonepileptic events, postictal confusion is short term or absent unless the patient simulates an ongoing caricature of confusion.

In addition to the common behaviors, other *diagnostic clues include a past or immediate history of emotional, interpersonal, or affective disturbance; weeping during the event; avoidance, for example, to visual threat or arm drop maneuvers; visual fixation on the examiner; and such goal-directed behaviors as a painful hand-grip on the arm of an observer.*

The differential diagnosis includes syncope, cataplexy, parasomnias, sleep attacks, migraine, panic attacks, psychotic hallucinations, hypoglycemia, paroxysmal dystonia, pheochromocytoma, third ventricular cysts, and Arnold-Chiari malformation.

2. *Laboratory and neuropsychological tests.*
The EEG is completely normal in 50% of patients; background and temporal slowing is frequently reported. The most definitive diagnosis is made by simultaneous video and EEG monitoring, which are available in major medical centers. Some investigators support the diagnosis by finding no elevation in serum prolactin level after a nonepileptic seizure, but such neurohormonal measurements are too insensitive to be used for routine diagnostic purposes.

No one cognitive or personality profile predicts nonepileptic seizures; these patients perform within normal limits on neuropsychological tests. Somatization and psychosomatic symptoms may be more common in patients with nonepileptic seizures.

3. *Epidemiology and risk factors.*
Patients with nonepileptic seizures make up 12% of refractory epilepsy clinic patients, 75% are female, and patients with a first episode after the age of 55 are rare. Risk factors include somatization or personality disorder, history of childhood loss or abuse, history of contact with a model for seizure symptoms, and history of or concurrent major depression with or without anxiety features. In our experience, chronic interpersonal conflict around goals, limited intellectual abilities, nonassertiveness, and various forms of depression are most frequently associated with nonepileptic seizures.

4. *Treatment.*
A lengthy history of nonepileptic seizures, a poor work history, and the patient's satisfaction with, and adoption of, an epileptic lifestyle are features that generally make a patient almost untreatable. Such patients usually remain disabled. The chances for change are greatly increased by a family and support system that values independence and has the curiosity to seriously investigate the possibility of nonepileptic seizures and is willing to make lifestyle changes when indicated. *Treatment is usually successful when the nonepileptic seizures occur in a young person and are of recent onset, and the nonepileptic seizures are concurrent with loss, bereavement, guilt, depression, or a change in personal direction* (Case Study).

The "good news!" strategy is one method for treating nonepileptic seizures; other possible strategies are described in Chapter 6. If the good news strategy is used, the physician needs to be reasonably certain that the problem is nonepileptic seizures.

Case Study

Tom is 17 years old, and he recently began driving independently. He has taken the driver's education course in his high school, and his easily angered father, who has high expectations, has given Tom hours of on-road instruction. Because they often argue, Tom's father wants to better the relationship and feels that they might "bond better" if he helps teach Tom how to drive. Unfortunately, Tom crashes the family's late-model car in an accident that brings Tom to the hospital semiconscious with minor lacerations and a closed head injury. Tom begins to regain consciousness in the ambulance, and by the time he arrives at his hospital room, he has a normal mental status on bedside testing. While his parents are on the way to the hospital, Tom has two "seizures." On arrival, Tom's mother is thankful that her son is alive, and Tom's father is beside himself, seemingly not knowing whether to "kill that damn kid" or be understanding and grateful. At the bedside, the doctors feel that Tom's father's behavior is hard to read; "he is obviously trying hard to contain his emotions." Tom continues to have "seizures" that are quickly diagnosed as nonepileptic.

Tom's physician uses the good news strategy by first telling Tom's parents that Tom is really lucky: he has nonepileptic seizures. The physician is careful to tell Tom's mother and father that *nonepileptic seizures are real;* the "good news" is that they are motivated by emotions and not by electrical events in the brain. The better news is that nonepileptic seizures are highly treatable, not with drugs, but with counseling.

Physician: *Why would Tom be upset?*

Father (angrily): *He almost lost his life; isn't that enough?*

Physician: *Maybe. But we see a lot of kids who could have died, and Tom is the first one I've seen recently with nonepileptic seizures.*

Mother: *Tom has to be afraid (his father) is going to kill him. Mother (to her husband): You just won't let Tom make a mistake; you're always on his case.*

Physician: *Let me talk to Tom, but for the moment let's not be angry with him or each other. This isn't the time for anger.*

The doctor makes sure she has a half hour to be alone with Tom. Tom receives the "good news." He is told that nonepileptic seizures are a real illness, but an illness caused by emotions.

Physician: *Nonepileptic seizures are very common. (pause) Is something bothering you, Tom?*

Tom is evasive.

Tom: *I was really scared that I was going to die. I don't know. Things seem pretty crazy lately. I guess I'm bummed out from studying so much. I never have any time to go out with my friends.*

Physician: *These are good thoughts, but you haven't mentioned Mom and Dad.*

Eventually, the doctor learns all about Tom's father's anger and expectations.

Tom: *I just know he is real pissed about the accident and the car.*

Physician: *Maybe I can help.*

Thereafter, Tom and his parents are brought together, the situation is re-explained, and the various emotional triggers are described—Tom's fear of the father's reaction and "understandable" anger and Tom's worries about school. At some point, Tom's father says, "Tom I love you. Of course, I was angry, that's me, but I feel so lucky you're alive, son, and that's all that counts now." The doctor reinforces these themes, and says, "I hope the seizures will become more infrequent," Tom has no more seizures, and the family is referred to a psychologist to better deal with the recent events and to make sure the nonepileptic seizures do not recur.

Discussion of case example.

The diagnosis was reframed and legitimized as being caused by emotions. Everyone was told that the problem is usually quite treatable. In a nonjudgmental way, the doctor dealt with the emotional issues and seemingly ignored the behavior. Note that the first, easy causal answers (e.g., Tom's nearly dying) were not the real motivators of the behavior. Tom was never told to give up the behavior; he was told that he would get better, and counseling, rather than pharmacologic treatment, was the path. Tom was allowed to "save face." There was a subtle shift in the family's "balance of power"; Tom and his mother were given some new means of control, and Tom's father was counseled to not be quite as critical, yet was told that his anger was "understandable." Thus, Tom's father, too, could save face. Could it be that the crash was motivated in part by Tom's anger at himself, his father, and his worries about school underperformance? These are all themes that could be usefully explored in continued counseling.

VIII. Counseling guidelines across disorders.

A. Recommended approach for patients and caregivers.

Neuropsychiatric illnesses are much the same as any chronic or progressive illness. The overall goal is improvement of the relationship between the illness and the emotional and behavioral responses of a particular patient and his or her caregivers. This goal is reached by use of one or many of the following approaches.

1. *Providing coping strategies and psychosocial support.*
Any chronic or progressive illness is a stress, and the patient's and caregiver's subsequent behaviors may be seen as reactions to stress. Such reactions are influenced by coping strategies, the availability and quality of social supports, the explanatory beliefs and attitudes, the perceptions of control, and the patient's self-image. By examining each of these variables separately, identifying the dysfunctional components of each one, and taking corrective action, the physician can sometimes help to make improvements.
The patient and family often view their circumstances as some sort of catastrophe. Every disaster that has ever been reported to be associated with their illness is perceived to be the definite immediate and long-term consequences of their condition. The *physician's approach is to "decatastrophize" the circumstances by fostering coping skills and by dealing with inflated probability estimates of threatening disaster and the underestimation of problem-solving skills and better outcomes.* Reframing tools are used to accomplish this goal.

2. *Reframing in terms of handicap.*
The conceptual tools for reframing are based on the following hierarchical set of ideas: (1) *Impairment* references a specific brain-related function, such as memory or motor control, and leads to statements about memory impairment and so forth. (2) *Disability* references a specific activity or behavior; for example, motor impairment may cause disabilities in walking or talking. (3) *Handicap* references a specific biopsychosocial disadvantage; for example, a memory or walking disability may prevent independent grocery shopping or self-care, resulting in a diminished quality of life. Rather than catastrophizing, successful handicapped patients and their caregivers focus on maximizing quality of life by isolating and prioritizing specific tasks, identifying those that can be accomplished, and using a device or strategy to achieve the desired outcome. Patients and caregivers should be counseled to reframe their thinking and behavior along these lines.
For example, the mild-to-moderately impaired patient with AD cannot function in most kitchens because the location of various items cannot be recalled. That same patient may be able to make or to help make coffee (i.e., the desired outcome) if all the necessary ingredients are in one location and in plain sight (i.e., the strategy). Being able to do something for others (like make coffee) is, after all, one meaning of fulfillment and one way to add quality to life. This person may also wish to wash and dry dishes, but a visuoperceptual impairment and a disability of hand-eye coordination may make him or her likely to drop and break a dish. This problem can be solved by the purchase of inexpensive plastic dishes at a resale shop. These examples illustrate the need for everyone involved with the patient to make a commitment to making accommodations and changing behaviors. Often, there is no lack of creativity; there *is* an unwillingness to give up a former lifestyle, and this, too, is a subject for counseling.
With progressive impairment and disability, former strategies for overcoming a handicap may no longer work. Some outcomes may no longer be possible. For this dilemma, the process of engagement, disengagement, and alternative re-engagement needs to be taught as part of the natural course of the disease. Specifically, when it becomes necessary to disengage from making the coffee, an alternative task must be found for re-engagement. If the coffee cannot be made, maybe the (plastic) coffee cups can be moved from the counter to the table, or the clean towels can be folded. Whatever specific tasks are

used, the idea is to provide a means for the patient to make a contribution and for the caretaker to be able to display enthusiasm and appreciation. None of these strategies work when caretakers are bitter and angry.

3. *Reframing in terms of "excessive" disability.* A neuropsychiatric illness, such as depression, makes every disability worse. Depression further disables the patient with Parkinson's disease (PD) and thereby makes dressing slower and talking more difficult. The depressed patient with AD has even more difficulty with attention and concentration and, as a result of depression, may be unable to make coffee. The point is that depression or other neuropsychiatric disorders make existing disabilities worse. The doctor's task is to acknowledge the reality of the permanent disability and then maintain that the depression adds unnecessary or excessive additional disability. Moreover, with successful treatment for depression, improvements in task performance and outcome are often possible.

4. *Considering the obvious but overlooked. A patient with a chronic progressive disease needs a safe, predictable, uncluttered, and well-lighted environment that is relatively free of unanticipated intrusions from noise, visitors, and events.* Often, such problems as agitation can be solved by inquiry about, and attention to, changing these factors.

   Caregiver burden and burnout need to be addressed by motivational counseling concerning the need for personal time, permission to ask for and accept help from others, and permission to make mistakes. No correct answers exist to these problems; there are only reasonable answers, and a mind open to advice and a spirit able to sustain disappointments are assets. In most communities, social workers or other professionals specialize in making resources available. Respite care and a Hoyer lift may be more helpful than counseling sessions.

B. Common pitfalls.

1. *"You would be depressed too if you had (insert name of disease)."* This is a common patient or family response to the doctor's recommendations for treatment of depression concurrent with neuropsychiatric or medical conditions. The assumptions behind this assertion are that all patients would be depressed under similar circumstances, that depression and suffering are to be expected, and that the situation is hopeless or unlikely to improve—it is just going to get worse. Moreover, the doctor may be easily persuaded to have the same opinion. Certainly, there are dying patients for whom all these assumptions apply, but for others, many or all are simply wrong. For each patient, these assumptions need to be carefully examined and reconsidered in light of the aforementioned approach.

2. *"My father (with AD) will learn to spell better (or master another task) if we do lots of practice drills."* This is a conviction about dementia that is held by many caregivers. After all, it is common experience that difficult memory tasks are accomplished by drilling and hard work—not so for a demented person with significant memory impairment. Caregivers should be informed that these unrealistic beliefs are a source of frustration and friction that may lay the foundation for depression. Caregivers would not ask a person with a broken leg to practice jogging. Caregiver efforts would be better spent being creative about how to compensate for handicaps.

3. *"Why should I set goals? There is no way to enjoy life."* These are common assertions that require the following direct answers:

   These statements are a form of catastrophizing or "awfulizing." Experience is not made up of all-or-none events. Patients can be less sad and more happy. Goals are needed, and plans must be made to ensure the best quality of life possible. Your life will be improved by taking a more positive attitude and an active role in your day-to-day activities and medical care.

4. *"We (the caregivers) cannot say or do anything that might hurt." "I (the patient) want my caregivers to try harder and be more considerate."* It is important for caregivers, friends, and colleagues to feel comfortable expressing their concerns and feelings, to have expectations of appropriate behavior in return, and to use assertive strategies to request behavioral change. It is unrealistic for the patient to expect everyone to behave sympathetically at all times. The patient needs to take some responsibility; if the patient insists on forcing his or her problem on others, those others will become angry and begin to withdraw. The doctor can be of considerable assistance by counseling the patient and family to help them understand these points and to help them change their behavior accordingly.

Case Study

After a bad flair, Mrs. M., a patient with MS, decides to return to work. Unfortunately, her condition is now worse and necessitates the use of a three-legged cane. Initially, colleagues at work are sympathetic and accommodating. In time, however, these same colleagues begin to have less time to talk about Mrs. M.'s rough life. Moreover, less help is spontaneously offered, and

Mrs. M. finds that she has to ask for assistance. A subtle atmosphere of mutual resentment exists.

During a primary care office visit, the doctor complements Mrs. M. on having the courage to go back to work so soon. "Nobody cares" and "I'm about to quit" are the replies. The doctor says "Can we talk about it first?" and a half-hour appointment is scheduled. At the subsequent meeting, the doctor gets a description of what's going on, listens to Mrs. M.'s perception of the events, and discusses how awful and unbearable the situation must be for her. Then, the doctor asks Mrs. M. to look at things through the eyes of the coworkers. The following conversation ensues:

Physician: *How would you feel at work if you had to go out of your way all the time for a handicapped person?*

Mrs. M.: *I'd do my best to help!*

Physician: *How would you feel after a month of doing your best?*

Eventually, the point is made that regardless of what is moral and right, people are going to resent having to stop their work for a handicapped person who too often wants to talk about the difficulties in his or her life.

Physician: *It's good therapy for you to keep working, but you may have to do some things to encourage your colleagues to make it possible for you to continue work and be happy.*

The doctor kindly suggests more expressions of "thank you," less talk about the difficulties of Mrs. M.'s life, and more talk about how tough it is for the patient's office mates and suggests that Mrs. M. bring in some cookies for her coworkers at the office. At every future office visit, the doctor helps Mrs. M. cope with the reality of her situation.

Selected References

Alzheimer's Disease

Knesper DJ. The depressions of Alzheimer's disease: Sorting, pharmacotherapeutics, and clinical advice. J Geriatr Psychiatry Neurol 1995; 8(Suppl.1):S40–S51.

McGovern RJ, Koss E. The use of behavior modification with Alzheimer patients: Values and limitations. Alzheimer Dis Assoc Disord 1994; 8(Suppl. 3):82–91.

Robinson A, Spencer B, White L. Understanding Difficult Behaviors. Ann Arbor: Geriatric Education Center of Michigan; 1990.

Parkinson's Disease

Huber SJ, Cummings JL, Editors. Parkinson's Disease: Neurobehavioral Aspects. New York: Oxford University Press; 1992.

Weiner WJ, Lang AE, Editors. Advances in Neurology: Behavioral Neurology of Movement Disorders Vol 65. New York: Raven Press; 1995.

Human Immunodeficiency Virus and Acquired Immunodeficiency Syndrome

Cohen MAA, Alfonso CA. Psychiatric manifestations of the HIV epidemic. AIDS Reader 1994; 4(3):97–106.

Janicak PG. Psychopharmacotherapy in the HIV-infected patient. Psychiatric Ann 1995; 25:609–613.

Perry SW. HIV-related depression. Res Publ Assoc Res Nerv Ment Dis 1994; 72:223–238.

Stroke

Laidler P. Stroke Rehabilitation: Structure and Strategy. San Diego: Singular Publishing Group; 1994.

Lazarus LW, Winemiller DR, Lingam VR, et al. Efficacy and side effects of methylphenidate for poststroke depression. J Clin Psychiatry 1992; 53:447–449.

Multiple Sclerosis

Grant I. Psychosomatic-somatopsychic aspects of multiple sclerosis. In: Halbreich U, Editor. Multiple Sclerosis: A Neuropsychiatric Disorder. Washington, DC: American Psychiatric Press; 1993.

Minden S, Schiffer R. Depression and affective disorders in multiple sclerosis. In: Halbreich U, Editor. Multiple Sclerosis: A Neuropsychiatric Disorder. Washington, DC: American Psychiatric Press; 1993.

Whitham RH. Cognitive and emotional disorders in multiple sclerosis. In: Herndon RM, Seil FJ, Editors. Multiple Sclerosis: Current Status of Research and Treatment. New York: Demos Vermande; 1994.

Epilepsy

Perrine K, Congett S. Neurobehavioral problems in epilepsy. Neurol Clin 1994; 12:129–152.

Smith DB, Treiman D, Trimble M. Advances in Neurology: Neurobehavioral Problems in Epilepsy Vol 55. New York: Raven Press; 1990.

Appendix

Mini-Mental State Exam (MMSE)*

The MMSE is, perhaps, the most widely used screening instrument for cognitive dysfunction. It can be administered in less than 10 minutes. Scores are primarily used for identifying dementia; a score of 23 or below (out of a possible 30) is consistent with dementia, and scores of 18 or less suggest significant impairment. For well-educated persons, a score of 25 or below is considered by some to be consistent with dementia. Sensitivity for non-dominant, hemispheric lesions or frontal lobe impairment is limited; the MMSE is not designed to distinguish delirium from dementia. The MMSE is less likely to pick up dementia in patients with mild impairment, and it is unlikely to pick up dementia in patients with a prior superior intellect who have become demented after a decline to "average" performance.

Registration and recall testing uses three simple items, such as apple, nickle, and bug. Standard practice is to begin serial 7 subtraction with "100 subtract 7." If the patient was really never good at mathematics, asking the patient to spell "world" backwards is a standard substitute.

For reading and obeying the command "close your eyes," the patient is presented with the written command "close your eyes," and the patient is simply asked to read and follow the instructions on the page. Somewhat involved procedures are available for scoring the patient's drawing of the interlocking pentagons. In practice, the "eyeball method" works well (e.g., a point is given if the patient's drawing is far worse than the doctor's).

*From Folstein MF, Folstein SE, McHugh PR. Mini-Mental State: A practical method for grading the cognitive state of patients for the clinician. J Psychiatr Res 1975; 12:189–198. Elsevier Science Ltd, Oxford, England, with permission.

Mini-Mental State Exam and Instructions

Patient
Examiner
Date

Mini-Mental State Exam

Maximum score	Score	
		Orientation
5	( )	What is the (year) (season) (date) (day) (month)?
5	( )	Where are we: (state) (county) (town) (hospital) (floor)?
		Registration
3	( )	Name 3 objects: 1 second to say each. Then ask the patient all 3 after you have said them. Give 1 point for each correct answer. Then repeat them until he learns all 3. Count trials and record. Trials
		Attention and Calculation
5	( )	Serial 7s. 1 point for each correct. Stop after 5 answers. Alternatively spell "world" backwards.
		Recall
3	( )	Ask for the 3 objects repeated above. Give 1 point for each correct.
		Language
9	( )	Name a pencil, and watch. (2 points) Repeat the following "No ifs, ands, or buts." (1 point) Follow a 3-stage command: "Take a paper in your right hand, fold it in half, and put it on the floor." (3 points) Read and obey the following: Close your eyes. (1 point) Write a sentence. (1 point) Copy design. (1 point) Total score
30	( )	Assess level of consciousness along a continuum:

Alert	Drowsy	Stupor	Coma

Orientation

1. Ask for the date. Then ask specifically for parts omitted, e.g., "Can you also tell me what season it is?" One point for each correct answer.
2. Ask in turn "Can you tell me the name of this hospital?" (town, county, etc.). One point for each correct answer.

Registration

Ask the patient if you may test his memory. Then say the names of 3 unrelated objects, clearly and slowly, about 1 second for each. After you have said all 3, ask him to repeat them. This first repetition determines his score (0–3) but keep saying them until he can repeat all 3, up to 6 trials. If he does not eventually learn all 3, recall cannot be meaningfully tested.

Attention and Calculation

Ask the patient to begin with 100 and count backwards by 7. Stop after 5 subtractions (93, 86, 79, 72, 65). Score the total number of correct answers.

If the patient cannot or will not perform this task, ask him or her to spell the word "world" backwards. The score is the number of letters in correct order, e.g., dlrow = 5, dlorw = 3.

Recall

Ask the patient if he can recall the 3 words you previously asked him to remember. Score 0–3.

Language

Naming: Show the patient a wrist watch and ask him or her what it is. Repeat for pencil. Score 0–2.

Repetition: Ask the patient to repeat the sentence after you. Allow only one trial. Score 0 or 1.

3-Stage command: Give the patient a piece of plain blank paper and repeat the command. Score 1 point for each part correctly executed.

Reading: On a blank piece of paper print the sentence. "Close your eyes", in letters large enough for the patient to see clearly. Ask him to read it and do what it says. Score 1 point only if he actually closes his eyes.

Writing: Give the patient a blank piece of paper and ask him to write a sentence for you. Do not dictate a sentence; it is to be written spontaneously. It must contain a subject and verb and be sensible. Correct grammar and punctuation are not necessary.

Copying: On a clean piece of paper, draw intersecting pentagons, each side about 1 in., and ask the patient to copy it exactly as it is. All 10 angles must be present and 2 must intersect to score 1 point. Tremor and rotation are ignored.

Estimate the patient's level of sensorium along a continuum, from alert on the left to coma on the right. (The MMSE is reliable only when it is administered to alert subjects.)

13

ALAN B. DOUGLASS, MD

MICHAEL S. ALDRICH, MD

Insomnia and Sleep Disorders

I. Evaluation and diagnostic overview.

Many sleep disorders are not obvious to the patient or bed partner because awareness is a product of the awake state. Current scientific knowledge about sleep disorders is younger than 15 years old, and new disorders are still being discovered. A large number of patients in primary practice have minor conditions that can be given a trial of treatment before sleep laboratory referral is considered.

Several commonly used terms have a specific meaning in sleep medicine. The term *insomnia* is a general concept that is akin to *fever*—it is not a sleep disorder diagnosis unless a cause is specified. Likewise, *narcolepsy* has been used for decades as a medical synonym for "excessive daytime sleepiness," but it is now known to be a specific inherited neurologic disorder that can be diagnosed by use of sleep laboratory analysis and human leukocyte antigen (HLA) tissue typing. The term *arousal* has the special meaning of an awakening from sleep (i.e., it has no sexual connotation).

Two major texts show the classification of the many sleep disorder diagnoses: the American Psychiatric Association's *Diagnostic and Statistical Manual of Mental Disorders, Fourth Edition* (DSM-IV)[1] and the *International Classification of Sleep Disorders*.[2] The DSM-IV classifies the major subtypes as

- *Dyssomnias:* disorders caused by pathology of the sleep mechanism itself, leading to trouble getting to sleep, staying asleep, or excessive daytime sleepiness.
- *Parasomnias:* disorders that intrude into sleep, such as unusual waking or motor activity.
- *Disorders related to another mental disorder:* disorders including disturbed sleep in major depression or anxiety disorders.
- *Disorders due to a general medical condition:* disorders such as chronic pain or chronic obstructive pulmonary disease, which interrupt continuous sleep by their own physiologic symptoms.

Most physicians in primary practice should have some understanding of the following conditions (prevalences in brackets):

- Narcolepsy (0.04%, same in males as in females).
- Obstructive sleep apnea (OSA) (3%).
- Periodic limb movements in sleep disorder (PLMD) and the restless legs syndrome (about 5%).
- Psychophysiologic insomnia, "primary insomnia" in DSM-IV (about 10%).
- Substance abuse insomnia, largely alcohol (about 15%?).
- Insomnia due to psychiatric disorders of mood or anxiety (4% to 6%).
- Insufficient sleep syndrome (about 30%).
- Delayed sleep phase syndrome (unknown).

A. The sleep history and differential diagnosis.

Psychiatric sleep disorders are diagnosed by history and by exclusion of physiologic sleep disorders. The latter can be identified objectively by use of polysomnographic monitoring in a sleep laboratory or by ambulatory equipment. A sleep history should be the first step in the assessment of a patient who has excessive sleepiness in the daytime, or insomnia. *The physician's questions should lead the patient through their usual 24-hour day with such questions as "What time do you usually go to bed?"* Then, the physician should ask "After you turn out the lights, how long does it take to get to sleep?" (10 to 15 minutes would be normal). To determine pattern of poor ability to sleep in the last third of the night, a characteristic of major depression, the physician should ask "Do you ever wake up during the night? How many times? Is this mainly after 3:00 a.m.?" Asking about pain or other attributable causes for waking at this point helps determine whether medical illnesses, such as paroxysmal nocturnal dyspnea, nocturnal angina, and gastroesophageal reflux, contribute to sleep disturbance. Next, the physician asks about waking up: "Do you use an alarm to wake up at the proper time?" "Do you sleep through your alarm?" "Do you use two or more alarm clocks to be sure of waking?" These questions assess the severity of excessive sleepiness. Some people arise with the alarm but are physically clumsy and uncoordinated for a while *(sleep drunkenness),* a symptom that can occur in OSA, narcolepsy, idiopathic hypersomnia, or delayed sleep phase syndrome.

Next, the physician assesses daytime sleepiness: "Do you fall asleep at your desk?" "Do you have near-miss accidents while driving?" "Have you ever fallen asleep at a stoplight?" If the sleepiness gradually clears by late morning, delayed sleep phase syndrome is a likely cause. If the daytime sleepiness is constant but relieved considerably by a 20-minute nap, narcolepsy or insufficient sleep syndrome are more likely diagnoses. Sometimes the daytime impairment is one of poor concentration, and the patient does not actually fall asleep. Good questions to ask are "Do you read a paragraph and then are not clear on what you just read?" "Do you have to reread entire pages before you comprehend simple explanations?"

Some other key signs and symptoms of the more serious sleep disorders are

- Loud snoring with breathing pauses (OSA).
- Obesity with new-onset hypertension or right-sided heart failure (OSA).
- Cataplexy—the sudden loss of motor tone on strong emotional expression (narcolepsy).
- Sleeping while driving (obstructive sleep apnea, narcolepsy, severe nocturnal sleep interruption).
- Day and night restless legs or cramps (restless legs syndrome).
- Initial insomnia caused by the patient's "mind being full of thoughts" (anxiety, psychophysiologic insomnia).
- "Early morning wakening," that is, the last third of the night (depression).
- Short weekday sleep period but much longer sleep period on weekends (insufficient sleep).
- Increasing demands for sedative-hypnotic prescriptions (substance abuse insomnia).
- Difficulty falling asleep at night and awakening in the morning (delayed sleep phase syndrome).

B. Laboratory tests.

A sleep laboratory is available at most referral centers. Two different tests are available. The *nocturnal polysomnogram* (NPSG) is an 8-hour all-night electroencephalographic test, with added measurements of breathing (air flow at nose, chest expansion, abdomen expansion), eye movements, muscle tone in the chin and legs, transcutaneous oximetry, electrocardiography, and other specialized measures as required. The NPSG results in a sleep graph that shows stages of sleep plus abnormalities in breathing or motor activity. The *multiple sleep latency test* is a daytime test, consisting of four or five naps of 20 minutes' duration each, that is usually performed on the day after the NPSG is completed. It tests the rapidity with which the patient falls asleep (sleep latency [SL]; Fig. 13–1), if at all. The average of all nap SLs provides an objective measure of daytime somnolence *(mean sleep latency)*. It is chiefly used to detect narcolepsy, which is the only major disorder that generates frequent episodes of rapid eye movement (REM) sleep in the daytime. In narcolepsy, HLA testing in an immunology laboratory is sometimes useful; virtually all patients with classical narcolepsy have HLA-DR15,DQ6 antigens. This is currently the highest association of HLA antigens with any known disease.

One practical problem in referring patients for multiple sleep latency testing is the persistence of REM-suppressing drugs, such as monoamine oxidase inhibitors, other antidepressants, and stimulants. The effects of antidepressants can persist for several weeks after their administration is discontinued, and the presence of traces of these drugs can invalidate the results of the multiple sleep latency test. Unfortunately, the patient may not be clinically stable without the drugs during the withdrawal period.

II. Epidemiology and pathophysiology.

A. Narcolepsy.

Narcolepsy affects males and females equally, with a 0.04 prevalence. It has a teenaged, postpubertal onset with a lifelong course. NPSG results may be normal or may show fragmented sleep. Multiple sleep latency testing usually shows a mean sleep latency of less than 7 minutes, with two or more naps containing REM sleep. Cataplexy—brief episodes of weakness triggered by emotion—is essentially REM sleep breaking through into the daytime and virtually clinches the diagnosis by history alone.

B. Obstructive sleep apnea.

The male-to-female ratio is approximately 2:1, and the prevalence is approximately 2% in women and 4% in men. It has a middle-age onset, and the condition worsens over time or as weight increases. The airway collapses at the base of the tongue or in the hypopharynx on an attempt at inspiration. The chief reasons for airway compromise are obesity, retrognathia, or simply an inherited geometry of the upper airway. Apneas may last up to 3 minutes and produce life-threatening hypoxia. The usual pattern is hundreds of 10- to 30-second apneas with short arousals after each.

C. Periodic limb movements in sleep disorder.

In PLMD, males and females are affected equally. The population prevalence is not well established but may be 5%, with most cases occurring in the older age groups. It is a central nervous system disorder that produces 2-second spasms of limb muscles every 20 or 30 seconds during sleep, with brief arousals after each spasm. The spasms are commonest in anterior tibial muscles. Subjective symptoms are largely caused by sleep loss. A related condition is the restless legs syndrome, which occurs in the daytime or during waking periods at night.

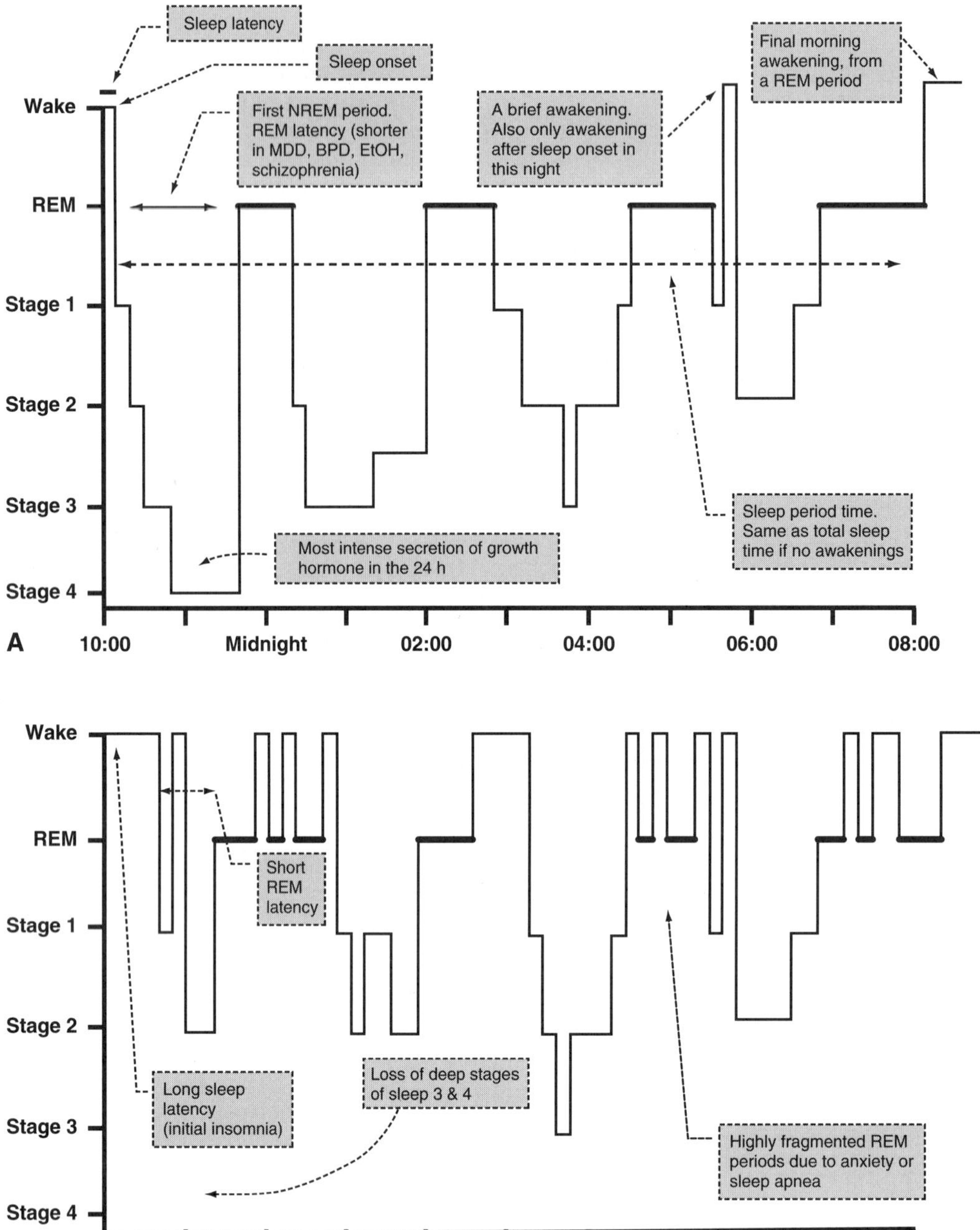

Figure 13–1.
How to Read a Sleep Study Report. This graph depicts sleep studies from two different patients. *A,* Most textbook examples of a sleep histogram show an idealized young healthy normal person, like this one. Note the clear, sequential transitions from stage 1 through stage 4 sleep, intact rapid eye movement (REM) periods and few awakenings. Note also the normal REM latency of about 90 minutes. *B,* This person has mild sleep apnea and moderately severe major depression. Note the short REM latency, the fragmented REM periods resulting from apnea, many minutes of "wake after sleep onset," and loss of the deeper stages of sleep. A short REM latency occurs in some apnea patients because of REM deprivation from the apneas, which are nearly always worse in REM than in non-REM (NREM) sleep. Short REM latency has also been reported in numerous psychiatric disorders. MDD = major depressive disorder; BPD = bipolar disorder; EtOH = ethanol (alcoholism).

D. Primary insomnia.

In primary insomnia, there is a mild female predominance, and the prevalence is high—about 10% of the population has had an episode. The primary care physician usually sees chronic sufferers of this condition. The NPSG may show increased muscle tone after the patient goes to bed, with a long *sleep latency* (time from lights out to first detection of sleep) and increased amounts of interspersed wakefulness. *REM latency* (time from sleep onset to first REM period) is normal, and sleep architecture for the remainder of the night is otherwise normal.

E. Substance abuse insomnia.

In this condition, there is a moderate male predominance. Prevalence could be as high as that of alcoholism in the general population. The substances abused may be sedatives (alcohol, barbiturates, benzodiazepines), opiates, or stimulants (caffeine, cocaine, amphetamines, appetite suppressants). The complaint of insomnia occurs either during intoxication with the substance or after withdrawal. NPSG findings of sedative abuse include loss of deep sleep stages, sleep fragmentation, and some REM suppression. Stimulants produce virtual sleeplessness with strong suppression of REM.

F. Insomnia due to psychiatric mood or anxiety disorders.

Nocturnal polysomnographic findings in depression include long sleep latency, short REM latency, intense eye movement activity in REM periods *(REM density)*, and shallow, fragmented, unrestful sleep. Intense REM activity is concentrated in the last third of the night and is often associated with early morning awakening. NPSG findings in anxiety disorders are largely normal, except for a long sleep latency and an increase in muscle tone. Excess alpha waves are seen on electroencephalography. Panic disorder may cause panic awakenings from non-REM sleep. Post-traumatic stress disorder causes intense nightmares in REM sleep, often with confusional awakenings in which the patient believes that the dream material is real for a few minutes. See the chapters on these topics for a full description of symptoms and prevalence.

G. Insufficient sleep syndrome.

Insufficient sleep syndrome is by far the commonest sleep disorder; the prevalence may be more than 30% of the population, with males and females being affected equally. Sleep need varies from individual to individual, averaging about 7.5 hours, but a range of 5 to 10 hours is not pathologic in adults. The syndrome usually results from staying awake late for the purposes of work, study, or recreation, despite a fixed waking time required for work or school. A *sleep debt* is built up over the working week, resulting in a decrease in productivity that peaks on Friday afternoon. In a related condition, *delayed sleep phase syndrome,* the patient habitually goes to bed late as a result of a lack of sleepiness, but the patient is sleepy until noon or later the next day. Acutely, such a condition can be produced by eastward air travel across many time zones, but it also exists in some persons who have not traveled.

III. Specific diagnoses.

A. Diagnosis and behavioral description.

1. *Narcolepsy.*
   Vivid dream images (hypnagogic hallucinations) occur at the onset of naps or at bedtime; these dreams can be mistaken for psychotic hallucinations. Severe daytime sleepiness is the rule. The *narcolepsy tetrad* of symptoms also includes *sleep paralysis, daytime attacks of sleep in inappropriate situations,* and *cataplexy.* Cataplexy is the most characteristic symptom.

2. *Obstructive sleep apnea.*
   Hypertension and right-sided heart failure can result from this condition. Loud snoring, with breathing pauses witnessed by others, is common. Mental effects include sleepiness, cognitive failure, and confusion. Extreme sleepiness in the daytime is the rule, but physical fatigue is also substantial.

3. *Periodic limb movements in sleep disorder.*
   Each leg jerk causes an arousal that interrupts sleep. The bed partner may report being kicked repetitively. Daytime symptoms may include a feeling of total fatigue and exhaustion rather than sleepiness. Daytime restless legs may be reported, but this phenomenon is not universal.

4. *Primary insomnia.*
   A common but benign form of primary insomnia follows obvious situational upset (e.g., death in family, major household move, job loss) and is limited to a week or two. Subjective complaints include a fear of not being able to go to sleep, "I can't turn my mind off to go to sleep," and a fear of poor performance at work the next day that results from the failure to sleep. The condition is a somatized tension resulting from environmental stress that the patient conceives of as a treatable medical condition. In fact, the opposite is true—reduction of life stress and relaxation would be the best treatment. Mental symptoms fall short of meeting criteria for DSM-IV anxiety disorders. Patients with primary insomnia resist the idea that their condition may have an emotional or behavioral cause.

5. *Substance abuse insomnia.*
Withdrawal is often worse than intoxication. Stimulating substances produce insomnia during use and hypersomnia plus depression symptoms in withdrawal. Sedatives produce the inverse. Withdrawal of either can produce vigorous REM rebound in the form of visual hallucinosis and confusion. Differential diagnosis is made largely on the basis of patient history and urine toxicology screens.

6. *Insomnia due to psychiatric mood or anxiety disorders.*
Diagnosis of the psychiatric disorder is made on the basis of patient history. The characteristic insomnia of major psychiatric disorders should respond to treatment for that disorder. An organic sleep disorder, such as narcolepsy or OSA, could be present in addition to a psychiatric illness and should be considered as a possible explanation for failure to respond to customary psychiatric care. Some psychiatric disorders, such as bipolar disorder and cyclothymia, produce severe insomnia, even when the main diagnosis is regarded as mild or in partial remission.

7. *Insufficient sleep syndrome.*
The weekend is marked by long sleep periods (10 to 12 hours' duration) in an effort to make up the sleep debt. Symptoms may include falling asleep while in class or while driving. Cognitive and memory abilities are blunted during sleep deprivation. A feeling of physical fatigue or weakness develops in severe cases, but these effects can be reversed with a day or two or normal sleep. *Particularly dangerous is the increased somnolent effect of alcohol when one is sleep deprived; alcohol can make the drive home from Friday afternoon "happy hour" a time of extreme risk for accidentally falling asleep.*

IV. General management guidelines.

A. Prevention.

Narcolepsy and PLMD are likely organic illnesses that are not preventable per se. OSA is most sensitive to increases in body weight, so maintenance of ideal body weight is of major importance. Psychophysiologic insomnia is worsened by cognitive factors such as apprehension, by impending stressful events, and by poor sleep hygiene (i.e., using the bedroom for many activities unrelated to sleep—watching TV, reading, telephoning). Insufficient sleep syndrome is a by-product of trying to do too much in too short a time, and advice to the patient is in order. Substance abuse insomnia and insomnia secondary to psychiatric illnesses wax and wane with the severity of the underlying disorder; therefore, adequate prophylaxis of psychiatric illness is of primary importance.

B. Medication and behavioral management.

1. *Narcolepsy.*
Once diagnosed properly in the sleep laboratory, the sleepiness of narcolepsy responds well to stimulants such as methylphenidate (Ritalin), 10 mg or more in the morning and at noon. A dose of 60 mg/d should not be exceeded without expert consultation. Dextroamphetamine (Dexedrine) is also effective. *Often, the cataplexy symptom requires its own separate treatment, usually an antidepressant drug.* Clomipramine (Anafranil), 25 to 50 mg in the morning, proptriptyline (Vivactil) 10 mg in the morning, and venlafaxine (Effexor), 37.5 mg in the morning have all shown good effect. In all cases, a nap can usually take the place of a medication dose, and many patients nap at work at lunch time or more frequently on the weekend.

2. *Obstructive sleep apnea.*
This problem is usually treated at the sleep disorders center by means of a continuous positive airway pressure device set at 5 to 15 cm H_2O. Home care companies rent or sell continuous positive airway pressure machines to the patient and maintain them. The largest problem is compliance over time; in this area, the primary physician is in the most powerful role to encourage the patient. *If hypertension and right-sided heart failure are part of the OSA illness, continuous positive airway pressure can bring about a dramatic recovery.*

3. *Periodic limb movements in sleep disorders.*
This problem has been treated with bedtime doses of numerous drugs, including clonazepam (Klonopin), baclofen (Lioresal), and levodopa-carbidopa (Sinemet). Levodopa-carbidopa is probably the most effective agent; the regimen begins with one tablet, 25 mg/100 mg, at bedtime. Anemia and iron deficiency, which may worsen periodic limb movements, should be corrected.

4. *Primary insomnia.*
This disorder sometimes responds to a few sessions of counseling by the primary care physician. The physician should encourage (1) good sleep hygiene, (2) avoidance of variable bedtime, and (3) dealing with impending stressors while awake rather than going to bed to think them over. Often, becoming more assertive with peers and supervisors during the day avoids "rehashing" of the day's events once in bed. Sleeping pills are generally not advisable, because they allow an avoidance of lifestyle changes. They can be used sparingly, however, to help the patient in times of added stress so that the insomnia does not cause panic for the patient.
Behavioral strategies include Bootzin's *stimulus control* and Spielman's *sleep restriction ther-*

apy.[3] Stimulus control involves using the bedroom only for sleep, so that it does not become psychologically associated with alerting recreational or business activities or eating. If sleep does not occur within 10 minutes of the lights being turned off, the patient is told to get out of bed and do something else until he or she feels sleepy, at which point, another attempt is made. *Sleep restriction* involves the use of a sleep log or diary for estimating the average number of hours of sleep obtained over a 2-week period of insomnia (e.g., 5 hours per night). The patient would then be told to set his or her alarm for 6:00 a.m. and to *not even try to go to bed until 1:00 a.m.*; this strategy allows the patient the 5 hours of sleep that the patient has demonstrated that he or she can achieve. Altering the bedtime in 15-minute increments enables the sleep period to be made progressively longer until the patient achieves a fully restful sleep without periods of insomnia.

5. *Substance abuse insomnia* and *insomnia due to psychiatric disorders.*
   These problems are responsive to adequate treatment of the underlying disease.
6. *Insufficient sleep syndrome.*
   This syndrome may be among the hardest sleep disorders to treat. People with insufficient sleep syndrome are often highly productive, driven individuals who have consciously chosen to adopt this lifestyle because of what they perceive as its greater rewards. These "workaholics" run a long-term risk of "burnout" but are hard to convince of this until they have reached middle age. More immediate concerns for the patient are falling asleep while driving late in the evening, experiencing excessive sedation from antihistamines or alcohol because of the patient's pre-existing sleep debt, and experiencing personality and/or family relationship changes because of the chronic sleepiness. Physician's advice is the best medicine. *The physician should not agree to requests for stimulants for such persons because these agents only worsen their tendency to avoid sleep and may result in addiction.*

C. Statements to the patient and family.

In general, a full disclosure of the sleep findings is helpful for the whole family. In the case of a 13- to 15-year-old patient with new-onset narcolepsy, teachers, peers, and family must become aware that the patient's sleepiness is a disease, not laziness. Naps must be allowed, perhaps at school in the nurse's office. Although narcolepsy is the rarest disorder mentioned in this chapter, it is the one most often misdiagnosed (as behavior disorder, thyroid illness, drug abuse, depression) and the one most responsive to medication treatment.

Self-help groups exist for narcolepsy, apnea, and restless legs syndrome/PLMD. Meeting fellow sufferers of these poorly known disorders can be very helpful for patient and family alike.

For primary insomnia patients, reassurance is important.

D. Relapse prevention.

In most of the illnesses described in this chapter, the most common cause of relapse is noncompliance with the indicated treatment. *The practitioner must stress that sleep is a basic part of physiology, like proper diet, and that its disorders have a disorganizing effect on many different aspects of life.*

V. Caregiver assistance: Coping suggestions.

Many patients are not aware of their sleep disorder, usually because they are asleep when the signs of the disorder are displayed. This fact makes the report of a spouse or family member very important in the diagnosis. Many wives of snoring husbands with OSA have tried for years to have the husband assessed by a physician, but because snoring is widely regarded by the general population as normal, the snorers often minimize the potential danger of OSA. Adequate interest in the snoring symptoms by the primary practitioner is the best assistance the spouse can have. The role of the spouse in facilitating alcoholic behavior is well known, and the spouse should be counseled to be firm with the alcoholic and to seek assistance from an alcohol counselor (see Chapter 17). In the other disorders, sleeping in separate beds or rooms may be needed in order for the spouse to sleep adequately.

VI. Practicalities and special situations.

A. Treatment modifications for rural and low-income patients.

The use of portable electronic diagnostic devices for sleep disorders is increasing. Although most sleep specialists still regard the sleep laboratory, with its continuous visual and polygraphic monitoring by a trained technician, as the gold standard for diagnosis, the portable systems are much cheaper. Often, a sleep laboratory offers both in-house and ambulatory recordings. Medicaid now pays for studies for apnea and narcolepsy.

B. Balancing cost and effectiveness.

The treatments for sleep disorders are economical when the morbidity of the untreated disorders is considered. Apart from the use of generic medications versus brand names, not many cost savings are to be realized. Again, compliance over the long term is the key to adequate treatment.

VII. When to refer.

All patients with suspected OSA, narcolepsy, or PLMD should undergo a sleep study in order to substantiate the diagnosis and its severity. Substance abuse insomnia and insomnia due to psychiatric disorders may require referral to a psychiatrist for a proper differential diagnosis and treatment plan, but these conditions can usually be managed by the primary care physician. Primary insomnia and insufficient sleep syndrome are the two disorders in which the primary care physician is in a better position than a specialist to implement behavior change in the patient.

References

1. American Psychiatric Association. *Diagnostic and Statistical Manual of Mental Disorders. Fourth edition.* Washington DC: American Psychiatric Association; 1994.
2. International Classification of Sleep Disorders: Diagnostic and Coding Manual. Diagnostic Classification Steering Committee; Thorpy MJ, Chairman. Rochester, Minnesota: American Sleep Disorders Association, 1990.
3. Hauri PJ, Editor. Case Studies in Insomnia. New York: Plenum Publishing Corp.; 1991.

Suggested Reading

Kryger MH, Roth T, Dement WC, Editors. Principles and Practice of Sleep Medicine. Second Edition. Philadelphia: WB Saunders Co.; 1994.

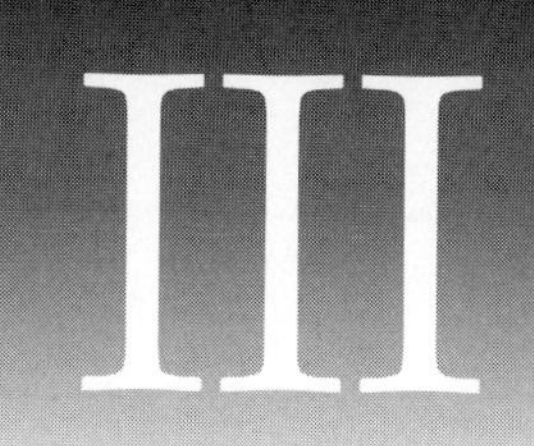

Neurobehavioral Medicine

14

N. CARY ENGLEBERG, MD

MARK A. DEMITRACK, MD

Chronic Fatigue Syndrome and Fibromyalgia

I. Evaluation and diagnostic overview.

A. Differential diagnosis.

Fatigue is one of the most common complaints encountered in general medicine. Most fatigued patients have a transient, self-limited illness or have a medical illness underlying their fatigue. In a small proportion of patients, the symptom persists for 6 months or longer and may be sufficiently severe to interfere with work or social activity. The medical and psychiatric disorders that can produce cryptic fatigue of this long a duration are numerous; a partial list is shown in Table 14–1. In the absence of any of these disorders as a cause for symptoms, patients are said to have *chronic idiopathic fatigue.* Many patients also have other troubling symptoms in addition to fatigue (Table 14–2). By convention, those patients with four or more specific, additional symptoms are said to have the *chronic fatigue syndrome* (CFS).

Fibromyalgia (FM) is a pain-defined condition that occurs with CFS in many patients. Based on the American College of Rheumatology's definition, the diagnosis of FM is considered when (1) the complaint of pain is generalized (both sides of the body, above and below the waist, and (2) the patient reports pain at 11 or more of the 18 classic tender points (Fig. 14–1). Both CFS and FM share prominent symptoms of fatigue, joint and muscle pain, sleep disorder, and neuropsychological symptoms, and many patients meet the criteria for both. These two entities may reflect the clinical spectrum of a single psychophysiologic disorder, although their relationship is not fully understood at present. However, whereas the current definition of CFS requires the symptoms not be explainable by any coexisting medical or psychiatric process, the FM syndrome can be diagnosed as a secondary process that complicates an underlying medical condition (e.g., rheumatoid arthritis, systemic lupus erythematosus).

B. Relevant laboratory orders and other diagnostic testing.

Chronic fatigue syndrome is a diagnosis of exclusion. Therefore, a careful and thorough history and physical examination are essential. A basic laboratory evaluation should include complete blood count, erythrocyte sedimentation rate, serum chemistry determinations (including alanine transaminase, total protein, albumin, globulin, alkaline phosphatase, calcium, phosphate, glucose, electrolyte, blood urea nitrogen, and creatinine levels), thyroid-stimulating hormone, and urinalysis. Additional laboratory evaluation may be warranted, depending on the patient's complaints and the physical findings. Prominent articular complaints or sicca syndrome may warrant further rheumatologic, serologic, or radiographic study. Tests for specific viruses (e.g., Epstein-Barr virus, human herpesvirus 6, human spumavirus, human T-cell lymphotropic virus, type II, or other retroviruses) have no role in the diagnosis or evaluation of CFS. Adult patients may have serologic evidence of indeterminate past exposure to these viruses, but these findings do not distinguish them from healthy individuals. Laboratory tests for other infectious diseases may be indicated if there is a relevant exposure history and compatible symptoms or signs. Although chronic fatigue may be a symptom of neuroborreliosis, a positive serologic result for Lyme disease does not establish this infection as the cause of the fatigue, nor does a negative result rule it out entirely. (A full discussion of this controversial topic is beyond the scope of this chapter; however, a study evaluating the value of empiric Lyme disease therapy in chronic fatigue states is provided by Lightfoot and associates[1]). Certain neurologic symptoms or objective neurologic findings on the physical examination may warrant an evaluation for multiple sclerosis; however, fleeting paresthesia and muscle fasciculations are commonly experienced in CFS. Although subtle brain abnormalities have been visualized in some patients by magnetic resonance imaging and single-photon emission computed tomography, these findings are neither specific nor universal for CFS, and their meaning is unknown. Therefore, these expensive tests are not useful for establishing the diagnosis of CFS, and they should

Table 14–1
Some Medical Conditions That May Present with Chronic Fatigue

Endocrine diseases
Diabetes mellitus
Hyperthyroidism
Hypothyroidism
Hyperparathyroidism
Addison's disease
Cushing's disease
Hyperaldosteronism
Panhypopituitarism
Infections
Tuberculosis
Lyme disease
Brucellosis
Chronic sinusitis
Bacterial endocarditis
Chronic pyelonephritis
Mononucleosis and other nonspecific viral infections
  Epstein-Barr virus
  Cytomegalovirus
  Toxoplasmosis
  Enteroviruses (e.g., coxsackievirus A5, A6, B5)
  Human herpesvirus #6
Chronic hepatitis
  Hepatitis B virus (± delta agent)
  Hepatitis C virus
  Human immunodeficiency virus
  Chronic rubella syndrome
Rheumatologic disorders
Systemic lupus erythematosus
Polymyositis
Sjögren's syndrome
Other
Other medical conditions
Occult or disseminated malignancy
Cardiac insufficiency
Starvation or nutritional deficiencies
Hepatic or renal dysfunction
Alcoholism
Chronic caffeine use (withdrawal)
Drugs (particularly beta blockers, antihistamines, and benzodiazepines)
Chronic electrolyte disorders

be used only for the confirmation of an alternate diagnosis. Occasionally, a primary sleep disorder (e.g., obstructive apnea, restless legs syndrome, and narcolepsy) may present as CFS. When the history raises a reasonable suspicion, a formal sleep evaluation is warranted.

II. Epidemiology.

Although CFS occurs in both sexes and over a large age range, the disorder as encountered in most medical practices occurs most commonly in women during the middle decades of life. In our clinic population, the female-to-male ratio is 4:1. It is not known whether this predominance reflects patterns of health service utilization or the true age-specific and sex-specific incidences in the population at large. Population-based studies, which have been hampered by methodologic difficulties, have varied considerably in their estimations of the prevalence of CFS. A study by the Centers for Disease Control and Prevention estimated the point prevalence of CFS to be 4.6 to 11.3 cases per 100,000, based on surveillance from four sites. In contrast, a study based in a large Pacific Northwest health care system placed the community prevalence at 75 to 267 cases per 100,000.[2] With FM, the proportion of females is even greater than with CFS (female-to-male ratio, 8 to 10:1). The prevalence of FM in the United States general medical clinics ranges from 2% to 6%, whereas in rheumatology clinics, the prevalence may be as great as 20%.[3] Population-based studies reveal a 1% to 3% prevalence of FM in the community. The public health cost of these syndromes is not trivial. CFS patients are over-represented among the high-utilizers of outpatient medical care. Recently, a large Canadian database study of 260 patients with FM revealed that 15% were receiving disability compensation. From this prevalence figure, the financial burden related to FM disability in Canada was estimated at $200 million per year.[4]

III. Pathophysiology.

The precise etiology of CFS is unknown. Various infectious, immunologic, toxic, nutritional, and psychiatric explanations for the syndrome have been advanced, but none has survived scientific scrutiny. Although approximately two thirds of patients with CFS have current or past psychiatric disorders, the notion that CFS is simply a variant of major depression is probably incorrect because at least 25% patients with clear diagnostic criteria for CFS lack any of the diagnostic criteria for depression. In addition, recent studies have demonstrated subtle and similar neuroendocrine changes in patients with CFS and FM (e.g., relative hypocortisolism, autonomic dystonia). Similar studies in depressed patients show strikingly different neuroendocrine features (e.g., sustained hypercortisolism during the active phases of the disease). However, the CFS and FM findings do suggest that a dysfunction within the central nervous system may account for the symptoms or may accompany them.

Chronic fatigue syndrome may follow different precipitating events (e.g., infection, trauma or surgery, childbirth, emotional distress); however, the reported symptoms are remarkably similar in different patients, regardless of the precipitant. Considering the heterogeneity of these precipitants and our limited understanding of the biology of the disorder, CFS is perhaps best conceptualized as a common, dysfunctional response to stressors of various kinds. Like CFS, FM may also follow discrete precipitating events.

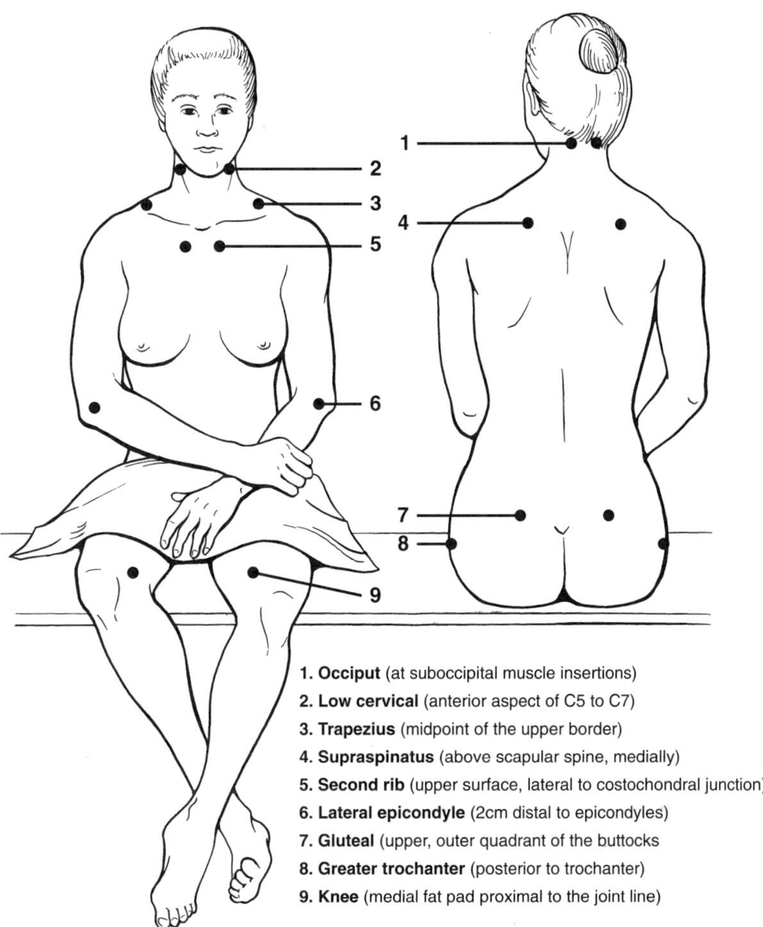

Figure 14–1
Fibromyalgia tender points.

IV. General management guidelines.

A. What to tell the patient and family.

Many patients seen for CFS and FM are told by less sensitive physicians that their illnesses are purely psychological or imaginary. Apart from being untrue in most cases, this posture simply increases the patient's anxiety that a serious disease state is being overlooked or ignored. The physician should validate the reality of the patient's symptoms while making clear that the available evidence makes it impossible to attribute them to any specific organic cause. In fact, the evidence suggests that both CFS and FM are the result of multiple biologic, social, and psychological factors that may differ among individuals. A conceptualization of the illness that resorts to a single causation model is rarely useful and may be counterproductive.

In order to know how to frame a discussion of CFS with a new patient, the primary care physician should know the level of knowledge or misinformation that the patient already has about the subject. It is therefore useful to ask the patient if they have read or heard anything about CFS and, if so, from what source. If the patient has any preconceptions about the diagnosis, the physician may begin by asking the patient to articulate his or her own notions about CFS and the sources of this information. At this point, the physician often hears ideas about Epstein-Barr virus or other viruses, the immune system, or "stress" of various kinds. Even the best-informed patients find these notions confusing and typically terminate their response with a question. The physician may then continue as follows:

I think that the proper name for your illness is "chronic fatigue syndrome." Let me tell you what this means and what its relationship to [the patient's stated concepts] is. You've been fatigued for a long time, and you've experienced a number of other symptoms as well. When patients have an illness like yours and we cannot find any common medical or psychiatric disorder to account for their fatigue, we diagnose it as chronic fatigue syndrome. We don't know what causes chronic fatigue syndrome, but we now know that it is unlikely to be explained by a single factor alone, such as a virus. In fact, most people working in this field would emphasize that chronic fatigue syndrome is probably a final common outcome from the interaction of several different factors, some of them biologic, such

Table 14–2
Definition of Chronic Fatigue Syndrome

Chronic fatigue syndrome—clinically evaluated, unexplained, persistent or relapsing chronic fatigue (>6 mo duration) that is of new or definite onset (has not been lifelong), is not the result of ongoing exertion, is not substantially alleviated by rest, and results in substantial reduction in previous levels of occupational, educational, social, or personal activities

Plus

Four or more of the following symptoms are concurrently present for > 6 mo:
- Impaired memory or concentration
- Sore throat
- Tender cervical or axillary lymph nodes
- Muscle pain
- Multijoint pain
- New headaches
- Unrefreshing sleep
- Postexertion malaise

Exclusionary clinical diagnoses:
- Any active medical condition that could explain the chronic fatigue
- Any previously diagnosed medical condition whose resolution has not been documented beyond reasonable clinical doubt and whose continued activity may explain the chronic fatiguing illness
- Psychotic major depression, bipolar affective disorder, schizophrenia, delusional disorders, dementias, anorexia nervosa, bulimia nervosa
- Alcohol or other substance abuse within 2 years before the onset of the chronic fatigue and at any time afterward

Adapted from Fukuda K, Straus SE, Hickie I, et al. The chronic fatigue syndrome: A comprehensive approach to its definition and study. Ann Intern Med 1994; 121:953–959.

as an infection, a serious accident, or surgery, and some of them situational, such as work or home problems. The particular factors can vary widely from person to person. Thinking about it from this perspective, we should treat your chronic fatigue syndrome by carefully understanding which factors are relevant to your situation and by helping you to draw reasonable connections among them in order to help you take charge of your own recovery.

Because this is not very encouraging news, it is important to reassure the patient that their condition is not a total mystery and that it can be treated.

Even though we don't fully understand what causes CFS, we do know from experience what to expect when people have this disorder, and there are some things you and I can do to make it better. This is common in medicine. There are many illnesses that doctors treat successfully, even though they don't know the real cause. So even though we don't know the cause of CFS, we do know certain important things about it. For example, we know that it is not a fatal illness, and we know that you are not any more likely than anyone else to get other diseases, such as cancer or multiple sclerosis. We also know that you cannot "catch" CFS from someone close to you, so you don't have to worry about giving it to anyone else. There is no evidence that it is contagious.

Rare intrafamilial clusters are more likely the result of a shared predisposition to the syndrome.

We know that by the time most patients are diagnosed with this condition, the worst part of their illness is usually behind them. Most patients gradually improve, although a return to relatively normal health can take a lot of time—months, or even years. When patients are recovering from CFS, the severity of their symptoms changes considerably on a day-to-day basis. As you get better, you can expect to have bad days and good days and some relapses. This is normal during recovery, and an increase in your symptoms does not mean that you are starting to get sick all over again. In fact, the most likely outcome is that you will recover completely or reach a level of symptoms that you can live with. Occasionally, patients with CFS do not recover and become permanently disabled. Fortunately, this outcome occurs in only a small number of patients, usually among those who have unmanageable medical or psychiatric problems complicating their chronic fatigue illness.

At this point, the physician can either reassure the patient that he or she does not have any such complicating problems or, if appropriate, can identify any other medical or psychiatric problems the patient has and outline what can be done for them.

Eventually, the physician must return to the patient's own concepts about their illness, correct misinformation, and place these notions into the proper perspective. It is useful in this context for the physician to have some familiarity with antiviral serologies (particularly Epstein-Barr virus serology) because many patients will have been told that these tests have meaning with respect to their chronic fatigue. In fact, although a small proportion of CFS cases follow primary Epstein-Barr virus infection, no correlation exists between the serologic titers and the severity of the illness or the prognosis. Patients can be told that no single virus or other infectious agent has been shown to cause any significant proportion of CFS cases. With regard to immune, neuroendocrine, and vasomotor irregularities found commonly in CFS, patients can be told that

These findings are helping us to understand better what's wrong in CFS patients. However, they are not present in all patients with CFS, and they also occur in other medical and psychiatric disorders. We don't know whether any of these subtle abnormalities have anything to do with producing the symptoms you have. Trying to correct them hasn't been very helpful either. They may be nothing more than another indicator that you have an illness.

Some authorities believe that the primary care physician can play a critical role in determining the prognosis by making a clinical diagnosis, limiting an otherwise endless evaluation, and providing a framework for the patient's understanding of the illness (see section I.B.).

Treatment is ultimately facilitated by a gradual reorientation of patients' beliefs about their illness.

Much of what can be said about CFS can also be applied to FM. The pathophysiology of FM is also not well understood; however, there is no compelling historical association of this disorder with specific chronic infections or immune dysfunction, as there has been with CFS. However, like CFS, FM often occurs as a secondary disorder in association with other medical problems. The data on long-term prognosis with FM are less optimistic than the data on CFS. However, patients can be reassured that they may recover completely from the FM. If the patient continues to have symptoms, he or she can significantly reduce their severity and improve his or her quality of life with a regimen of proper exercise, sleep habits, and some medications.

B. Goals of treatment.

Treatment for CFS is based on the notion that the illness is usually self-limited but can be exacerbated by external stresses. Therefore, the role of the treating physician is to promote activities and therapies that lead toward normal functionality and to instruct the patient to avoid stressors that may facilitate or prolong the illness. Because the true cause of CFS is unknown, treatments (e.g., antiviral drugs, immunomodulating drugs, nutritional supplements) directed at presumed causes are generally ineffective. A more rational approach to treatment focuses on the management of individual symptoms. Relief of symptoms allows the patient to engage in rehabilitative activities more easily and presumably to recover faster. However, the patient must understand this rationale and the goals of the treatment plan, and the treatment rationale should be compatible with the patient's own model of his or her illness. Dissonance between the physician's therapeutic intent and the patient's expectations inevitably results in frustrating treatment failures. The approach to the treatment of FM is philosophically similar to that of CFS, consisting of symptom management and rehabilitative activities.

1. *Behavioral management.*
   Some models for CFS place strong emphasis on an external cause for the syndrome (e.g., attack by a virus) and thereby put the illness outside of the patient's control. Because the engagement of the patient in treatment is essential, the rigid belief in an external cause may be counterproductive. Indeed, a recent follow-up study of CFS patients showed a strong correlation between the belief in a viral cause and the long-term persistence of symptoms. For this reason, a gradual reorientation of thinking about the nature of the illness is helpful in recruiting the patient to become his or her own best ally in recovery.

   The patient should be enlisted in a program of gradual return to functionality. This program invariably includes graded exercise, attention to sleep hygiene, and normal diet. All such behavior modifications should be accomplished slowly and should involve a reassessment of progress with the patient at each step. At the same time, the patient should be provided with rationales for discontinuing certain dysfunctional behaviors that may actually perpetuate the symptoms or amplify the patient's disability (e.g., bed rest, extensive napping, fad diets, self-overmedication).

2. *Medications.*
   Any medical intervention should have an outcome that is empirically verifiable by the patient and the physician, it should be medically and psychiatrically safe, and it should not incur unjustified financial cost. Two classes of medications are particularly useful in this regard—pain relievers and antidepressants. Antidepressants may provide beneficial effects on pain, sleep disorder, headache, and mood disturbances, all of which are prominent complaints in CFS and FM. However, the responses to these medications are highly individualized. Treatment trials should therefore be guided by two simple principles: (1) only one medication should be added, removed, or dose-adjusted at a time because no independent means exists for assessing the response to a given manipulation, apart from the patient's assessment of symptoms, and (2) assuming that the drug does not make the patient feel subjectively worse, the trial should be of sufficient duration and dose to determine whether the drug has any effect (i.e., 4 to 6 weeks for most antidepressants).

   Some patients may wish to experiment with medications that are not part of the usual formulary but are available through health food stores and mail order companies (e.g., coenzyme Q10, dihydroepiandosterone, suma, evening primrose oil, melatonin). The patient should be encouraged to inform the physician of any unconventional medications and to make no new additions while conventional medication trials are in progress. Thereafter, the physician should help the patient assess the potential hazard and cost-benefit of such unproven therapies.

C. Return visits and general follow-up care.

An early investment of time with patients with CFS or FM at the initial evaluation is usually rewarded. Well-oriented patients are often able to develop useful symptom management strategies on their own once they have the proper cognitive framework. Follow-up appointments may be scheduled at monthly intervals during medication trials, less frequently as the patient begins to show progress or to plateau. At these visits, the status of the principle symptoms, fatigue, pain, sleep disorder, impaired cognition, and mood changes should be reviewed. In selected circumstances, it may be helpful to have the patient keep diaries documenting one or more of these symptoms over time so that an objective record of symptom occurrence is available.

Follow-up should also include evaluation of any new symptoms, particularly if they are not part of the usual complex experienced in CFS and FM. The danger of attributing all new symptoms to a heterogeneous, idiopathic disorder is that an emerging organic illness might be overlooked.

D. Relapse prevention.

Unresolved medical problems that coexist with CFS and FM may serve as perpetuating factors in these syndromes. Common minor problems, such as sinusitis, gastroesophageal reflux, recurrent urinary tract infections, and temporomandibular joint syndrome, should be addressed and optimally managed. Although patients with CFS or FM are probably not more susceptible to acquiring common infectious illnesses, they may be more seriously affected and for longer periods. It has been our policy to immunize all patients with CFS annually against influenza.

As mentioned earlier, minor relapses are common in CFS. Some patients may place undue significance on minor variations in symptoms. They must be reminded that such temporary setbacks rarely presage a return to severe symptoms and disability.

V. Fatigue.

A. Assessing the symptom.

Patients with CFS or FM perceive a sensation of being "completely drained of all energy." Some report the perception of an increasing lack of energy as the day progresses. Analogies to "spent batteries" or to "running out of gas" are common. As a consequence, patients may feel the need for prolonged rest in preparation for anticipated activity. In addition, most report postexertional malaise, an accentuation of fatigue after activity that may persist for days. This latter symptom may lead to a state of exercise phobia, which may further decondition the patient and contribute to the illness.

In CFS and FM, fatigue is believed to be central in origin rather than myopathic. Formal studies of muscle strength, endurance, and recovery, as well as biochemical, electrophysiologic, and microscopic studies, have failed to reveal a major disturbance of muscle function in patients with CFS. On the other hand, studies of exercise tolerance to aerobic work have shown physiologic measures compatible with prolonged physical inactivity, in conjunction with a discrepancy in the conscious perception of the degree of physical effort relative to the workload performed. The presence of objective muscle weakness or atrophy in a patient with CFS or FM should suggest an alternate diagnosis. Likewise, limitation of activity by breathlessness or tachycardia is not a direct consequence of CFS or FM per se but rather results from subsequent deconditioning or a confounding medical condition. Finally, anxiety and mood disorders are often accompanied by fatigue. Patients who experience symptoms of anxiety or depression may experience improvement in their physical stamina with control of these emotional symptoms, even when they are perceived as secondary to CFS or FM.

B. Behavioral management.

All patients with CFS and FM should be encouraged to exercise within certain limits. Although activity may exacerbate symptoms in the short term, there is no evidence to suggest that it impairs recovery. Moreover, a graded exercise program has been demonstrated to be of value in patients with FM. The alternative, bed rest and inactivity, tends to reinforce invalidism and a sense of helplessness.

The type and amount of exercise should be individualized according to the patient's disability and available resources. The exercise should be quantifiable (e.g., walking or swimming a fixed distance, exercise on a metered exercise machine) rather than indeterminate (e.g., most competitive sports). It should not involve significant tension or impact on tendons and joints, such as occurs with jogging, weight lifting, or power aerobics. Initially, the patient should be encouraged to find a quantifiable level of exercise that will not induce prolonged postexertional fatigue and that can be repeated five to seven times per week. As the program becomes routine, the amount of exercise can be increased slowly.

In severely affected patients, a minimal exercise program is a walking program complemented with stretching exercises or yoga. Videotapes of appropriate exercise regimens are available through the Fibromyalgia Association.

C. Medication management.

No specific therapy for fatigue exists per se. However, antidepressants may be helpful for several reasons. Several case reports have suggested that some patients may benefit from the activating effects of selective serotonin reuptake inhibitors, although one recent controlled trial was unable to find a systematic benefit from the use of these agents. Our experience suggests that some patients may feel increased energy when depression or anxiety symptoms are brought under control. In addition, pain reduction and improved sleep associated with antidepressant therapy may facilitate adherence to an exercise program in some patients and thus have an indirect beneficial effect on fatigue. Some patients are confused by the suggestion to use an antidepressant because they perceive their illness to be purely physical in origin. The physician can make two important points that may help the patient understand this therapy. First:

The antidepressant is not being used to treat the *cause* of the disorder, but rather the symptoms. The CFS (or FM) will get better on its own. The medicine is being used to make you feel better and more normal while this healing process takes place.

Second, antidepressants can be characterized as multifunctional drugs:

Antidepressants have many different effects on the nervous system. They can improve a depressed mood to be sure, but they also relieve pain and they regularize sleep. That is why they are often used for conditions that have nothing to do with depression, such as migraine headaches, sleep disorders, chronic pain after shingles, or even bed wetting.

The physician and patient should identify which symptoms the patient has that might be expected to benefit from antidepressant therapy.

1. *Suggested protocols.*
   Patients with CFS or FM tend to have an exaggerated response to many medications. Administration of selective serotonin reuptake inhibitors (SSRIs) or other antidepressants should be started at very low doses and gradually increased to standard treatment doses as tolerated, for instance, fluoxetine (Prozac) therapy could begin with 10 mg (or less if the liquid suspension is used), sertraline (Zoloft), with 25 mg, or paroxetine (Paxil), with 10 mg each day. All three drugs are usually given in the morning. A treatment trial with one of these agents (or with any antidepressant) should be continued for at least 4 to 6 weeks before the effects can be adequately evaluated.

2. *Medications to avoid.*
   Central nervous system stimulants, intravenous immunoglobulin, immunomodulators, and antivirals should be avoided.

3. *Innovative protocols.*
   Recently, patients with CFS, FM, or both have been found to have hypotension or syncope inducible by tilt-table testing. Reasoning that this response was similar to that observed in patients with vasodepressor syncope, treatment with a mineralocorticoid, such as fludrocortisone (Florinef), plus dietary salt, atenolol, or disopyramide was administered to some patients. Forty-one percent of patients improved with this therapy in one nonblinded, uncontrolled study. Until several gaps in our understanding of these autonomic phenomena are better understood and the efficacy of therapy is confirmed in a placebo-controlled trial, this mode of diagnosis and therapy cannot be recommended without serious reservations.

VI. Pain.

A. Assessing the symptom.

Pain is a nearly universal symptom in CFS and is the defining symptom of FM. Patients with FM have generalized tenderness that can be quantified by the tender point examination. Patients with CFS may also have several tender points, even if they do not meet the formal criteria for FM. In both disorders, tender point examination is a useful way to monitor the degree of pain over time and with treatment.

Neither CFS nor FM is associated with inflammation at a painful location. Therefore, although articular or periarticular pain may be reported, joint swelling or erythema never occurs, and when it is present, it should suggest an alternate diagnosis. Moreover, highly localized pain or "trigger points" may suggest concurrent tendonitis, bursitis, or myofascial pain syndromes, which required other specific therapies not outlined in this chapter.

In severely affected patients, pain may be compounded by the effects of profound inactivity. It is important to help the patient distinguish painful symptoms that are secondary in origin.

B. Behavior management.

Patients with intermittent pain should be encouraged to identify specific precipitants. Sometimes, it is useful for the patient to keep a diary to assist the patient in discovering painful stimulants. Exercise and stretching are critical for the prevention of secondary painful symptoms. A physical therapy referral may be considered for some patients. Patients with myofascial pain can be taught to stretch and use ice on painful joints.

C. Medication management.

1. *Suggested protocols.*
   Amitriptyline (Elavil) has been shown to be of benefit in controlling the pain of FM in double-blind, placebo-controlled trials. Undoubtedly, other tricyclic antidepressants with less anticholinergic activity and SSRIs are also effective in FM and CFS. If a tricyclic agent is preferred to an SSRI, we prefer to use nortriptyline (Pamelor), beginning at 25 mg at bedtime and increasing by increments of 25 mg to 75 mg over several weeks as tolerated.

   Tramadol (Ultram), is a nonaddictive narcotic agonist that has remarkable activity in some patients. It can be given at a dose of 50 mg three times a day as needed for persistent pain or 100 mg at bedtime for patients whose sleep disruption can be attributed to nocturnal pain. Nonsteroidal anti-inflammatory drugs may be used; however, the response to these agents is often disappointing. An NSAID taken 30 minutes before exercise may be helpful for patients who report increased pain after exercise.

Muscle relaxants, such as cyclobenzaprine (Flexeril), can be helpful, particularly if muscle spasms are present. Ten to 20 mg at bedtime may be helpful for nocturnal pain, and the sedative effect of this drug may facilitate sleep. The anticholinergic side effects of cyclobenzaprine are additive to those of tricyclics.

2. *Medications to avoid.*
Systemic corticosteroids have no proven benefit in CFS, and they may worsen the symptoms of fibromyalgia. Because of the high potential for tolerance and addiction, narcotics should not be used in this chronic pain condition.

VII. Sleep problems.

A. Assessing the symptom.

Patients with CFS may complain of excessive sleepiness or insomnia. Insomnia occurs in various forms, although middle insomnia and fragmentation of sleep are the most common problems. A sense that sleep has not been restorative is reported by many CFS patients and most FM patients.

Whether sleep is excessive or fragmented, many patients seek to resolve the problem by napping. This behavior is actually counterproductive because it disturbs nocturnal sleep architecture even further.

Some patients with primary sleep disorders present with fatigue. Patients or their bed partners should be questioned about snoring, nocturnal breathing, and leg movements, or sudden, uncontrollable urges to sleep. If the history suggests the possibility of obstructive apnea, restless legs syndrome, or narcolepsy, a formal polysomnographic study may be warranted.

B. Behavioral management.

Patients should be advised to keep regular sleep hours, to sleep during nighttime hours in a darkened room, and to avoid napping, if possible. If napping is unavoidable, the patient should be instructed to limit naps to 30 to 60 minutes by setting an alarm clock. Often, the restoration of normal sleep hygiene cannot be accomplished immediately, and the physician has to set goals and limits for the patient to achieve over time.

C. Medication management.

1. *Suggested medications.*
The choice of an antidepressant should be made with the patient's specific sleep disorder in mind. In patients who have significant depression as a component of their sleep disorder, any antidepressant that restores their mood typically corrects the sleep problem. Patients without significant depression who have excessive sleepiness may profit from an SSRI taken in the morning. In contrast, patients without significant depression who have onset or middle insomnia may respond to a tricyclic antidepressant or trazodone (Desyrel).

Zolpidem tartrate (Ambien) is a short-acting agent that is occasionally useful for onset insomnia in a dose of 5 to 10 mg.

2. *Medications to avoid.*
Central nervous system depressants are best avoided. Benzodiazepines may facilitate sleep, but they also contribute to fatigue. They may be useful in the short term when initial therapy with an SSRI causes a transient insomnia, but the patient should be promptly weaned off of the drug as he or she becomes adjusted to this drug effect. Because of their potential for habituation, barbiturates should not be prescribed. Likewise, alcohol is best avoided as a sedative. Most patients with CFS do not tolerate alcohol well in any case.

VIII. When to refer.

Effective management of CFS and FM is a time-consuming process. The initial evaluation is extensive, given all of the diagnostic possibilities that must be considered, and the required patient education and training is a lengthy and ongoing process. Primary care physicians who follow these guidelines and make the necessary time available for their patients may be able to treat this chronic illness without the need for referral. Given the demands of the managed care setting, many physicians may be unable to commit the required time. Under these circumstances, it is preferable to refer the patient to a specialist experienced in the care of these disorders rather than to simply medicate the patient without also providing the appropriate cognitive framework. The prescription of an antidepressant is misunderstood by many patients as a sign that the physician believes the illness to be psychosomatic or that the patient is depressed even though he or she perceives no mood disturbance. When this happens, the physician is an unwitting contributor to the pernicious problem of misattributing the cause of the illness. The patient may reject the prescribed treatment and continue to pursue answers elsewhere, adding to the chronicity and the cost of the disorder.

Of course, referral is also appropriate when the clinical diagnosis is still in doubt or when the patient does not respond to treatment attempts and when a reasonable specialist or program is available to treat these disorders. Primary care physicians are advised to investigate carefully the practices and treatment philosophy of specialists to whom they refer. We believe that the best management for CFS and FM is achieved in a program that involves both an internist and a psychiatrist in evaluation and therapy. In our experience, legitimate specialists in this area typically adhere to the conservative, cognitive symptom-directed approach described earlier. They reinforce the patient's health behavior, rather than his or her illness behavior, and they are willing to provide the patient with the necessary education about their illness and to address their questions and concerns. Clinical services that are overpriced, that offer treatments with unlicensed or investigational drugs at great cost to the patient, or require extensive and expensive laboratory testing in order to "diagnose" CFS or FM are exploitative and should be avoided.

Some patients may wish to consult "alternative" healers who specialize in acupuncture, naturopathy, homeopathy, massage therapy, therapeutic touch, or other methods. These alternative treatments usually cannot be formally recommended, because their value is unknown. To the extent that these services are safe, not excessively costly, and lead to symptomatic relief, we do not discourage patients from trying them. We do, however, insist that our patients refrain from using alternative treatment modalities during trials of prescribed medications so that confusion about their benefits or untoward effects does not occur.

Organizations

The Centers for Disease Control, "The Facts About Chronic Fatigue Syndrome," on-line at: http://www.cdc.gov/ncidod/diseases/fatigue/fatigue.htm

The National CFS Association, 919 Scott Avenue, Kansas City, KS. 66105. Tel. (913) 321-2278.

References

1. Lightfoot RW Jr, Luft BJ, Rahn DW, et al. Empiric parenteral antibiotic treatment of patients with fibromyalgia and fatigue and a positive serologic result for Lyme disease: A cost-effectiveness analysis. Ann Intern Med 1993; 119:503–509.
2. Buchwald D, Umali P, Umali J, et al. Chronic fatigue and the chronic fatigue syndrome: prevalence in a Pacific Northwest health system. Ann Intern Med 1995; 123:81–88.
3. Goldenberg DL. Fibromyalgia, chronic fatigue syndrome, and myofascial pain syndrome. Curr Opin Rheumatol 1991; 3:247–258.
4. McCain GA, Cameron R, Kennedy JC. The problem of long-term disability payments and litigation in primary fibromyalgia. J Rheumatol 1989; 16(Suppl 19):174–176.

Suggested Reading

Bates DW, Schmitt W, Buchwald D, et al. Prevalence of fatigue and chronic fatigue syndrome in a primary care practice. Arch Intern Med 1993; 153:2759–2765.

Cope H, David A, Pelosi A, Mann A. Predictors of postviral fatigue. Lancet 1994; 344:864–868.

Demitrack MA, Abbey SE, Editors. Chronic Fatigue Syndrome: An Integrative Approach to Evaluation and Treatment. New York: Guilford Publications; 1996.

Fukuda K, Straus SE, Hickie I, et al. The chronic fatigue syndrome: A comprehensive approach to its definition and study. Ann Intern Med 1994; 121:953–959.

Sharpe M, Hawton K, Simkin S, et al. Cognitive behaviour therapy for the chronic fatigue syndrome: A randomised controlled trial. BMJ 1996; 312:22–26.

Straus SE, Editor. Chronic Fatigue Syndrome. New York: Marcel Dekker; 1994.

Wessely S, Chalder T, Hirsch S, et al. Postinfectious fatigue: Prospective cohort study in primary care. Lancet 1995; 345:1333–1338.

Wilson A, Hickie I, Lloyd A, et al. Longitudinal study of outcome of chronic fatigue syndrome. BMJ 1994; 308:756–759.

15

RANDY S. ROTH, PhD

BARBARA KAMHOLZ, MD

Major Pain Syndromes and Chronic Pain

I. Introduction.

A. The treatment of pain is one of the most daunting challenges for the primary care physician because it is often a meaningful sign of somatic illness. However, pain often persists despite negative results on diagnostic work-up or effective treatment of disease or injury. The symptoms may become diffuse and ambiguous, and when pain and dysfunction appear to be out of proportion to an identified somatic cause, the physician becomes suspicious that psychological variables are at work.

B. The issues relating to human pain are fraught with misunderstanding, stereotypes, and prejudices. This chapter provides a means of addressing this complex clinical situation. *A major conceptual theme of this chapter is that the successful management of pain syndromes and chronic pain requires the primary care physician to match the patient to a pain syndrome. Distinguishing the nature and the cause of different pain syndromes is important because each syndrome has specific treatments. Chronic pain syndromes share persistent pain as a defining characteristic but are not all alike.*

C. Because a comprehensive review of chronic pain management is beyond the scope of a single chapter, the major pain syndromes that are most common and that are particularly challenging for the primary care physician are highlighted. These syndromes include pain of neurologic, musculoskeletal, and sympathetic origin as well as common headache disorders. The relationship between chronic pain and psychological disturbance is discussed, with particular reference made to the frequently encountered problems of substance abuse, depression, anxiety, and somatoform disorders. Medical and psychiatric strategies for the management of chronic pain are reviewed, with an emphasis on the classes of medications available for the treatment of various pain syndromes. A glossary of pain terms is available at the end of this chapter.

D. An extensive review of the neurophysiology of pain has been included to illustrate recent advances in elucidating the mechanisms of pain perception and the implications of these data for enhancing the effectiveness of clinical pain management. *Evidence of plasticity and sensitization of neural structures responsible for pain transmission and endogenous mechanisms of pain modulation indicate the need for a new paradigm for understanding persistent pain and the patient with chronic pain.*

II. Definitions of pain.

A. Pain is "an unpleasant sensory and emotional experience associated with actual or potential tissue damage or described in terms of such damage."[1]

1. Pain is always subjective and occurs within a psychological state.
2. Pain is no longer defined in terms of an identifiable physical cause (e.g., noxious stimulus) or activity in nociceptors.
3. Pain has three processes:
   a. *Sensory-descriminative:* provides information on the time course and topographic pattern of sensory disturbance.
   b. *Affective-motivational:* accounts for the unpleasantness of painful sensory changes; provides the motive to avoid or escape noxious stimuli.
   c. *Cognitive-evaluative:* describes the "meaningfulness" of the pain experience for the individual; also includes various pain-specific beliefs (e.g., "no pain, no gain," "hurt is harm") and the individual's interpretation of disturbed somatic experience.

B. Acute pain has a time course of seconds to weeks.

1. It is almost always associated with tissue damage and evoked by a noxious stimulus.
2. It serves a protective signaling function to alert the patient of potential harm or danger to biologic integrity.
3. *It is rarely due primarily to psychological or envi-*

ronmental factors but can be influenced by psychological factors.

4. Its psychological profile is typically one of heightened autonomic arousal.

C. Chronic pain has a time course 3 months to years.

1. It may be the result of ongoing nociception caused by tissue damage or physiologic impairment, it may develop as the result of alterations in neurophysiologic sensory processes following prolonged nociception (e.g., sensitization), or it may be due to psychological and/or environmental factors (e.g., depression, social reinforcement).
2. It does not serve a biologic function.
3. Its psychological profile usually involves a diminution of autonomic responses concurrent with a progressive onset of vegetative signs of depression.
4. It imposes serious and severe emotional, functional, economic, and social hardships for patients and their families and constitutes a major health crisis for society.

D. Treatment considerations are as follows:

1. Acute pain states should be treated promptly and adequately; *prolonged acute pain can promote changes in the peripheral nervous system and the central nervous system (CNS), producing heightened sensitivity to pain for both noxious and innocuous stimuli.*
2. Chronic pain may require treatment by multiple medical specialties in order to address complex and multifactorial problems; treatment goals focus on improved function, adaptive psychological coping, and enhanced quality of life.

III. Epidemiology.

A. Epidemiologic studies of chronic pain are limited because a significant proportion of patients avoid or delay medical attention for pain. Nearly 60% of Americans are unwilling to seek treatment for persistent pain rated as "mildly" severe, and nearly 20% are similarly reluctant, even when their ongoing pain is considered "severe." Individuals who do seek pain therapy believe that their pain may be life threatening and that their physician is capable of providing an accurate diagnosis and effective therapy.

B. Estimates of the prevalence of chronic pain in the United States suggest that

1. One in three individuals has persistent pain that requires medical attention.
2. More than 50 million people are either partially or totally disabled by chronic pain.
3. By pain condition:
   a. Twenty-one million people have low back pain.
   b. Forty million have recurring headache.
   c. Twenty-four million have various arthritic conditions.
   d. Twelve million have assorted musculoskeletal disorders.
   e. Eleven million have other chronic pain conditions (e.g., visceral, neurologic, cardiac, and orofacial).

C. Between 1960 and 1980, the awarding of social security disability for low back pain increased 3000%, compared with a 500% increase for lung cancer. For society, a major issue pertaining to chronic pain is the ever-growing epidemic of disability attributed to persistent pain states.

IV. A selective review of recent advances in neurophysiologic mechanisms of pain.

A. The traditional view of basic mechanisms of pain perception.

1. Pain is fundamentally a one-way sensory phenomenon at the physiologic level.
2. Biologic ("real") pain has a one-to-one relationship with tissue damage.
3. Pain experience in the absence of identifiable tissue disturbance is fundamentally "psychogenic."

B. The modern view of basic mechanisms of pain perception.

1. Peripheral and central mechanisms devoted to pain perception are dynamic and mutually interactive.
2. In response to persistent nociceptive input, the nervous system biases toward *enhancement* of nociception and pain by
   a. Prompting functional and morphologic changes in neurologic mechanisms.
   b. *Sensitizing* peripheral and central pain mechanisms by lowering the activation threshold in nociceptors or responding to constancy of noxious stimulation with *enhancing central neuronal discharge* (e.g., wind-up).
3. The nervous system possesses an extraordinary capability to modulate and suppress pain transmission via peripheral (e.g., counterstimulation) and central (e.g., descending inhibition from supraspinal structures) activation.
4. Excessive pain behavior, including allodynia (i.e., pain caused by a stimulus that does not normally evoke pain) and hyperalgesia (i.e., exaggerated pain response to a stimulus that is normally painful), in the absence of an appar-

ent physiologic cause, is now believed to be caused by *neurophysiologic plasticity and sensitization* rather than exclusively by psychogenic factors.

C. Basic pain physiology.

1. *Pain pathways in the peripheral nervous system:* three major groups of peripheral primary afferents exist: axons are diverse in diameter and presence or absence of myelin sheath; they subserve motor and autonomic control as well as sensory transmission.
   a. *A-alpha, A-beta:* large-diameter, myelinated, high–conduction-velocity mechanoreceptors.
      (1) They are motorneurons and include muscle proprioceptors.
      (2) They do not differentially respond to noxious stimuli.
      (3) Stimulation of A-beta afferents is known to modulate nociceptor transmission in the dorsal horn of the spinal cord by activating inhibitory spinal neurons; pain modalities involving counterstimulation, such as massage, heat and cold, transcutaneous electrical nerve stimulation (TENS), and dorsal column stimulators are thought to work by stimulating A-beta afferents.
   b. *Nociceptor:* primary afferent neuron with peripheral terminals that respond differentially to noxious stimuli; transduce mechanical, thermal, and/or chemical activity to electrochemical nerve impulses; transmit coded information to the CNS.
      (1) *A-delta:* small diameter, myelinated, slower conduction velocity; both mechanoreceptor and thermoreceptor.
         - Activated by noxious and innocuous stimuli.
         - Increase discharge as stimulus intensity increases into a range that produces tissue damage.
         - Stimulation associated with sharp, intense pain or tingling.
      (2) *C-fiber:* small diameter, unmyelinated, slowest conduction velocity; respond to mechanical, thermal, and chemical stimul(1) (C-polymodal nociceptors respond to all three)
         - The "workhorse" of nociceptors: unmyelinated afferents make up 80% of axons in human cutaneous nerve.
         - Its stimulation produces intense, prolonged, burning pain.

2. *Sensitization and hyperalgesia resulting from persistent activity in nociceptors following noxious stimulation:*
   a. *Sensitization:* with repeated stimulation, nociceptors exhibit increased sensitivity and lowered threshold to activation and prolonged and enhanced response to stimulation (afterdischarge).
   b. Sensitization likely related to three sources of nociception-inducing substances.
      (1) Damage to cell produces leakage of intracellular contents, including
         - Potassium and histamine—both excite C-polymodal nociceptors.
         - Acetylcholine, serotonin, and adenosine triphosphate also known to activate nociceptor.
      (2) Substances are released by damaged tissue or enter damaged area secondary to plasma extravasation or lymphocyte migration.
         - One of the most important pain-producing substances found in damaged tissue is *bradykinin,* which is known to activate nociceptors.
         - Also synthesized in region of tissue damage are metabolic products of arachidonic acid, including prostaglandins and leukotrienes; both are known to be powerful inflammatory mediators and to sensitize nociceptors.
      (3) Nociceptors release substances known to enhance nociceptor discharge, such as substance P and calcitonin gene-related peptide.

3. Pain pathways in the CNS.
   a. Primary afferent nociceptors (PANs) terminate in the dorsal horn, and their cell bodies are located in dorsal root ganglion (DRG).
      (1) Primary afferent nociceptors synapse directly on three cells in the dorsal horn.
         - *Projection neurons:* relay nociception to higher brain structures.
         - *Excitatory interneurons:* relay nociception to projection neurons, other interneurons, or motoneurons that mediate spinal reflexes.
         - *Inhibitory interneurons:* contribute to reduction of nociceptive transmission.
      (2) Spinal neurons receive input from both A-beta and nociceptor afferents; there is also convergence of input from viscera, somatic structures, and sympathetic pathways; *with prolonged nociceptor input, spinal neurons can become sensitized and, as a result can be activated by low-threshold A-beta afferents, resulting in pain to innocuous stimuli.*
   b. Ascending pathways for pain are as follows:
      (1) *Neospinothalamic tract* (lateral): has few synapses, projects almost directly to thalamus; responsible for *sensory-discriminative* component of pain.
      (2) *Paleospinothalamic tract* (medial): collateralizes to medulla and pons with projections to hypothalamus and limbic system; responsible for *motivational-affective* component of pain.
   c. Central nervous system mechanisms for control of pain: descending inhibitory modulation.

(1) Activation of the periaqueductal gray (PAG) in the midbrain, the rostral ventral medulla at the medullary level (including the nucleus rapha magnus), and the dorsolateral pontine tegmentum contributes to inhibition of pain as their descending pathways terminate in the dorsal horn at the synapse of PANs and spinal neurons.

(2) Role of biogenic amines.
- Dorsolateral pontine tegmentum pathway: mediated by norepinephrine
- PAG–rostral ventral medulla pathway: mediated by serotonin
- *Both norepinephrine and serotonin are plentiful in inhibitory descending pathways of pain modulation; they are also known to be important in mood and sleep disorders.*

(3) Opioid activation of pain modulation.
- Opioids are believed to at least partly activate descending pathways via the PAG, the rostral ventral medulla, and the dorsolateral pontine tegmentum.
- Endogenous opioids include: enkephalin distributed widely throughout CNS (amygdala, hypothalamus, PAG, rostral ventral medulla, and dorsal horn); and β-endorphin densely organized in hypothalamus, PAG, dorsolateral pontine tegmentum, spinal interneurons, medulla, and pituitary.
- A high correlation of presence of endogenous opioids, opiate receptors, and nociception/pain modulation pathways implicates opioid activation as a contributing factor in the promotion of analgesia.
- Factors that activate the pain modulation system include: stress; intense, prolonged pain; restraint; and fear.

4. Up-regulation in the nervous system after *nerve injury* (how the nervous system becomes more sensitive to stimuli causing pain).
   a. *"Wind-up"*: spinal neurons' increasingly exaggerated discharge in response to repetitive, fixed stimulation of PANs.
   b. Sprouting of large diameter afferents centrally: within 14 days of nerve injury, there is evidence for A-beta sprouting into the dorsal root entry zone and the dorsal horn, which contain nociceptor terminals; *thus, A-beta afferents may synapse with and stimulate high threshold nociceptors after A-beta activation, leading to allodynia, hyperalgesia.*
   c. Spinal reflexes activated by nociception.
      (1) Reflex efferent activity to skeletal muscle causes muscle spasm, continued nociception from muscle, and maintenance of efferent reflex (e.g., pain-spasm–pain cycle).
      (2) Sympathetic efferent activity that facilitates inflammatory response may lead to C-polymodal nociceptor sensitization as a result of release of local factors (e.g., bradykinin, prostaglandin, substance P)
   d. Role of sympathetic nervous system
      (1) Normally, there is some postganglionic sympathetic innervation of DRG, but with nerve injury, there is proliferation of sympathetic innervation of DRG and broader communication with PANs; this reflects postganglionic *coupling,* or *ephapsis* of the sympathetic nervous system and the DRG.
      (2) Sympathetic nervous system efferent–somatic afferent coupling may occur at the site of nerve injury that produces neuroma or neuronal sprouting distal to DRG.
      (3) Evidence indicates that alpha-adrenergic transmitters activate C-fibers in injured nerves: thus, peripheral nerve injury induces adrenergic excitation of C-fibers; *alpha-adrenergic transmitters are released by stress and negative emotional states.*

D. A clinical strategy for understanding the patient with chronic pain.[2]

1. A clinical model (Fig. 15–1) useful for evaluating the patient with chronic pain separates chronic pain into four constituents arranged hierarchically and defines it as follows:
   a. *Nociception:* Nociceptors being activated by thermal, mechanical, or chemical noxious stimuli.
   b. *Pain:* sensory transmission of nociception to the CNS and registering in supraspinal centers involved in processing of noxious afferent impulses.
   c. *Suffering:* unpleasant affective response resulting from activation of higher nervous system centers of pain interpretation.

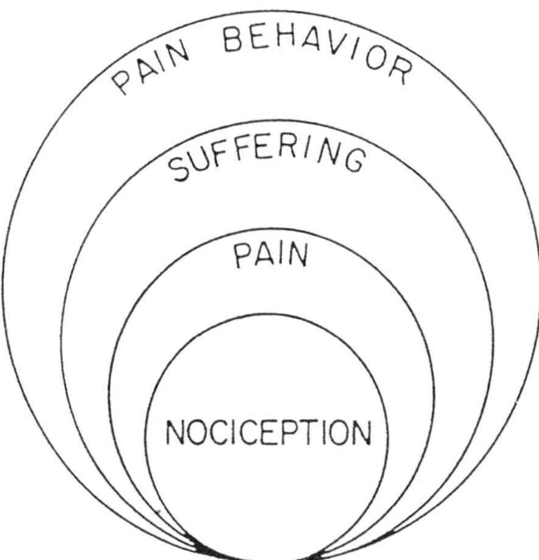

Figure 15–1
Fordyce's revised clinical model of pain to assist in the assessment of the chronic pain patient. (From Fordyce WE. Environmental factors in the genesis of low back pain. In: Bonica JJ, Liebeskind JC, Albe-Fessard DG (eds.). Advances in Pain Research and Therapy. New York: Raven Press, 1979, p. 659–666.)

d. *Pain behavior:* public display by the individual that communicates the subjective experience that reflects nociception.

2. The correlation between adjacent levels in this model can be affected by intervening factors, such as
   a. The degree of nociception that gains access to the CNS and higher centers may be influenced by
      (1) *Modulation* of pain in spinal cord by peripheral counterstimulation or descending inhibitory activation.
      (2) *Enhancement* of pain, caused by nociceptor sensitization, central facilitation, or absence of normal inhibitory controls.
   b. The degree of suffering may be negatively influenced by factors beyond pain processing:
      (1) Mood disorders, such as depression, anxiety.
      (2) Guilt-ridden, dependent, or obsessive personality style.
      (3) Developmental history associated with abuse, trauma, and child-parent bonding involving themes of punishment.
      (4) Biogenetic factors suggested by a family history of depression or substance abuse.
   c. The exhibition of pain behaviors may be affected by factors beyond suffering:
      (1) Secondary gain to obtain positive consequences (e.g., financial incentives, social sanctioning of dependency or disability) or to avoid negative encounters (e.g., work or interpersonal responsibilities).
      (2) Health care seeking for psychosocial reasons.
   d. In the typical clinical setting, the physician attempts to draw a direct relationship between nociception (e.g., tissue damage, physiologic impairment) and pain behavior, but
      (1) By arranging these component levels hierarchically, the clinician can more clearly distinguish those factors relevant to a patient's pain symptoms.
      (2) *Adjacent levels* of the model are likely to be the most strongly related (e.g., nociception-pain; suffering-pain behavior), whereas *causal inferences drawn from nonadjacent levels* (e.g., nociception-suffering, nociception/pain–pain behavior) *may be misleading* because of the intervening factors mentioned earlier.

V. Major pain syndromes and associated treatments.

A. Pain of neurologic origin.

1. *Peripheral neuralgias and neuropathies.*
   a. *Neuropathy* is a disturbance of function or pathologic change in a nerve, often, but not always, associated with pain; *neuralgia* is pain in the distribution of a nerve or nerves.
   b. Common causes of neuropathic pain include trauma, surgery, neural compression, systemic disorders (e.g., hypothyroidism, diabetes), vitamin deficiency, toxic exposure, and metabolic disorders; longstanding alcohol abuse is a common origin of peripheral neuropathy.
   c. Clinical features are as follows:
      (1) Pain is typically described as sharp, stabbing, burning, and stinging and is often superimposed on a background of constant pain. Transient recurrent episodes of severe, *paroxysmal lancinating* pain occur, and patients may also report parasthesias, including numbness and tingling.
      (2) In cases of neuralgia, pain is circumscribed to the distribution of a single nerve, either confirmed by physical examination, by differential nerve blockade with local anesthetic, or by electromyography.
      (3) In cases of neuropathy and polyneuropathy, neurologic symptoms include numbness, distal sensory loss, hyperesthesia and burning pain; loss of proprioception due to profound sensory impairment may be evident in severe cases.
   d. Treatment.
      (1) Address underlying cause of the neuralgia/neuropathy when possible (e.g., surgically treat nerve entrapment, maximize diabetes management).
      (2) Prescribe pharmacologic therapy (Tables 15–1 to 15–3; see also medication section).
         - Antidepressants, particularly tricyclics, should be the first choice for the treatment of neuropathic pain.
         - Anticonvulsants can be additionally helpful, especially for patients who report paroxysmal lancinating pain episodes.
           Phenytoin (Dilantin) may be effective for lancinating pain attacks.
           Carbamazepine (Tegretol) has been found to be particularly effective for trigeminal neuralgia.
           Gabapentin (Neurontin) has shown particular promise for various neuropathic pain syndromes.
           Clonazepam (Klonopin).
         - Mexilitene (Mexitil), an oral lidocaine analogue has been helpful for some patients, starting dose is 200 mg three times a day, and the dosage is increased to 300 to 400 mg three times a day.
         - Maintenance opioids may be considered for selected patients.
      (3) Transcutaneous electrical nerve stimulation and physical therapy.
      (4) Nerve blockade.
         - A series of nerve blocks with or without

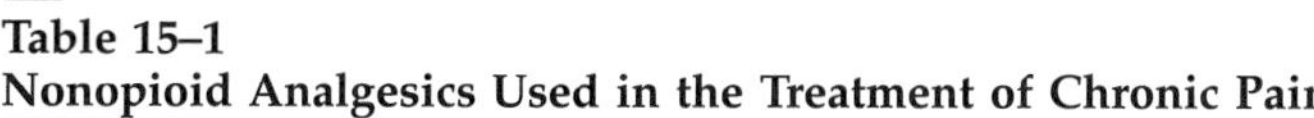

Table 15–1
Nonopioid Analgesics Used in the Treatment of Chronic Pain

Drug Name (Trade Name)	Usual Adult Dose	Comments
Acetaminophen (Tylenol, other brands)	650–975 mg q4h	Analgesic and antipyretic that lacks anti-inflammatory properties. High doses may cause toxicity in the form of liver damage; hepatic coma can occur.
Salicylates		
Aspirin	650–975 mg	Aspirin (650 mg) is the standard against which all other oral analgesics are compared. Rate of gastric distress is high. Interferes with coagulation and causes irreversible inhibition of circulating platelets. Possesses analgesic, anti-inflammatory, and antipyretic effects.
Choline magnesium (Trilisate)	1000–1500 mg bid	
Diflunisal (Dolobid)	500 mg bid	Acts like aspirin but has prolonged duration of action with fewer GI side effects.
NSAIDs		NSAIDs were originally introduced for arthritis treatment. Action is both peripheral and central. All NSAIDs share the side effect of gastric distress and can increase liver enzyme levels. They may also cause a variety of renal complications.
Propionic acids		
Fenoprofen (Nalfon)	200 mg tid	Relatively short acting, e.g., 6 h.
Ibuprofen (Advil, Nuprin—QTC) (Motrin, Rufen—Rx)	200–800 mg qid	Relatively short acting, e.g., 6 h.
Naproxen (Naprosyn)	250–500 mg bid	Relatively rapid therapeutic onset.
Naproxen sodium (Anaprox)	275–550 mg bid	
Ketoprofen (Orudis)	25–75 mg tid	Relatively rapid therapeutic onset.
Indole derivatives		
Sulindac (Clinoril)	150–200 mg bid	
Tolmetin (Tolectin)	400 mg qid	Analgesic effect is weak.
Fenamates		
Mefenamic acid (Ponstel)	250 mg	Not recommended for use over 7 d. Primarily for dysmenorrhea.
Meclofenamate (Meclomen)	50 mg qid	May cause diarrhea.
Oxicams		
Piroxicam (Feldene)	20 mg qd	Once a day dosing for maintenance. Avoid using in persons with liver or kidney dysfunction because accumulation may be toxic. Causes considerable GI distress.
Acetic acids		
Ketorolac (Toradol)	10 mg tid oral dose	Oral dose not to exceed 7 consecutive days.
Indomethacin (Indocin)	50–75 mg bid–tid	Particularly effective for paroxysmal hemicrania headache.
Diclofenac sodium (Cataflam, Voltaren)	50–75 mg bid	
Etodolac (Lodine)	200–400 mg tid	Relatively lower rate of GI distress.
Nabumetone (Relafen)	1000–1500 mg qd	Relatively lower rate of GI distress.

NSAIDs, nonsteroidal anti-inflammatory drugs; GI, gastrointestinal; OTC, over the counter; TLx, prescription; qd, every day; bid, twice a day; tid, three times a day; qid, four times a day.

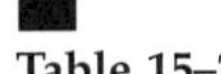

Table 15–2
Common Antidepressants Used in the Treatment of Chronic Pain

Drug Name (Brand Name)		Inhibition of Reuptake: *Serotonin*	Inhibition of Reuptake: *Norepinephrine*	Side Effects: *Anticholinergic*	Side Effects: *Sedation*	Side Effects: *Cardiac conduction*	Dose (mg/d)	Comments
								General comments: low doses may be adequate for analgesia; higher doses may be necessary if coexistent depression and sleep disturbance are present; tricyclics have highest analgesic potency.
Tricyclics								
Tertiary amines								
Amitriptyline	(Elavil, Endep)	+ + + +	+ +	+ + + + +	+ + + + +	+ + + + +	10–200	"Gold standard," high incidence of side effects
Doxepin	(Adapin, Sinequan)	+ +	+	+ + +	+ + + + +	+ + + +	10–200	Equivalent to amitriptyline, but with fewer side effects.
Imipramine	(Tofranil)	+ + + +	+ +	+ + + +	+ + + +	+ + + + +	25–150	
Clomipramine	(Anafranil)	+ + + + +	+ +	+ + + +	+ + + +	+ + + +	25–200	
Secondary amines								
Desipramine	(Norpramin)	+ +	+ + + +	+ + +	+ + +	+ + +	10–150	Few side effects, less sedating
Nortriptyline	(Pamelor, Aventyl)	+ + +	+ +	+ +	+ +	+ +	10–150	Equivalent to amitriptyline, but with fewer side effects.
SSRIs								
Fluoxetine	(Prozac)	+ + + + +	±	0	±	±	10–80	SSRIs tend to be less reliably analgesic but effective in individual cases.
Sertraline	(Zoloft)	+ + + + +	±	0	±	±	50–200	
Paroxetine	(Paxil)	+ + + + +	±	+	+	±	20–40	
Other*								
Bupropion	(Wellbutrin)	±	±	±	−	+	75–450	

SSRI, selective serotonin reuptake inhibitor; −, reverse effect; bupropion produces stimulation; 0, no known effect; ±, equivocal or sporadic effect; +, minimal effect; + +, mild effect; + + +, moderate effect; + + + +, strong effect; + + + + +, marked effect.

*Newer agents, such as venlafaxine (Effexor) and nefazodone (Serzone), are not included because available data are inadequate.

corticosteroids to the affected nerve may produce lasting relief in some patients.
- Sympathetic blockade may afford some value for patients in whom the neuropathy contains a sympathetic component.

(5) Psychological intervention in cases of unrelenting severe pain and marked emotional or behavior disturbance.

2. *Radiculopathy.*
   a. *Radiculopathy* implies a disturbance of function or a pathologic change in one or more nerve roots, typically associated with pain that follows the discrete distribution of the affected root or roots; *radiculitis* implies inflammation in one or more nerve roots in which no mechanical lesion or anatomic alteration in the nerve root is evident; disc herniation is the most common origin for radicular pain, but other sources include disease (e.g., diabetes), tumor, and spinal anomalies (e.g., spinal stenosis, compression fractures).
   b. Pathophysiology.
      (1) Disruption of normal nerve function by mechanical or chemical irritation produces pain in a dermatomal distribution, with associated localized inflammation.
      (2) The injured nerve root may become increasingly mechanosensitive whereby mild traction on the nerve produces exaggerated neural firing and afterdischarge with a sharp, stabbing, shooting pain perceived along the nerve distribution.
      (3) With persistent nociceptive input, spinal neurons that synapse with PANs may become sensitized, leading to lowered thresholds for activation and a wider receptive field of pain.
   c. Clinical features.
      (1) Dermatomal distribution of pain.
      (2) Diminished sensation, muscle strength, and reflex in the distribution of the affected nerve.
      (3) Pain described as shooting, stabbing, electrical; extremity pain usually described as more problematic than trunk pain.
      (4) Abnormal diagnostic findings, including electromyography, magnetic resonance imaging, computed tomography, myelography.

Table 15–3
Oral Opioid Analgesics Used in the Treatment of Chronic Pain

Drug Name (Trade Name)	Active Ingredients*	Peak Effect	Duration	Comments
Weak opioids				
Propoxyphene napsylate				
(Darvon N)		2 h	3–4 h	Structurally related to methadone.
(Darvocet N-50, 100)	100 mg + 325/650 mg Acet			
Propoxyphene HCl				
(Darvon Compound 65)	65 mg + 389 mg ASA + 32.4 mg caffeine	2 h	2–4 h	
(Darvon)	65 mg			
Codeine sulfate		2 h	3–4 h	Same as morphine, but weaker.
(Tylenol No. 3)	30 mg + 300 mg Acet			
(Tylenol No. 4)	60 mg + 300 mg Acet			
Hydrocodone		2 h	2–4 h	
(Vicodin, Zydone, Lorcet, Anexsia)	5 mg + 500 mg Acet			
Lorcet Plus, Anexsia 7.5/650,	7.5 mg + 650 mg Acet			
Vicodin ES	7.5 mg + 750 mg Acet			
Lorcet 10/650	10 mg + 650 mg Acet			
Azdone	5 mg + 500 mg ASA			
Strong opioids				
Oxycodone HCl		1 h	3–4 h	
Percodan	4.5 mg + 325 mg ASA			
Percocet	5 mg + 325 mg Acet			
Tylox	5 mg + 500 mg Acet			
Oxycontin				Sustained release.
Pentazocine HCl		1 h	3–4 h	Mixed agonist-antagonist may cause emotional or behavioral side effects. Use with caution in patients with cardiac abnormalities.
(Talwin)		2 h	3–4 h	
Meperidine HCL (Demerol, Pethadol)		2 h	3–4	Causes CNS excitation ranging from irritability to seizures. Not for long-term administration to patients with renal dysfunction or to those taking an MAOI.
Methadone HCl (Dolophine)		2 h	4–5 h	Same precautions as with morphine.
Morphine sulfate		2 h	4–5 h	May cause oversedation confusion, visual disturbances, urinary retention. Contraindicated in patients with impaired ventilation, asthma, increased intracranial pressure, liver failure.
(MS Contin, Roxanol SR)		4–5 h	8–12 h	Sustained release.
Hydromorphine HCl (Dilaudid)		1 h	3–4 h	Quick onset of action. Same precautions as with morphine.
Levorphanol tartrate (Levo-Dromoran)		2 h	4–5 h	Same precautions as with morphine.

CNS, central nervous system; MAOI, monoamine oxidase inhibitor; qid, four times a day; HCl, hydrochloride; Acet, acetaminophen; ASA, acetylsalicylic acid.

*Active ingredients are listed for products that contain more than one analgesic. Single constituent products come in several dosages, none of which are listed.

From Fields HL, Liebeskind JC (eds): Pharmacological Approaches to the Treatment of Chronic Pain: New Concepts & Critical Issues. (Progress in Pain Research and Therapy Ser.: Vol. 1), Chapter 16. Seattle, IASP Press; 1994.

d. Treatment.
 (1) *Acute radiculopathy* is often time limited and responds to conservative measures, including:
 - Brief bed rest not to exceed 1 week.
 - Epidural steroid injection.
 - Physical therapy, including emphasis on extension or flexion exercises, whichever produces less pain initially; patient is trained in exercise and postural strategies to maximize neutral spine position, including lower abdominal strengthening; TENS; traction.
 - Analgesic medications, including nonsteroidal anti-inflammatory drugs (NSAIDs).

 (2) If conservative measures fail, surgical consultation is advisable.
 (3) In *chronic radiculopathy,* persistent radicular pain may be related to permanent alter-

ation in the nerve root (e.g., surgically induced epidural fibrosis; diabetes-induced radiculopathy); treatment strategies include

- Physical therapy to maintain maximum mobility and strength and prevent secondary musculoskeletal and arthropathy pain.
- Transcutaneous electrical stimulation.
- Nerve blockade with corticosteroids—epidural or caudal injection.
- Pharmacologic therapy (see Tables 15–1 to 15–3 and Medication section for dosing schedules).
  Antidepressants.
  Anticonvulsants.
  Nonsteroidal anti-inflammatory drugs.
  Maintenance opioids.
- Psychological intervention.
- Neurosurgical consultation for consideration of surgically implantable spinal cord stimulator or morphine pump.

3. *Postamputation pain.*
   a. Pain following amputation may arise for many reasons, including
      (1) Local tissue changes at the site of amputation (e.g., stump), including bone and soft tissue abnormalities.
      (2) Alterations in neurologic functioning as a result of disruption of normal afferent processing or neuroma formation.
      (3) Postamputation pain may have both peripheral nervous system and CNS components.
   b. Epidemiology.
      (1) The incidence of persistent stump pain after surgery may be between 15% and 25%.
      (2) Phantom pain that is severe and requires medical treatment occurs in 7% to 10% of amputees, although some studies suggest that the prevalence of postamputation pain may be much higher.
   c. Clinical features.
      (1) Stump pain.
         - Localized tenderness with discrete "trigger points" (TPs) representing myofascial pain or evidence of neuroma.
         - Signs of vascular insufficiency or impairment.
         - Distal tenderness along the scar formation.
         - Bony prominences overlying soft tissue.
         - Evidence for localized infection.
      (2) Phantom pain.
         - Continuous or intermittent pain is experienced in the lost limb, generally of neuropathic character (e.g., burning, electrical) or described as squeezing or clenching.
         - Phantom pain should be distinguished from *phantom sensations;* the latter are regarded as a normal sequela of surgery in which the lost body part is perceived, albeit with distorted sensation, and gradually resolves over weeks or months by "telescoping" or shrinking progressively into the stump.
         - The occurrence and severity of phantom pain may correlate with the duration and severity of preamputation limb pain.
   d. Treatment.
      (1) Stump pain.
         - Local infiltration into trigger areas with local anesthetic and/or corticosteroids.
         - Physical therapy modalities, including massage and TENS.
         - Modify prosthesis.
         - Pharmacotherapy appropriate for chronic neuropathic pain, including antidepressants, anticonvulsants, NSAIDs, and opioids (see Tables 15–1 and 15–2 and Medication section.)
      (2) Phantom pain.
         - Pharmacotherapy.
           Antidepressants as a first treatment with anticonvulsant agents added secondarily.
           Beta blockers have been of value in selected patients; propranolol (Inderal), starting dose 40 mg twice a day, titrating to a maximum of 240 mg/d; sustained-release agent can be considered when a therapeutic level is achieved.
           Mexilitene, starting at 200 mg three times a day, titrating to 300 to 400 mg three times a day.
           Maintenance opioids in carefully selected patients.
         - Sympathetic blockade may be significantly beneficial in some patients.
         - Surgical consultation for consideration of surgical sympathectomy when indicated or spinal cord stimulator implant.

4. *Postherpetic neuralgia.*
   a. *Postherpetic neuralgia* is pain that persists after resolution of the acute phase of herpes zoster outbreak (e.g, vesicular rash); it distributes along the affected dermatome; pain is constant, with superimposed spontaneous paroxysmal attacks; pain is described as severe, stabbing, and sharp.
   b. Epidemiology.
      (1) Herpes zoster is common in the elderly; the incidence is 5 to 10 per 1000.
      (2) Postherpetic neuralgia occurs in approximately 10% of all patients, and the rate increases to 50% after the age of 50.

c. Clinical picture.
   (1) Pain in dermatomal distribution with associated hyperesthesia and hyperalgesia.
   (2) Common dermatones include thoracic (> 50% of cases) and ophthalmic division of the trigeminal nerve.

d. Treatment.
   (1) In acute herpes zoster, aggressive intervention may prevent the occurrence of postherpetic neuralgia. Interventions include
      - Antiviral agents, such as acyclovir (Zovirax) or amantadine hydrochloride (Symmetrel)
      - *Sympathetic blockade,* initiated within the first 2 weeks of onset of disease, repeated several times per week until pain resolves.
      - Oral corticosteroids: Prednisone (Deltasone) 60 mg daily for 3 to 5 days, tapered over 2 weeks.
      - Opioid analgesia, especially during the acute phase of illness, and NSAIDs.
   (2) For postherpetic neuralgia, the following therapies may be considered:
      - Sympathetic/nerve blockade.
      - Antidepressants.
      - Anticonvulsants.
      - Phenothiazines, particularly fluphenazine (Prolixin) 1 to 2 mg three times a day, and perphenazine (Trilafon), 1 to 2 mg three times a day in combination with antidepressants.
      - Maintenance opioids.
      - Psychological therapy.

5. *Central pain syndromes.*

a. *Central pain* is a generic term that describes pain that arises after injury or disease in the CNS; historically, central pain has been associated with thalamic lesions (e.g., thalamic pain syndrome), but it is now recognized to result from a lesion *at any level of the CNS,* including the spinal cord, brain stem, or brain.
   (1) Central pain as a diagnostic entity should not be confused with psychogenic pain or pain associated with peripheral neuropathy.
   (2) Central pain may be associated with, and in the distribution of, somatosensory deficits noted on examination, *but it may occur in the absence of such deficits.*
   (3) The most common causes of central pain include vascular insult to the CNS (*note:* only half of cerebrovascular accidents leading to central pain involve the thalamus), head trauma, spinal cord injury, surgical ablation of the nervous system, syringomyelia, disc disease, and neurologic diseases, such as multiple sclerosis.
   (4) Central pain may also result from impairment of the peripheral nervous system that disturbs normal afferent input to the CNS, so-called *deafferentation pain.*

b. Epidemiology: estimates of the prevalence of central pain resulting from spinal cord injury vary from 7% to 40%.

c. Pathophysiology: the mechanisms underlying various central pain disorders are not well understood, but attention has focused on
   (1) The effect of CNS lesions on pathways of pain transmission and perception.
   (2) The loss of inhibitory modulatory mechanisms of pain control resulting from disruption of normal afferent stimulation to the CNS and ascending sensory pathways.

d. Clinical presentation.
   (1) Pain is described in neuropathic terms: intense, burning, lancinating, stabbing, shooting, or cramping; deep or superficial; of varying intensity or constant. Paroxysmal episodes of severe, bursting pain may be present.
   (2) Pain may occur immediately after CNS injury or its onset may be delayed for weeks or months.
   (3) Pain may be exacerbated by minor activity, weather changes, or emotional distress.
   (4) Allodynia (i.e., pain in response to an innocuous stimulus) and hyperalgesia (i.e., enhanced pain in response to a noxious stimulus) are common.
   (5) Distribution of pain may vary from localized (e.g., portion of limb) to diffuse (e.g., hemibody).
   (6) Signs of sympathetic dystrophy may be present in an affected limb.

e. Treatment.
   (1) The management of central pain is problematic and frequently disappointing.
   (2) Pharmacotherapy is the first-line approach for treatment.
      - Antidepressants, particularly the tricyclics, have been of considerable value for many patients, although pain relief is usually moderate.
      - Of anticonvulsants, carbamazepine has been most efficacious, particularly for symptoms of paroxysmal pain; phenytoin, clonazepam, divalproex sodium (Depakote), and gabapentin (Neurontin) should also be considered.
      - Phenothiazines, such as fluphenazine, 1 to 2 mg three times a day, or perphenazine, 1 to 2 mg three times a day, in combination with the antidepressants may provide added relief.
      - Mexiletine, 200 to 300 mg three times a day, was shown to be effective in one clinical study.
      - Baclofen (Lioresal), 10 to 20 mg four times a day.
      - Opioids have limited potency to decrease central pain but may offer relief for selected patients.

(3) Nerve blockade may be used.
- Sympathetic blockade may be of diagnostic benefit for determining whether a sympathetic component to the pain exists, especially if vasomotor and sudomotor signs are evident; repeat sympathetic blocks may be therapeutic if the patient has a positive response to initial blockade.
- Peripheral nerve blockade has generally been ineffective for long-term management.

(4) Surgical therapy may be used.
- *Neuroablative procedures, such as cordotomy, cordectomy, rhizotomy, and dorsal root entry zone lesions, which are designed to interrupt known pain pathways, have proved disappointing.*
- More recent neuromodulation techniques, such as deep brain and dorsal column stimulation, have shown some promise and should be considered in cases of severe pain in which alternative, conservative measures have been exhausted.

(5) Psychological intervention may be necessary because central pain is often inadequately controlled by medical therapy and can cause devastating emotional and behavioral invalidism.

B. Myofascial pain syndrome.

1. *Myofascial pain syndromes* (MPSs) represent a common form of chronic pain, particularly in cases of trauma to spinal structures and in the absence of neurologic disturbance.
   a. Myofascial pain has been synonymous with various pain diagnoses, including myositis, myofascitis, idiopathic myalgia, nonarticular rheumatism, myogelosis, and interstitial myofibrositis.
   b. More importantly, the terms *fibrositis* and *fibromyalgia* have been considered as a form of myofascial pain; *fibrositis/fibromyalgia has distinct diagnostic criteria and should be considered as a separate pain entity.*

2. No reliable data are available regarding the prevalence of MPS. However, pain clinicians and published reviews attest to the widespread occurrence of MPS as the most common cause of spinal (e.g., neck, back) and extremity pain.

3. Pathophysiology.
   a. The basic mechanisms underlying MPS remain obscure.
   b. The lack of a viable pathophysiologic model for MPS has been a major hindrance to wider acceptance and recognition of MPS as a legitimate cause of chronic pain.

4. Clinical presentation.
   a. Myofascial pain syndrome is characterized by muscle aching and tenderness, restricted range of motion, and the presence of trigger points (TPs), which, when activated, give rise to a characteristic pattern of *referred* pain; TPs are activated by palpation of the TP and stretching or contraction of the affected muscle.
      (1) A TP is a palpable nodule located in a tense fibrous band within a muscle that is shortened and weak.
      (2) Myofascial pain syndrome is often associated with pseudoneurologic symptoms (e.g., subjective numbness, tingling, paresthesias), often resulting from nerve entrapment by muscle.
      (3) Myofascial pain syndrome often includes autonomic concomitants, such as sweating, local vasoconstriction, pilomotor activity, dermatographia, in the referred pain zone.
   b. Clinical signs of MPS are as follows:
      (1) The results of neurologic examination and diagnostic and radiographic work-up are normal, although subjective sensory disturbances and reduced maximum muscle contractile force may be evident.
      (2) Myofascial pain syndrome may be a simple syndrome involving few muscle groups or, in longstanding cases, may present in multiple muscle groups with their associated pain referral patterns; *rarely is MPS limited to a single muscle.*
      (3) Because referred pain follows a nondermatomal distribution, it is often construed as *nonanatomic,* or *nonphysiologic,* and is consequently *interpreted as evidence for psychogenesis.*
      - Familiarity with the characteristic referred pain patterns associated with each muscle allows the clinician to identify the offending muscle based on the patient's pain description.
      - *Myofascial pain syndrome–related referred pain is often mistaken for neuropathy, radiculopathy, or other pain syndromes* as a result of its radiating pattern; common examples follow:
        Anterior scalene MPS mimics cervical radiculopathy.
        Piriformis MPS mimics lumbosacral radiculopathy.
        Anterior scalene/pectoralis minor MPS mimics thoracic outlet syndrome or brachial plexopathy.
        External oblique MPS mimics ilioinguinal neuralgia.
        Upper trapezius MPS mimics migraine headache.
        Abdominal rectus MPS mimics chronic pelvic pain.
        Iliopsoas MPS mimics lumbar radiculopathy.
   c. Common causes of MPS are as follows:
      (1) Acute muscle strain or trauma (e.g., "whiplash").

(2) Repetitive muscle overuse or overload.
(3) Chronic muscle strain (e.g., poor posture).
(4) Fatigue or overexertion.
(5) Sustained or recurrent psychological tension.
(6) Myofascial pain syndrome may also be evident secondary to other medical disorders, such as disc disease, inflammatory disease, nerve root irritation or compression, dental occlusive disease, and failed back syndrome.

d. Treatment for MPS is as follows:

(1) Identification of perpetuating factors: in chronic MPS, muscle pain and TPs are often maintained by the continuing contribution of perpetuating factors; their identification and control may be critical to management of MPS. Common perpetuating factors include:
- Excessive physical activity beyond muscle tolerance.
- Abnormal posturing and adaptive, compensatory body mechanics (e.g., antalgic gait, slumped shoulders).
- Psychological stress, emotional lability, anger.
- Prolonged immobilization, such as bed rest.
- Structural asymmetries, such as leg length discrepancy, small hemipelvis.
- Nutritional inadequacies, such as vitamin B_1, B_6, B_{12}, and C and folic acid deficiencies.

(2) Education.
- Patients need to understand the musculoskeletal origins of their pain; it should be distinguished from neurologic and arthritic pain.
- Patient's role in managing perpetuating factors and compliance with therapeutic exercises should be emphasized.

(3) Physical therapy: therapeutic exercise is the mainstay of treatment for MPS.
- Initial intervention directed at restoration of range of motion by stretching exercises; flexibility can further be facilitated by therapeutic massage, such as myofascial release technique.
- Therapeutic modalities, including ice massage, heat, ultrasound.
- Trichloromonofluoromethane; dichlorodifluoromethane (Fluori-Methane) spray applied to affected muscle or muscles in long strokes, distal-to-proximal and parallel to muscle fibers; muscle placed in taut position before application and repeated several times as range increases; heat and gentle active stretching follow.
- Education in proper posture and body mechanics.
- Progressive, graded strengthening program to restore strength while continuing to *maintain flexibility* with stretching regimen.
- Aerobic conditioning.
- Transcutaneous electrical nerve stimulation.

(4) Trigger point injections.
- Judicious use of several milliliters of local anesthetic (e.g., .5% procaine or lidocaine, longer-acting 0.25% bupivacaine) infiltrated into TP to restore range of motion and reduce TP tenderness.
- Trigger point injections should be administered in the context of stretching program to facilitate flexibility training, *not to replace it.*
- The addition of steroids appears to offer no therapeutic advantage beyond local anesthetic.
- Trigger point injection should be followed by gentle, passive stretching, Fluori-Methane spray and stretching, heat and/or active stretching.

(5) Psychological intervention.
- Relaxation training and stress management.
- Emotional adjustment counseling to address reactive mood disturbances, anger/frustration, fear of reinjury, obsessive worry.

(6) Medications
- No specific drug regimen is consistently effective for MPS.
- Antispasmodics or muscle relaxants may be helpful in acute MPS but are generally ineffective for sustained muscle shortening associated with chronic MPS.
- Nonsteroidal anti-inflammatory drugs are of benefit for some patients and should be routinely considered.
- Opioids have a limited role for selected patients with chronic MPS.
- Antidepressants may provide analgesia and symptomatic treatment (e.g., sleep and mood disturbance) in some patients.

e. Somatic dysfunction.

(1) *Somatic dysfunction* is a malfunction or malalignment of a segment or segments of the spinal column, pelvis, or extremities that may produce limited motion in an area, muscle spasm, pain, and tenderness.
(2) Somatic dysfunctions are frequently a contributing factor to, or are maintained by, restricted muscle function associated with MPS.
(3) Many patients who present with chronic MPS also have evidence for somatic dysfunctions; failure to address and resolve

these musculoskeletal dysfunctions results in ineffective treatment and continued pain.

(4) Manual therapy techniques (e.g., osteopathic manipulation, muscle energy technique) are typically necessary to resolve dysfunctions.

C. Reflex sympathetic dystrophy (RSD) and causalgia/complex regional pain syndromes (CRPS).

1. *Reflex sympathetic dystrophy* refers to a variety of disorders in which an apparent neurovascular pain complex is present, usually affecting a limb; the *causalgia* described by wounded soldiers who, after peripheral nerve injury, were observed to manifest symptoms of severe burning pain associated with hyperesthesia, allodynia, and hyperpathia along with vasomotor and sudomotor disturbances, represents on early description of RSD.
   a. Evidence that sympathetic blockade could eradicate the limb pain in patients with causalgia drew attention to the link between peripheral nerve injury and sympathetic activation.
   b. The term *RSD* has come to encompass pain disorders (e.g., Sudeck's atrophy, sympathalgia, shoulder-hand syndrome) in which sympathetic hyperactivity was felt to be etiologic, whether or not nerve injury was associated with the onset of pain.
   c. The nature of the relationship between sympathetic activation and RSD is complicated by the evidence that the associated autonomic disturbances appear to fluctuate over time and become less prominent and by the decreasing effectiveness of sympathetic blockade to arrest the pain and accompanying vasomotor symptoms as the syndrome becomes chronic.
   d. Some investigators have suggested that a distinction be made between sympathetically maintained pain and sympathetically independent pain in RSD patients.
   e. Recently, a taxonomy has been proposed that categorizes RSD and causalgia based on history, symptoms, and clinical findings, irrespective of pathophysiology (i.e., contribution of sympathetic nervous system); *CRPS I (RSD) and II (causalgia)* make up this new taxonomy.[3]
   f. This taxonomy redefines sympathetically maintained pain as the aspect of pain that is attributable to the sympathetic nervous system; a sympathetic pain component may be present in different painful conditions (e.g., phantom pain, neuralgias, metabolic neuropathies) in addition to CRPS but is not pathognomonic of them.

2. Epidemiology.
   a. The CRPS/RSD can occur in children but is most common among adults.
   b. Women appear to suffer more than men (3:1 ratio).
   c. Estimates of the percentage of patients sustaining injury who develop the syndrome vary from 0.05% to 15%.

3. Pathophysiology.
   a. No accepted model adequately explains the complexities of CRPS/RSD.
   b. Most theories focus on the development of an abnormal reverbatory circuit between afferent (nociceptive) input and efferent sympathetic hyperactivity; this conceptualization presupposes a dysregulatory reflex in the normal outflow of sympathetic impulses that facilitate healing after injury in post-traumatic cases.

4. Clinical presentation.
   a. The term *CRPS* describes a variety of painful conditions that are usually the result of injury, although they may be idiopathic; it is regional, with a predominance of distal abnormal findings; *it exceeds both in magnitude and duration the expected clinical course of the inciting event.*
   b. Typically, evidence for autonomic dysregulation, sensory abnormalities, motor changes, trophic changes, and reactive psychological disturbance is present.
   c. *Both CRPS I (RSD) and CRPS II (causalgia) share identical symptoms and clinical findings, with the exception that CRPS II develops after nerve injury.*
   d. Pain may be initiated by a noxious event that is severe (e.g., crush injury) or minor (e.g., limb sprain or surgery), a benign cut or contusion, neurologic disease (e.g., brachial plexopathy, stroke, infiltrating tumor), infection, or vascular disease, or it may be idiopathic.
   e. Sensory symptoms.
      (1) Pain that is described as diffuse, burning, aching, or throbbing; may occur spontaneously; allodynia to mechanical or thermal stimuli; hyperesthesia, hyperpathia usually present.
      (2) Pain distribution not consistent with peripheral nerve or dermatome.
      (3) Pain either intermittent or constant, exacerbated by physical activity, environmental stimuli, or psychological distress.
   f. Autonomic symptoms.
      (1) Vasomotor instability, including alterations in blood flow; usually vasodilation in early stages followed by or alternating with vasoconstriction; red, blue, mottled, or blanched appearance; resultant hyperthermia or hypothermia.
      (2) Edema (pitting, brawny).
      (3) Sudomotor dysfunction (e.g., hyperhidrosis).
   g. Motor symptoms.
      (1) Weakness, tremor, joint stiffness.
      (2) Dystonias and contractures in later stages.
      (3) Protective postures.
   h. Trophic symptoms.

(1) Muscle atrophy.
(2) Osteopenic arthropathy.
(3) Glossy skin.
(4) Altered hair and nail growth.

5. Course of CRPS/RSD.
   a. Stage 1: *acute phase.*
      (1) Signs of sympathetic denervation result in vasodilation, hyperthermia, hyperemia, edema, and increased nail and hair growth.
      (2) Burning pain is aggravated by light touch and environmental factors, such as cold, draft, loud noise, or motion.
      (3) Pain is typically responsive to sympathetic blockade.
   b. Stage 2: *dystrophic phase.*
      (1) Within 2 to 3 months, vasoconstriction generally predominates, with skin that appears pale, glazed, cyanotic, mottled, and hypothermic; edema may lessen or become brawny.
      (2) Nails become cracked and brittle, and hair loss is common.
      (3) Joint stiffening and contractures, muscle atrophy, and osteoporosis typically ensue secondary to disuse and abnormal posturing.
      (4) Sympathetic blockade may be only partially or temporarily effective in reducing pain.
   c. Stage 3: *atrophic phase.*
      (1) Over months and years, classic sympathetic signs may be less evident and replaced by increasing motor disturbances, diffusion of symptoms proximally and to other body parts, greater functional disability, and severe psychological decompensation.
      (2) Increasing CNS involvement is suggested by the failure of sympathetic blockade to alter CRPS symptoms in longstanding cases.

6. Graded presentation of CRPS: although most clinicians acknowledge the classic CRPS presentation, *milder forms of the disorder are common in which a slow onset, only mild vasomotor/sudomotor symptoms, and a dull, aching pain are evident.*

7. Role of psychological factors.
   a. Many authors have suggested a prevailing role for psychological factors in explaining why some patients develop RSD after minor trauma while others do not.
   b. Psychological studies of RSD patients have been retrospective and confounded by the presence of pain, thus limiting the inference of psychological disturbance as a precursor of RSD.
   c. Clinical experience suggests that RSD patients may be "sympathetic reactors."
   d. *It is incontrovertible that the severe, relentless pain of RSD can promote devastating psychological invalidism.*

8. Treatment.
   a. Mild cases of RSD may resolve spontaneously or respond to conservative measures; *however, the severe morbidity of chronic RSD demands that early identification of symptoms results in immediate referral for sympathetic blockade; aggressive sympathetic blockade with an active mobilization program is the most effective strategy for resolving acute RSD and preventing chronicity. All therapeutic measures become less effective as the course of symptoms extends to months.*
   b. Sympathetic blockade may be used.
      (1) Local anesthetic sympathetic block repeated several times per week until symptom relief plateaus.
         - Stellate ganglion block, lumbar sympathetic, epidural, or spinal block.
         - Intravenous regional infusion of ganglionic blocking agents, such as guanethidine, bretylium.
      (2) In patients in whom sympathetic blockade provides excellent but consistently transient relief, surgical or chemical sympathectomy should be considered.
   c. Pharmacologic agents found helpful in selected RSD patients include
      (1) Systemic corticosteroids administered in short bursts; prednisone, 15 to 20 mg four times a day for 2 to 4 days, then tapered over 10 to 14 days, or moderate doses over longer duration, such as 10 mg three times a day for 1 to 3 months.
      (2) Oral nifedipine (Procardia), 10 to 30 mg three times a day. This agent is a calcium chemical blocker that relaxes smooth muscles, raises peripheral blood flow, and antagonizes the effect of norepinephrine.
      (3) Adrenergic blocking agents (sympatholytics), such as prazosin (Minipress), 5 mg twice or three times a day; propranolol (Inderal), 120 to 240 mg a day; clonidine (Catapres), 0.2 to 0.6 mg twice a day.
      (4) Antidepressants.
      (5) Anticonvulsants, particularly gabapentin (Neurontin).
      (6) Maintenance opioids.
   d. Physiotherapy.
      (1) *Physical therapy and occupational therapy are critical components in the treatment of RSD and may suffice for mild cases; however, vigorous passive range of motion or excessive strengthening may retrigger RSD.*
      (2) Tactile skin desensitization of the affected limb may be attempted across different sensory modalities (e.g., temperature, light touch, textures).
      (3) In more severe cases, physical therapy may need to occur in conjunction with analgesia, either by oral agents or nerve blockade.
   e. Psychological intervention.
      (1) Instruction in relaxation strategies (e.g., biofeedback, hypnosis) to reduce sympathetic activation.
      (2) Cognitive-behavioral strategies for pain control and improved coping.
      (3) Address reactive mood disturbances, such

as depression, anger, and anxiety, as well as adjustment issues in chronic cases.

D. Headache.

- Headache is one of the most common reasons for medical consultation and the most common pain complaint.
- Headaches may be primary, as in migraine or tension-type, or, in rare instances, secondary to more serious organic disease, such as brain tumor or subdural hematoma.
- Although headache has been historically viewed as primarily of psychosomatic origin or stress induced, *recent evidence suggests that headache is a biogenetic malady that is readily exacerbated by emotional and behavioral factors.*

1. Epidemiology.
   - **a.** Ninety percent of Americans have at least one headache per year.
   - **b.** Forty million Americans experience recurring headaches.
   - **c.** Approximately 25 million people experience migraine headaches.
   - **d.** Six percent of males and 15% to 17% of females have migraine headaches.
   - **e.** Sixteen percent of the general population have cervicogenic headaches at any one point in time.
   - **f.** Patients who have migraines use between two and five times more health care services than nonmigraineurs.
   - **g.** Chronic headache accounts for 150 million lost work days and $57 billion in lost productivity each year.
   - **h.** Significant comorbidity exists between migraine and tension-type headaches and psychiatric diagnoses, particularly with depression, anxiety, and panic disorders.

2. Vascular headache syndromes.
   - **a.** *Migraine:* a severe and potentially incapacitating headache that represents an inherited disposition for neurovascular instability and is associated with dysregulation of brain chemistry and regional alterations in blood flow.
     - **(1)** Pathophysiology.
       - Although traditionally viewed as primarily a disorder of intracranial and extracranial blood flow, increasing attention is being given to central mechanisms of pain physiology to explain migraine pain and associated symptoms.
       - Particular attention focuses on the trigeminovascular reflex as a central mediator of migraine.

         Activation of the trigeminal nerve produces vasodilation; efferent innervation from the reflex may activate the locus coeruleus and dorsal raphe nucleus, which are known to produce vasoconstriction and vasodilation, respectively.

         Disturbance in neuropeptide activity is suggested by evidence that calcitonin gene-related peptide, vasoactive intestinal peptide and substance P—all known nociception-inducing substances—produce vasodilation and are released by trigeminal activation; resultant perivascular inflammation induced by peptide release (e.g., prostaglandins, bradykinin) may lead to cranial vessel sensitization and associated nociceptive input to brain stem, completing a vicious cycle of pain and vascular disturbance.

         Alterations in serotonergic regulation are associated with migraine, and selective serotonin agents, such as sumatriptan (Imitrex) and methysergide (Sansert), can promote effective migraine control.

         Hypothalamic dysregulation appears to be related to premonitory symptoms of migraine; hypothalamic projections to the locus couruleus and the dorsal raphe nucleus may initiate vascular disturbances.

         The aura of migraine appears to be related to a focal reduction in occipital/frontal blood flow followed by progression of reduced blood flow across the cerebral cortex (oligemia).
     - **(2)** Migraine types.
       - *Migraine with aura* ("classic migraine"). Headache is preceded by reversible prodrome, including one or more symptoms suggesting cerebral cortical or brain stem dysfunction.

         Duration of aura symptoms is typically 4 to 60 minutes; headache follows within 60 minutes of aura.

         Aura symptoms include scotoma (scintillating), visual field cuts, and photophobia; motor disturbances, weakness, and dysarthria; and unilateral numbness, paresthesias, dizziness, nausea, and vomiting.
       - *Migraine without aura* ("common migraine").

         Headache lasting 4 to 72 hours.

         Usually unilateral but not necessarily; pulsating, throbbing pain; moderate to severe intensity; pain aggravated by activity.

         Presence of nausea, vomiting, photophobia, or phonophobia.

- *Basilar migraine.*
  - Migraine with aura symptoms that originate in the brain stem or occipital lobes.
  - Meets criteria for migraine with aura.
  - Includes two or more aura symptoms of the following: visual disturbance (e.g., hemianopia, temporary blindness), dysarthria, vertigo, tinnitus, impaired hearing, diplopia, ataxia, bilateral parasthesias and/or paresis, decreased level of consciousness.
- *Ophthalmoplegic migraine.*
  - Repeated headaches consisting of unilateral eye pain associated with paresis of one (usually third) or more (fourth, sixth) cranial nerves in absence of a cranial lesion.
  - Headache may last hours to months.
  - Most common in children.
- *Menstrual migraine.*
  - Headache only, beginning 1 to 3 days before and after the onset of menses; when headache occurs only during ovulation, it is termed *menstrually related* migraine.
- *Abdominal migraine.*
  - Paroxysmal or recurrent abdominal pain or vomiting, associated with headache or not, preceded by prodrome of yawning, fatigue, or other aura symptoms.

(3) Clinical features.

- Female-to-male ratio, 3:1.
- Prevalence of migraine increases from adolescence and peaks between 35 and 45 years, then steadily drops.
- Seven percent to 18% of children experience migraines.
- Common prodromal signs that precede aura include changes in mental state (e.g., depression, euphoria, irritability, restlessness), neurologic status (e.g., yawning, poor concentration, dysphasia), and other features (e.g., stiff neck, appetite disturbance, chills, sluggishness).

(4) Common triggers of migraine.

- Variations in sleep pattern.
- Foods containing a vasodilating amine (e.g., tyramine, phenylethlamine, dopamine), monosodium glutamate, caffeine, nitrate compounds; examples of food group triggers: chocolate; ripened cheese; alcoholic beverages; meats with nitrates; fermented, pickled, or marinated foods; fruits and their juices; yeast products (e.g., fresh bread, doughnuts).
- Lights.
- Fasting.
- Changes in barometric pressure.
- Hormonal changes, especially estrogen in women.
- Physical exertion.
- Stress.

(5) Treatment of migraines.

- Intervention strategies.
  - Preventive, including identification of and management of migraine triggers, medication prophylaxis if headache frequency exceeds one to two times per week, modification of lifestyle habits (e.g., sleep, diet, exercise, stress), education of patient.
  - Abortive: use of medications or other modalities (e.g., oxygen, relaxation) after the onset of early headache symptoms.
- Drug prophylaxis.
  - Antidepressants are first choice agents. Tricyclics appear to be most effective, but selective serotonin reuptake inhibitors have demonstrated efficacy.
  - Beta blockers, such as sustained-release propranolol, 80 to 240 mg once daily.
  - Calcium channel blockers such as sustained release verapamil (Calan), 80 to 320 mg in divided doses.
  - Methysergide (Sansert) 2 mg three times a day, although retroperitoneal, pleural, or pericardial fibrosis is a serious potential complication.
  - Nonsteroidal anti-inflammatory drugs, such as naproxen (Naprosyn) or indomethacine (Indocin) daily.
  - Divalproex sodium (Depakote), with a starting dose of 250 mg twice a day, to a maximum of 1800 mg/dL.
  - Monoamine oxidase inhibitors, such as phenelzine (Nardil), 15 to 30 mg three times a day, although important dietary restrictions apply.
- Abortive agents, to be taken at the earliest sign of headache.
  - Ergotamine preparations (Ergostat) or in combination with caffeine (Cafergot, Wigraine), phenobarbital (Bellergal-S), or both (Cafergot P-B and Wigraine PB suppository).
  - Dihydroergotamine mesylate (DHE 45) infusion.
  - Isometheptene-dichloralphenazone-acetaminophen (Midrin), two tablets at onset, one tablet every

hour to maximum of five tablets per day.
Aspirin, caffeine, butalbital (Fiorinal, Fioricet), 1 to 2 tablets every 4 hours, not to exceed 6 tablets per day.
Nonsteroidal anti-inflammatory drugs, particularly naproxen (Anaprox), ketoprofen (Orudis).
Opioids, administered judiciously.
Often require antiemetic agents to control nausea and vomiting; suppository administration may be necessary in severe cases.
All abortive agents except NSAIDs must be limited in use to twice within 7 days to avoid development of "rebound" headaches.

b. *Cluster:* unilateral (temporal, forehead, eye) headache, severe in intensity; occurs with periods ranging from one to several months, usually followed by periods of remission varying from months to years; *chronic cluster headache* characterizes pattern in which remissions are less prolonged.
   (1) Clinical features.
   - Male-to-female ratio is 5:1.
   - During cluster episodes, headaches last up to 1 hour, typically several times per day.
   - Cluster episodes often occur during fall and spring seasons.
   - They are commonly triggered by alcohol, awakening from sleep, or other migraine triggers during cluster periods.
   - Associated symptoms include ipsilateral lacrimation, rhinorrhea, nasal congestion.

   (2) Treatment.
   - Prophylaxis (during cluster period).
     Methysergide.
     Prednisone, starting at 40 mg/d and then down tapered over the following three weeks.
     Lithium (Eskalith), 300 mg, two to four times a day, to maintain a serum level of 0.8 to 1.2 mg/dL.
     Ergotamine.
   - Abortive therapy.
     Oxygen (7 to 10 L/min) for 15 minutes.
     Ergotamine, 2 mg, administered 2 hours prior to headache recurrence.

c. *Paroxysmal hemicrania:* a variant of cluster headaches, with attacks more frequent per day but of shorter duration (10 to 20 minutes).
   (1) More common in females.
   (2) Can be triggered by cervical motion.
   (3) Treatment: particularly responsive to indomethacin, 25 to 50 mg three times a day.

d. *Chronic daily headache:* daily headache with mixed tension and vascular symptoms, without typical migraine features but may include superimposed migraine attacks.
   (1) Chronic daily headache has two types:
   - *History of intermittent migraines in which, over time, headache frequency increases until headaches occur daily ("transformed migraine")*
   - *History of increasing use of abortive agents for acute migraine such that patient develops "rebound headache," which represents physiologic dependence and abstinence syndrome manifesting as migraine.*

   (2) Treatment.
   - Transformed migraine should be treated as a chronic migraine variant, and the emphasis is on prophylaxis and abortive intervention, the latter limited to twice per week in order to avoid rebound.
   - Rebound headache requires *withdrawal from abortive medications for 4 to 6 weeks;* often, headache severity improves or resolves after detoxification.

3. *Tension-type headache syndromes.*
   a. Headaches that arise from musculoskeletal structures in or of the face (e.g., temporomandibular joint syndrome), head and cervical spine *(cervicogenic headache).*
   b. Pathophysiology.
      (1) Little is known regarding the mechanisms of pain from tension headaches.
      (2) Data are equivocal on the causal relationship between increased tension in skeletal muscles and pain.
      (3) *Many tension and cervicogenic headaches are referred from myofascial trigger points (TPs) of the face and neck.*
   c. Clinical features.
      (1) More common in women.
      (2) Pressing, bandlike character, unilateral or bilateral, lasting 30 minutes to several days.
      (3) Often precipitated by or associated with stress, depression.
      (4) Variable location but commonly involves frontalis, occiput, temporalis, cervical spine with related restrictions in range of motion and tenderness/TPs evident on palpation.
   d. Treatment (see Myofascial Pain Syndrome section for additional information).
      (1) Physical therapy: primarily consists of stretching to restore cervical and jaw range of motion, eradicate TPs, posture education.
      (2) Trigger point injection.
      (3) Pharmacologic therapy.
      - Antidepressants.
      - Nonsteroidal anti-inflammatory drugs.
      - Muscle relaxants/antispasmodics in acute cases.

      (4) Psychological therapy.

- Stress management/relaxation training.
- Cognitive behavior therapy.
- Electromyographic biofeedback.

4. *Occipital neuralgia.*
   a. Occipital headache in the distribution of the lesser or greater occipital nerve.
   b. Pathophysiology: nerve irritation as a result of trauma or nerve compression between the atlas and the axis or entrapment by the cervical myofascial muscles.
   c. Clinical features.
      (1) Pain can be intermittent or persistent.
      (2) Palpation of occipital nerves reproduces pain in expected distributions.
   d. Treatment.
      (1) Occipital nerve blockade with local anesthetic.
      (2) Treatment of myofascial restrictions in cases of nerve entrapment.
      (3) Antidepressants.
      (4) Anticonvulsants.

5. *Post-traumatic headache syndromes.*
   a. Headache after minor or severe head trauma, usually with an onset within days of injury but may be delayed for months; *no correlation between the severity of head trauma and the severity of headache.*
   b. Pathophysiology.
      (1) The pathogenesis of post-traumatic headache may relate to a variety of neurophysiologic sequelae of head injury.
      (2) Mechanical forces to the head and neck may result in nerve fiber degeneration and damage particularly in the brain stem, neuronal disturbance resulting from axonal sheering, slowed cerebral circulation, and/or altered neurotransmitter function.
   c. Clinical features.
      (1) Post-traumatic headache is similar to other types of chronic headache and most commonly include symptoms compatible with a mixed migraine-tension headache.
      (2) Circumscribed migraine episodes may be superimposed on a chronic, daily headache of mixed features.
      (3) Post-traumatic headache is frequently associated with cervicogenic and myofascial sources of pain.
      (4) Common associated symptoms include dizziness, vertigo, tinnitus, alcohol intolerance, syncope, decreased alertness, and fatigue.
      (5) Cognitive impairment includes reduced attention span and poor short-term memory.
      (6) Alterations in mood, stress tolerance, and personality may occur.
   d. Treatment.
      (1) Management is approached symptomatically, based on the mix of headache symptoms.
      (2) Use of migraine prophylaxis, primarily tricyclic antidepressants, beta blockers, or calcium channel blockers, can be effective in treating daily headache, even if formal migraine signs are not prominent.
      (3) Migraine abortive agents are indicated for recurrent migraine attacks.
      (4) Medical and physical therapy interventions should be used if there is evidence of myofascial pain syndromes of the face, neck, and upper back.
      (5) In cases of superficial hyperesthesia at the site of injury, anticonvulsants such as phenytoin (Dilantin) may be effective in reducing neuropathic pain from entrapment of sensory nerve endings (by local scar formation or trauma-induced sensitization of sensory nerves).
      (6) Psychological treatment if headache management is inadequate or emotional, cognitive, and behavioral disturbance is formidable.

VI. Pain, emotions and comorbid psychiatric disorders.

A. When is chronic pain a psychiatric disorder?

1. *Conceptualizing chronic pain and psychological impairment.*
   a. *Pain and the emotional reaction to pain are intimately linked along a biopsychosocial continuum.*
   b. Common neurologic structures that are innervated by pain pathways (e.g., limbic system, reticular formation) and shared neurotransmitters systems (e.g., serotonin, norepinephrine) are responsible for these associations and interact with the environmental context in which pain occurs.
   c. Pain, depression, and anxiety have complex interrelationships, and it is frequently very difficult, and often fruitless, to decipher which came first.
   d. *Pain is most often not initiated or sustained by psychological processes alone,* and there is no specific personality profile associated with chronic pain.

2. *"Shared responsibility."*
   a. Pain syndromes tend to be chronic, relapsing disorders that often require a long-term interaction between an internist and a psychiatrist or psychologist for adequate management.
   b. *Shared responsibility* provides a mechanism to address a physician's discomfort with treating a highly disabling disorder that has no measurable end-organ dysfunction and also allows for a "checks and balances" approach by integrating medical and psychiatric findings in management.

B. Specific psychiatric disorders comorbid with chronic pain.

1. *Substance abuse.*[4]
   a. Studies reveal a varying prevalence of concurrent or pre-existing substance abuse disorders in patients with chronic pain; certain aspects of substance abuse have significant relevance to the treatment of chronic pain.
   b. Effect of substance abuse on pain.
      (1) *Withdrawal:* patients with substance dependency or abuse may actually worsen their pain experience by intermittent withdrawal.
         - Opioid withdrawal (which may occur intermittently if long-acting and short-acting substances are used, or if the patient has had difficulty maintaining intake of the substance) is well known to produce headache.
         - Pain may actually be disinhibited by the sympathetic arousal that is related to episodic withdrawal or that is part of the clinical effects of substances such as cocaine; this disinhibition may occur as a result of alterations in pain pathways and inhibitory mechanisms.

      (2) *Sleep disturbance:* commonly known to exacerbate pain and is closely associated with addictive disorders.
      (3) *Depression:* often found in the circumstance of cocaine withdrawal, alcohol abuse, and dependence; depression is known to decrease pain tolerance.
      (4) *Lifestyle:* secondary physical illnesses and the financial and social disruption caused by addictive illness tend to worsen the distress and disability often associated with pain.
   c. Efficacy of rehabilitation treatment for substance abuse.
      (1) Chronic pain and addictive disease often appear similar clinically.
      (2) Syndrome of pain facilitation or disinhibition may occur in the presence of the two syndromes; patients often feel that they abuse substances to treat pain; however, it is notable that after *treatment for addiction, pain is often reduced, and only rarely does it increase; further, after detoxification, a clearer locus of pain may emerge, as may an augmented response to nonpharmacologic treatments of pain.*
   d. Treatment of pain in patients vulnerable to substance abuse.
      (1) When opioids are indicated for pain, *the addicted patient can be considered for opioid therapy if he or she is closely supervised.*
      (2) Opioids should be continued for a reasonable amount of time (given the nature of the injury), and then the treatment course can be re-evaluated.
      (3) *Long-acting opioids (e.g., methadone [Dolophine], levorphanol [Levo-dromoran], and morphine [MS Contin]) are preferred* over the reinforcing "rush" of shorter-acting medications.
      (4) When a patient addicted to an opioid requires pain management, it is important to provide baseline opioid requirements; thereafter, incremental opioid can be added in order to treat the patient's pain, along with any helpful adjunctive treatments, such as regional analgesia, TENS, physical therapy, and nonopioid medications.
      (5) Gradual tapering of medications to baseline is important in order to avoid rebound pain when the injury or illness has sufficiently resolved.
      (6) If the patient becomes resistant to tapering, a thorough search for other causes of pain is indicated; the physician should seriously consider treatment for anxiety, with agents such as buspirone (BuSpar), 40 to 80 mg/d; an antidepressant such as sertraline (Zoloft), 50 to 100 mg/d; or a benzodiazepine, such as clonazepam (Klonopin), 1 to 4 mg/d.
      (7) Addicted patients may become anxious at the thought of potential withdrawal symptoms or recurring pain during tapering, and an anxiolytic may smooth the process; a longer-acting benzodiazepine, such as clonazepam, 0.5 mg twice a day to 1 mg three times a day, is preferred. This practice will avoid the episodic "miniwithdrawals" of the shorter-acting benzodiazepine agents (e.g., alprazolam [Xanax]). Then, the longer-acting benzodiazepine can be carefully tapered.
      (8) Signs of new addiction to the pain medication include
         - Resistance to tapering.
         - Denial of pain relief by any medication other than opioids.
         - Preference for short-acting high-dose analgesics.
         - Repeated requests for medications.

      (9) Medication scheduling: *time interval* dosing rather than "as needed" dosing is recommended.
         - As needed dosing may cause friction with medical personnel, leading to suspicions regarding the patient's motives for requesting medication.
         - Routine dosing, *guided by an adequate understanding of the half-life and pharmacokinetics* of the analgesic drug,

greatly minimizes interdose withdrawal symptoms.

- *Administration of the medication on a regular dosing schedule is dependent on the schedule, not the pain,* thus, reinforcement of the symptoms of pain is avoided.
- The addicted pain patient should be included in the decision-making process to determine when pain medication should be given; this involvement may significantly allay the patient's anxiety about receiving adequate medications to avoid withdrawal or pain.

2. *Depression.*
   a. Prevalence: depression is highly associated with pain syndromes; epidemiologic studies note a prevalence of depression in patients with chronic pain to range from 35% to 100%.
   b. Phenomenology.
      (1) For most patients, depression follows in response to pain, particularly as pain becomes persistent.
      (2) As in other medical conditions, at any given level of disability, the treatment of depression improves clinical function and outcome.
   c. Treatment.
      (1) The rigorous treatment of depression with a medication compatible with the patient's pain regimen is advised; nearly all current antidepressants are compatible with most pain regimens, with the following provisos:
         - Monoamine oxidase inhibitors are contraindicated in conjunction with meperidine (Demerol); deaths from this combination have been reported.
         - Antidepressants and pain medications can both suppress level of consciousness.
         - Highly bound antidepressants may alter anticonvulsant levels.
3. *Anxiety disorders.*
   a. Prevalence: anxiety disorders are highly prevalent in chronic pain patients; these include generalized anxiety disorder, agoraphobia with panic attacks, and adjustment disorder with anxious mood.
   b. Phenomenology.
      (1) The high prevalence of anxiety disorders in this population may be partly the result of sympathetic activation mediated hypothalamically in response to nociception.
      (2) It is often very difficult to separate anxiety from depression in clinical settings—*what the patient describes as anxiety may well represent significant depression instead.*
      (3) Anxiety may significantly confound medical diagnoses; nearly 50% of emergency room visits for noncardiac chest pain are due to panic disorder.[5]
   c. Treatment.
      (1) Effective management of pain is the best solution for the patient's anxiety.
      (2) If anxiety continues to be severe, a nonbenzodiazepine agent, such as sertraline (Zoloft), up to 50 mg twice a day or paroxetine (Paxil), 10 to 20 mg twice a day may be safely added to most regimens.
4. *Somatoform disorders and the pain-prone patient.*
   a. This is a complex group of disorders with varying contributions from "emotional pain"; patients are often demanding and have much anxiety regarding their physical health; somatizing patients make up about 36% of patients on psychiatric disability and 48% of sick leave requests.[6]
   b. Not every patient with an unexplained pain warrants a psychiatric diagnosis; patients with pain have no greater prevalence of comorbid psychiatric illness than do other medical patients[7]; *what distinguishes this group of patients is their preoccupation with physical symptoms and the role such symptoms play in their lives.*
      (1) *Somatization disorder.*
         - Five to 15% of patients with chronic pain have somatization disorder[8]; there is a high comorbidity of somatization disorder with depression and anxiety disorders. Anxiety is often focused on medical concerns.
         - These individuals suffer from four or more different pain complaints over time, with an onset before the age of 30 years; somatization disorder is usually associated with complaints in multiple organ systems (not necessarily pain); the patient's suffering is out of proportion to what would be expected from physical findings.
         - Frequently, the patient has a history of multiple doctor visits and high utilization of health care services.
      (2) *Conversion disorder.*
         - One or more symptoms affect voluntary motor or sensory function, suggesting a neurologic condition, but the symptoms are nonanatomic or nonphysiologic; pain, numbness, and weakness are the most common complaints.
         - Often, a temporal association exists between a significant stressor and the onset of symptoms.
         - *If pain is the only symptom, the diagnosis of a pain disorder rather than a conversion disorder diagnosis is made.*

(3) *Hypochondriasis.*
- A firm, fixed, and intractable conviction of illness or disease exists for 6 months or longer, regardless of objective findings and physician reassurance.
- New physical signs or symptoms are often incorporated into the belief.
- Head, facial, cardiac, or abdominal pain is common, as are numbness and burning pain.

(4) *Pain disorder.*
- Pain is the patient's primary somatic focus.
- Pain is not fully explained by the observable pathology.
- Pain causes significant impairment in function or is the cause of significant distress.
- Psychological factors play a primary role in the onset or continuation of pain.
- Past history often reveals physical abuse, family history of depression and/or alcoholism, or dependent personal relationships.

(5) *Malingering.*
- The patient consciously produces symptomatology with clear rewards in mind, such as monetary reward, avoidance of criminal charges, or to obtain medications.
- Patients do not present with signs of intrapsychic conflict or emotional pain, and they specifically avoid psychiatric referral.
- Actual pain is probably very rare in this disorder.
- Diagnosis may be suggested by certain clinical findings:[7]
  Lateral anesthesia ending at midline.
  Astasia/abasia gait with upper body lurching.
  Nonanatomic vibratory sensation cutoffs.
  Also common in pain disorder, somatization disorder, and conversion disorder.

(6) *Factitious disorder/Munchausen's syndrome.*
- Distinguishable from those with malingering by the presence of an intrapsychic need for the sick role; may result in the patient's seeking or acquiescing to physically invasive procedures or commiting self-inflicted injury to mimic physical illness; not due to psychosis.
- Three subtypes exist:
  With predominantly physical signs or symptoms.
  With predominantly psychological signs or symptoms.
  Combined.
- Seeking of narcotics.
- Complex history of multiple prior hospitalizations and surgeries.
- Avoidance of psychiatric consultation.

VII. Physicians' reactions to the patient with pain.

A. Stigma.

Much stigma is attached to pain behavior. It is often the practitioner's feeling that this behavior is, on some level, under the patient's control. However, as was noted earlier, pain and the autonomic, anxious reaction to it are often intimately linked and not easily controlled.

B. Psychological magnification.

At times, clinicians suspect that the experience of bodily pain may be significantly magnified by psychological need or conflict, but

1. *Individuals who are capable of assessing and verbalizing psychological needs generally do so without a somatic focus.* Conversely, individuals who have difficulty with, or are unable to, verbally express their distress (e.g., alexithymia) are prone to somatization.
2. In cases with significant psychological underpinnings, *pain is the psychological expression of need. Until the needs are addressed (or met), pain persists, even if its somatic source has been addressed.*
3. Unfortunately, it is not often easy to meet the wide-ranging psychological needs of patients with pain, and clinicians frequently feel frustrated and helpless. Four common elements have been found to characterize chronic pain patients' relationship with their physicians:
   a. Muted anger.
   b. Demands to personalize the relationship or that are inconsistent with professional, ethical practice.
   c. Covert depression.
   d. Unrequited wishes for nurturance and dependency.

C. Frustration and helplessness.

1. Patients often feel frustrated and helpless in the face of overwhelming illness.
2. Clinicians derive satisfaction from helping people and solving medical problems. They are invariably frustrated by patients who do not respond to treatment whose clinical presentation is ambiguous, confusing, and complex.
   a. Frustration may lead a clinician to unintentionally prescribe larger doses of medications than indicated; the clinician may

also experience significant conflict about physician-patient encounters, causing the physician to change regimens inappropriately or to provide therapeutic measures to afford quick, albeit temporary, relief but ignore realistic and long-term treatment goals.

b. The clinician may feel himself or herself caught in an overwhelming struggle with a given patient; in such a case, the clinician would be wise to step back and ask himself or herself if the particular case has more personal meaning for the physician, perhaps recalling a frustrating, emotionally charged personal experience or prior clinical dilemma.

3. A potential solution exists:
   a. Certain patients may be so difficult to treat that any one clinician may have insufficient resources to deal with the complexities and emotional demands of the situation.
   b. When strategies such as structured, regularly scheduled visits have failed, the clinician may need to invoke a treatment team approach to diffuse the effort by soliciting assistance from a pain clinic or available mental health resources.

VIII. Treatment guidelines for patients with chronic pain.

A. Basic guidelines for the management of chronic pain.

1. *Convey to patients you believe their pain is real.* Do not question the veracity of the patient's pain complaint. *Regardless of the cause of the pain, whether physiologic or unconsciously motivated, the patient's suffering is real and merits confirmation.* Few patients deliberately fake a pain problem. A therapeutic physician-patient alliance begins with mutual trust and respect. The primary care physician must adopt a posture of genuine concern coupled with a realistic medical approach.

   These concepts might be conveyed to the patient by using the following script:

   I know that your pain is significant and real, even though we are not exactly sure what is causing it. Medical specialists are discovering that the nervous system can sometimes produce pain, even when an injury has healed or an illness has resolved. For example, a person still feels a foot or arm even after it has been amputated. This is not a psychological problem but a function of the nervous system that we do not yet quite understand. I will continue to work with you to get to the bottom of this, but we have to accept the possibility that you may continue to experience discomfort, even if no cause for it can be found. Our goal is to help you to be as comfortable and active as possible, but we must be realistic.

2. *Distinguish acute from chronic pain and provide treatment recommendations accordingly.* Clarify for the patient that an *acute* pain approach—with goals of cure and emphasis on rest, medication, and time to heal—*is inappropriate for long-standing pain and should be replaced by a rehabilitation approach emphasizing increase in function, improved quality of life, self-reliance, adaptive psychological coping, and realistic goal setting.*

   These concepts might be conveyed to the patient by using the following script:

   It is important to understand that the pain you are experiencing is chronic pain and not acute pain. Chronic pain and acute pain have quite different treatments. Most often, chronic pain is managed because a cure is simply not possible. You and I need to manage it in the best way possible. Most of the time, pain is a signal that we have suffered some type of injury or have developed an illness. In these cases, the pain tells us that something is wrong in the body. It is like the fire alarm that signals to the fire department that there is a fire. However, sometimes, pain does not go away, even though the body has healed. It is as if, after the fire department has put out the fire, the alarm continues to ring. When pain becomes chronic, it is no longer signaling danger, even though it still hurts very much. At this point, waiting for healing to eliminate the pain is rarely successful. We must work together to help you to learn to deal with and manage this discomfort while, at the same time, you get back to doing the things you like to do and have to do. We manage chronic pain by rehabilitation. If you were to badly break your ankle, it may never work exactly right again, yet, rehabilitation would enable you to walk again, sometimes with a limp. Just like the badly broken ankle may never be perfect again, some of your pain feelings may never go away completely.

3. *Educate the patient.* Review diagnostic tests and their circumscribed purpose in diagnosing or ruling out specific pain conditions. When appropriate, clarify that normal test results do not imply that the patient does not experience pain. Address patient's fear of illness, disease, or physical impairment, if evident.

   These concepts might be conveyed to the patient by using the following script:

   I have good news for you. Your tests have come back, and they don't indicate the presence of any serious disease or neurologic disorder, such as a tumor, fracture, or herniated disc. This does not mean that your pain is not real but simply that it is not due to a tumor or neurologic disease. In fact, most of the time results of tests such as x-ray studies, magnetic resonance imaging, electromyography, and bone scanning or other fancy tests are normal when we evaluate people who suffer with pain. Unfortunately, we are as yet unable to objectively measure pain through our tests, even when we know that the patient with pain is being honest and genuine. The good news is that, at least, we know that your pain is not being caused by something that is life threatening or dangerous.

4. *Inquire about the patient's understanding of his or her problem.* Patients maintain numerous ideas and beliefs about the nature of their pain and illness. *Erroneous pain beliefs* (e.g., "pain = harm"; "one should always be afraid of pain"; "it is impossible to function with pain") *can be critical impediments to increasing functional independence.* Inform patients about their diagnosis, clarify normal test findings that rule out certain pain disorders, and *encourage patients' competence to acquire control over their pain and function.*

   These concepts might be conveyed to the patient by using the following script:

   It is important for me to know what you actually think about your pain, what you think is causing it, if you are frightened that your pain may represent a serious disease or be a danger to you, or if you are afraid that your pain means that you are causing more harm or damage to your body. (These items are most often explored one at a time.) We have performed several tests, and we know that your pain is not being caused by something that is life threatening or dangerous. You don't have to worry that something bad is wrong with you, even though we know that you are still uncomfortable. It is okay to slowly increase your activity without worrying that you are hurting something. Many people, such as those with arthritis, live with pain every day. Our job is to help you learn to cope with your discomfort by slowly and progressively returning you to your regular activities and not be afraid.

5. *Periodically ask the patient about his or her emotional and behavioral status.* Specifically assess for symptoms of depression, anxiety or panic or repressed anger; feelings of self-blame for causing or perpetrating his or her pain and disability; changes in the quality of social, family, or marital relationships; and present or pending life or work stresses. Solicit information from family members concerning the psychological adjustment of the patient. Refer the patient for appropriate psychiatric or psychological intervention when indicated.

   These questions might be discussed with the patient by using the following script:

   I want to know how things have been going for you. I know that your pain is still a real problem. Every person who has to cope with chronic pain has, at one time or another, had to deal with the anxieties and frustrations caused by pain and the way it interferes with his or her life. Sometimes, it can even lead a person to become sad, angry, discouraged, and even depressed, or it can cause a person to be less interested in his or her family and friends. I need to know if you have been feeling this way so that we don't let this pain disrupt the quality of your life.

6. *Prescribe medications on a time-interval rather than as needed basis.*
7. *Encourage modulation of physical activity within pain or functional tolerance* and outline a graded, progressive increase in activity level (e.g., home chores, leisure, social).
8. *Maintain support and contact.* Reassure the patient that you will continue to monitor his or her medical status and potential causes of pain. *Schedule regular (e.g., monthly, bimonthly) appointments to eliminate the need for the patient to have a "pain crisis" in order to receive medical attention.* Routine contact may not be curative, but it can help to prevent doctor shopping, emergency department visits, iatrogenic complications, psychological decompensation, and unnecessary misuse of health care resources.
9. *Refer to a specialized, interdisciplinary pain center for consultation as soon as you suspect that an acute pain episode may become chronic invalidism.* Chronicity begets chronicity—the earlier the symptoms of disability and psychological impairment are addressed, the brighter the prognosis.

B. Medications used to treat pain.

1. *Placebos.*
   a. The placebo response is common; up to one third of all patients with pain respond to a placebo challenge.
   b. Because the placebo response is based on conditioning, it *cannot differentiate "functional" from "organic" pain.*
   c. Some clinicians may feel that it is more ethical to use a less toxic placebo if it will treat pain as effectively as a more active drug, such as an opioid; if a patient learns that he or she has been treated with a placebo, vital rapport between patient and clinician most likely will be lost.
   d. *We do not recommend the use of placebos for patients with pain.*
2. *Nonsteroidal anti-inflammatory drugs* (see Table 15–1).
   a. Highly useful for both acute and chronic pain.
   b. Side effects common to all NSAIDs include bronchospasm in sensitive patients, gastric ulcers, possible renal failure with long-term use.
   c. Recent data suggest that NSAIDs may have more than a peripheral anti-inflammatory action and that they may affect prostaglandin synthesis in pain-relevant spinal neurons; NSAIDs with demonstrated central analgesic effect include ibuprofen (Motrin), and ketoprofen (Orudis).
   d. If a patient fails to respond to a drug of one

class of NSAIDs, switching to another class may provide effective treatment.

e. Nonsteroidal anti-inflammatory drugs that may be especially *useful in patients who cannot tolerate gastrointestinal side effects* include diflunisal (Dolobid), etodolac (Lodine), and nabumetone (Relafen).

3. *Anticonvulsants: may be useful for central or neuropathic pain.*
   a. *Gabapentin* (Neurontin): usual dose is 300 mg at bedtime on the first day, 300 mg twice a day on the second day, and 300 mg three times a day on the third day; slowly increased over several weeks to a maximum of 2400 mg/d.
   b. *Carbamazepine* (Tegretol): is generally more effective than phenytoin and may be particularly helpful in trigeminal neuralgia, postherpetic pain, diabetic neuropathy, multiple sclerosis, and neuralgia.
      (1) This agent must be used cautiously because it may cause bone marrow suppression with resulting aplastic anemia or suppression of white blood cell count; it may also cause significant liver damage.
      (2) Usual starting dose is 100 mg twice a day, with an increase to 200 mg three to four times a day; blood level should be checked to determine if therapeutic range has been approached and to avoid toxicity.
   c. *Phenytoin* (Dilantin): starting dose, 100 mg three times a day and titrated to 300 to 500 mg/d.
   d. *Divalproex sodium* (Depakote): usual starting dose is 250 mg twice a day, with an increase over 10 days to 2 weeks up to approximately 1500 to 1800 mg/d; blood levels can assist in determining whether the patient has reached adequate nontoxic therapeutic levels.
   e. *Clonazepam* (Klonopin): usual dosing starts at 0.5 mg twice a day and increased to 1 to 4 mg/d.
   f. *Phenobarbital is not useful in this context.*

4. *Antidepressants* (see Table 15–2).
   a. Pain relief is often independent of antidepressant effect, and these drugs may well be effective in patients with pain who are not depressed.
   b. Tricyclic antidepressant–responsive pain syndromes include terminal cancer, neuropathy, postherpetic neuralgia, vascular and tension headache, and facial pain; both tertiary and secondary amine tricyclics are effective.
   c. Tricyclic antidepressants appear to be more reliably analgesic than selective serotonin reuptake inhibitors or other antidepressants.
   d. Low-dose antidepressants may be adequate for the treatment of chronic pain syndromes; *higher doses may be necessary for the treatment of patients who also exhibit evidence for depression and sleep disturbance.*
   e. Rheumatologic pain is inconsistently responsive to antidepressants.
   f. Antidepressants may be particularly analgesic for patients who report a personal or family history of mood and substance abuse disorders.

5. *Stimulants.*
   a. These are effective adjuvants to other analgesics; they offer few side effects and provide reversal of the sedation and impaired cognition caused by agents such as opioids.
   b. Postoperative pain and pediatric cancer pain respond well to analgesic-stimulant combinations.
   c. Dextroamphetamine (Dexedrine), 5 to 10 mg/d, or methylphenidate (Ritalin), 5 to 15 mg/d, may be used as adjuncts to other analgesic agents.

6. *Opioids* (see Table 15–3).
   a. Controversy surrounds the increasing use of opioids for the management of chronic nonmalignant pain, especially for patients whose pain behaviors appear to be motivated by emotional and psychological needs.
      (1) Many patients needlessly suffer treatable pain because of withholding or undermedication of opioid analgesics that results from inadequate knowledge of pharmacology, misconceptions and stereotypic beliefs about the use of opioid analgesics, and fear of promoting drug abuse/addiction.
      (2) Erroneous beliefs regarding opioid analgesia derive in part from laboratory studies with human volunteers and animals.
         - In laboratory studies, adverse effects of opioids, such as the development of tolerance and respiratory depression, are commonly observed.
         - In patients with pain, tolerance and respiratory depression are uncommon complications of treatment; the presence of pain appears to explain these differences.
      (3) The risk of promoting drug addiction in patients with pain treated with maintenance opioids is not supported by epidemiologic studies and results from physicians confusing pain patients with "street addicts" and failing to distinguish physical dependence, psychological dependence, and drug abuse.
         - *Physical dependence:* a physiologic

phenomenon characterized by development of an abstinence (withdrawal) syndrome after abrupt discontinuation of opioid therapy; this is a characteristic of opioids and should be presumed for all patients; it is not evidence for psychological dependence or drug abuse.
- *Psychological dependence/addiction:* a psychological and behavioral process that includes loss of control over drug use, compulsive drug use, and persistent drug use, despite evidence of increasing physiological and psychosocial harm and encouragement to desist; does not occur solely based on the administration of opioids but rather the interaction of the drug with predisposing physiologic (biogenetic), psychological, and social factors.
- *Drug abuse:* use of a particular drug outside of social norms.

b. General principles of opioid therapy.
  (1) There is considerable opioid variability.
  - One opioid is not inherently more efficacious than another.
  - *Patients have variable responses to different opioids.*
  - Several different opioids should be used before a patient's pain is deemed not responsive to opioids.
  - When switching opioids: a dose reduction of one third to one half should be calculated for the newly prescribed opioid and then titrated empirically; this reduces the incidence of avoidable side effects and recognizes variations in cross-tolerance among opioids.

  (2) *Not all pain is equally opioid responsive;* for instance, bone pain from metastases and neuropathic pain may be less amenable then visceral pain; however, opioids may provide partial benefit.
  (3) Patients generally exhibit increased tolerance to adverse effects of opioids (e.g., sedation, cognitive interference, behavioral) more quickly than to the analgesic effect. Constipation and miosis may persist as adverse effects; *patients should be considered for a prophylactic bowel regimen when opioids are administered;* methadone (Dolophine) has been associated with sexual dysfunction, insomnia, and sweating.
  (4) Opioids demonstrate few differences in speed of onset; generally 20 to 30 minutes.
  (5) Opioids vary in duration of effect, from 2 to 3 hours to 8 to 12 hours.
  (6) Opioids vary in their bioavailability by oral administration (e.g., oxycodone is two-thirds available, compared with morphine, which is one-third available, rendering oxycodone and morphine approximately equipotent when given orally); meperidine (Demerol) provides poor opioid analgesia orally.
  (7) Younger patients (< 40 years) eliminate opioids more rapidly, and the duration of analgesia is reduced; thus, they may require more frequent dosing.
  (8) Little evidence exists for major organ toxicity with administration of opioids; some evidence indicates decreased immune function.

c. Prescription of opioid therapy.
  (1) Opioids are classified in terms of receptor site affinity.
  - Most clinically used opioids are predominantly mu agonists.
  - Mixed agonist-antagonist opioids (e.g., pentazocine [Talwin]) should not be prescribed concurrently with mu agonist opioids.

  (2) Opioids are classified as weak (e.g., propoxyphene, codeine, hydrocodeine) and strong (e.g., morphine, oxycodone).
  - Weak opioids have a dosage ceiling effect as with increasing doses there is an increased incidence of side effects and the toxicity associated with aspirin and acetaminophen contained in most preparations.
  - Strong opioids have wider range of efficacy and can relieve severe pain.

  (3) Prescription of analgesia can be standardized in a stepwise manner of administration.
  - Nonopioid (aspirin, acetaminophen, or nonsteroidal anti-inflammatory drug) + adjuvants.
  - Weak opioid + nonopioid + adjuvants.
  - Strong opioid + nonopioid + adjuvants.

  (4) After increase of opioid level to therapeutic efficacy, the opioid requirement stabilizes in most patients; a *dramatic change in opioid needs usually reflects progression of disease or change in psychological functioning.*
  (5) If patient exhibits inadequate relief with opioid regimen, the following should be considered
  - Increase the dose of current opioid.
  - Decrease the interval between doses or change the regimen to a longer-acting opioid.
  - Switch to an alternative opioid.

  (6) *Most complaints of persistent pain or evidence of drug-seeking behavior are best*

understood in terms of inadequate opioid responsiveness and not as signs of addiction.

d. Bonica has proposed the following guidelines in the management of opioid maintenance therapy for nonmalignant pain.[9]

(1) Opioid maintenance therapy should be considered only after all reasonable attempts at analgesia have failed.

(2) A history of substance abuse, a severe personality disorder, and a chaotic home environment should be reviewed as *relative* contraindications.

(3) A single practitioner should take primary responsibility for treatment.

(4) Patients should give informed consent before the start of therapy; points to be covered include recognition of the low risk of true addiction, potential for cognitive impairment from the drug alone or from coadministration of sedative-hypnotics, likelihood that physical dependence will occur, and understanding by female patients that children born when the mother is receiving opioid drugs will likely be physically dependent at birth.

(5) After drug selection, doses should be given on an around-the-clock basis; several weeks should be agreed on as the period of initial dose titration, and although improvement in function should be continually stressed, all parties should agree to at least partial analgesia as the appropriate goal of therapy.

(6) Failure to achieve at least partial analgesia at relatively low initial doses in the nontolerant patient raises questions about the potential treatability of the pain syndrome with opioids.

(7) Emphasis should be given to attempts to capitalize on improved analgesia by gains in physical and social function; opioid therapy should be considered complementary to other analgesic and rehabilitative approaches.

(8) Initially, patients must be seen and drugs prescribed at least monthly. When the dose level stabilizes, less frequent visits may be acceptable.

(9) At each visit, assessment should specifically address:

- Comfort (degree of analgesia).
- Opioid-related side effects.
- Functional status (physical and psychosocial).
- Existence of aberrant drug-related behaviors.

(10) Evidence of drug hoarding, prescription forgery, selling or borrowing of drugs, repeated seeking of prescriptions from other physicians or emergency rooms, multiple dose escalations and other signs of noncompliance, concurrent abuse of alcohol or other illicit substances, or evidence of deterioration in vocational and psychosocial functioning may constitute the need to discontinue opioid therapy. Consultation with a mental health or substance abuse specialist should be considered.

References

1. Merskey H. Pain terms. Pain 1979;6:249–252.
2. Fordyce WE. Environmental factors in the genesis of low back pain. In: Bonica JJ, Liebeskind JC, Albe-Fessard DG (eds.). Advances in Pain Research and Therapy. New York: Raven Press; 1979, pp. 659–666.
3. Stanton-Hicks M, Jänig W, Hassenbush S, et al. Reflex sympathetic dystrophy: Changing concepts and taxonomy. Pain 1995; 63:127–133.
4. Savage SR. Management of acute and chronic pain and cancer pain in the addicted patient. In: Miller NS (ed.): Principles of Addiction Medicine. Washington, DC: American Society of Addiction Medicine, 1994, pp. 1–16.
5. Eisendrath SJ. Psychiatric aspects of chronic pain. Neurology 1995; 45(Suppl. 9):S26–S34.
6. Sigvardsson S, von Knorring AL, Bohman M, et al. An adoption study of somatoform disorders: The relationship to somatization of psychiatric disability. Arch Gen Psychiatry 1984; 41:853–859.
7. Bouckoms AJ. Chronic pain: Neuropsychopharmacology and adjunctive psychiatric treatment. In: Rundell JR, Wise MG (eds.). Textbook of Consultation-Liaison Psychiatry. Washington, DC: American Psychiatric Press; 1996, pp. 1006–1036.
8. Bouckoms AJ, Hackett TP. The pain patient: Evaluation and treatment. In: Cassem NH (ed.). Massachusetts General Hospital Handbook of General Hospital Psychiatry, 3rd ed. St Louis: Mosby–Year Book, 1991, pp. 39–68.
9. Portnoy RK. Opioid therapy for chronic nonmalignant pain: Current status. In: Fields HL, Liebeskind JC (eds.). Pharmacological Approaches to the Treatment of Chronic Pain: New Concepts and Critical Issues. Seattle: International Association for the Study of Pain Press; 1994, pp. 247–287.

Suggested Reading

Bonica JJ. The Management of Pain, Vols. 1 and 2, 2nd ed. Philadelphia: Lea & Febiger; 1990.

Fields HL. Pain. New York: McGraw-Hill; 1987.

Raj PP. Pain Medicine: A Comprehensive Review. St. Louis: Mosby–Year Book, 1996.

Travell JG, Simons DG. Myofascial Pain and Dysfunction: The Trigger Point Manual, Vols. 1 & 2. Baltimore: Williams & Wilkins, Vol. 1, 1983; Vol. 2, 1992.

Wall PD, Melzack R. Textbook of Pain, 3rd ed. Edinburgh: Churchill Livingstone; 1994.

Warfield CA. Principles and Practice of Pain Management. New York: McGraw-Hill; 1993.

Glossary of Pain Terms*

Algology—the science and study of pain phenomena. An algologist is a student, investigator, and practitioner of algology.

Allodynia—pain due to a stimulus that does not normally provoke pain.

Analgesia—absence of pain in response to stimulation that would normally be painful.

Analgesic—an agent that produces analgesia.

Anesthesia—absence of all sensory modalities.

Anesthesia dolorosa—pain in an area or region that is anesthetic.

Arthralgia—pain in a joint, usually caused by arthritis or arthropathy.

Causalgia—a syndrome of sustained burning pain, allodynia, and hyperpathia after a traumatic nerve lesion, often combined with vasomotor and sudomotor dysfunction and later trophic changes.

Central pain—pain associated with a lesion of the central nervous system.

Deafferentation pain—pain due to loss of sensory input into the central nervous system, as occurs with avulsion of the brachial plexus or other types of lesions of peripheral nerves or as a result of pathology of the central nervous system.

Dermatome—the sensory segmental supply to the skin and subcutaneous tissue.

Dysesthesia—an unpleasant abnormal sensation, whether spontaneous or evoked.

Hyperesthesia—increased sensitivity to stimulation, excluding special senses.

Hyperalgesia—an increased response to a stimulus that is normally painful.

Hyperpathia—a painful syndrome, characterized by increased reaction to a stimulus, especially a repetitive stimulus, as well as an increased threshold.

Hypoalgesia—diminished sensitivity to noxious stimulation.

Hypoesthesia—diminished sensitivity to stimulation, excluding special senses.

Neuralgia—pain in the distribution of nerve or nerves.

Neuritis—inflammation of a nerve or nerves.

Neuropathy—a disturbance of function of pathologic change in a nerve; neuropathy in one nerve is *mononeuropathy;* in several nerves, *mononeuropathy multiplex;* if symmetrical and bilateral, *polyneuropathy.*

Nociceptor—a receptor that is preferentially sensitive to a noxious stimulus or to a stimulus that would become noxious if prolonged.

Noxious stimulus—a stimulus that is potentially or actually damaging to body tissue.

Pain threshold—the least experience of pain that a subject can recognize.

Pain tolerance level—the greatest level of pain that a subject is prepared to tolerate.

Paresthesia—an abnormal sensation, whether spontaneous or evoked.

Radiculalgia—pain along the distribution of one or more sensory nerve roots.

Radiculopathy—a disturbance of function of pathologic change in one or more nerve roots.

Radiculitis—inflammation of one or more nerve roots.

Somatic—derived from Greek word for "body."

Somatosensory input—sensory signals from all tissues of the body, including skin, viscera, muscles, and joints. However, the term is usually used for input for body tissue other than viscera.

Trigger point—a hypersensitive area or site in muscle or connective tissue, usually associated with myofascial pain syndromes.

*From Bonica JJ. The Management of Pain, Vol 1, Second edition. Philadelphia, 1990; pp. 20–21.

16

MINDY SMITH, MD, MS

OVIDE F. POMERLEAU, PhD

WILLIAM WADLAND, MD, MS

Nicotine and Smoking

I. General approach.

Why should health providers get involved in helping patients stop smoking? The reasons are numerous. First, most patients state that they would consider quitting if advised by their doctor and that firm, supportive messages from physicians can act as an important motivator in smoking cessation. Health providers also have frequent contact with smokers. Up to 70% of the 45 million smokers in America have at least one office visit with a physician every two years. Smokers visit their doctors an average of four times a year.

There is also very persuasive evidence that physician-provided smoking cessation techniques are helpful. The most common interventions are brief advice, self-help materials, and nicotine replacement therapy. When these methods are used in actual practice settings, cessation rates of up to 15% are reported. *The largest impact on smoking cessation rates is achieved when physicians become active in the intervention process, using chart stickers or computerized reminders to routinely identify smokers at each visit and providing appropriate brief advice, written materials, or counseling.* Patients who receive routine physician reminders are up to six times more likely to quit than are patients who receive "usual care," meaning sporadic or no reminders.

Despite this encouraging evidence, many physicians identify numerous barriers to providing this type of care. Discouraging experiences with patients, belief that nothing can be done, competing demands, and lack of formal training, time, and reimbursement are reasons often cited. These perceived barriers, however, can be minimized by the creation of a *team approach,* in which nurses and other office personnel are involved and some changes in office procedures are made (described in section III.B). This type of coordinated effort has substantial benefits for patients and has been shown to be more cost effective than other important preventive practices, including the treatment of hypertension and increased cholesterol level.

A. Identification of patients.

The first step in any intervention for smoking is the identification of smokers. The term *the fifth vital sign* has been used to highlight the need to *identify smoking behavior on a routine basis.* Many authors have suggested office systems that facilitate routine assessment. Opportunities for identification include having the patient sign in (through the use of an updated health form) or, at the time of nursing assessment, having the office nurse ask all patients during their vital sign checks if they currently smoke, never smoked, or did smoke. *The nurse should mark the progress note at each visit with an "S+" (current smoker), "So" (never smoked), or "Sx" (ex-smoker), and the nurse may attach a sticker to the charts of patients who smoke.* The clinician should record plans to manage the smoking status in the progress notes and list tobacco use/abuse in the problem list as a true medical problem, if so identified. Special chart markers, stamps, or labels can be ordered or developed by the practice. These materials can also be obtained by contacting the American Academy of Family Physicians (AAFP Stop Smoking Kit; 1-800-274-2237), the American Cancer Society (Tobacco-Free Young America: A Kit for the Busy Practitioner; 1-404-320-3333 or 1-800-ACS-2345), or the National Cancer Institute (Quit for Good Kit and the manual for physicians entitled How To Help Your Patients Stop Smoking; 1-800-4-CANCER). The NCI reference manual for physicians contains appendices that list questions and concerns of smokers, smoking cessation tips, and self-help materials. Including smoking status as a vital sign has been shown to greatly increase the likelihood of smoking-related discussions between smoking patients and their physicians.

Adolescence is perhaps the most important time to identify cigarette smoking. *Behavioral cues* include low levels of academic achievement and little school involvement. Nearly all first use of tobacco occurs before high school graduation, and people who smoke at an early age are most likely to develop severe nicotine addiction. Approximately one fourth of 12 to 14 year olds report having smoked cigarettes at some time, and 4% to 6% of these adolescents are current smokers. *Because passive smoke also has negative health consequences, the question about smoking must be raised with all patients.*

B. Assessment of receptivity and cofactors.

Once patients are identified, most experts in smoking cessation strategies suggest that *two parameters be assessed:* the *level of nicotine dependence* and the patient's *willingness to quit* smoking. The level of dependence can be approximated by the number of cigarettes smoked each day; 20 cigarettes (one pack) or more per day are indicative of a need for nicotine replacement therapy. The original formal assessment of dependence was the Fagerström Tolerance Questionnaire, which contained eight questions and was scored with a range of zero (indicating minimum nicotine dependence) to 11 (indicating maximum dependence). Most studies confirmed an association between scores on this questionnaire and measures of tolerance, withdrawal, nicotine self-administration, and cessation success. A shorter assessment form, the Fagerström Test for Nicotine Dependence, which captures the essence of the Fagerstrom Tolerance Questionnaire but has greater predictive ability, has been suggested as the best screening instrument for the identification and treatment of smokers (Table 16–1).

The Fagerström Test for Nicotine Dependence may be given to identified smokers while they wait in an examination room to see their provider. Fagerström indicates that patients scoring greater than 5 points usually benefit from nicotine replacement therapy (personal communication, 1995). Smoking more than one pack per day, smoking more in the morning than at other times of the day, smoking within 30 minutes of arising, having difficulty refraining from smoking in forbidden places, and smoking even when ill are key characteristics of nicotine dependence and have been found to discriminate between lighter and heavier smokers on biochemical measures.

Willingness to quit is usually described according to three stages: precontemplation, contemplation, and action. Precontemplators are smokers who have no thoughts of stopping. Contemplators are smokers who are considering quitting but have no concrete plans about how to quit. Smokers in the action stage are ready to quit and are often prepared to discuss treatment options and proceed. The stages can then be used, as described later, to better tailor messages and treatment plans to patient needs and receptivity.

Patients with known psychiatric (history of depression, anxiety disorder, attention-deficit disorder) or drug and alcohol problems often need specific psychiatric or substance abuse treatment before they attempt smoking cessation. Studies have shown that smokers with such cofactors are less likely to successfully stop smoking in the absence of adequate treatment for and resolution of these problems. Smokers who have failed previous attempts to quit should be screened for the presence of psychiatric, drug, and alcohol problems because the prevalence of these difficulties is higher in smokers than in nonsmokers, and there is some potential for precipitating psychiatric distress from smoking cessation in patients with a history of psychiatric disorders. However, *most smokers make three or four attempts before they quit smoking,* and quit attempts should be viewed positively in the process of successful cessation.

Table 16–1
Items and Scoring for Fagerström Test for Nicotine Dependence

Questions	Answers	Points
1. How soon after you wake up do you smoke your first cigarette?	Within 5 minutes	3
	Within 6–30 minutes	2
	Within 31–60 minutes	1
	After 60 minutes	0
2. Do you find it difficult to refrain from smoking in places where it is forbidden (e.g., in church, at the library, in cinema, etc.)?	Yes	1
	No	0
3. Which cigarette would you hate most to give up?	The first one in the morning	1
	All others	0
4. How many cigarettes/day do you smoke?	10 or less	0
	11–20	1
	21–30	2
	31 or more	3
5. Do you smoke more frequently during the first hours after waking than during the rest of the day?	Yes	1
	No	0
6. Do you smoke if you are so ill that you are in bed most of the day?	Yes	1
	No	0

From Heatherton TF, Kozlowski LT, Frecker RC, Fagerström KO. The Fagerström test for nicotine dependence: a revision of the Fagerström Tolerance Questionnaire. Addiction 1991; 86:1119–1127.

C. Relevant laboratory studies.

Few specific tests are recommended for the assessment of patients who smoke. In the context of the periodic health examination, aspects of the screening that are relevant to smokers are (1) attention to the interval history of cigarette smoking (at the very least asking questions about current smoking and number of cigarettes), (2) complete oral examination, (3) auscultation for carotid bruits and an electrocardiogram for those with two or more cardiovascular risk factors (smoking, hypertension, diabetes mellitus, increased cholesterol level, or family history of early coronary artery disease), and (4) counseling in smoking cessation. The performance of these tests is supported by the United States Preventive Services Task Force and the American Academy of Family Physicians.

Peak flow measures can be used as a simple office screen for obstructive lung disease and can be additional motivating information for the patient. The measurement of carbon monoxide (CO) levels has also been suggested as a means of encouraging smoking cessation and providing positive reinforcement for quitting (levels decrease appreciably after 1 day of abstinence). Although used for many years in the research setting, experience using expired CO levels in the clinical setting has only recently been reported by clinicians at the Mayo Nicotine Dependence Center in Rochester, Minnesota. The CO level appears to correlate well with blood carboxyhemoglobin level and number of cigarettes smoked, but it has been found to be inadequate in detecting occasional and light smokers (CO has a 3 to 5 hour half-life, depending on activity level and other factors). Units for measuring CO cost less than $1000 and can be used for thousands of tests. With ambient CO contamination being taken into account, a good cut-off for CO level in the detection of smoking is 10 ppm or greater. Sputum cytology samples are useful for the early detection of carcinoma of the lung in especially high-risk smokers (those with a family history of lung cancer, industrial exposure, and/or heavy dependence). Cytology may also be useful in recalcitrant smokers, in whom subsequent samples can be compared with baseline samples in order to document improvement or deterioration associated with smoking.

Preliminary evidence now supports the use of a urine dipstick for the detection of nicotine and its metabolites. The kit, called NicCheck™ by DynaGen, Inc. changes color to indicate three gradations (negative, low-moderate, and high), with the high level being used to identify failure to abstain from smoking.

D. Presentation of information to patients and families.

Although messages about the adverse effects of smoking and the need for cessation must be clear, patient receptivity should alter the approach used by the clinician. An algorithm for physician-based treatment for smoking cessation has been developed by Hughes.[1] It is based on the stage of readiness to quit and provides guidance on the need for pharmacotherapy. The algorithm is presented in Figure 16–1.

Suggested script for a precontemplator:

Physician: *Do you intend to quit smoking in the next several months?*

Patient: *No, not at all. I haven't even thought about it. I like smoking. It relaxes me. I need it, and I don't want to quit.*

Physician: *As your physician, it is my responsibility to be concerned about your overall health. I feel that quitting smoking is the best thing you could do for your health. Although I respect your choice, here is some information on smoking risks and suggestions for quitting. We can discuss it at follow-up visits.*

For precontemplators, a discussion of personal reasons for cessation and barriers to cessation should be attempted. Material specifically designed to motivate patients not yet ready to stop may be obtained from the American Academy of Family Physicians, the American Cancer Society (The Fifty Most Often Asked Questions About Smoking and Health and the Answers, How Can We Reach You, Why Start Life Under a Cloud?), the American Dental Association (38 Million People Have Quit Smoking. You Can Too), and the NCI (Why Do You Smoke).

Suggested script for a contemplator:

Patient: *I would like to quit in the next several months, but I don't know exactly when or how. I am afraid I might get lung cancer like my father did.*

Physician: *I'm glad that you are interested in quitting, and I can help you. If you quit, you can reduce the risks of getting lung cancer greatly. The best way to quit is to set a quit date. If you are nicotine dependent, then the nicotine patch or gum may help.*

Patient: *I don't want to quit now, but my 50th birthday is in 2 months. I want to be quit by then.*

Physician: *I suggest that you decrease smoking and try to avoid key cigarettes. By this I mean the most important cigarettes of the day; an example is the cigarette you smoke with your morning cup of coffee, an activity that is almost automatic. I would like for you to return before your birthday and read this literature on suggestions for quitting. I am very pleased that you are considering quitting.*

For contemplators, reasons to quit and barriers can also be discussed. A more detailed discussion about difficulties with previous attempts to quit may be useful, and patients should be encouraged to work on future plans to quit. Motivational materials, as listed earlier, may be used, or materials from the kits listed later may be started, in which suggestions for preparing to stop smoking, a daily smoking record, identification of

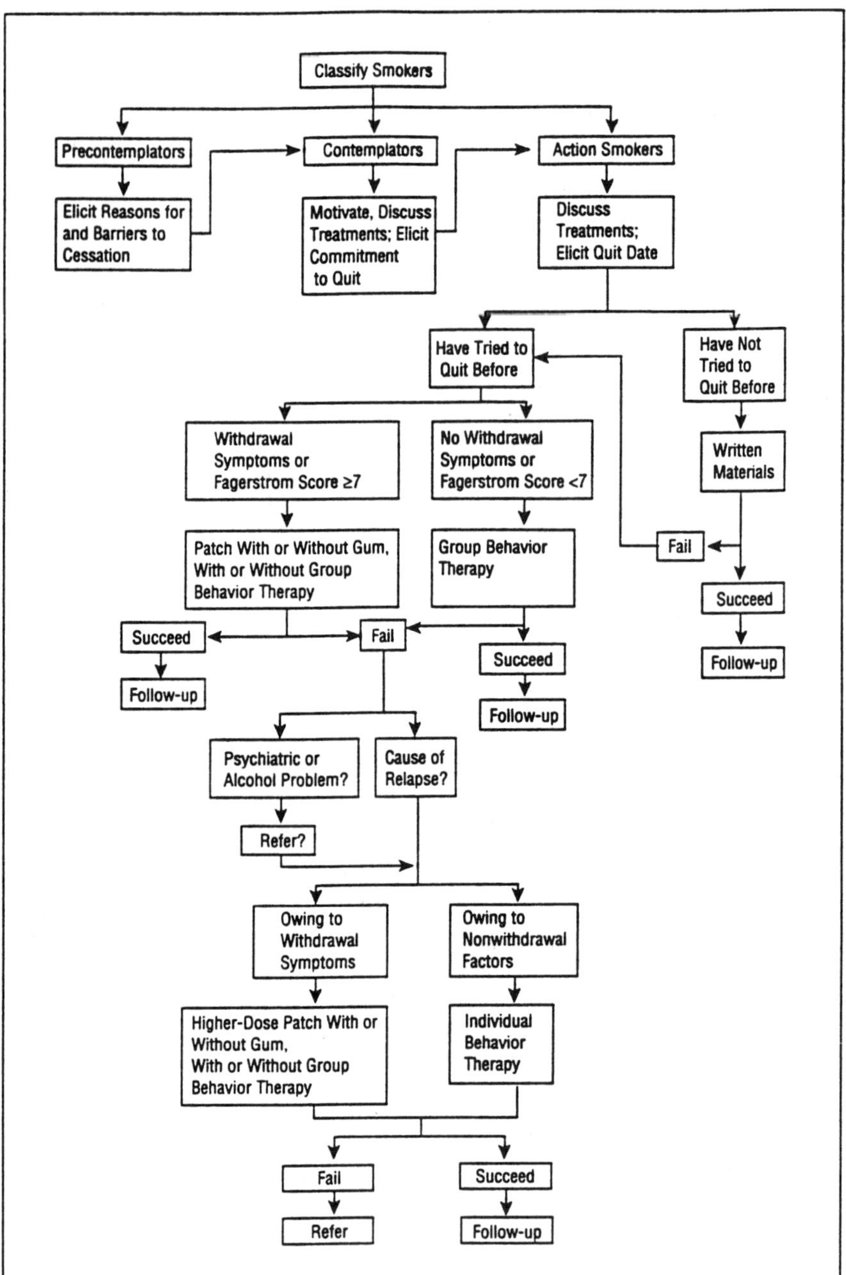

Figure 16–1
An algorithm for smoking cessation. (From Hughes JR. An algorithm for smoking cessation. Arch Fam Med 1994; 3:280–285.)

key cigarettes and smoking cues (e.g., particular locations and accompanying foods and drinks that trigger smoking), and lists of personal reasons to quit are the focus.

Suggested script for a patient in the active stage:

Patient: *I want to quit smoking tomorrow. I can't afford it anymore, and my son has asthma.*

Physician: *Good! Quitting will definitely help your son and your pocketbook. Do you smoke within 15 minutes of awaking? Do you get irritable and restless and have difficulty sleeping if you have not smoked for a long period?*

Patient: *Yes, smoking is the first thing I do in the morning, even before showering. I get real restless without a regular cigarette.*

Physician: *I think that you will probably benefit from the nicotine patch or gum. They will help buffer withdrawal symptoms so that you can focus on changing your behavior around smoking. You can't smoke while using them. First, I would like to assess whether you have any risks for side effects from the nicotine patch or gum. Second, I want you to keep a diary of symptoms and situations where you may slip. I would like to review it within 1 to 2 weeks after your quit date.*

With smokers in the action stage, treatment options should be reviewed, and a specific date to quit smoking (quit date) should be set in writing. The development of a specific plan and quit date have been shown to be extremely helpful. For patients who respond to written information, instructions on how to prepare for quitting can be provided with the self-help materials listed below. Patient handouts on tips for smoking cessation are provided at the end of this book. For smokers who are nicotine dependent, several pharmacologic agents can be presented and discussed to assist with the cessation effort. These are reviewed in section III.B.3.

Providing a *clear, strong message* that advises all patients to quit smoking is essential. *Personalizing the message* (tying it to the patient's present condition, family history, impact on others, and so on) increases the effectiveness of the advice. Table 16–2 can be used to help patients identify reasons to quit that are meaningful to them.

In addition to this personalized advice, the *provision of self-help materials* is often useful. A national survey of adult smokers in the United States found that approximately 90% of people who successfully quit smoking used self-help methods rather than an organized program. The American Cancer Society (I Quit Kit, Smart Move), the National Cancer Institute (Quit for Good), and the American Lung Association (Freedom from Smoking in 20 Days, A Lifetime of Freedom from Smoking) have created a number of materials for smokers, including motivational pamphlets and quitting aids. The program tested by the University of Michigan called Patch Plus is another resource that can be purchased from Homewood Health Services (telephone: 1-519-824-1010, or fax: 1-519-824-1813). Office personnel should become familiar with at least one set of these materials and make them available to patients.

E. Special considerations for adolescent smokers.

Reaching out to the adolescent smoker can be difficult. Most adolescent smokers, however, report that they want to quit but are unable to do so. Evidence of nicotine addiction is present in this group, and reported relapse rates and withdrawal symptoms are similar to those in adults. Advice regarding smoking cessation for the adolescent patient should begin with a clear message to quit and appropriate health risk information. Although most young people believe that smoking a pack or more a day is a serious health risk, three of 10 high school seniors surveyed in 1991 still did not believe that heavy smoking posed a serious health threat. *Emphasis on current symptoms and immediate consequences* may be particularly relevant for this age group. For example, even occasional smokers report having more shortness of breath when they are not exercising, more colds, coughing spells and sore throats, and poorer overall physical health than do nonsmokers. There is also an increasing perception by peers that smoking is a dirty habit (e.g., bad breath, clothes smell), and most adolescents (94% of those who have never smoked and 51% of current smokers) prefer to date nonsmokers.

Table 16–2
Estimated Relative Risks of Selected Conditions Among Smokers and Former Smokers (Versus Never Smokers) and Smoking-Attributable Mortality

	Relative Risk Among Smokers*		Mortality Attributable to Smoking†	
Condition	*Current*	*Former*	*Percent*	*Total‡*
Ischemic heart disease				
Age 35–64 y				
Male	2.8	1.8	45	
Female	3.0	1.4	40	34,132
Age >65 y				
Male	1.6	1.3	20	
Female	1.6	1.3	10	64,789
Cerebrovascular disease			50	
Age 35–64				
Male	3.7	1.4		
Female	4.8	1.4		8671
Age >65 y				
Male	1.9	1.3		
Female	1.5	1.0		14,610
Chronic airway obstruction			81.5	
≥21 cig/d				
Male	13.5	12.6		
Female	17.1	8.3		48,982
Cancer				
Lung				
Male	22.4	9.4	90	
Female	11.9	4.7	79	116,920
Esophagus				
Male	7.6	5.8	78	
Female	10.3	3.2	75	7284
Pancreas				
Male	2.1	1.1	29	
Female	2.3	1.8	34	6114
Bladder				
Male	2.9	1.9	47	
Female	2.6	1.9	37	4026

*Data from Chronic Disease and Health Promotion—Adapted from the MMWR. Tobacco Topics 1990–1993. Atlanta, GA: Public Health Service, Centers for Disease Control and Prevention, National Center for Chronic Disease Prevention and Health Promotion; 1994. US Department of Health and Human Services.

†Data from The Health Benefits of Smoking Cessation: A Report of the Surgeon General. Rockville, MD: Public Health Service, Centers for Disease Control, Center for Chronic Disease Prevention and Health Promotion. 1990. US Department of Health and Human Services.

‡Total smoking-attributable mortality for men and women combined.

Relatively few studies have examined adolescent smoking cessation. Traditional smoking cessation programs appear to have low success rates, and the impact of smoking prevention programs on regular smokers appears to be small. School-based cessation programs have had modest success, but recruitment efforts are difficult, partly because of concerns about disclosure and confidentiality. More work in this area is clearly needed. Efforts toward primary prevention, as opposed to secondary smoking cessation, appear to be far more fruitful in this age group.

II. Biobehavioral impact of cigarette smoking.

A. Epidemiology.

Cigarette smoking is the principal preventable cause of chronic disease and death in the United States and is responsible for one of every five deaths each year. The prominence of tobacco as a contributor to mortality prompted former Surgeon General C. Everett Koop to state that cigarette smoking is the most important public health issue of the time. Table 16–2 lists many of the diseases associated with cigarette smoking and both the relative risks and smoking-attributable mortality in current and former smokers compared with those in nonsmokers.

Prevalence of smoking in the United States peaked in the 1960s, when 41% of the adult population smoked, and it declined steadily up to the early 1990s; it now seems to have reached a plateau, at 25% of the United States adult population. This figure includes 24 million men (28% of the total) and 22 million women (23%), with the highest prevalence occurring in persons 25 to 44 years of age. Paradoxically, the percentage of smokers who report that they are heavy smokers (20 or more cigarettes per day) has not changed between 1974 (26%) and 1985 (27%). Possible reasons for the recent slowing of the rate of decline in the prevalence of smoking and for the lack of change in heavy smoking are discussed later.

B. Pathophysiology.

Cigarette smokers inhale deeply to bring nicotine-containing smoke into intimate contact with the small alveoli of the lungs. Pulmonary absorption factors include inhalation amount, depth, and duration; pH of the smoke; and characteristics of smoke constituents: Tobacco smoke contains about 4000 pyrolysis products, many of which have been found to be pharmacologically active, toxic, mutagenic, or carcinogenic. In addition to harmful volatile constituents, such as CO, the particulate phase of cigarette smoke contains nicotine, water, and "tars." Tars include radioactive compounds and numerous aromatic hydrocarbons known to be carcinogenic, such as nitrosamines, aromatic amines, and benzopyrene. The pathophysiologic consequences of bringing products of combustion into such close contact with pulmonary tissue are well documented.

1. *Cancer.*
   In addition to causing over 85% of lung cancers, smoking is associated with cancer of the mouth, pharynx, larynx, esophagus, stomach, pancreas, uterine cervix, kidney, ureter, and bladder. Death rates from cancer are twice as high in smokers as in nonsmokers, and heavy smokers have rates that are four times greater than in nonsmokers (Table 16–2). In general, the greatest impact from tobacco is on tissues directly exposed to cigarette smoke, such as the bronchial lining of the lung. Cocarcinogens in cigarette smoke may interact with trace amounts of carcinogens from environmental sources to produce potentiation. For example, alcohol consumption and cigarette smoking together are associated with more than an additive increase in the incidence of esophageal, oral, and laryngeal cancer. Similarly, industrial workers who smoke and are exposed to asbestos or radioactive decay products have a markedly increased risk of developing lung cancer.
2. *Cardiovascular disease.*
   Cigarette smoking has been shown to increase the risk of peripheral vascular disease, myocardial infarction, aortic aneurysm, and sudden death. Quitting smoking is associated with reduced morbidity and mortality from cardiovascular disease. Nicotine promotes the release of epinephrine and norepinephrine, resulting in heightened sympathetic tone with vasoconstriction, increased peripheral resistance, increased arterial pressure, and enhanced cardiac output. For these reasons, smoking by people with atherosclerotic disease may result in increased angina or myocardial infarction.

   Smoking may contribute directly to the atherosclerotic process. Various constituents of cigarette smoke, including nicotine itself, have been shown to damage vascular endothelium. Smoking also has adverse effects on platelet aggregation and vasomotor reactivity. The net result of these various events is promotion of endothelial cell injury and interference with vascular repair mechanisms. In addition, smoking is a major risk factor for coronary vasospasm, and smoking a single cigarette can cause profound disturbances in regional coronary blood flow in patients with angina and coronary artery disease. Smoking can cause significant increases in premature ventricular contractions, contributing greatly to the risk of sudden death caused by a lethal arrhythmia.
3. *Pulmonary disease.*
   Cigarette smoking is the leading cause of pulmonary illness and death in the United States, mainly as a result of pneumonia, influenza, bronchitis, emphysema, and chronic airway obstruction. Smoking accounts for 81.5% of chronic obstructive pulmonary disease mortality (Table 16–2) and results in destruction of peribronchiolar alveoli, alterations in central and peripheral airways, reduction in the number of small arteries, and diminished microbicidal ac-

tivity. In particular, smokers with severe chronic airflow obstruction have been found to have inflammation, atrophy, goblet cell metaplasia, squamous metaplasia, and mucous plugging in terminal and respiratory bronchioles.

C. Neuroscience.

The acute psychoactive effects of inhaled cigarette smoke are largely attributable to nicotine. One fourth of the nicotine taken into the lungs reaches the brain in about 15 seconds, producing nearly immediate effects. Although potent peripheral actions occur, the weight of the evidence shows that the reinforcing effects of nicotine from smoking are centrally mediated. Nicotine (through stimulation of cholinergic neurons) temporarily enhances visual surveillance, reaction time, mental efficiency, rapid information processing, and memory recall. Nicotine has been found to act on dopamine pathways in the ventral tegmental ("brain reward") area in a manner similar to that experienced with heroin, cocaine, and amphetamines. This phenomenon may be partially responsible for the addictiveness of nicotine.

Nicotine's ability to alter the bioavailability of neuroregulators (neurotransmitters and neurohormones) suggests that it may be used by smokers both to regulate physiologic mechanisms, such as by providing relief from withdrawal, and to alter psychological function, such as by providing temporary improvements in performance or affect. Ordinary activities, such as socializing, finishing a meal, and driving an automobile, as well as activities that demand focused attention and vigilance, such as test taking, and dysphoric states (e.g., anxiety and sadness) eventually become powerful cues for smoking. The number of affective states or performance demands that function as cues for smoking is potentially large, explaining the thorough interweaving of the smoking habit into the fabric of daily living.

D. Nicotine dependence and cofactors for smoking.

In the past 30 years, the prevalence of smoking in adults in the United States has decreased by nearly a third, and nearly half of all people who ever smoked have quit. With such numbers of people defecting from the ranks of tobacco users, it has become apparent that smoking is no longer randomly distributed throughout the population. As the "easy quitters" and casual smokers are eliminated from the smoker pool, smokers who remain can be characterized by greater dependence on nicotine. These individuals may be genetically hypersensitive to nicotine, or more favorably disposed to its effects, or both.

Many of the remaining smokers also exhibit cofactors for smoking, that is, factors that increase the likelihood of starting and/or decrease the likelihood of stopping. Cofactors associated with smoking include depression, premenstrual syndrome, eating disorders, anxiety disorders, alcohol dependence, adult-attention deficit hyperactivity disorder, and schizophrenia. Recent findings suggest that when such smokers attempt to quit, cofactor symptomatology is unmasked or exacerbated and persists well beyond the duration of nicotine withdrawal symptoms, which usually peak 2 to 3 days after smoking cessation. Although manipulation of social and environmental factors that promote smoking has achieved dramatic success in smoking reduction over the past 3 decades, at this juncture, interventions need to be directed at the cofactors that promote smoking by providing treatment for these conditions before smoking cessation is attempted. Also, the potential of nicotine replacement vehicles for managing these cofactors has yet to be fully exploited. Although still well in the future, focused interventions involving nicotine anologues or even gene therapy may help alter susceptibility to nicotine dependence.

III. General management guidelines.

A. Prevention.

1. *Adolescents.*
Every day an estimated 3000 adolescents and children begin smoking. Physicians who care for children or parents of young children have both the opportunity and the obligation to offer anticipatory guidance in an attempt to prevent young people from smoking. *Stages of smoking* initiation in children and adolescents have been identified: (1) a preparatory stage, in which attitudes and beliefs about the utility of smoking are formed; (2) a trying stage, in which the first few cigarettes are smoked; (3) an experimental stage, in which smoking is repeated but irregular; and (4) the regular use stage, in which smoking occurs at least weekly across various situations and personal interactions. The time from the first cigarette to regular use takes an average of 2 to 3 years, and considerable individual variation exists.

   Many factors have been identified that influence the adolescent progression into adult smoking. At the earliest stage, *advertising and the behavior of adult and older sibling role models* are considered important. In well child and routine visits with parents of young children, physicians should ask about smoking in the home and explain the relationship between smoking and the child's health as well as the influence on the child's subsequent smoking behavior. Advice, assistance, and follow-up can then be targeted at parents. Posters depicting positive role models speaking out against smoking and examples of the negative consequences of smoking can be placed in waiting areas or patient rooms, and magazines advertising tobacco can be removed. These materials can be obtained from the American Lung Association (215-315-8700) and the National Cancer Institute (800-4-CANCER).

As the child matures, the *availability of cigarettes and peer pressure* become strong influences. Parents of prepubertal children should be counseled that cigarette smoking begins in grade school in some communities, and that children observe their parents' own behavior. Children should be included in discussions about smoking and asked in private about their own use and about use by any friends. Children should be warned about both short-term and long-term negative effects of smoking and should be advised to refuse offers or to stop if he or she is already experimenting with cigarettes. *If the child believes that tobacco use is harmful but is uncertain about how to refuse, role playing is a technique that can be used to practice this skill. Phrases like "No thanks, it makes my clothes smell" or "My boyfriend/girlfriend doesn't like it" can be offered.*

Community and school interventions likely to be helpful at this stage include bans on smoking on school grounds, stricter enforcement of restrictions on tobacco sales to minors, and peer-resistance training. Parents should be assisted in smoking cessation and children can be involved in supporting the attempt.

For adolescents, physicians should *ask about smoking attitudes and behaviors and availability of cigarettes.* In a summary of findings from 27 prospective studies on smoking initiation, Conrad and colleagues[2] found that factors such as peer use and approval, high normative estimates of smoking by peers, and offers and availability of cigarettes were strong predictors of smoking onset. Other risk factors are low levels of academic achievement and school involvement, lack of skills to resist peer influences, and low self-image. Physicians should ask adolescents about smoking, *discuss the health risks, and explore situations that promote tobacco use.* As with adults, personalizing messages and correcting misperceptions is helpful. Physicians should *encourage school involvement and provide external validation of the adolescent's self-worth.* Emphasizing cost and social unacceptability are additional strategies.

2. *Adults.*
Primary care physicians should be role models in *advocating smoke-free environments and counter advertising* in combating tobacco use and promotion. Physicians should clear their offices of magazines that promote tobacco use, and they should post office policies against smoking and remove ashtrays from waiting rooms. Doctors Ought to Care (DOC, 1-404-721-2739) provides counter advertisements and warning labels, which can be placed on common magazines (Newsweek and Time) that contain tobacco promoting ads. Other means of limiting access to tobacco (increasing the cost and restricting the places in which cigarettes can be used, e.g., airline flights and work settings) should be supported, and physicians should advertise (by placing smoking information and cessation pamphlets in the patient areas) that they are actively involved in preventing initiation of smoking and promoting quit attempts in active smokers.

B. Behavioral management and medication.

Each primary care practice should develop its own comprehensive approach for preventing and treating nicotine addiction. The entire practice, including all providers and staff, should be committed to the approach. *The main steps for an office-based smoking cessation program include (1) select an office smoking cessation coordinator, (2) create a smoke-free office, (3) identify all smoking patients, (4) develop patient smoking cessation plans, and (5) provide follow-up support.*

Specific tasks might be assigned as follows: (1) patients are systematically identified by the nurse, (2) advice and nicotine replacement systems, as appropriate, are provided by physicians, (3) self-help information is provided by staff as the patient exits, and (4) a system of follow-up calls and/or visits can be scheduled for patients who set a quit date by the office coordinator.

1. *Brief office counseling.*
The National Cancer Institute's manual for clinicians to help patients stop smoking proposes the *four "As" of office based interventions,* which are: (1) *ask* about smoking at every opportunity, (2) *advise* all smokers to stop, (3) *assist* patients in cessation effort, and (4) *arrange* follow-up. The first step, to identify all smokers in the practice, was reviewed in section I.A. Smokers can then be classified, as shown in Figure 16–1, as precontemplators (those not considering to quit), contemplators (those considering to quit in the future but no plans), and action smokers (those ready to quit soon). Fewer than 20% of smokers are contemplating or are ready to take action to quit in primary care practice.

The second step, to advise patients to quit smoking, should be delivered in a concerned, nonjudgmental fashion by the clinician. It is important to personalize the message, such as, "I am concerned about your overall health and recommend that you quit smoking. You will begin to feel better, even within a few weeks after quitting." Even the precontemplator (one who does not consider quitting) should be advised but not badgered. Providing written handouts can serve as motivators.

Smokers who are ready to quit should be encouraged to set a quit date, when they will eliminate all smoking. They can prepare for the quit date by keeping a diary, enlisting support of friends and family, and attempting to decrease smoking before the quit date. It is important to secure the patient's commitment to the cessation program and to the quit date. Having the patient sign a commitment statement in the medical record enhances compliance and commitment to medications and follow-up care.

The third step is to assist patients throughout the smoking cessation process. Patients should be informed that they will have the primary care physician, the physician's trained staff, or a special consultant or group arranged for patients to cope with the transition from smoking to abstinence from smoking. Richards[3] identified *patient blockers, ways that patients avoid dealing with tobacco use,* such as highlighting previous failed attempts, emphasizing the beneficial effects of smoking on anxiety and coping with problems, accentuating smoking benefits and minimizing smoking risks, blaming the spouse's smoking for continued smoking, believing that it is too late to quit, and worrying about the consequences of quitting. Health providers need to familiarize themselves with these "blockers" and prepare to respond in a way that moves the patient beyond this behavioral block. This strategy may include pushing patients to explain their reasoning, dispelling misconceptions, and offering other options. Many examples of physician responses are provided by Richards. The following phrases may be tried:

- What specifically have you tried that didn't work before?
- Smoking will not improve your problems. Would you like to discuss them?
- Help me to understand what you enjoy about smoking? Is there something else that you might enjoy more? Is it worth the risks?
- If your partner is the problem, why don't I meet with you both?
- From the moment that you quit, your health will improve.
- Let's discuss what you can do to avoid gaining weight.

Techniques of behavior therapy may also be useful and include the following: (1) determine potential relapse situations and avoid or decrease the frequency of them, when possible, (2) enhance the motivation to quit by announcing the intention to quit to others and keeping a list in writing of the reasons to quit and the consequences of smoking, and (3) prepare for withdrawal symptoms. *In order to improve the chances that a smoker will quit smoking and avoid relapse, preparation is strongly encouraged.* Maintenance of a *smoking diary* before the quit attempt helps establish the pattern of smoking and helps identify key smoking events that prompt and maintain the behavior. Once habits are identified, an attempt can be made to disrupt the smoking rituals (e.g., moving a favorite "smoking" chair, eliminating the first morning cup of coffee, and avoiding alcohol) before the cessation attempt. Understanding situations that have caused relapse in the past and discussing avoidance or management of these situations can also be of great help. Cigarettes should be removed from the house, car, office, and so on, in order to decrease the availability of cigarettes, and friends should be asked to refrain from offering cigarettes. A common concern among smokers is that quitting will be associated with weight gain. Advice can include having low-calorie foods and snacks available, such as sugar-free hard candies, and beginning an exercise program before quitting. These behavioral techniques are based on the observation that smoking is a learned behavior that is controlled by antecedents (situations that prompt smoking) and consequences (events that either reinforce or punish smoking). If all of the physician's suggestions are to no avail, the physician should offer to make a referral to someone who specializes in smoking treatment.

2. *Suggestions for family.*
   Family involvement is often helpful in a successful attempt to quit smoking. Although social support interventions have not been shown to improve cessation rates, smokers often attribute failure to the smoking behavior of their partner. It may be possible to encourage a smoking partner to also attempt to quit or to ask the patient to identify a "buddy" to use for support. The patient can also be encouraged to involve family members by giving them specific tasks (to do or to stop doing) in order to assist the patient in the attempt to quit smoking.

3. *Nicotine pharmacotherapies.*
   Most current smokers seen in the office setting have tried to quit before and failed. Smokers should be asked if they have had common nicotine withdrawal symptoms (craving for nicotine, irritability, frustration, anger, anxiety, difficulty sleeping at night, depression, poor concentration, restlessness, and hunger) when they decreased smoking or attempted to quit in the past. Smokers should be asked if they have characteristics of nicotine dependency or addiction, including smoking within 30 minutes of arising, difficulty refraining to smoke in forbidden places and during illnesses, enjoying the first cigarette of the day the most, and smoking more than a pack per day. If withdrawal symptoms and addictive character-

istics are experienced, the patient is probably a candidate for nicotine replacement therapy.

Relative contraindications to nicotine replacement therapy are active cardiovascular disease, peptic ulcers, skin sensitivity to nicotine, and pregnancy. *With respect to pregnancy, nicotine chewing gum (polacrilex) is in pregnancy category C and the transdermal nicotine patch is in pregnancy category D.* A conservative approach might be to start with nonpharmacologic treatment for smoking cessation; if that fails, although nicotine replacement is not without risk, replacement is safer than cigarette smoking. The chewing gum is preferable to the patch because dosing is more time limited and ceases at night. The patch is also considered to pose a greater risk to the fetus because it more readily provides doses equivalent to those that have adverse effects in animals. In general, nicotine replacement may be viewed more favorably than continued smoking for women smoking more than 10 to 15 cigarettes a day who have failed attempts to quit without medication.

For *patients with cardiovascular disease,* both types of nicotine replacement cause fewer cardiovascular effects than nicotine delivered by tobacco smoke. Although one study demonstrated no adverse effects of transdermal nicotine in patients with active heart disease, the safety of nicotine replacement systems in such patients has yet to be established. Again, the risks of continued smoking without the potential benefits on smoking cessation of the patch must be carefully considered. Finally, tobacco use and nicotine replacement should not be mixed, so that toxic addictive effects are prevented.

a. *Transdermal nicotine.* Products vary in nicotine dose and recommended weeks of use. All brands recommend higher doses for the first weeks of therapy. The amount of nicotine delivered by typical dosages of transdermal nicotine is equivalent to about 30% to 50% of the nicotine derived by usual smoking. Four patch products are approved by the United States Food and Drug Administration (Table 16–3).

Although manufacturers may draw distinctions between their products, all meet Food and Drug Administration standards for clinical safety and effectiveness. Meta-analysis studies conclude that (1) subjects using the active patch are twice as likely to quit than those using a placebo (22% versus 9% at 6 months), (2) effectiveness is consistent across patch-use strategies (either part-time or full-time use, and with/without tapering), and (3) effect is present at both low-intensity and high-intensity counseling.

Information about use of the patch is provided in Table 16–4. *Use of the patch for at least 8 weeks has the greatest likelihood for success.* The highest available dose (21 mg) should be used for people who smoke more than 10 cigarettes a day. Weaning should begin after 3 to 8 weeks (with the longer duration used for more heavily addicted smokers), and each of the lower doses (14 mg and 7 mg) should be used for 2 to 4 weeks. Patients with cardiovascular disease or weighing less than 100 pounds may initially be given a lower nicotine dose (14 mg). Patients who are heavy smokers may benefit from higher doses of nicotine replacement. A recent report of high-dose patch therapy found that better relief of withdrawal symptoms and higher rates of short-term abstinence (but similar long-term cessation rates) occurred in patients treated with a 44-mg/d patch dose. Although this dose was found to be relatively safe in this study, (only one patient experienced nicotine toxicity), myocardial infarction was reported in a man (later found to be free of coronary artery disease) who used routinely prescribed doses of the patch.

Patients should be advised to discontinue tobacco use before using first patch. Only one patch per day should be used; it should be applied to a nonhairy, clean, dry skin surface (including upper arm or upper body). The same skin site should not be used more than once in a week, in order to prevent skin irritation. Used patches should be folded over, and they should be disposed of away from pets and children.

Local dermatologic reactions are the most common side effects (occurring in up to 50% of users of the patch) and include erythema, burning, and itching. These effects are often managed by application of a mild hydrocortisone cream and avoidance of the use of this site until the condition resolves. Sleep disturbance, including vivid dreams, is encountered in up to 20% of patients. This phenomenon may be caused either by nicotine withdrawal from smoking cessation (possibly inadequate nicotine replacement) or by nicotine dosing from the patch (possibly excessive nicotine replacement). Although these problems generally subside with continued use, the latter

Table 16–3
Nicotine Patch Systems Approved by the FDA

Product	Company	Duration of Action	Doses
Habitrol	Basel Pharmaceutical	24 h	7, 14, 21 mg
Nicoderm	SmithKline Beecham	24 h	7, 14, 21 mg
Nicotrol	Parke-Davis	16 h	5, 10, 15 mg
Prostep	Lederle	24 h	11, 22 mg

Table 16–4
Information About Nicotine Patch Use

Preparation	Patients should stop smoking before beginning to use the nicotine patch and be involved in a smoking cessation program under the care of a physician or other health care provider. Although the patches have proved to be beneficial even in the absence of supportive care, they are much more effective when used in conjunction with a smoking cessation program.
Dosage	All patch manufacturers recommend an initial treatment dosage, followed by one or two weaning dosages. Most manufacturers advise starting administration at the highest dosage patch available, except with small patients (weighing <100 pounds) and those with a history of cardiovascular disease.
Administration	The patch should be applied only once a day to a clean, dry, and nonhairy site on the trunk or the upper arm. The patch should be applied promptly on removal from its protective pouch in order to prevent evaporative loss of nicotine from the system. Application sites should not be reused for at least a week in order to prevent skin irritation. For all-day systems, the used patch should be removed after 24 h and a new one applied to another site. For the 16-h system, the patch should be applied on waking and removed at bedtime.
Duration of therapy	Depending on the type of patch, the recommended duration of therapy ranges from 10 to 16 wk.
Adverse reactions	The most common side effect of the nicotine patch is a mild, transient (15–60 min) itching or burning at the site after application. Erythema, sometimes accompanied by edema, also occurs frequently at the patch site. Other common side effects include contact sensitization (rare), headache, vertigo, insomnia, somnolence, abnormal dreams, myalgia, arthralgia, abdominal pain, nausea, dyspepsia, diarrhea, and nervousness. Anxiety, irritability, and depression may also occur but are more often symptoms of nicotine withdrawal than patch toxicity.
Contraindications	Contraindications to nicotine patch use include serious cardiac arrhythmias, severe or worsening angina, recent myocardial infarction, hypersensitivity or allergy to nicotine, and pregnancy. The patch should be used with caution in patients with psoriasis, dermatitis (atopic or eczematous), active peptic ulcers, severe renal impairment, accelerated hypertension, hyperthyroidism, pheochromocytoma, or insulin-dependent diabetes mellitus.

Adapted from Glynn TJ, Mantley MW. How to Help Your Patients Stop Smoking: A National Cancer Institute Manual for Physicians. Bethesda, MD: National Institutes of Health, 1989. DHHS publication NIH 89-3064.

problem may be relieved by removal of the patch at night. Less common side effects include dry mouth, dyspepsia, nervousness, arthralgias, and myalgias.

b. *Nicotine chewing gum.* Information about use of the nicotine chewing gum is provided in Table 16–5. Gum replacement therapy is available over the counter in 2-mg doses, and by prescription in 4-mg doses. Patients who cannot afford transdermal nicotine, have severe skin irritation from the patch, prefer an oral treatment, and are willing to comply to self-dosing may be candidates for nicotine gum therapy. The 1-year efficacy of nicotine polacrilex 2 mg gum is approximately 10% when it is administered with a physician's brief advice, compared with a rate of about 5% for physician's advice alone. A meta-analysis of 14 controlled trials showed a success rate of 27% at 6 months in nicotine chewing gum users who attended cessation group therapy, compared with 11% in a placebo group.

A starting dose can be estimated by use of one dose of 2 mg for every 2 cigarettes smoked per day. Nicotine gum in the 4-mg dose is suggested for heavily dependent smokers (those smoking more than 20 cigarettes, or 1 pack, per day, or scoring > 6 on the Fagerström Tolerance Questionnaire), with a starting dose of 4 mg in place of every three to four cigarettes per day. Patients should be advised to chew the gum slowly until a stinging sensation is experienced (the "chew and park" method), to avoid drinking acidic beverages (coffee, juices, colas) while chewing, and to chew for 20 to 30 minutes when the urge to smoke arises. Regular dosing of the gum appears to be an important determinant of success. Patients experiencing inadequate relief of withdrawal symptoms should increase the number of doses per day. Use of inadequate amounts and an inadequate duration are the main reasons for nicotine chewing gum failures. Patients should be advised to use sufficient amounts (even ≥ 20/d) to decrease the urge to smoke and to use the gum for approximately 10 to 12 weeks. After 1 or 2 months, weaning by one unit dose (2 or 4 mg) per week may be initiated. Although nicotine gum is available over the counter, patients should be advised to use these products under professional supervision for the greatest efficacy.

Side effects of nicotine gum include gastrointestinal upset, jaw pain, hiccups, diarrhea, and mouth sores. These can be mostly eliminated by slowing of the chewing rate. Nicotine replacement therapy via nasal spray has

Table 16–5
Information About Nicotine Chewing Gum Use

Preparation	Patients should stop smoking before beginning to use nicotine chewing gum and should be involved in a smoking cessation program under the care of a physician or other health care provider.
Dosage	Patients should use one piece of gum whenever they have the urge to smoke. Patients should be instructed not to exceed 30 pieces of 2-mg gum/d. For patients who have trouble with an as-needed approach, a fixed dosing schedule (e.g., one piece every 60 to 90 min) may be more appropriate. At least two boxes (192 pieces) of the 2-mg gum should be prescribed at the initial visit. A common problem is that patients use the gum too sparingly in the first few days after quitting, and then relapse occurs because of lack of nicotine.
Administration	Each piece of nicotine gum should be chewed slowly and intermittently for about 30 minutes. Chewing quickly can release the nicotine too rapidly and reduce the effect of the gum. Each piece of gum should be chewed enough to soften it or until the taste or "tingling" from the nicotine is felt. Then it should be "parked" in contact with the oral mucosa so that the nicotine can be absorbed. The gum should be rechewed gently every few minutes in order to release more nicotine.
Duration of therapy	The need for refills should be assessed at follow-up visits. The dosage of nicotine gum should be tapered after about 3 mo. Use of the gum for more than six mo is not recommended.
Adverse reactions	Potential side effects of nicotine gum use are sore jaw, mouth irritation, heartburn, nausea, sore throat, and palpitations.
Contraindications	Nicotine gum is contraindicated for patients who have had a recent myocardial infarction, severe or worsening angina, or life-threatening arrhythmias. It is also contraindicated for patients who are pregnant, nursing, or unable to chew.

Adapted from Glynn TJ, Manley MW. How to Help Your Patients Stop Smoking: A National Cancer Institute Manual for Physicians. Bethesda, MD: National Institutes of Health, 1989. DHHS publication NIH 89-3064.

shown even greater efficacy than the patch or chewing gum in controlled trials but is pending approval for use by the Food and Drug Administration. Because the pharmacokinetics of this preparation are similar to those of tobacco smoking, the potential adverse effect on patients with cardiovascular disease should be considered in the selection of this form of therapy and in its dosing.

c. *Combined nicotine replacement therapy.* As with all nicotine replacement therapies, patients should be counseled to *stop smoking before they initiate therapy.* This is important not only because of safety but also because patients must be aware that relief from withdrawal symptoms is most effectively obtained from exclusive reliance on the nicotine replacement product.

Recently, numerous clinical investigators have explored the use of high doses of the patch or the chewing gum (or the patch plus the gum) and reported better outcomes in highly nicotine dependent smokers. For people who experience withdrawal symptoms (see Fig. 16–1, *bottom panel*) or for those who are highly addicted and/or have failed previous attempts with replacement therapy, combined therapy may be indicated. This may be an indication for referral.

4. *Nonnicotine pharmacotherapies.*
Several agents may be considered for patients with contraindications to nicotine replacement. Clonidine (Catopres) appears to be advantageous for a select group of smokers, particularly women who do not wish to undergo nicotine replacement therapy. It may be used with a test dose of 0.05 mg, given on the first evening, followed by a 0.1-mg pill or patch for 7 days. Side effects of hypotension and dizziness may occur, and the United States Food and Drug Administration has not approved its use for smoking cessation. The use of antidepressants (e.g., selective serotonin reuptake inhibitors) should be reserved for patients with major depressive disorders. Benzodiazepines have no proven efficacy in smoking cessation. Several limited trials have been conducted with buspirone (BuSpar) that show promise for use of this agent for smoking cessation.

5. *Combined approaches.*
Smokers who are willing to be referred to intensive group counseling and to undergo nicotine replacement therapy (< 5% in general medical practice) have the highest long-term success rates (35% to 40% at 1 year). In addition, a meta-analysis of studies of smoking cessation interventions showed that the *most effective interventions* used teams of providers (physicians and nonphysicians) and multiple intervention modalities and included discussions over several visits. Because most smokers rely on the services available to them during the primary care office visit, office practices that develop a systems approach to smoking cessation, including routine identification, repeated smoking cessation messages, provision of self-help materials, nicotine replacement, and scheduled follow-up are likely to

have the greatest impact on reducing smoking among their patients.

C. Return visits and general follow-up care.

The fourth step recommended by the National Cancer Institute program is to arrange follow-up care. *Returning to smoking during the first week after quitting is the greatest predictor of failure to abstain in the long term. Therefore, close follow-up within the first week after quitting is recommended.* Patients should be contacted by telephone or scheduled for a return office visit within 1 to 2 weeks so that the physician can evaluate medication usage and effects. They should be asked to report any use of cigarettes and any mood changes that may be related to withdrawal symptoms or medication side effects. Personalized coping methods should be offered. Frequent follow-up visits are correlated with greater success. Typically, patients are scheduled for a 4- to 6-week follow-up visit. Telephone reminders, personalized mailing, and nurse-assisted counseling sessions enhance smoking cessation success in the practice setting.

D. Relapse prevention.

Most (80% to 90%) smokers who attempt to quit with brief advice and nicotine replacement therapies in primary care medical practice experience relapse. The clinician should be prepared to retreat smokers who have relapsed. If withdrawal symptoms are present during the relapse, then higher dosages of nicotine replacement may be needed, such as 4 mg versus 2 mg of nicotine chewing gum, or transdermal nicotine plus 2 mg of gum if withdrawal symptoms occur despite use of the transdermal patch. Psychological triggers, such as negative moods or stresses, should be documented. Specific coping strategies should be offered. Concurrent psychological or psychiatric illnesses, such as alcoholism and depression, should be identified. Primary care clinicians should become familiar with, and offer common coping strategies for, patients who have experienced relapse or should offer referral to trained counselors in smoking cessation.

IV. Special programs for smoking cessation and when to refer.

Although most smokers quit independently, many (particularly those who are heavily addicted to nicotine), seek out formal programs for assistance. Many voluntary and commercial programs are available, and listings can be found in most cities and in many smaller communities in the yellow pages. *Voluntary agencies* include the American Cancer Society program Freshstart (four 1-hour group sessions covering reasons for smoking, withdrawal symptoms, stress management, and coping strategies), the American Lung Association Freedom from Smoking program (seven sessions aimed at reducing the stress of quitting), and the Seventh Day Adventist Church program Breath-Free (eight sessions emphasizing behavior modification). Many states support organizations that provide information and resources for quitting smoking. For example, in Michigan, information can be obtained through the Michigan Health Promotion Clearinghouse in Lansing (telephone: 1-800-537-5666). To find out about similar organizations in other states, providers should contact the United States Office on Smoking and Health, Centers for Disease Control and Prevention (1600 Clifton Rd. N.E., Atlanta, Georgia 30333; 404-488-5701).

Several commercial programs are also available, although they have become less available in recent years. The more well-known programs include SmokEnders (6 weekly sessions emphasizing positive reinforcement and changing attitudes), the Schick centers for the Control of Smoking (5 days of aversive conditioning [smoke satiation/low-grade shocks] followed by 6 weekly sessions), Smokeless, and Smoke Stoppers. The last two programs license their programs to hospitals and businesses. The format is four sessions in the first week before smoking cessation, followed by 2 or 3 weeks of maintenance.

The effectiveness of any single program, however, is not a key factor in successful smoking cessation for the individual patient; the number of previous attempts to quit greatly influences subsequent success. The message for patients is that regardless of the method used, they should keep trying until they stop smoking.

V. Benefits of quitting and implications for managed care (Table 16–6).

Even though success rates for brief counseling with nicotine replacement therapy are as low as 10% to 20% in primary care practice, *smoking cessation intervention is perhaps the most cost-effective primary care prevention activity.* Studies have shown that the cost per year of life saved for smoking cessation in primary care is approximately $4000 to $10,000, compared with $10,000 to $30,000 for common hypertension therapies and $50,000 to $100,000 for hyperlipidemia therapies. Although third-party payers have been slow to support such an approach, the aforementioned observations clearly support the appropriateness of investing in smoking cessation. Staff model health maintenance organizations should have trained staff in smoking cessation, along with accessible, practical methods that are easily applied to the routine office practice. Primary care providers should be required to complete continuing medical education training in smoking cessation in order to maintain staff privileges in health maintenance organizations.

Transdermal nicotine is effective, even with minimal or no counseling. Therefore, third-party payers, including Medicaid, should offer coverage of transdermal nicotine as an effective medication. *Requiring patients to attend intensive behavior therapy programs in order to re-*

Table 16–6
Benefits of Smoking Cessation

A few years after quitting, risk of cervical cancer is less than risk in a continuing smoker.
Stroke risk reduced 5 to 15 years after quitting to that of a person who never smoked.
Five years after quitting, rates of cancers of the mouth, throat, and esophagus risk half those of a continuing smoker.
After quitting, risk of cancer of the larynx less than that of a continuing smoker.
One year after quitting, excess risk of coronary heart disease half that of a continuing smoker; risk returns to that of a person who has never smoked after 15 years.
After long-term quitting, risk of death from chronic obstructive pulmonary disease less than that of a continuing smoker.
Ten years after quitting, lung cancer risk as little as half that of a continuing smoker.
Ten years after quitting, pancreatic cancer risk less than that of a continuing smoker.
After quitting, ulcer risk less than that of a continuing smoker.
A few years after quitting, bladder cancer risk half that of a continuing smoker.
After quitting, risk of peripheral artery disease less than that of a continuing smoker.
In women who quit before pregnancy or during first trimester, risk of low-birth-weight baby reduced to that of one who never smoked.

Adapted from Health Benefits of Smoking Cessation: A Report of the Surgeon General, 1990 at a Glance. Rockville, MD: Centers for Disease Control, 1990. DHHS publication CDC 90-8419.

ceive transdermal nicotine, as is done by some health maintenance organizations, is a huge barrier to effective care for a large number of smokers who visit primary care practices and are interested in quitting. A stepped care approach may be more appropriate. In summary, the evidence clearly supports the idea that reimbursement for the treatment of nicotine dependency constitutes a sound investment in health promotion and disease prevention, both for fee-for-service and managed care systems.

References

1. Hughes JR. An algorithm for smoking cessation. Arch Fam Med 1994; 3:280–285.
2. Conrad KM, Flay BR, Hill D. Why children start smoking cigarettes: Predictors of onset. Br J Addict 1992; 87:1711–1124.
3. Richards JW. Words as therapy: Smoking cessation. J Fam Pract 1992; 34:687–692.

Suggested Reading

Adlkofer FX. Involvement of nicotine and its metabolites in the pathology of smoking-related diseases: Facts and hypotheses. In: Clarke PBS, Quick M, Adlkofer F, Thurau K, Editors. Effects of Nicotine on Biological Systems: II. Boston: Birkhauser Verlag; 1995.

Dale LC, Hurt RD, Offord KP, et al. High-dose nicotine patch therapy. JAMA 1995; 274:1353–1358.

Fagerstrom K-O. Measuring degree of physical dependency to tobacco smoking with reference to individualization of treatment. Addict Behav 1978; 3:235–241.

Fiore MC, Editor. Cigarette smoking. Med Clin North Am 1992; 76(2).

Fiore MC. The new vital sign: Assessing and documenting smoking status. JAMA 1991; 266:3183–3184.

Fiore MC, Novotny TE, Pierce JP, et al. Methods used to quit smoking in the United States. JAMA 1990; 263:2760–2765.

Glassman SH. Cigarette smoking: Implications for psychiatric illness. Am J Psychiatry 1993; 150:546–553.

Glynn TJ, Manley MW. How to help your patients stop smoking: A national cancer institute manual for physicians. Public Health Service, National Institutes of Health; 1989. US Department of Health and Human Services, NIH publication 89-3064.

Glynn TJ, Manley MW, Solberg LI, Slade J. Creating and maintaining an optimal medical practice environment for treatment of nicotine addiction. In: Orleans CT, Slade J, Editors. Nicotine Addiction: Principles and Management. New York: Oxford University Press; 1993, pp. 162–180.

Henningfield JE. Nicotine medications for smoking cessation. N Engl J Med 1995; 333:1196–1203.

Kottke T, Battista R, DeFriese G, et al. Attributes of successful smoking cessation intervention in medical practice: A meta-analysis of 39 controlled trials. JAMA 1988; 259:2882–2889.

Lam W, Sze PC, Sacks HS, et al. Meta-analysis of randomized controlled trials of nicotine chewing gum. Lancet 1987; 2:27–30.

MacKenzie TD, Bartecchi CE, Schrier RW. The human costs of tobacco use. N Engl J Med 1994; 330:975–980.

Pomerleau OF, Pomerleau CS. Neuroregulators and the reinforcement of smoking: Towards a biobehavioral explanation. Neurosci Biobehav Rev 1984; 8:503–513.

Prochaska JO, DiClemente CC. Stages and processes of self-change of smoking: Toward an integrative model of change. J Consult Clin Psychol 1983; 51:390–395.

Sigagy C, Mant D, Fowler G, Lodge M. Meta-analysis on efficacy of nicotine replacement therapies in smoking cessation. Lancet 1994; 343:139–142.

Solberg LI, Maxwell PL, Kottke TE, et al. A systematic primary care office-based smoking cessation program. J Fam Pract 1990; 30:647–654.

US Department of Health and Human Services. Preventing Tobacco Use Among Young People: A Report of the Surgeon General. Atlanta, GA: Public Health Service, Centers for Disease Control and Prevention, National Center for Chronic Disease Prevention and Health Promotion, Office of Smoking and Health, 1994. US Department of Health and Human Services, Publication No. 192.

17

KIRK J. BROWER, MD

JOHN D. SEVERIN, MD

Alcohol and Other Drug-Related Problems

I. Introduction.

Substance abuse and dependence affect between 17% and 27% of Americans over their lifetime. Twenty percent of out-patients in primary care clinics have alcohol disorders. Higher rates are found in hospitalized patients and in those in emergency department settings. Unfortunately, substance use disorders remain largely undetected and underdiagnosed. The stigma and shame associated with substance problems cause the patient and the family to hide the problems. Physicians may collude with patients in keeping substance problems hidden because of negative attitudes, stereotypes, and past experiences associated with difficult, treatment-resistant patients, yet *up to two thirds of patients improve after specialized treatment, and many more get better after brief counseling by their primary care physicians.* Moreover, primary care practitioners have an important role in identifying and intervening with at-risk patients before they have problems, as well as with patients manifesting mild-to-moderate problems. Early identification and treatment enhance outcomes, which reward clinicians' efforts and balance the more challenging cases clinicians encounter. Knowledge and skills as outlined in this chapter are easily learned and readily applied.

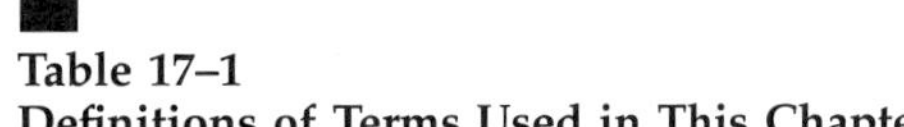

Table 17–1
Definitions of Terms Used in This Chapter

Hazardous drinking or substance use: a pattern of drinking or other drug use that places an individual at increased risk for adverse consequences.

Substance abuse: the persistent use of a substance, despite adverse consequences. Impaired control, tolerance, and withdrawal are not present. Abuse may lead to substance dependence, but the diagnosis is not made if the criteria for dependence have ever been met.

Substance dependence: the essential features are (1) a compulsion to take a substance for its psychological effects despite recurrent, adverse consequences and (2) impaired control over use. Tolerance and withdrawal may or may not be present, depending on the particular substance used and the severity of the dependence.

Physical, physiologic, or pharmacologic dependence: the occurrence of withdrawal symptoms after stopping or reducing substance use. Neither necessary nor sufficient for a diagnosis of *substance dependence* as defined above.

Alcoholism: "a primary, chronic disease with genetic, psychosocial, and environmental factors influencing its development and manifestations. The disease is often progressive and fatal. It is characterized by impaired control over drinking, preoccupation with the drug alcohol, use of alcohol despite adverse consequences, and distortions in thinking, most notably denial. Each of these symptoms may be continuous or periodic" (Morse and Flavin, 1992). By this definition, alcoholism is a severe form of alcohol dependence.

II. Diagnoses of abuse and dependence.

The diagnoses of substance abuse and substance dependence are based on signs and symptoms that can be elicited during the patient interview. Whereas the phrase *substance abuse* is often used generically to refer to any substance problem, it has a more specific definition when it is used as a diagnosis (Table 17–1). Likewise, the term *dependence* is often used to refer simply to physical dependence. In this section, physical dependence as a limited syndrome is distinguished from the full syndrome of substance dependence or addiction. Finally, substance abuse is a milder and earlier disorder than substance dependence. Patients with mild-to-moderate problems usually qualify for a diagnosis of substance abuse, whereas those with moderate-to-severe problems typically meet the criteria for substance dependence (Fig. 17–1). Mild-to-moderate problems often respond to brief interventions conducted in the primary care setting. Moderate-to-severe problems are best treated in a specialized treatment setting.

A. Signs and symptoms.

1. Patients with *impaired control* take more substance than they intend, try to make rules about their use that they are unable to keep, or are unable to decrease their use despite wanting or trying to.
2. *Continued use despite recurrent problems* is easily remembered by the UCR mnemonic: *u*se, followed by adverse *c*onsequences, followed by

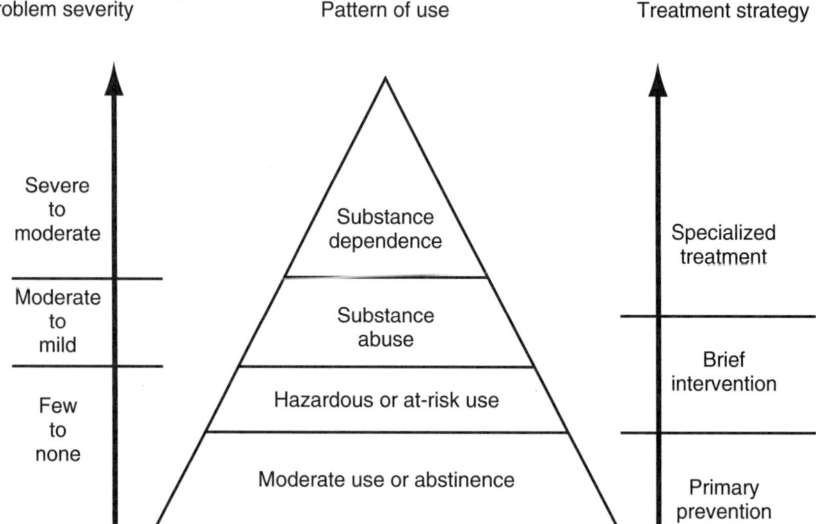

Figure 17–1
The relationship between problem severity, pattern of use, and treatment strategy. Increasing intensity is indicated by the arrows. The diagnostic assessment establishes the pattern of use and the problem severity. Primary care physicians conduct brief interventions for patients with hazardous use, substance abuse, and problems that are not severe. Patients with substance dependence, severe problems, significant psychosocial comorbidity, or problems resistant to brief interventions should be referred for specialized treatment.

repetition. Adverse consequences may be biomedical, psychological, or social.

3. *Tolerance and withdrawal.* Tolerance is defined as the need for larger amounts of a substance to achieve a desired effect or the occurrence of a diminished effect with the same amount. Withdrawal refers to characteristic, new-onset signs and symptoms that occur when substance use is reduced or stopped. The acute withdrawal period is time limited and rarely lasts more than 1 to 3 weeks. Both tolerance and withdrawal are evidence of physiologic adaptations to long-term substance exposure.

B. Substance abuse.

Substance abuse is defined as continued use despite recurrent problems (UCR). Patients who repeatedly drive while intoxicated in the absence of other problems qualify for a diagnosis of substance abuse. Patients with mild-to-moderate problems usually qualify for a diagnosis of substance abuse, and they often respond to brief interventions by the primary care practitioner.

C. Substance dependence.

Substance dependence is a more severe diagnosis than substance abuse, in which patients manifest impaired control and continued use despite recurrent problems. The usual notion of alcoholism (see Table 17–1) is a form of substance dependence. Some patients with moderate problems and most patients with severe problems qualify for a diagnosis of substance dependence. Patients with substance dependence usually require a referral to specialized treatment (Fig. 17–1), although some respond to brief intervention, and others quit on their own without treatment. Tolerance and withdrawal may or may not be present with substance dependence as defined here. However, when withdrawal symptoms are present, *substance dependence is distinguished from physical dependence (see below) by a compulsion to use or a tendency to relapse, even after withdrawal symptoms have abated.* Some authors refer to substance dependence as *psychological dependence* or *addiction* in order to distinguish it from physical dependence.

D. Physical dependence.

Physical dependence, also called *physiologic* or *pharmacologic dependence,* is diagnosed by the occurrence of withdrawal symptoms. Patients given therapeutic doses of benzodiazepines or opioids for several months may manifest physical dependence in the absence of substance abuse or substance dependence. Patients with physical dependence alone should not be considered addicted, nor should they be denied prescription medication for legitimate indications, such as the treatment of cancer pain. Physically dependent patients are important to identify because they require a tapering of their medications for safety and comfort when their medications are no longer clinically indicated. Patients with physical dependence only who lack other medical and psychiatric problems usually respond to a simple tapering of their medications, which can be readily managed by the primary care physician, often in an out-patient setting (see section V.H.2).

E. Hazardous use.

This type of use is also called *at-risk use.* Some patients are at high risk for developing problems such as abuse or dependence because of their pattern of consumption. For example, a patient's level of consumption may exceed general norms for moderate use, even though the physician can detect few or no problems. Patients with hazardous use benefit from education and brief interventions in the primary care setting.

III. Identifying and assessing substance problems.

A. Risk factors.

Although all patients should be screened for substance problems, some patients are at higher risk than others based on the following:

1. *Level of consumption.*
   Moderate use is defined as a level of consumption associated with a low risk for developing problems. *Hazardous use* exceeds moderation and is associated with a high risk for developing problems (see Table 17–1).
   a. For *alcohol,* varying definitions exist as to what constitutes hazardous drinking. The United States Department of Health and Human Services (DHHS) defines *moderate drinking as no more than two drinks a day for men and one drink a day for women.* Exceptions would include pregnant women, individuals younger than 21 years, people taking medications that interact with alcohol, and people with medical conditions, such as liver disease, for whom abstinence might better be recommended. *For elderly individuals aged 65 years and older, no more than one drink a day for men and women constitutes moderate drinking.* The DHHS recommends the following screening guidelines for at-risk drinking: *more than three drinks in a day for women, four drinks in a day for men, seven drinks in a week for women, and 14 drinks in a week for men (the 3-4-7-14 rule).* Another commonly used guideline for screening for hazardous drinking is more than three drinks a day for women, four drinks a day for men, or 12 drinks in a week for either gender *(the 3-4-12-rule).* These numbers are based on dose-related consequences of drinking, such as increased mortality in those drinking more than 4 drinks a day.
   b. For *prescription drugs,* hazardous consumption can be defined as use of more drug than prescribed, escalation of dose, or use of the medication for reasons other than prescribed, such as to get high. In either case, hazardous consumption implies that substance-related problems have yet to occur.
   c. For *illicit drugs,* any use is considered hazardous because of the legal risk and the unknown composition of illicitly sold substances.
2. *Family history and genetics.*
   For example, biologic sons of alcoholics have a twofold to fourfold greater risk of alcoholism than biologic sons of nonalcoholics, even when the sons are adopted at birth.
3. *Comorbid psychiatric disorders.*
   A lifetime history of a mental disorder increases the risk of substance abuse and dependence nearly threefold. Childhood diagnoses that predispose to substance disorders include attention-deficit disorder, conduct disorder, and other behavioral problems. Approximately 50% of patients with schizophrenia, manic-depressive illness, or bulimia have a comorbid substance disorder. Antisocial personality disorder increases the odds of a substance disorder by 30-fold. Patients with other depressive or anxiety disorders are two to three times more likely than patients without a mental illness to have a substance disorder.
4. *Other substance disorders.*
   Having one substance disorder increases the likelihood of having another substance disorder. For example, individuals with an alcohol disorder (abuse or dependence) have about a sixfold greater prevalence of another drug disorder than do individuals without an alcohol disorder. Likewise, *risk factors for prescription drug abuse include a current or past history of alcohol or other drug abuse. Therefore, the physician should carefully screen for substance problems before prescribing sedatives, hypnotics, or narcotic analgesics.* Finally, tobacco consumption is highly correlated with heavy drinking, and alcoholics are more likely than nonalcoholics to be heavy smokers (>1 pack per day).
5. *Demographic correlates.*
   Demographic correlates of alcohol and other drug disorders include male gender, younger age, lower income, and lower educational level. Obviously, people without these demographic correlates are not immune to the development of substance problems. For example, some elderly persons have late-onset drinking problems after the death of a spouse or retirement.
6. *Adolescent risk factors.*
   a. Family history of drug or alcohol addiction.
   b. Permissive home attitudes regarding smoking or alcohol use.
   c. Peers who use.
   d. Criminal behavior.
   e. Mood disorder.
   f. Selling or delivery of drugs.
   g. Physical or sexual abuse.
   h. Low self-esteem.

B. Screening for alcohol problems.

Screening should be conducted for all patients seen in a primary care practice. *Interviews and questionnaires are by far the best approach to screening* because of their higher sensitivity and specificity than those of physical and laboratory examinations. In interviews, screening questions can be introduced during a discussion of other personal health habits, such as wearing of seat belts or diet, or they can be easily introduced in the family history. An example question is *"Do you think anyone in your family has ever had a problem with alcohol?"* (Follow this with screening questions). Written questionnaires can be readily self-administered while a patient is waiting to be seen. Written questionnaires can be either administered alone or preferably embedded into general health questionnaires. For alcohol screening, many good questionnaires are outlined later and in Table 17–2. When interviewing, we generally begin with the CAGE questions and follow with quantity-frequency questions (Table 17–3), but many clinicians prefer to reverse this sequence, starting with quantity-frequency questions and following with the CAGE questions. Whichever order is used, quantity-frequency questions provide the best screen for hazardous or at-risk drinking, whereas the CAGE questions are most useful for screening for abuse and dependence.

1. The *CAGE questions* (Table 17–3) are probably the briefest and simplest screening tool for alcohol abuse and alcohol dependence. The sensitivity and specificity of the CAGE questions are generally good. If a patient answers "yes" to a CAGE question, then the patient should be prompted to elaborate: "Tell me more about that." When asking any questions about substance abuse, the physician wisely pays attention to both the content of the answers and the manner in which the patient responds. If the patient manifests defensiveness or anger, then the question about feeling annoyed is already answered. Maintaining rapport and a nonjudgmental attitude are critical to the screening process. Two or more "yes" responses indicate a positive result on the screening for alcohol problems. However, even one "yes" response may indicate hazardous drinking that may result in problems over time.

2. The CAGE questions need to be supplemented because they do not assess *level of consumption*, hazardous drinking, or use of other drugs. Regarding alcohol, the physician should ask about frequency:
   - How many days in a week do you typically have something to drink?
   - How many days in the past 4 weeks have you had something to drink?

   Then, the physician may inquire about quantity:
   - On days that you drink, how many drinks do you typically have? On days when you drink more than that, how much do you drink?

   Finally, the physician asks about heavy consumption or binge drinking:
   - What is the most you have had to drink in any one day during the past month?

   The physician should avoid asking, "How much do you drink?" as the first screening question or else be prepared for such vague answers as, "Not that much." Rather, specific questions that focus on frequency, then quantity, and finally on heavy consumption are more likely to evoke meaningful responses. *In asking about quantity, the physician should define what is meant by a drink (a 12-ounce beer = a 5-ounce glass of table wine = a shot or 1.5 ounces of 80-proof liquor = approximately 0.5 ounces or 12 g of absolute ethanol).* For patients who use different frames of reference ("I go through half a fifth a week"), general equivalencies are given in Table 17–4.

3. The *Alcohol Use Disorders Identification Test* (AUDIT) is a self-administered, 10-item screening instrument that assesses both level of alcohol consumption and related problems, including symptoms of dependence (see Appendix). The AUDIT screens for hazardous drinking as well as for alcohol abuse and dependence. The score ranges from zero to 40, and a score of 8 or more indicates problem drinking and the need for further assessment. Unlike the CAGE questions, the wide scoring range on the AUDIT allows the physician to determine the severity of drinking problems; higher scores indicate greater severity. Feedback about the score can be given in a manner similar to that used in informing patients about their laboratory values. The authors favor the AUDIT over the Michigan Alcoholism Screening Test (MAST) because the AUDIT is briefer, determines quantity and frequency, and screens for a broader range of alcohol problems (see Table 17–2).

4. *Special populations.*
   a. *Elderly patients.* The Michigan Alcoholism Screening Test—Geriatric Version (MAST-G) is a 24-item, yes-no, self-administered questionnaire that is designed specifically for adults aged 55 years and older (see Table 17–2 and Appendix). The score ranges from zero to 24, and 5 or more "yes" responses indicate an alcohol problem. Unlike the regular version of the MAST, questions about fights, work difficulties, and arrests have been eliminated because these events occur less often in the elderly. Instead, questions about skipped meals, loss of interest in hobbies, and effects on sleep appear. *We recommend using the MAST-G to screen for alcohol problems in geriatric patients,* although few data comparing the MAST-G with other screening instruments in the elderly are available at this time.
   b. *Obstetric patients.* The TACE and the TWEAK questions may perform better than the CAGE, from which they are derived. The TACE is similar to the CAGE except that it replaces the question about guilt with a

Table 17–2
Screening Tools for Alcohol and Drug Problems

Instrument	Items	Scoring Range*	Cut-Off Score	Comments	Source†
Alcohol					
CAGE	4	0–4	2	Recommended for brevity. (See Table 7–3)	Ewing JA. Detecting alcoholism: the CAGE questionnaire. JAMA 1984; 252:1905–1907.
Alcohol Use Disorders Identification Test (AUDIT) (see Appendix)	10	0–40	8	Screens for past 1 year only.	Saunders JB, Aasland OG, Babor TF, Unreal N. Development of the Alcohol Use Disorders Identification Test (AUDIT): WHO collaborative project on early detection of persons with harmful alcohol consumption. Addiction 1993; 88:791–804.
Michigan Alcoholism Screening Test (MAST)	24	0–53	5	Lifetime screen for alcoholism. Several versions and scoring protocols available, including the simpler 13-item Short MAST.	Hedlund JL, Vieweg BW. The Michigan Alcoholism Screening Test (MAST): A comprehensive review. J Operational Psychiatry 1984; 15:55–65.
MAST-Geriatric Version (MAST-G) (see Appendix)	24	0–24	5	For older adults aged 55 years and older	Blow FC, Brower KJ, Schulenberg JE, Demo-Dananberg LA, Young JP, Beresford TP. The Michigan Alcoholism Screening Test—Geriatric Version (MAST-G): A new elderly-specific screening instrument. Alcohol Clin Exp Res 1992; 16:372. Available from the University of Michigan Alcohol Research Center, 400 E. Eisenhower Pkwy, Suite 2A, Ann Arbor, MI 48108. Telephone: 313-998-7952
TACE	4	0–5	2	For pregnant women. (See section III.B.4.b)	Russel M, Martier SS, Sokol RJ, et al. Screening for pregnancy risk-drinking. Alcohol Clin Exp Res 1994; 18:1156–1161.
TWEAK	5	0–7	2	For pregnant women. (See section III.B.4.b)	Ibid.
Drugs					
CAGE Adapted to Include Drugs (CAGEAID)	4	0–4	2	Parallels the 4 CAGE questions. (See section III.C.1)	Fleming MF, Barry KL. Addictive Disorders. St. Louis: Mosby–Year Book; 1992.
Risk Prediction Scale for Drugs	14	0–42	10	Part of the Substance Abuse Subtle Screening Inventory.	Cooper SE, Robinson DAG. Use of the Substance Abuse Subtle Screening Inventory with a college population. J Am Coll Health 1987; 36:180–184.
Drug Abuse Screening Test (DAST-10) (see Appendix)	10	0–10	3	Contains questions 1, 3, 5, 8, 9, 10, 15, 21, 23, and 24 from the 28-item version.	Skinner HA. The Drug Abuse Screening Test. Addict Behav 1982; 7:363–371.
Both					
Problem-Oriented Screening Instrument for Teenagers (POSIT)	16	0–16	1	For adolescents. 16-item subscale of a larger instrument.	Rahdert ER. The Adolescent Assessment/Referral System Manual. Rockville, MD: US Department of Health and Human Services; 1991. DHHS Publication No. (ADM) 91-1735. Available from the National Clearinghouse for Alcohol and Drug Information. Telephone: 800-729-6686.

*Tests with broad scoring ranges (≥10 points) are useful to assess problem severity as well as to screen for problems. Higher scores indicate greater severity.

†Source specifies either a reference that contains the instrument or an address where instrument can be obtained.

Table 17–3
Screening for Alcohol Problems

Ask the CAGE questions*

1. Have you ever felt you should *c*ut down on your drinking?
2. Have people *a*nnoyed you by criticizing your drinking?
3. Have you ever felt bad or *g*uilty about your drinking?
4. Have you ever had a drink first thing in the morning to steady your nerves or get rid of a hangover (*e*yeopener)?

Ask about level of consumption

1. How many days in a week do you typically have something to drink? (quantity)
2. On days that you drink, how many drinks do you typically have? (frequency)
3. What is the most you had to drink in any one day during the past month? (maximum)
4. When was your last drink? *(Most patients with a problem will know exactly)*

If quantity × frequency > 7 drinks a week for women and > 14 drinks for men, or if maximum is > 3 for women and > 4 for men, then patient exceeds criteria for low-risk drinking.

If CAGE or consumption questions are positive, then assess for consequences, dependency symptoms, and severity (see text, section III.D)

*Scoring: 2 or more "yes" answers is a positive result for an alcohol disorder, but one "yes" answer indicates hazardous drinking.

question about tolerance: "How many drinks does it take to make you feel high?" An answer of three or more drinks is considered positive for tolerance in a woman and is scored as 2 points. On the other three questions, 1 point is scored for each "yes" response. Thus, scores on the TACE range from zero to 5, with 2 or more points indicating a positive result. The TWEAK borrows questions from the MAST as well as from the CAGE. The questions are:

- *T*olerance (T): How many drinks can you hold? (>5 drinks without falling asleep or passing out is scored as 2 points)
- Have close friends or relatives *w*orried (W) or complained about your drinking in the past year? (a "yes" response is scored as 2 points)
- *E*yeopener (E): Do you sometimes take a drink in the morning when you first get up? (a "yes" response is scored as 1 point)
- *A*mnesia (A): Has a friend or family member ever told you about things you said or did while you were drinking that you could not remember? (a "yes" response is scored as 1 point)
- Do you sometimes feel the need to *c*ut (K[C]) down on your drinking? (a "yes" response is scored as 1 point)

The TWEAK score ranges from zero to 7, with 2 or more considered a positive result for an alcohol problem.

c. *Adolescents and other children.* Unlike adults, for whom a few screening tests have emerged as preferred methods, no consensus exists about optimal screening tools in children. Although the CAGE questions, the AUDIT, and the Risk Prediction Scale for Drugs (see section III.C.2) may be used, children are less likely than adults to manifest physical dependence and other symptoms appearing on questionnaires designed for adults. Adolescent-specific questionnaires are available (see Table 17–2), but a skillfully performed interview by someone the patient views as caring, trustworthy, and credible may be more useful than screening questionnaires for children.[1, 2] Finally, children suffer not only from their own use, but also from that of their parents.

Table 17–4
General Equivalencies of Alcoholic Beverages*

Hard liquor (approximately 40% alcohol or 80 proof)	
1 shot or highball (1.5 ounces)	= 1 drink
1/2 pint of liquor	= 6 drinks
1 pint of liquor	= 12 drinks
1 fifth of liquor	= 20 drinks
1 quart of liquor	= 24 drinks
Wine (11% to 12% alcohol)	
1 glass of wine (5 ounces)	= 1 drink
1 bottle of wine (750 mL)	= 6 drinks
1 gallon of wine	= 30 drinks
Beer (4% to 5% alcohol)	
1 12-ounce bottle or can	= 1 drink
1 40-ounce container	= 3.3 drinks
1 6-pack of beer	= 6 drinks
1 case of beer	= 24 drinks
Wine Coolers (5% alcohol)	
1 wine cooler (12 ounces)	= 1 drink

*One drink contains approximately 0.5 ounces or 12 g of absolute ethanol.

C. Screening for drug problems.

1. The *CAGEAID questions* are the CAGE questions that have been *a*dapted to *i*nclude *d*rugs:
   - Have you felt you ought to Cut down on your drug use?
   - Have people *A*nnoyed you by criticizing your drug use?
   - Have you felt bad or *G*uilty about your drug use?
   - Have you ever used drugs the first thing in the morning to steady your nerves or to get the day started? (*E*yeopener)
2. The *Risk Prediction Scale for Drugs*, part of the Substance Abuse Subtle Screening Inventory, is a 14-item self-administered questionnaire with scores ranging from zero to 42. Scores of

10 or more constitute a positive result, and higher scores indicate a greater problem severity (see Table 17–2).

3. The *Drug Abuse Screening Test (DAST-10)* is a 10-item, yes-no, self-administered questionnaire (see Appendix). It is a shortened version of the original 28-item DAST (see Table 17–2). Scoring ranges from zero to 10. Guidelines for scoring are:
1 to 2 = low level of problems
3 to 5 = moderate level of problems
6 to 8 = substantial level
9 to 10 = severe level.

D. Assessment.

A positive result from screening is followed by an assessment. Whereas the purpose of screening is to *identify* a possible problem; *the purpose of an assessment is to confirm the problem and determine its extent, which guides treatment planning*. The assessment establishes (1) the diagnosis, (2) the severity of problems, and (3) the motivation for change.

1. *Assessing signs and symptoms of substance abuse and dependence.*
Conceptually, the important diagnostic issues are what happens when the patient uses a substance (impaired control, adverse consequences, and tolerance) and what happens when the patient tries to stop (unsuccessful attempts and withdrawal symptoms).
   a. *Adverse consequences*. The following areas are assessed: medical, psychiatric, and social (job, school, family, other relationships, financial, legal). Medical problems are determined by the history and physical examination. Two approaches exist for eliciting social consequences.
      (1) *Use direct questioning*:
         - Have substances caused any problems for you or your family? For you emotionally? At your job or school? For your social life? For your finances?
         - Do you have any legal problems?

         This approach is effective for patients who admit that they have a problem and want help. However, the questions may evoke resistance in other patients, and they are easy to deny.
      (2) *Assess problem areas first, then link them to substances*. A psychosocial history is obtained and is empathically related back to substances. An example is
         - How are things on the job? At home? With your family?

         An empathic response is
         - It sounds like things are pretty difficult right now, and you are feeling frustrated. I want to help in whatever way I can. How does your use of substances fit in with this?
   b. *Impaired control.*
      - Do you use more than you intend to?
      - Have you tried or wanted to cut down? What happened?
      - Do you ever make rules for your drinking or drug use? Do you always keep them? (e.g., the patient decides to drink only four beers in the evenings on weekends and eventually drinks hard liquor throughout the week.)
   c. *Tolerance.*
      - Do you need more to get the same effect?
      - Do you get less of an effect with the same amount? (Determine what the desired effect is: getting high, reducing anxiety, getting to sleep, or pain reduction.)
   d. *Withdrawal.*
      - Do you ever feel sick when you try to stop or cut down your use? What symptoms do you have?

      Compare symptoms with characteristic withdrawal symptoms listed in section V.

2. *Assessing problem severity.*
Questionnaires are a simple way to assess problem severity. The AUDIT or MAST-G for alcohol problems and the DAST-10 or Risk Prediction Scale for drug problems are recommended (see sections III.B and III.C and Table 17–2).

3. *Assessing motivation.*
   - How do you feel about your substance use?
   - Do you have any concerns we have not talked about?
   - Are you interested in changing?

E. Physical examination.

The physical examination may provide clues to intoxication, withdrawal, or long-term substance use. Although the physical examination is not sensitive as a screening test for substance use, positive findings require treatment. Equally important, when the patient is counseled, objective findings should be linked to the substances used as the practitioner expresses concern for the patient's health. Nevertheless, an absence of findings on the physical examination does not imply an absence of a substance problem, because *most of the early manifestations of substance abuse and dependence are psychosocial.*

1. *General appearance.*
Weight loss and an *emaciated appearance* can be seen in chronic alcoholics and result from poor nutrition. In chronic cocaine and stimulant users, these manifestations are caused by anorexic effects. Long-term users of other substances may neglect their health and also appear poorly nourished. By contrast, anabolic steroid users show evidence of *muscular hypertrophy* and an athletic appearance. Female anabolic steroid users manifest signs of masculini-

zation. *Shivering* and huddling for warmth may be seen during opioid withdrawal. The smell of alcohol on a patient's breath during a primary care visit is highly suggestive of impaired control over drinking.

2. *Vital signs.*
   One or more vital signs are generally increased during intoxication with cocaine, stimulants, hallucinogens, phencyclidine (PCP), and marijuana and during withdrawal from alcohol, sedatives, and opioids. Marijuana intoxication typically increases heart rate without affecting other vital signs. Respirations may be depressed with opioid intoxication. Mild increases in blood pressure may be seen with anabolic steroid use. Although nitrite inhalants can lower blood pressure and increase heart rate acutely, these effects last only for 5 minutes and so are unlikely to be observed during an office physical examination.

3. *Skin.*
   a. *Associated with injectable drug use. Needle tracks* along the forearm and other veins (e.g., in the hands, feet, and groin) are visible with intravenous drug use (most often heroin or cocaine). *Thrombosed or hardened veins* may be palpable beneath the skin in intravenous users, and it may be difficult to find viable veins from which blood can be drawn. Subcutaneous injections ("skin popping") may leave circumscribed, *pocklike depressions* in the skin. Anabolic steroid users typically inject into large muscle groups, such as the deltoids or gluteals, with a preference for the gluteals so that marks are hidden during body-building competitions. *Abscesses, cellulitis,* and other infections are possible with parenteral drug use.
   b. *Other cutaneous signs. Diaphoresis* accompanies intoxication with stimulants, cocaine, or hallucinogens and withdrawal from alcohol, marijuana, sedatives, or opioids. *Piloerection* is seen during opioid withdrawal. *Self-induced excoriations* may result from cocaine-induced or stimulant-induced formication, the sensation of bugs crawling under the skin. *Abnormal vascularization of the facial skin* is seen in chronic alcoholics, including spider angiomas when liver disease is present. *Jaundice* may result from alcohol-related liver disease, steroid-related liver disease, or viral hepatitis transmitted from contaminated needles. *Acne* can be seen with anabolic steroid use. *Hirsutism* in females and male pattern *baldness* in males may be associated with anabolic steroid use. *Burns,* especially on the fingers may be associated with smoking drugs. *Traumatic bruises* may result from falls, accidents, or fights while intoxicated. *Flushing* can be seen with alcohol, hallucinogen, and opioid intoxication.

4. *Eyes.*
   Dilated pupils are seen during intoxication with cocaine, stimulants, and hallucinogens and during opioid withdrawal. *Pinpoint pupils* are seen with opioid intoxication. *Lacrimation* is seen during opioid withdrawal. *Conjunctival erythema* is seen with marijuana or inhalant intoxication and with chronic alcoholism. *Nystagmus* is seen during intoxication with alcohol and other sedatives, PCP, and some inhalants. *Vertical nystagmus* is more specific for PCP use. Nystagmus is also part of Wernicke's encephalopathy in thiamine-deficient alcoholics. *Jaundiced eyes* may result from substance-related liver disease.

5. *Nose, mouth, and throat.*
   Rhinorrhea is seen during opioid withdrawal. An *infected, ulcerated, or perforated nasal septum* may be seen with intranasal cocaine use. *Glue sniffer's rash* may occur around the nose and mouth. *Dry mouth* may occur with marijuana intoxication. Excessive salivation occurs in PCP intoxication. *Pharyngeal erythema* may occur with smoking drugs (tobacco, marijuana, cocaine, PCP). *Oral cancers* may occur with heavy alcohol and tobacco use. *Coated tongue* may be seen in chronic alcoholism. *Poor dentition* may be seen in chronic substance users who neglect their health. *Deepened voice* is heard in female anabolic steroid users. *Yawning* is observed during opioid withdrawal but may also occur during cocaine or stimulant withdrawal as a result of sleep deprivation after a multiple-day binge.

6. *Chest.*
   Rhonchi associated with upper airways irritation and coughing may occur in long-term smokers of marijuana or cocaine. *Gynecomastia* with painful lumps is seen with anabolic steroid use. Alcoholics with significant liver disease may also manifest gynecomastia.

7. *Abdomen.*
   Hepatomegaly and *right upper quadrant tenderness* may occur in alcohol-related liver disease and with anabolic steroid use. Later signs of alcoholic cirrhosis include *ascites, dilated periumbilical veins,* and a *venous hum* heard by auscultation over those veins (caput medusae). *Diffuse abdominal tenderness* accompanied by nausea, vomiting, and diarrhea may occur during withdrawal from opioids, alcohol, and sedatives.

8. *Genitourinary system.*
   Testicular atrophy may be seen with chronic, heavy alcohol or anabolic steroid use. *Clitoral hypertrophy* and *prostatic hypertrophy* occur in female and male anabolic steroid users, respectively.

9. *Neurologic examination.*
Slurred speech, ataxia, or incoordination occur during intoxication with alcohol, sedatives, marijuana, opioids, hallucinogens, PCP, and inhalants. Persistent ataxia and incoordination may occur with alcohol-related or inhalant-related cerebellar degeneration. *Tremor* occurs during intoxication with cocaine, stimulants, hallucinogens, and inhalants and during withdrawal from alcohol, sedatives, and opioids. *Hyperreflexia* occurs during intoxication with cocaine, stimulants, PCP, and hallucinogens and during withdrawal from alcohol and sedatives. In some instances, hyperreflexia precedes *seizures. Depressed reflexes* are seen during inhalant intoxication. *Diminished response to pain* and *numbness* is seen, especially with PCP intoxication, because of its anesthetic properties, but it may also be seen with alcohol, sedative, and opioid intoxication. *Peripheral neuropathies* are seen with long-term alcohol and inhalant use.

F. Relevant laboratory orders.

1. How long a substance can be detected in *urine* depends on the amount, frequency, and duration of use; the individual's metabolism; the pharmacokinetics of the particular substance; and the sensitivity of the assay. General guidelines appear in Table 17–5.

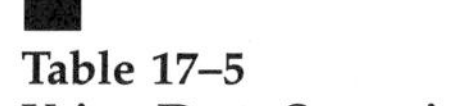

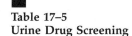

Table 17–5
Urine Drug Screening

Substance	Duration in Urine*
Alcohol	1 d
Amphetamines	1–3 d
Barbiturates	
Short-acting	3–5 d
Long-acting	10–14 d
Long-term phenobarbital use	Several wk
Benzodiazepines	
Long-acting, long-term use	Several wk
Cannabinoids (THC)	
Short-term use	2–8 d
Long-term daily use	14–42 d
Cocaine (benzoylecgonine)	
Single dose	1–3 d
Repeated high doses (possibly)	7–12 d
LSD†	2–4 d
MDMA†	2–4 d
Methaqualone	7–14 d
Opioids (except methadone/LAAM)	1–2 d
Phencyclidine (PCP)	
Single dose	2–8 d
Prolonged or high doses	Several wk

*Duration depends on the individual's level of consumption and metabolism, the pharmacokinetics, and the sensitivity of the assay. Longer durations may not be detected by less sensitive assays. Therefore, these guidelines are designed for general clinical assessments rather than for forensic testing linked to specific laboratories.

†Must be specially ordered; not included in most routine drug screens.

THC = Δ-9-tetrahydrocannabinol; LSD = lysergic acid diethylamide; MDMA = methylenedioxymethamphetamine; LAAM = levo-alpha-acetylmethadol.

2. *Blood alcohol levels* are highly correlated with breath analyses and with behavioral manifestations of alcohol intoxication. However, in long-term drinkers with tolerance to alcohol, their appearance may be normal at alcohol levels usually associated with intoxication. Some alcoholic patients manifest withdrawal signs at levels ordinarily associated with intoxication. (*Note*: 100 mg% = 100 mg/100 mL = 100 mg/dL = 0.1 g/dL = legal limit for intoxication or drunk driving in many parts of the United States.) Alcohol is eliminated from the bloodstream by zero-order kinetics (i.e., at a constant rate) down to a level of 20 mg/dL. The rate of elimination above this threshold is about 15 to 20 mg/dL/h. Metabolism varies across individuals, and heavier people have faster rates of elimination. Thus, if an individual presents to the office with a blood alcohol level of 115 mg/dL, he or she cannot legally drive home for at least 1 hour in many states.

3. *Liver function tests* should be performed.
   a. γ-*Glutamyltransferase* (GGT), also called gamma-glutamyltranspeptidase, is the most sensitive blood test for screening for long-term heavy drinking. However, false-positive increases can result from the use of anticonvulsants, barbiturates, or anticoagulants; nonalcoholic liver disease; some heart and kidney diseases; trauma; and obesity. Still, the test is useful as an adjunct to other screening tools, and positive results can be used for feedback during brief interventions. Increased GGT levels from drinking begin to decrease within the first week of abstinence in most patients. Accordingly, GGT level is a useful monitor during treatment for sustained abstinence versus relapse.
   b. Increases in serum levels of the liver enzymes *aspartate transaminase* (AST) and *alanine aminotransferase* (ALT) have a low sensitivity for detecting alcohol problems. However, when AST and ALT levels are increased because of liver causes, it becomes important to advise abstinence and to monitor the enzyme levels over time. The enzymes, also released by muscle tissue, are at increased levels in steroid users because of intramuscular injections and intensive weight training.

4. Elevated *mean corpuscular volume* is another

indicator of heavy drinking. It returns to normal with abstinence more slowly than liver enzymes.

5. Patients with substance disorders have an increased risk for tuberculosis and infections with human immunodeficiency virus (HIV) and hepatitis B and C.

6. In summary, *a recommended laboratory battery for assessing substance problems in someone with a positive screening interview includes a urine drug screen; a blood or breath alcohol level; GGT, AST, and ALT levels; and mean corpuscular volume.* As in any patient, other tests are ordered as indicated from the history and physical examination. Testing for human immunodeficiency virus, hepatitis B, and hepatitis C is indicated, especially for patients who share needles or engage in high-risk sexual practices. In addition, a tuberculosis skin test is recommended for confirmed cases of substance problems because of the association between tuberculosis and substance abuse. The absence of laboratory abnormalities should not deter one from diagnosing substance abuse and dependence, because laboratory tests have only low-to-moderate sensitivity as screening tests. For alcoholic patients who have increases in GGT, AST, and ALT levels without other causes, periodic monitoring provides a measure of abstinence. In other drug users, random urine drug screens can be used to monitor abstinence.

G. Differential diagnosis.

1. *Other mental disorders.*
Substances can induce reversible mood and anxiety disorders; psychosis; delirium; memory disturbances, including dementia; sexual dysfunction; and sleep disorders. For example, *all of the symptoms of major depression can be mimicked by alcohol dependence and withdrawal.* Furthermore, intoxication and withdrawal can exacerbate symptoms of comorbid mental disorders. Thus, *substance-related disorders should always be included in the differential diagnosis of other mental and behavioral problems.* One distinguishes between substance-related disorders and other mental disorders based on the chronology of onset, the family history, and the presence of mental symptoms during previous periods of sustained abstinence. Although the duration of abstinence required for facilitating differential diagnosis can vary, depending on the individual, the substance, and the complexity of symptoms, *psychiatric symptoms that persist for 4 weeks or longer of continuous abstinence are unlikely to result from acute intoxication or withdrawal.* In such cases, the diagnosis of a comorbid mental disorder should be strongly considered. Nevertheless, some authors describe a so-called *protracted withdrawal syndrome*, in which anxiety and depressive symptoms (including sleep disturbance) may last for several months after the initiation of abstinence. A consultation with an addiction psychiatrist may be helpful for distinguishing between protracted withdrawal symptoms and a comorbid mental disorder and for recommending appropriate treatment.

2. *Other medical conditions.*
Intoxication and withdrawal must be distinguished from many neurologic, metabolic, and infectious conditions that can cause slurred speech, tremor, incoordination, and altered mental status. Alcoholic patients, for example, are prone to head injuries, vitamin deficiencies, and liver dysfunction.

H. Family involvement.

Involving family and other significant others in the assessment is invaluable for gathering information, corroborating the patient's history, fostering motivation, and providing support for treatment recommendations.

1. *When a family member is the identified patient.*

Case Study
Charlene is a 53-year-old woman who presents for recurrent abdominal pain for which no physical cause can be found. The physician initiates a discussion of possible stressors.

Doctor: *Is there anyone in your family whom another person in the family would say has a problem with alcohol?*
Patient: *Yes. My father drank too much. He died of lung cancer at 63.*
Doctor: *How is your marriage?*
Patient: *We tolerate each other.*
Doctor: *Any children?*
Patient: *No.*
Doctor: *How much does your husband drink?*
Patient: *Well . . . I think too much.*
Doctor: *I'd like to give you a test called the AUDIT and have you answer the questions as if you were answering for your husband.* (After 5 minutes, a score of 24 is obtained.)
Doctor: *Charlene, a score of 8 indicates a harmful level of alcohol use, and David scored 24 out of a maximum of 40 points. This indicates a significant alcohol problem. I like to see the whole family whenever I can. If David is due for a physical examination or needs a doctor, I would be glad to see him.*
Patient: *He doesn't go to the doctor unless he's sick.*
Doctor: *Well, that screening test you took for him indicates he may be sick, and it makes sense to have a regular doctor and, at his age, a routine physical examination anyway.*

Patient: Well, I'll mention it to him. Thanks.
Doctor: (Returning focus to the patient). *I don't know why this is, but women often marry people with alcohol problems when they have grown up with it in their homes. In any case, it can be stressful for you, which may contribute to your stomach pain. I think it would be helpful for you to have some support in this from the experts. Have you ever been to Al-Anon?*
Patient: No.
Doctor: (After an explanation of Al-Anon). *I would like you to attend a meeting before our next appointment.* (Doctor writes a prescription with the Al-Anon resource number, which is available from most telephone books. Consider offering names of contact people in your practice with Al-Anon experience.)

The patient does not go to Al-Anon, but several months later, the patient's husband comes in for a physical examination and agrees to enter a specialized treatment program. This case demonstrates how the AUDIT can be used with a relative as a proxy. It helps to have a dispassionate piece of paper make the "diagnosis" because the patient may feel less accused, and the physician may have more confidence reporting the objective results of a validated instrument.

IV. Treatment.

A. General management guidelines.

Many treatments for substance disorders have been proven effective in controlled clinical trials, but no single treatment is effective for everyone. Therefore, the assessment results are used to guide the selection of treatment strategies, a process known as *treatment matching*. The primary care physician is most involved in the first level of treatment matching: matching to brief intervention or to specialized treatment (see Fig. 17–1). *Patients with either hazardous patterns of use or mild-to-moderate problems can be treated with brief interventions.* Brief interventions are conducted by the primary care physician or by a trained member of the primary care team, such as an office nurse or a social worker. Referral to specialized treatment is indicated for moderate-to-severe problems, substance dependence, or problems complicated by significant psychiatric or medical comorbidities.

1. *Empathy and the therapeutic alliance.*
Empathy and therapeutic alliance are essential for effective treatment. Empathy conveys that the physician truly understands the patient's experience and point of view. When the physician reflects the patient's point of view back to the patient, empathy has occurred. Empathy makes the patient feel understood; it is the foundation of the therapeutic alliance. Without this rapport between the patient and the physician, the physician is unlikely to help the patient change. *Patients must feel that the physician is on their side rather than pressuring them to change.* For example, "You're not sure you have a problem" is more empathic than "You have a problem whether you see it or not!"

2. *Family involvement.*
National health statistics indicate that 43% of Americans have had a family member with alcoholism. Whenever possible, the family or significant others should be involved in the assessment and the treatment plan. At best, the family can be extremely supportive of a patient's efforts to change. However, family members can also influence the patient in negative ways, either directly or unwittingly. For example, family members themselves may have substance problems that require intervention. Some family members may even resent the time patients spend away from home attending treatment or meetings of *Alcoholics Anonymous* (AA). Families may also become overwhelmed by frequent relapses and treatment failures. The impact on the family system is similar to that seen in other chronic diseases. Family members may feel guilty, ashamed, fearful, and angry, and they may adopt a codependent role to cope. *Codependency* refers to a style of relating to the addicted person, not to a diagnosis or to substance dependence. *The codependent family member takes over responsibilities for the patient and "enables" the patient's use by protecting the patient from the consequences of the addiction.* By taking such "good care" of the addict, codependent individuals sacrifice their own needs in the process. In these cases, family members may benefit from a referral to their own therapy in order to help them cope better with the stresses of living with an alcoholic or addict. Referral to Al-Anon or Nar-Anon may be especially helpful. Al-Anon and Nar-Anon are 12-step groups in which family members learn that they did not cause the patient's problems, they cannot control the problem, and they cannot cure it (see section IV.G.2). The message of Al-Anon and Nar-Anon frees the family members to focus on their own well-being and to allow the patient to be responsible for his or her own recovery.

3. *Treatment goals.*
The goal in most treatment programs has traditionally been abstinence. *Abstinence is clearly recommended for patients with severe problems or dependence and for those who use any illicit substances.* The increased focus on primary and secondary prevention of alcohol problems, that is, intervening before diagnostic criteria for alcohol abuse or dependence are met, means that many patients are managed expectantly with controlled drinking or reduction trials

(the 3-4-12 rule or threshold for hazardous drinking). *Research supports moderate drinking goals for patients with hazardous drinking patterns or mild-to-moderate drinking problems.* Moreover, when patients are made partners in the selection of treatment goals, outcomes are improved. Therefore, the wise physician negotiates the treatment goal with the patient in a way that does not jeopardize the patient's health, rather than prescribes a rigid goal that the patient rejects. *Nevertheless, patients who are able to abstain entirely for a 2-week period at the beginning of treatment are more likely to attain their ultimate goal, whether abstinence or moderate drinking.* Moreover, this initial period of abstinence allows the physician and patient to assess further the effect of alcohol on the patient's well-being as the alcohol is eliminated. Situations that trigger urges to use also become more apparent during abstinence and can be targeted for treatment purposes. Finally, when assessing patients who appear to be good candidates for a goal of moderate drinking, the practitioner must be aware of significant hidden consequences that the patient may not consciously acknowledge; these consequences may move him or her into a far more serious diagnostic category. *The importance of corroborative history from significant others cannot be overemphasized.*

B. Brief interventions.

Brief interventions are conducted in the primary care setting for the following indications: hazardous consumption, mild-to-moderate problems, and some cases of substance abuse (see Fig. 17–1). Before a brief intervention is attempted, a patient's commitment to change should be assessed (see Assessing Motivation, section III.D.3.). In addition to empathy, the components of effective brief interventions include all of the following:

1. *Feedback.*
   After the assessment, the physician provides feedback from the screening tests, history, physical examination, and laboratory tests. When normative scores and laboratory values are available, these should be presented to the patient and the patient's score compared to them:
   - The level of your liver enzyme, known as GGT, was increased to 128, and the normal range is zero to 30. (Show patient the actual laboratory report). This occurs when the liver is exposed to too much alcohol.
   - Your blood pressure was 150/90, which increases your risk for heart disease. It should be less than 140/90, and drinking is one of the things that can cause this type of increase.
   - The AUDIT is a test that screens for alcohol problems. Your score on the AUDIT was 23, and the cut-off for low-risk drinking is 8.

   The strategy of feedback is to present the patient with the facts in a nonjudgmental fashion, along with information that allows the patient to understand the personal implications of those facts. Scare tactics are avoided because they may increase the patient's defensiveness. Rather, the discrepancy between the normal range and the patient's status helps to build motivation for change. The patient's response to the feedback should be elicited and responded to empathically:
   - What do you think about this?
   - How are you feeling about this information?
   - You seem uncomfortable. This is not easy for you to hear.

2. *Advice.*
   The physician advises the patient to make a change:
   - I would like you to stop drinking altogether for the next 2 weeks so that I can recheck you and see what effect stopping may have on your blood pressure.
   - I would like for you to limit your drinking to no more than two drinks a day. I will see you in a month, and we will talk about how it went.
   - I would like you to see a specialist for your cocaine problem.

3. *Choices.*
   Whenever possible, *offer the patient a choice of goals or strategies.* Offering choices enlists the patient as a partner in the decision making, which reduces the patient's resistance to change.
   - We can try a number of options to help you stop drinking. You can simply try it on your own. You can attend some AA meetings. You can use a self-guided manual, which will help you track your tendencies to drink and come up with alternatives to drinking.
   - You can stop drinking altogether, or you could limit yourself to no more than two drinks a day.

4. *Therapeutic optimism.*
   The physician conveys a sense of hope and optimism that positive change is possible. Even patients who know they should change their substance use do not if they believe that they cannot. Some authors discuss the need to reinforce a patient's sense of self-efficacy, which is the patient's belief that he or she can do something about a problem.

5. *Responsibility.*
   Both the physician and patient must be clear that the patient is responsible for changing or not changing.

   It's up to you whether you change or not. I hope that you do, and if you decide to, I will do everything in my power to help you.

6. *Follow-up.*
   Brief interventions can be performed in one or more visits. Arrange a follow-up visit in 2 to 4 weeks to monitor the patient's progress and to assess the need for further intervention.

Case Study

A 57-year-old woman presents for a preoperative physical examination for a steel plate removal from her chronically painful ankle. Her examination is unremarkable except for a blood pressure of 180/100 mm Hg. She has no family history of alcohol problems. She scores zero on the CAGE questions. She did not experience withdrawal symptoms when she stopped drinking during a hospital admission one year previously. She admits drinking two to four drinks daily, or 21 drinks per week. Her GGT level is 60 IU/L (normal, 0 to 30 IU/L) and her ALT level is 63 IU/L (normal, 0 to 45 IU/L).

Doctor: I'm concerned that your drinking may be harming you in several ways. One, your blood pressure is increased. Two, your liver is affected, and there appears to be some dysfunction. Three, you are exceeding the recommended limits of moderate drinking, which puts you at risk for other problems.
Patient: I don't think so, I can take it or leave it.
Doctor: That's good. I think you can, too. I propose that you "leave it," or stop drinking for the next month. We'll delay your surgery. If you have withdrawal symptoms, call me. Let's repeat your blood pressure measurement at that time and talk about a long-term plan.

The patient abstains, and her liver test results and blood pressure normalize. The brief intervention includes feedback, advice, support for self-efficacy, and follow-up. The doctor discusses cause and effect, risks, and safe drinking limits and institutes a plan to monitor her drinking, blood pressure, and liver function over time. Labels like alcoholism and substance abuse are not appropriate and are avoided.

C. Managing resistance.

Resistance is viewed as a dynamic, interactional process between the patient and the practitioner rather than as a rigid characteristic of the patient. As such, *resistance can be influenced by the practitioner's manner and approach during the interview.* The overt behaviors of resistance (denying, minimizing, changing subjects, blaming, arguing, or complying superficially) are easy to detect in the interview. Resistant behaviors occur because of underlying feelings of shame, guilt, anxiety, or pessimism about change. From an interactional viewpoint, the patient has probably practiced these resistant behaviors on others, particularly family. The re-emergence of resistant behaviors in the interview indicates that the practitioner is going too fast for the patient. As such, the practitioner needs to shift strategies and determine where the patient is. Either the patient is not ready to accept that a problem exists or the patient does not believe that change is necessary or possible. If the patient does not yet think that he or she has a problem, then the patient is in a stage of *precontemplation.* In this case, the task is simply to get the patient to *think* about it and to move the patient from precontemplation to *contemplation.* Once the patient recognizes the problem and expresses concern about it, then the strategy shifts to building commitment and optimism for change. In managing resistance, the practitioner should acknowledge the patient's point of view, reflect back both sides of the issue, provide education, reframe the problem, emphasize the patient's personal choice and responsibility, and involve others in the process who will be supportive of change. Although such strategies are best used selectively and sequentially, the following example illustrates their use in composite form:

Patient: I don't think I have a problem with drinking. I just don't like my wife's criticism of it. And even though you tell me my blood pressure is increased, I feel just fine.
Doctor: It's hard for you to see what all the fuss is about when you feel fine (acknowledging the patient's point of view). *On the other hand, you would like things to be different with your wife, and you know that the problem has something to do with your drinking* (reflecting the other side of the issue). *I'm also concerned that your blood pressure is increased, especially because you can't feel it. If you felt sick from your blood pressure, there would be no question. But you are walking around at a higher risk for heart disease or stroke, and you* won't *feel it until it's too late* (education about the risks of high blood pressure and reframing "feeling fine" as part of the problem). *It's entirely your choice. No one can force you to change against your will* (emphasizing personal choice). *You can change, though, if you would like* (expressing optimism for change). *Why don't I see you with your wife next time and we can talk more about this?* (involving supportive others)

D. Formal interventions.

When brief interventions are not successful, then referral to specialized treatment is indicated. When the patient appears unlikely to accept specialized treatment, then a more formal intervention by a trained therapist can be considered. Formal interventions are indicated for patients with severe problems of abuse or dependence, not for patients with hazardous use.

1. A group of five to seven participants are chosen who have first-hand knowledge of the patient's addictive behaviors and consequences, such as the primary care physician, spouse or partner, other family members, employer, friends, and a member of

the clergy. Intervention can be effective with even fewer participants.

2. A trained therapist who is experienced in the technique leads the group in conducting the formal intervention.
3. The leader gathers the participants without the patient for one to two meetings before the formal intervention to assess participants and rehearse what they will say.
4. Each participant prepares a script to be read to the patient, including what the participant has directly observed and when, how it made the participant feel, and how each participant cares about the patient. During the intervention, the patient is asked to listen to each participant in turn and afterward is given the opportunity to respond.
5. The tone of the intervention is nonjudgmental and caring, although often highly emotional.
6. The participants finally suggest a specific treatment plan or treatment facility that is arranged in advance.
7. A positive consequence for obtaining treatment or a negative consequence for not obtaining treatment adds extra force but also an element of coercion (e.g., continued employment or partnership contingent on acceptance of treatment). Thus, formal interventions should be reserved for severe problems that have not responded to other approaches.

E. Monitoring for relapse/relapse prevention.

Substance use disorders have been described as chronic, relapsing disorders. Even patients who have remained abstinent or problem-free for several years can relapse, although most relapses tend to occur in the first few months to 1 year. The primary care physician plays an important role in monitoring the patient for relapse. Liver function tests can help monitor relapse to alcohol (see section III.F.3). Relapse prevention refers to a treatment modality in which patients are instructed to identify the people, feelings, thoughts, and situations that precede and trigger their substance use. Patients are then guided to develop alternative coping strategies for dealing with the events that serve as triggers for the substance use. Such strategies might include avoiding people, places, and things associated with using; talking to a trusted friend when the patient feels angry; or going to an AA meeting when the patient feels urges to drink. One often-taught mnemonic for preventing relapse is HALT, which reminds the patient to avoid *h*unger, *a*nger, *l*oneliness, and *t*iredness as triggers to using substances.

Case Study

David is a 53-year-old loading dock worker who entered an alcohol program 18 months previously. Now, he presents with an overuse injury to his right bicipital tendon. He had stayed sober for 6 months. The physician uses this period of success as an opportunity to inquire about his drinking, and learns the patient has relapsed.

Doctor: How long have you been drinking again?
Patient: About a year.
Doctor: What are you up to in terms of numbers of beers?
Patient: About four to six beers a day.
Doctor: Do you want to do something about it? (assessing motivation)
Patient: I don't know—it's not as bad as it was.
Doctor: Good, we can do something now, before it gets worse. I'm worried about you, Dave. How can I help?
Patient: I don't know. (Patient looks ashamed, and physician pays attention to nonverbal cues.)
Doctor: The nature of your illness is for relapses to happen. You are not a bad person. You simply need additional help. Use this "slip" as an opportunity to make changes. You've changed before, and you can do it again (therapeutic optimism). *Let me make some suggestions* (doctor's advice) *and see what you are willing to do* (patient's responsibility). *The program you went through has a relapse program. Let's call the program together and find out what is available in terms of relapse support. Let's also have you stop drinking, start on Antabuse again, and start going to your AA meetings again.* (Patient calls the program from the doctor's office.)

The goals of relapse prevention are (1) to prevent any substance use and (2) to prevent a slip from developing into a full-blown relapse. More frequent follow-up contacts for patients entering treatment programs help to prevent such slips (e.g., monthly visits for the first 12 months), but in this case, the goal was to prevent a relapse from worsening. Patients may blame themselves for slipping and then use more of the substance in order to medicate their negative feelings. Thus, relapse should be normalized as part of the illness and then reframed as an opportunity to learn how to avoid slips in the future. A menu of options, an optimism for change, and the patient's self-responsibility are emphasized as in any brief intervention.

F. Detoxification.

The term *detoxification* implies the treatment of physical dependence. It is in effect the management of withdrawal symptoms and the transition to a drug-free state. Withdrawal is potentially life threatening in the case of sedatives such as alcohol, barbiturates, and benzodiazepines. Detoxification from these agents often *requires* pharmacologic support. Detoxification from opioids often *benefits* from pharmacologic support in that such support may enhance the addict's chances of abstinence and may decrease the considerable discomfort of withdrawal; however, opioid withdrawal is rarely life threatening, unless the patient is already severely medically compromised. Detoxification from agents such as marijuana, cocaine, amphetamines, and hallucinogens *does not require* pharmacologic support. Detoxification alone is never adequate treatment for patients with the full syndrome of substance dependence. Specific detoxification protocols are discussed in section V.

G. Treatment tools.

1. *Treatment plan and contract.*
Having the patient sign or agree to a written or verbal contract can be a helpful tool. For example,

 I, John Doe, agree to reduce my use of alcohol to no more than 12 standard drinks a week and no more than four in one day. Inability to keep to this level of use means I will agree to a comprehensive assessment and possible formal treatment for a presumed substance problem. I will also attend a drug and alcohol lecture series to improve my understanding of substances and their potential for harm.

 Signed and dated ______________________________

 This schema can be adapted to many clinical situations and consequences. Treatment contracts can include random urine drug screening, breath tests for alcohol, and liver function monitoring. A major principle of substance abuse treatment is accountability.

2. *Self-help groups.*
Addresses of organizations are included so that physicians can familiarize themselves with, and make available to patients, descriptive literature of various programs. Pertinent groups can be exceedingly helpful to patients as part of their menu of options to help them change.
   a. *Alcoholics Anonymous* was founded in 1935 as a fellowship of alcoholics who helped other alcoholics to stay sober by sharing their experience, strength, and hope. The only requirement for attending AA meetings is a desire to stop drinking. AA is based on spiritual (not religious) principles of accepting powerlessness over alcohol and recognizing the need for help from others and a "higher power" as each individual understands it. Despite the group's religious feel to some patients, *many atheists and agnostics are in AA who define AA itself as their higher power.* AA members are encouraged to attend meetings, work the 12 steps of the recovery program, and obtain a sponsor (a trusted AA member who has more than a year of sobriety). The contact number for AA is available in most local phone books.

      Alcoholics Anonymous
      P.O. Box 459, Grand Central Station
      New York, NY 10163
      212-686-1100

   b. *Al-Anon* is a 12-step group designed for the support and recovery of significant others who are affected by the person with alcoholism (see "Al-Anon: Is It For You?" in Appendix.) Alateen groups, similar to Al-Anon, are designed for teenagers. The contact number is in most local phone books.

      Al-Anon Family Group Headquarters, Inc.
      1600 Corporate Landing Parkway
      Virginia Beach, VA 23454-5617
      1-800-356-9996

   c. *Narcotics Anonymous* (NA) is a 12-step program that is often preferred by patients whose primary or preferred drug is not alcohol. *Nar-Anon,* which was modeled after Al-Anon, is the corresponding group for family members and concerned others.

      Narcotics Anonymous World Service Office, Inc.
      P.O. Box 9999
      Van Nuys, CA 91406
      818-780-3951

   d. *Cocaine Anonymous* (CA) is a 12-step program that is specific to cocaine users. Similarly, *Prescription Drug Anonymous* meets that special need. The lesser availability of these groups often leads patients to AA and NA for primary support.

      Cocaine Anonymous
      3740 Overland Avenue, Suite H
      P.O. Box 2000
      Los Angeles, CA 90034
      800-347-8998

   e. *Secular Organization for Sobriety* (SOS) and *Rational Recovery* (RR) are support groups that some patients find preferable to 12-step groups because they do not emphasize spiritual principles. The availability of these groups varies from region to region.

      Rational Recovery
      P.O. Box 800
      Lotus, CA 95651
      916-621-4374

      Secular Organization for Sobriety
      5521 Grosvenor Boulevard
      Los Angeles, CA 90066
      310-821-8430

H. Pharmacologic adjuncts.

Pharmacologic adjuncts constitute a small piece of the overall treatment strategy. Patients often request "quick fixes" in lieu of more time-consuming and difficult recovery activities. Patients should be counseled to view medication as an adjunct to their treatment rather than a cure.

1. *Disulfiram* (Antabuse) is best used in motivated patients with alcoholism who are involved in

other aspects of recovery. Disulfiram blocks the breakdown of ingested alcohol such that acetaldehyde accumulates in the system, causing hypotension, tachycardia, dizziness, weakness, flushing, sweating, nausea and vomiting, headache and neck ache, chest pain, palpitations, dyspnea, blurred vision, confusion, and syncope. The more alcohol consumed, the more severe the reaction, including unconsciousness, respiratory depression, convulsions, and cardiovascular collapse. Thus, the medication is contraindicated in patients with severe heart disease, for whom a reaction could be fatal. Minor side effects in the absence of alcohol include drowsiness, fatigue, headache, transient impotence, and garlic or metallic taste. These effects usually disappear during the first 2 weeks of treatment or after a reduction in the dose. Drowsiness and fatigue can be minimized by nighttime administration. Skin rashes usually respond to antihistamine therapy and do not necessarily contraindicate therapy. *Because disulfiram-induced hepatitis can be rapidly fatal, liver function (transaminase) results should be monitored at baseline, in 2 to 4 weeks, then monthly for 2 months, quarterly for 1 year, and then every 6 months while the patient takes the medication.* We withhold disulfiram if liver transaminase levels are more than three times normal levels. Other major side effects include optic neuritis and peripheral neuropathy. Psychosis is reported rarely when the agent is used in high doses (>500 mg) or when combined with metronidazole (Flagyl) or isoniazid (INH). Disulfiram may also increase phenytoin (Dilantin) levels and prothrombin time in patients taking oral anticoagulants, necessitating dosage adjustment. Patients must avoid topical use and ingestion of all alcohol-containing products. In order to avoid a delayed disulfiram-alcohol reaction, patients must also abstain from alcohol for 10 to 14 days after stopping disulfiram therapy. Dosing generally starts at 250 mg/d and can be reduced to 125 mg/d in patients who do not accommodate to minor side effects in 1 to 2 weeks. Disulfiram therapy should not be initiated until the patient's blood alcohol level is zero, which is usually reached 24 hours after the patient's last drink, unless the peak blood alcohol level was greater than 360 mg/dL. In some cases, disulfiram use can be monitored by a significant other, a treatment center, or the work place as a means of enhancing compliance during early recovery. Intradermal disulfiram implants have not been successful.

2. *Naltrexone* (formerly Trexan, renamed ReVia) is used as adjunctive treatment for either opioid dependence or alcohol dependence. Naltrexone acts like long-acting naloxone (Narcan), by competitively blocking opioid receptors. If an opioid addict relapses and uses impulsively, no euphoria is experienced, allowing the patient to call for help. It does not block the craving for opioids and precipitates acute opioid withdrawal in active opioid users. Therefore, *naltrexone must not be administered until the urine drug screening is negative for opioids*, usually 7 to 10 days after the last use of opioids. An initial test dose of 25 mg by mouth confirms the absence of withdrawal, although some treatment centers prefer to use the Narcan Challenge Test, as described in the *Physicians' Desk Reference*.[3] Usual dosage thereafter is 50 mg orally daily. Another dosing regimen used by programs that administer the naltrexone in conjunction with treatment visits is 100 mg each on Mondays and Wednesdays and 150 mg on Fridays, resulting in the same weekly dosage as the 50-mg daily regimen. Naltrexone is compatible with abstinence-oriented programs, but it has been demonstrated as efficacious for opioid dependence only in the highly motivated professional patient with easy access to opioids. Side effects include nausea and vomiting, abdominal pain, difficulty sleeping, anxiety, nervousness, low energy, headache, and joint and muscle pain. Because naltrexone can cause liver injury, liver function tests must be monitored at baseline and periodically thereafter. Use of naltrexone is contraindicated in patients with acute liver disease. Physicians should withhold naltrexone if liver transaminase levels are more than three times normal levels. Patients should be warned that naltrexone's blockade of opioid receptors can be overcome by high-dose opioid use, leading to a risk of overdose. *Naltrexone has also been shown to enhance recovery rates in the first 12 weeks for alcoholic patients when the regimen is combined with formal, specialized treatment.* The exact mechanism of action is unknown, but it may be related to a decrease in craving for alcohol and to an attenuation of the reinforcing effect of alcohol. In 1995, studies assessing the use of naltrexone as part of brief intervention trials in primary care settings were in progress, as were studies assessing the efficacy of naltrexone beyond the first 12 weeks of therapy.

3. *Opioid maintenance and detoxification with methadone* (Dolophine) or *levo-alpha-acetylmethadol* (LAAM) are specialized treatment approaches for opioid dependence that are legally available only through federally licensed programs. Buprenorphine (Buprenex) is another opioid being considered (but not yet approved) by the United States Food and Drug Administration for the treatment of opioid dependence. *The primary*

care physician incurs legal liability and should not prescribe any opioids for the purpose of treating opioid dependence. Of course, primary care physicians *may* prescribe methadone and other opioids in order to treat pain. They may also continue methadone or LAAM for an opioid-dependent patient *during* hospitalization for a medical condition, if the patient is already receiving methadone or LAAM as part of a specially licensed out-patient program. The primary care physician should obtain written consent from the patient to consult clinicians at the treatment program under these circumstances. Patients dependent on opioids for more than 1 year who have failed prior treatment attempts at detoxification and abstinence are candidates for opioid maintenance. Methadone doses ranging from 80 to 120 mg/d are associated with decreases in drug use, needle sharing, and criminality as well as an increase in employment. Methadone maintenance is a preferred approach during pregnancy because of the risk of fetal death if detoxification is attempted.

I. Referral to specialized substance abuse treatment.

The patient should be referred to specialized treatment when brief interventions are either ineffective or inappropriate (see Fig. 17–1). A situation that merits consideration of referral is a newly diagnosed substance abusing or dependent individual whose family and social situation need help that the primary care physician cannot provide. Patients with comorbid psychiatric disorders are also best referred. Finally, pregnant patients with opioid and other drug dependencies should be referred. Physicians should be aware of local treatment agencies to which they can refer with confidence. Specialized treatment programs are not allowed to disclose patient information to the referring primary care physician without written authorization from the patient. Treatment programs even require written authorization to disclose information to the patient's family, because of strict federal laws regarding patient confidentiality in addiction treatment settings. Primary care physicians should request patients to sign releases of information to facilitate communication and to coordinate care with the specialized treatment program. The following *levels of specialized care* are described in order of increasing intensity of service:

1. *Out-patient assessment* services conduct an initial consultation and evaluation to determine the appropriate level and type of care for each patient. Many health maintenance organizations have a center for diagnosis and referral that provides assessment services for patients with substance problems.
2. *Traditional out-patient care* consists of 1 to 3 hours a week of individual, group, and/or family therapy. Patients may enter this level of care initially or transfer to it after completing a more intensive level of care. Treatment duration varies from several months to more than 1 year.
3. *Intensive out-patient care and partial hospital care* usually involve patients in a minimum of 3.5 hours a day of treatment for 3 to 7 days a week for approximately 4 weeks. After the first 2 weeks, some programs stretch the duration of therapy to 8 weeks or more by decreasing the number of treatment days each week. Both daytime and evening programs are available in order to allow patients to continue other activities, such as work and child care. Programs provide education; individual, group, and family therapies; and a milieu in which patients and staff can interact less formally during a meal or a break. Patients typically sleep at home.
4. *Residential care* allows patients to spend 24 hours a day in a protected, safe setting in addition to providing the same services as in partial hospital care. Subacute detoxification using supportive care and oral medication therapy is often available. Duration of care typically varies from 1 to 4 weeks.
5. *In-patient care* is hospital-based treatment used for acute detoxification. Such care is indicated when detoxification either requires parenteral medication or is complicated by serious psychiatric or other medical illness.
6. *Long-term residential care* is more intensive than in-patient and short-term residential care in terms of duration, which typically ranges from 3 to 12 months, and often in terms of social structure. For example, traditional therapeutic communities are highly structured, long-term residential programs in which the community consists of peers in different stages of recovery, supervised by staff. Community members move through a hierarchical series of jobs, responsibilities, and increasing privileges; negative behaviors may result in losing privileges. Medical services, however, may be limited. Socially unstable patients without steady jobs or places to stay who have failed less intensive forms of treatment are usual candidates.

V. Specific substances.

This section describes the clinical manifestations and treatment of specific intoxication and withdrawal syndromes. Consistent with the book's focus on primary care psychiatry, the following descriptions emphasize psychiatric manifestations and treatment, while recognizing that overdoses, severe intoxications, and some withdrawal syndromes are best treated in medical emergency departments and other acute medical settings.

A. Alcohol

1. *Intoxication.*
   a. *Signs and symptoms.* These include slurred speech, incoordination, ataxic gait, nystagmus, impaired attention or memory, impaired judgment, emotional lability, possible aggressiveness, and in severe states, stupor or coma.
   b. *Treatment.* No treatments can reverse or quicken the course of intoxication. The blood alcohol level decreases between 15 to 20 mg/dL an hour. *Although the commonly applied "remedy" of caffeine may increase alertness and energy, it does not reverse impaired judgment or incoordination, so the patient remains a dangerous driver.*
2. *Alcohol withdrawal* (Table 17–6).
   a. The *stages of withdrawal* from alcohol or short-acting sedatives are as follows:
      (1) *Stage 1* (minor or uncomplicated withdrawal): restlessness, anxiety, sleeping problems, agitation, and tremor. The patient may have increased temperature, blood pressure, and pulse.
      (2) *Stage 2* (major withdrawal with hallucinosis): stage 1 signs and symptoms plus visual or auditory hallucinations, increased agitation and fright; tremor may involve the whole body. Nausea and vomiting may occur. Patients are not delirious and often know their hallucinations are not real.
      (3) *Stage 3* (delirium tremens [DTs]): the main diagnostic criterion is that the patient becomes delirious (global confusion and disorientation). Other signs and symptoms are more severe than during stage 2, including agitation, hallucinations, vomiting, hypertension, tachycardia, and increased temperature. Hallucinations are perceived as real, and patients may act accordingly. This is a medical emergency, and the mortality, even with treatment, is 2% to 5%. Intensive care unit admission is indicated. Other medical problems should be ruled out, including embolism, infection, meningitis, pancreatitis, and severe fluid and electrolyte imbalance.
      (4) *Withdrawal seizures* may occur during any stage but usually between 12 and 48 hours after the last drink. These are almost always grand mal and self-limited (not status epilepticus).
   b. *Risk factors* for developing alcohol withdrawal symptoms[4]:
      (1) Age greater than 40 years.
      (2) Male.
      (3) Daily consumption greater than one fifth of liquor (>20 drinks a day).
      (4) Drinking around the clock in order to maintain steady blood alcohol level.
      (5) Excessive drinking for longer than 10 years.
      (6) Tremors and anxiety appearing within 6 to 8 hours.
      (7) History of seizures, hallucinations, delusions, or DTs during previous episodes of alcohol withdrawal.
      (8) Presence of an acute medical problem, such as pneumonia.
      (9) Alcohol level of 250 mg/dL or greater on presentation.
      - Zero to two factors—low risk for severe withdrawal.
      - Three to six factors—moderate risk for severe withdrawal.
      - Seven to nine factors—high risk for severe withdrawal.
   c. Approximately 10% of currently alcohol-

Table 17–6
Alcohol Withdrawal Syndromes

Syndrome	Onset	Peak	Duration (when most symptoms are over)	Signs and Symptoms
Uncomplicated alcohol withdrawal (stage 1)	Within 4–12 h of last drink	1–2 d	5–7 d	Tremor, increased vital signs (*P*>100), sweating, nausea or vomiting, anxiety, irritability, depressed mood, headache, insomnia, hyperreflexia
Alcohol hallucinosis (stage 2)	2 d	—	7 d	Hallucinations in a clear sensorium; reality testing not always intact
Delirium tremens (DTs) (stage 3)	3–4 d	3–4 d	6–9 d	Marked confusion and disorientation, markedly increased vital signs and sweating, hallucinations and delusions, psychomotor agitation
Alcohol withdrawal seizures ("rum fits")	12–48 h	1–2 d	1–2 d	Few generalized tonic-clonic seizures

dependent patients require in-patient detoxification. Admission criteria for in-patient alcohol detoxification are one or more of the following:

- Onset or expectation of moderate-to-severe withdrawal based on observation and history.
- Other medical or psychiatric conditions that require close observation during withdrawal (e.g., seizures or history of seizures, pregnancy, heart disease, liver disease, suspected head injury, uncontrolled hypertension).
- Co-morbid drug dependence and withdrawal.
- Uncontrolled behavior endangering self or others.
- Suicide risk.
- Patient inability to care for his or her immediate needs.
- Failure of ambulatory detoxification.
- Lack of social supports or safe living environment to initiate out-patient detoxification.

d. The *Clinical Institute Withdrawal Assessment Scale for Alcohol—Revised* (CIWA-Ar Scale) can be used to determine the level of care and the need for pharmacologic detoxification (see Appendix). The 10-item scale takes 2 minutes to administer and can be readministered every 30 to 60 minutes as needed. One author uses the following scoring protocol:

- Zero to 8: no medications.
- 8 to 15: medications as an out-patient.
- >15: medications as an in-patient.

A less conservative scoring protocol follows:

- Zero to 10: no medications.
- 10 to 20: may benefit from pharmacotherapy based on clinical judgment and assessment of other risk factors in section V.A.2.b.
- 20 to 67: medication needed.

e. Patients who require *pharmacologic detoxification* can be treated with chlordiazepoxide (Librium), diazepam (Valium), phenobarbital, or any of a number of other benzodiazepines. The authors prefer to use chlordiazepoxide, oxazepam (Serax), and diazepam, but many sedative-hypnotics have utility and advantages in specific cases. Using long-acting agents, such as chlordiazepoxide, diazepam, and phenobarbital, results in gradual declines in physiological levels during the taper process. Diazepam and phenobarbital have greater anticonvulsant activity than chlordiazepoxide and oxazepam. The metabolism of oxazepam and lorazepam (Ativan) is simpler and less affected by liver disease and age than the metabolism of other benzodiazepines, making these two agents useful in elderly patients and in patients with acute liver disease. Lorazepam is more reliably absorbed after intramuscular injections than chlordiazepoxide and diazepam. Diazepam and lorazepam are preferred for intravenous administration in the treatment of DTs (Table 17–7), although chlordiazepoxide can also be used. Diazepam and lorazepam cross the blood-brain barrier faster than chlordiazepoxide and oxazepam, providing quicker symptom relief but also more feelings of euphoria. These particular advantages aside, one should use the agent with which one has the most experience.

f. *In-patient and out-patient treatment protocols* are given in Tables 17–7 and 17–8, respectively.

Table 17–7
Guidelines for In-Patient Alcohol Detoxification*

1. *Multivitamins:* 1 tablet daily.
2. *B complex vitamins and thiamine:* 100 mg IM every day for 3 d.
3. *Magnesium:* 2 Magnesium Plus tablets TID or magnesium sulfate 1 g IM every 6 h for 4 days if patient has a history of withdrawal seizures, is at high risk for stage 2 withdrawal, or has an initial serum magnesium level < 1.5 mEq/L.
4. *Antiemetics: hydroxyzine* (Atarax, Vistaril), 50 mg IM every 4 h PRN nausea.
5. *Seizure treatment: Diazepam* (Valium) and *carbamazepine* (Tegretol) are the drugs of choice for seizures. Patients with a history of withdrawal seizures may benefit from a loading dose of *carbamazepine*, 100 mg qh for 4 doses, then 200 mg q6h for 7 days.
6. *Patients in stage 1 withdrawal:* Load with 10–20 mg of *diazepam* PO q2h for three doses or until patient is sedated but arousable. Many patients require no more medication if treated early, because of the long half-life of diazepam.
7. *Patients in stage 2 or 3 withdrawal:* administer 10–20 mg of *diazepam* IV (at a rate of 5 mg/min) or PO every 30 min until symptoms are controlled. Patients who need more than 150 mg of diazepam for control of symptoms should be supplemented with *lorazepam* (Ativan) and/or *haloperidol* (Haldol).
8. *For patients not controlled with diazepam or with end-stage liver disease: lorazepam* 4–6 mg IV or IM every 30 min until symptoms reduced.
9. *Treatment of agitation and psychotic symptoms:*
   Haloperidol, 2–10 mg IM or IV q2h (20 mg of haloperidol in a 24-h period may be necessary). Haloperidol increases the risk of withdrawal seizures but may be needed in some situations.
   Benztropine (Cogentin) 2 mg PO or IM every 2 h PRN for extrapyramidal symptoms (maximum, 8 mg/24 h) is seldom necessary unless haloperidol is used for more than 72 h.

*Many of the medications in the table potentiate each other's effects, so routinely combining these medications is contraindicated.

Adapted from Project SAEFP Executive Committee: Project SAEFP Workshop Materials: Substance abuse education for family physicians. Kansas City, MO: The Society of Teachers of Family Medicine; 1991.

IM = intramuscularly; TID = three times a day; PRN = as needed; PO = by mouth; IV = intravenously.

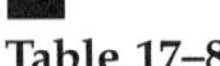

Table 17–8
Guidelines for Out-Patient Alcohol Detoxification

Day 1: Clinical history and physical examination Breath test or blood alcohol level. Laboratory tests: Urine drug screen and CBC, GGT, AST, ALT levels. Thiamine, 100 mg IM or PO for 3 d. If CIWA-Ar score ≥ 8 and positive risk factors for withdrawal are present, then treat with benzodiazepines. If CIWA-Ar score > 15 or patient has history of DTs or seizures, refer to in-patient treatment. Anticonvulsants have minimal preventive benefit. Start chlordiazepoxide (Librium) therapy, 25 mg PO QID or equivalent. Refer to AA, employee assistance program, or out-patient treatment program. **Day 2: Clinical re-evaluation** Breath or blood alcohol level. If positive, consider in-patient treatment. Benzodiazepines: decrease chlordiazepoxide dose to 25 mg PO q8h if patient is clinically better. Administer immediate dose if patient is clinically deteriorated; consider in-patient admission if patient has poor response. If patient is clinically improved with immediate dose, increase chlordiazepoxide dose to 25 mg PO q4h. Reinforce AA, EAP, or out-patient program.	**Day 3: Clinical re-evaluation, emphasizing abnormal laboratory tests** Breath/blood alcohol evaluation: if results are positive, consider in-patient admission. For patients who were improved on day 2, decrease chlordiazepoxide dose to 25 mg q12h for 3 doses, then discontinue. For those who required medication q4h on day 2: admit to in-patient facility if patient is not clinically improved; if patient is improved, then decrease dose to 25 mg PO q6h, and so on. Reinforce AA, EAP, or out-patient treatment. **Day 4: Clinical re-evaluation** Benzodiazepines: most patients require no medication after this day. Reinforce abstinence; schedule follow-up visit; monitor abstinence. **Alternative regimen** Oxazepam (Serax), 30 mg PO QID for 2 days; then 30 mg TID on day 3; 30 mg BID on day 4, and 15 mg BID on day 5; then discontinue. As with chlordiazepoxide, the daily dose is adjusted based on frequent clinical monitoring. An extra 30-mg PRN dose may be given for the first several days, necessitating a longer tapering when needed.

CBC = complete blood count; GGT = γ-glutamyltransferase; AST = aspartate transaminase; ALT = alanine transaminase; IM = intramuscular; PO = by mouth; CIWA-Ar = Clinical Institute Withdrawal Assessment for Alcohol; AA = Alcoholics Anonymous; QID = four times a day; TID = three times a day; DTs = delirium tremens; BID = twice a day; PRN = as needed; EAP = employee assistance program.

Adapted from Worner TM. New strategies in treating the alcohol withdrawal syndrome. Hosp Med 1995; 31(3):54–63.

The goals of treatment are safety; prevention of complications, such as seizures and DTs; comfort; and referral to rehabilitation. Although the in-patient guidelines include a protocol for seizure prophylaxis, anticonvulsants are usually not necessary when benzodiazepines are used sufficiently to suppress manifest withdrawal symptoms. Of course, patients with pre-existing seizure disorders should receive maintenance doses of their anticonvulsants. Magnesium supplementation may also reduce the risk of seizures. Even if the serum magnesium level is normal, supplementation is indicated in the presence of severe withdrawal symptoms, especially hyperreflexia or ankle clonus. Many of the medications in Table 17–7 potentiate each other's effects, so routinely combining these medications is contraindicated. Atenolol (Tenormin), 50 to 100 mg orally daily, is sometimes used adjunctively with benzodiazepines to decrease tremor, pulse, and blood pressure. We do not recommend its routine use because, unlike the benzodiazepines, it does not prevent seizures or DTs. Instead, atenolol may mask withdrawal symptoms that are better treated by the benzodiazepines. The precautions for atenolol also apply to the adjunctive use of clonidine for alcohol withdrawal.

B. Amphetamines and cocaine.

Amphetamines and cocaine are stimulant drugs that are discussed together in this section because their clinical effects, in terms of intoxication and withdrawal, are nearly identical. "Crack" cocaine is chemically identical to freebase cocaine and is a smokeable form of cocaine that is very short acting and rapidly addictive. Cocaine hydrochloride, the other major form of cocaine, is preferred by intranasal and intravenous users. "Ice" is a smokeable form of methamphetamine, which is longer acting than crack cocaine.

1. *Intoxication.*
   a. *Signs and symptoms.* Signs and symptoms of amphetamine or cocaine intoxication are euphoria, anxiety, anger, impaired judgment, hypervigilance, paranoia, stereotyped behaviors, tactile and other hallucinations, increased vital signs, dilated pupils, anorexia, nausea and vomiting, psychomotor agitation,

chest pain, arrhythmias, seizures, dyskinesias, dystonias, and in severe states, coma. Severe paranoia may put patients at risk for hurting themselves or others. Adverse effects are enhanced by the parenteral route of administration and by smoking.

b. *Treatment.* For acute anxiety and panic states, benzodiazepines may be used, such as lorazepam, 2 mg orally or intramuscularly every 6 hours. In severe cases of anxiety or in cases with psychotic symptoms (paranoia, hallucinations), an antipsychotic can be used in conjunction with lorazepam or by itself, such as haloperidol, 5 mg orally or intramuscularly every 4 to 6 hours. Panic attacks usually occur during active use or intoxication but may persist in some cases. Benzodiazepines may be used acutely, but antidepressants are preferred for the long-term treatment of panic disorder because patients with established histories of substance abuse are at greater risk for benzodiazepine abuse than other patients. Patients with persistent psychosis (more than 1 to 2 days) should be referred to a psychiatrist.

2. *Withdrawal.*

a. *Signs and symptoms.* Signs and symptoms of withdrawal are anxiety, irritability, depressed mood, fatigue, vivid unpleasant dreams, insomnia or hypersomnia, increased appetite, and psychomotor retardation or agitation. The symptoms of withdrawal, often referred to as "crashing" by stimulant users, generally dissipate within 4 to 7 days. Severe depression may put patients at risk for suicide.

b. *Treatment.* The management of cocaine withdrawal is supportive. Proper nutrition, rest, and a drug-free environment usually suffice. Educating patients about the course of withdrawal helps patients to understand their symptoms and plan for recovery. Because life-threatening physical symptoms do not occur as part of the stimulant withdrawal syndrome, pharmacotherapy is neither essential nor recommended for uncomplicated stimulant withdrawal. *The major complication of stimulant withdrawal is suicidal ideation.* Fortunately, suicidal thoughts usually diminish rapidly within several days of initiation of abstinence. When depressive symptoms are severe or persistent, then antidepressants may be considered. The clinician must weigh the lag time of 2 to 4 weeks for an antidepressant effect against the likelihood that depressive symptoms will abate in the first week of abstinence. When the primary care physician chooses an antidepressant, consideration should be given to agents that do not interact adversely with stimulants (monoamine oxidase inhibitors should be avoided) or have serious overdose potential (e.g., the tricyclic antidepressants). Thus, we prefer to use the selective serotonin reuptake inhibitors, such as sertraline (Zoloft), paroxetine (Paxil), and fluoxetine (Prozac).

3. *Pharmacotherapy.*

Numerous medications have been studied experimentally for the treatment of cocaine withdrawal and dependence in order to facilitate early abstinence during the first 4 to 12 weeks. These agents include amantadine (Symmetrel), bromocriptine (Parlodel), the antidepressants, carbamazepine (Tegretol), lithium, and amino acids. Study results have been mixed, and routine use of these medications is not recommended in the absence of another indication (e.g., a mood disorder).

C. Cannabis (marijuana and hashish).

Cannabis comes from the plants, *Cannabis sativa, Cannabis indica,* and hybrids. Slang terms for marijuana include pot, weed, and grass. Hashish or hash is a dried resinous exudate from the flowering tops. The street cost of marijuana in 1995 was $300 to $500 an ounce, an amount that could be made into approximately 60 marijuana cigarettes, or "joints," weighing 500 mg each. The psychoactive ingredient is Δ-9-tetrahydrocannabinol, which binds cannabinoid receptors concentrated in the brain's limbic system.

1. *Intoxication.*

a. *Signs and symptoms.* Signs and symptoms of cannabis intoxication are impaired motor coordination, sensation of slowed time, impaired judgment, euphoria, anxiety, altered perceptions including hallucinations with intact reality testing, conjunctival erythema, tachycardia, dry mouth, and increased appetite. Course of intoxication depends on the route of administration. Effects begin 30 to 60 minutes after oral use, peak at 2 to 3 hours, and last 3 to 5 hours. After the drug is smoked, effects start within minutes, peak in 20 to 30 minutes, and last 2 to 3 hours. However, performance of complex psychomotor tasks may be impaired for up to 24 hours after a single marijuana cigarette is smoked. Severe intoxications may manifest as delirium, paranoid psychosis, or intense anxiety or panic.

b. *Treatment.* Treatment is generally supportive. Benzodiazepines may be used acutely to treat panic reactions in an emergency situation, but take-home medication is generally contraindicated because of the abuse potential in patients already abusing other drugs. Delirium and psychosis respond to a short-term course of antipsychotics.

2. *Withdrawal.*

Irritability, insomnia (may last several weeks), restlessness, hot flashes, sweating, rhinorrhea, diarrhea, anorexia, hiccoughs, mild tremors, and nausea or vomiting may begin within 12 hours and last about 3 to 5 days after cessation of high-dose, long-term use of this drug. These symptoms are usually mild and do not require pharmacologic treatment.

D. Hallucinogens.

Hallucinogens are a heterogeneous group of substances, some plant derived and some synthesized, that are capable of altering perceptions and inducing hallucinations (Table 17–9). Also referred to as psychedelic (mind-manifesting), psychotomimetic (psychosis-mimicking), or psychotogenic (psychosis-generating) drugs, hallucinogens are broadly grouped as the *indolealkylamines* (including lysergic acid diethylamide [LSD], psilocybin, and dimethyltryptamine [DMT]) and the *phenalkylamines* (including mescaline, methylenedioxymethamphetamine [MDMA], methylenedioxyamphetamine [MDA], and dimethoxymethylamphetamine [DOM]). MDMA and MDA have been called "stimulant hallucinogens" and "designer drugs." Hallucinogens are taken orally, except for DMT, which is injected, sniffed, or smoked in marijuana and tobacco. Hallucinogens exert their psychoactive effects through the brain's serotonin system as serotonin (type 2) postsynaptic receptor agonists.

1. *Intoxication.*
   a. *Signs and symptoms.* Signs and symptoms of hallucinogen intoxication are intensified perceptions, illusions, hallucinations, synesthesias (e.g., "seeing" sounds or "hearing" colors), depersonalization, derealization, dilated pupils, tachycardia, sweating, palpitations, blurred vision, tremor, incoordination, hyperreflexia, and increased blood pressure. Jaw clenching and bruxism may occur with MDMA. Medical complications include seizures and hyperthermia. Nystagmus is not observed as in phencyclidine intoxication. The term "bad trip" was coined by users experiencing marked anxiety or depression, panic, fear of losing one's mind, and paranoia. This phenomenon can also take the form of a delirium, psychosis, or manic state. The duration of intoxication varies with the particular drug used (Table 17–9), although residual effects may persist.
   b. *Treatment.* Treatment consists of supportive measures, such as staying with the patient in a quiet room and providing reassurance and ongoing orientation. The patient should not be left alone, because of the potential for self-harm in response to psychotic symptoms. Severe anxiety and agitation may necessitate sedation with a benzodiazepine, such as lorazepam, 1 to 2 mg orally, intramuscularly, or intravenously every 1 to 2 hours, to a maximum of 10 mg. Psychotic symptoms can be treated with haloperidol (Haldol). Patients with persisting psychoses (>1 to 2 days) should be referred for psychiatric consultation.

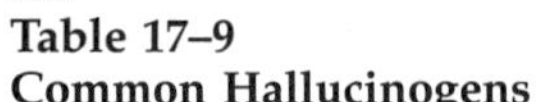

Table 17–9
Common Hallucinogens

Name	Other Names	Duration of Effects
LSD	Lysergic acid diethylamide, "acid"	8–12 h
Psilocybin	Derived from the mushroom, *Psilocybe mexicana,* "magic mushrooms," "shrooms"	5–6 h
DMT	Dimethyltryptamine, "businessman's high"	0.5–1 h
Mescaline	Derived from the peyote cactus, *Lophophora williamsii*	12 h
MDMA	Methylenedioxymethamphetamine, "ecstasy," "X," "XTC," "Adam"	3–4 h
DOM	Dimethoxymethylamphetamine, "STP"	7–8 h

2. *Withdrawal.*
   No withdrawal signs or symptoms have been reported for the hallucinogens, although a "hangover" after MDMA use, consisting of headache, fatigue, and sore jaw muscles, is possible.
3. *Flashbacks.*
   Flashbacks are transient, recurrent perceptual disturbances that are similar to those experienced during hallucinogen intoxication. Reality testing is intact. Flashbacks may recur from several months to more than 5 years after hallucinogens are used. Flashbacks do not require specific treatment other than reassurance unless they cause significant distress or impairment. Severe cases should be referred for specialized treatment with a psychiatrist or psychotherapist who is familiar with addiction treatment. Some authors recommend treatment with antipsychotics, carbamazepine (Tegretol), or benzodiazepines, but controlled studies are not available, and we avoid using benzodiazepines in patients with addiction histories.

E. Inhalants.

Inhalants are a diverse group of substances that include hydrocarbons (glue, paint thinners, acrylic and spray paints, gasoline, cleaning fluids, spray can propellants, typewriter correction fluid), ketones (nail polish remover), nitrites (amyl, *n*-butyl, isobutyl), and anesthetic gases (nitrous oxide or laughing gas, ether). With the exception of nitrites and possibly nitrous oxide, inhalants are used mostly by early adolescents. Indeed, inhalants are the only group of substances for which the prevalence of use declines from the eighth to the twelfth grade. Children are susceptible to use of inhalants because they are inexpensive, widely available in homes and stores, and legal to purchase at any age. Nitrous oxide is used as a whipping cream propellant, giving rise to its street name, "whippets." Street names for amyl nitrite include "poppers" and "snappers." Amyl nitrite is used to get high and to enhance orgasm.

1. *Intoxication.*
   a. Amyl nitrite intoxication causes euphoria and giddiness. Users report sensation of enhanced, prolonged orgasm due to a distorted perception of the slowing down of time. Vasodilation lowers blood pressure and causes tachycardia, dizziness, weakness, faintness, syncope, nausea, headache, and flushing of the neck and face. Onset of intoxication begins within 30 seconds and lasts for 5 minutes. Amyl nitrite may cause methemoglobinemia, resulting in cyanosis.
   b. Other inhalants (excluding nitrites and nitrous oxide) cause euphoria, disinhibition with belligerence, assaultiveness, apathy, impaired judgment, dizziness, nystagmus, incoordination, slurred speech, unsteady gait, lethargy, depressed reflexes, psychomotor retardation, tremor, generalized muscle weakness, blurred vision or diplopia, stupor, or coma. Death may occur from respiratory or cardiovascular collapse. The course of intoxication varies with the particular substance used. Intoxication with gasoline, for example, begins within 3 to 5 minutes and lasts for 5 to 6 hours. Inhalant intoxication may also manifest as delirium, psychosis, and mood or anxiety disorders. Delirium and psychosis may be treated with haloperidol, but benzodiazepines and other sedative-hypnotics may increase inhalant intoxication and respiratory depression.
2. *Inhalant withdrawal.*
   No signs or symptoms of inhalant withdrawal have been reported.
3. *Inhalant-related toxicity.*
   Signs and symptoms of toxicity are coughing, dyspnea, headache, nausea and vomiting, peripheral neuropathies, cerebral atrophy, dementia, cerebellar degeneration, hepatitis, renal failure, bone marrow suppression, and fatal arrhythmias.

F. Opioids, also called opiates.

1. *Intoxication.*
   Euphoria may be followed or accompanied by dysphoria, apathy, impaired judgment, poor attention and memory, constricted pupils, slurred speech, and drowsiness. Severe cases of opioid intoxication and overdose, as manifested by extreme somnolence, coma, or respiratory collapse, necessitate acute treatment with naloxone (Narcan), 1 to 2 mg intravenously, subcutaneously, or intramuscularly. This may be repeated every 2 to 3 minutes or given in a continuous drip in 5% dextrose in water or normal saline. Because naloxone is shorter acting than many opioids, the patient must be carefully observed, and repeat doses may be required, even after intoxication is completely reversed. Naloxone can precipitate acute withdrawal in dependent individuals and could be treated with the clonidine (Catapres) protocol (Table 17–10) as well as symptomatically.
2. *Withdrawal.*
   Symptoms of withdrawal are described in Table 17–11. Opioids are divided into long-acting (methadone, fentanyl [Duragesic] transdermal patches) and short-acting agents; the duration of action determines the duration of withdrawal symptoms. The longer the half-life of the opioid, the longer the duration of the withdrawal. The length of detoxification varies accordingly. Clonidine and adjunctive medications are preferred treatment in primary care settings (see Table 17–10) because detoxification with methadone and other opioids requires specialized licensing (see section IV.H.3).
3. *Pharmacotherapy.*
   Pharmacotherapy for long-term treatment of

Table 17–10
Sample Clonidine (Catapres) Protocol for Opioid Withdrawal

For days 1–5

1. Clonidine 0.1 mg PO QID for 5 days
2. Clonidine 0.1 mg PO q2–3h PRN for opioid withdrawal symptoms.
3. Total clonidine administration not to exceed 1.2 mg in 24 h (without contacting physician).
4. BP before each clonidine dose:
   Hold clonidine if systolic BP <90 or diastolic BP <60.
   If systolic BP is between 90 and 100, then give 0.05 mg of clonidine.

For days 6 and after*

1. *All opioids but methadone and fentanyl (Duragesic) patches:*
   Reduce dose by 0.1–0.2 mg/d.
2. *For methadone and fentanyl patch withdrawal:*
   On days 6–10: maintain maximum dose given on day 5.
   On days 11 to completion: reduce dose by 0.2–0.4 mg/d.

Other orders

1. Ibuprofen (Motrin), 400 mg PO q4h PRN for pain.
2. Loperamide (Imodium), 4 mg PO initially, then 2 mg PO PRN for diarrhea (maximum dose, 8 mg/d).
3. Trimethobenzamide (Tigan) suppository, 200 mg TID PRN for nausea or vomiting.
4. Trazodone (Desyrel), 50–100 mg PO at bedtime PRN for sleep.

*For days 6 and more, new clonidine orders should be written by the physician.

BP = blood pressure; PRN = as needed.

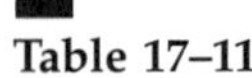

Table 17–11
Opioid and Sedative-Hypnotic Withdrawal Syndromes

Syndrome	Onset	Peak	Duration	Signs and Symptoms	Treatment
Methadone withdrawal and fentanyl (Duragesic) patch withdrawal	36–72 h	4–6 d	14–21 d	Increased BP and pulse, low-grade fever, yawning, diaphoresis, lacrimation, rhinorrhea, mydriasis, piloerection, nausea and vomiting, abdominal cramps, diarrhea, muscle twitches, shivering, hot or cold flashes, restlessness, anxiety, irritability, craving, musculoskeletal pain, insomnia, malaise	Clonidine and adjunctive medications per Table 17–10
Other opioid withdrawal (e.g., meperidine [Demerol], hydromorphone [Dilaudid], propoxyphene [Darvon], heroin, morphine, codeine)	4–24 h	1–3 d	5 10 d		
Sedatives with short half-lives	12–72 h	5–9 d	7–14 d	Increased pulse and BP, anxiety, irritability, depression, insomnia, restlessness, tremor, sweating, dizziness, headache, fatigue, decreased concentration, nausea, anorexia, depersonalization, derealization, increased sensory perception, abnormal perception of movement	Phenobarbital substitution and tapering per Tables 17–12 to 17–14
Sedatives with long half-lives	4–8 d	10–14 d	14–28 d		

BP = blood pressure.

opioid dependence includes naltrexone, methadone, and LAAM (see sections IV.H.2 and IV.H.3).

G. Phencyclidine.

Phencyclidine (PCP, angel dust, PeaCe pill) and the related compound ketamine are dissociative anesthetics. PCP may be used orally, intravenously, and intranasally, and via smoking.

1. *Intoxication.*
   a. *Signs and symptoms.* Signs and symptoms of PCP intoxication are belligerence, assaultiveness, impulsiveness, unpredictability, agitation, and impaired judgment, and are complicated by the patient's diminished response to pain. Consequently, combative patients are not easily deterred by pain or physical force, and they may unknowingly injure themselves. Patients may appear manic, panicked, depressed, psychotic, or delirious. Other physical effects include nystagmus, tachycardia, hypertension, ataxia, dysarthria, hyperacusis, muscle rigidity, seizures, and coma. Acute intoxication may last 4 to 12 hours with an extended "coming down" period, caused by PCP's long half-life of 1 to 3 days.
   b. *Treatment.* Treatment consists of supportive measures in a quiet, nonthreatening setting with minimal stimulation. Benzodiazepines, such as lorazepam, 2 to 4 mg intramuscularly, are used as needed for anxiety and agitation. High-potency neuroleptics, such as haloperidol (Haldol), 5 to 10 mg every 30 to 60 minutes, are used for psychosis and agitation that are not responsive to benzodiazepines. Some experts recommend urinary acidification to facilitate PCP excretion, but rarely, patients with severe rhabdomyolysis may require urinary alkalization.
2. *Withdrawal.*
   Withdrawal is not generally observed, although psychiatric symptoms, including depression, anxiety, and irritability, may persist for several weeks after acute intoxication. Some clinicians recommend antidepressants during the early recovery period, but few studies address outcomes of such treatment. Persisting psychotic symptoms require referral to a psychiatrist for differential diagnosis and neuroleptic treatment.

H. Sedative-hypnotics.

1. *Intoxication.*
   Symptoms are similar to alcohol intoxication and include mood instability, impaired judgment, inappropriate sexual or aggressive behavior, slurred speech, incoordination, unsteady gait, nystagmus, impaired attention and memory, and stupor or coma. Memory impairment

can resemble alcoholic blackouts. Respiratory depression is more commonly seen with barbiturates or combinations of alcohol and benzodiazepines than with benzodiazepines alone.

2. *Withdrawal.*
The sedative-hypnotics are divided into long-acting and short-acting agents (see Tables 17–12 and 17–13); the duration of the action determines the duration of the withdrawal symptoms (see Table 17–11). We use the CIWA-Ar for monitoring symptoms of sedative withdrawal because alcohol and other sedative withdrawal syndromes are similar (see Appendix). An objective instrument like the CIWA-Ar helps to monitor the withdrawal process and to make adjustments in the detoxification regimen as needed. Two general approaches to detoxification from sedative-hypnotics exist. For patients who are physically dependent on therapeutic doses without evidence of impaired control, adverse consequences, or other drug abuse, the agent is tapered weekly by 10% to 25% of the starting dose over a 4- to 12-week period. Weekly out-patient visits are useful to monitor the process and adjust the rate of tapering. For patients with a full dependency syndrome who use more than the prescribed dosage or abuse other drugs as well, the phenobarbital substitution and tapering technique is preferred (Table 17–14). In this way, the patient's preferred drug is withdrawn immediately, which attenuates drug-seeking behavior. Some specialists prefer to substitute and taper with long-acting benzodiazepines, such as chlordiazepoxide (Librium), clonazepam (Klonopin), and diazepam (Valium). The general principle is to substitute a long-acting sedative with low abuse potential and good antiseizure activity for the generally short-acting sedatives. The withdrawal phenomenon is characterized by the sudden unmasking of the sympathetic nervous system, which has been "up-regulated" to compensate for the chronic presence of the sedatives. This adaptation and the resultant "sympathetic storm" that occurs when the sedative is suddenly taken away is the main driving force for sedative withdrawal. Controlling the sympathetic storm before it starts by adding phenobarbital and tapering allows the sympathetic nervous system to gradually down-regulate. The exact time course of detoxification depends on the half-life of the patient's drug, the amount taken, and the duration of use. Shorter phenobarbital tapering (7 to 14 days) is tolerated in well-motivated patients who used short-acting sedatives in therapeutic doses for brief periods of time (3 to 6 months). Longer phenobarbital tapering (14 to 21 days) is preferred in patients who used long-acting sedatives, at supratherapeutic doses, or for long periods of time (>1 year). In addition, shorter phenobarbital tapering is tolerated better in in-patient settings than in out-patient

Table 17–12
Phenobarbital Substitution Doses* for Benzodiazepines

Drug	Dose Equal to 30 mg of Phenobarbital (mg)*
Drugs with short half-lives	
Alprazolam (Xanax)	1
Lorazepam (Ativan)	2
Oxazepam (Serax)	10
Temazepam (Restoril)	15
Triazolam (Halcion)	0.25
Drugs with long half-lives	
Chlordiazepoxide (Librium)	25
Clorazepate (Tranxene)	7.5
Clonazepam (Klonopin)	2
Diazepam (Valium)	10
Flurazepam (Dalmane)	15
Halazepam (Paxipam)	40
Prazepam (Centrax)	10

Adapted from Smith DE, Wesson DR. Benzodiazepines and other sedative-hypnotics. In: Galanter M, Kleber, H, Editors. Textbook of Substance Abuse Treatment. Washington, DC: American Psychiatric Press; 1994.

**Caution:* Phenobarbital doses are for short-term substitution and tapering only; i.e., for the purposes of detoxification. Using these doses as therapeutic equivalents may lead to accumulation of phenobarbital and toxicity.

Table 17–13
Phenobarbital Substitution Doses* for Short-Acting Nonbenzodiazepine Sedatives†

Drug	Dose Equal to 30 mg of Phenobarbital (mg)*
Barbiturates	
Amobarbital (Amytal)	100
Butabarbital (Butisol)	100
Butalbital (Fiorinal, Sedapap)	100
Pentobarbital (Nembutal)	100
Secobarbital (Seconal)	100
Other	
Chloral hydrate (Noctec, Somnos)	500
Ethchlorvynol (Placidyl)	500
Glutethimide (Doriden)	250
Meprobamate (Equanil, Equagesic, Miltown)	400
Methaqualone (Quaalude)	300
Methyprylon (Noludar)	200

Adapted from Smith DE, Wesson DR: Benzodiazepines and other sedative-hynotics. In: Galanter M, Kleber H, Editors. Textbook of Substance Abuse Treatment. Washington, DC: American Psychiatric Press, 1994.

**Caution:* Phenobarbital doses are for short-term substitution and tapering only; i.e., for the purposes of detoxification. Using these doses as therapeutic equivalents may lead to accumulation of phenobarbital and toxicity.

†These agents are relatively short-acting, and the course of withdrawal is similar to that with the short-acting benzodiazepines listed in Table 17–12.

Table 17–14
Phenobarbital Substitution Technique for Sedative Detoxification

1. Determine the dosage of sedatives used during the month before treatment and discontinue administration.
2. Calculate the phenobarbital substitution dose according to Tables 17–12 and 17–13, up to a maximum of 500 mg of phenobarbital.
3. Stabilize patient on phenobarbital substitution dose divided into 3–4 daily doses for first 2 days.
4. Consider 2 extra doses that may be given as PRN doses for withdrawal symptoms not responsive to aforementioned strategies.
5. Then decrease daily dose by an average of 10% per day for shorter-acting agents and by 5% per day for longer-acting agents.
6. Hold dose if sustained nystagmus, slurred speech, or ataxia occur. (Physician decreases that day's intended dose by 25–50% and adjusts tapering accordingly.)
7. If objective withdrawal signs emerge during tapering (e.g., CIWA-Ar >10), then the physician increases that day's dose by 50% and adjusts tapering accordingly.
8. Consider administering propranolol (Inderal), 20 mg PO QID for 2 wk for persistent withdrawal signs after the tapering or when the physician does not wish to prolong tapering by further dose increases (contraindicated in asthmatics and patients with heart failure; use with caution in patients taking haloperidol (Haldol) or calcium channel blockers or those with angina, diabetes, hyperthyroidism, or liver or renal dysfunction. Hold dose if pulse <60 or systolic BP <90 or diastolic BP <60.

PRN = as needed; BP = blood pressure; CIWA-Ar = Clinical Institute Withdrawal Assessment for Alcohol; PO = by mouth; QID = four times a day.

ones. The phenobarbital substitution doses are estimates for suppressing withdrawal symptoms and preventing seizures when tapering is initiated (Tables 17–12 and 17–13). They are not maintenance doses, because phenobarbital accumulates over time and causes toxicity (ataxia, slurred speech, nystagmus) because of its long half-life of 100 hours. The pentobarbital challenge test is another method for determining the phenobarbital substitution dose. By determining the patient's response and tolerance to a 200-mg test dose of pentobarbital, the phenobarbital substitution dose can be estimated. This method is most useful when the doctor is unable to determine from the patient's history how much sedative the patient was taking. In actual practice, we find that the substitution tables are sufficient. Rarely, patients may experience symptoms up to 3 months after stopping sedatives, the so-called protracted withdrawal syndrome. Propranolol (Inderal), 20 mg orally four times a day, may help during the first 2 weeks after the phenobarbital tapering is completed. Protracted withdrawal symptoms must be distinguished from a comorbid anxiety disorder or mood disorder, for which the patient may have been treated with sedative-hypnotics in the first place. Comorbid disorders in patients with a full dependency syndrome should be treated without the use of sedative-hypnotics. Antidepressants may be used for both depression and anxiety disorders. Trazodone (Desyrel), 50 to 100 mg at bedtime, often helps with insomnia without the risk of dependence. Antihistamines such as hydroxyzine (Atarax, Vistaril) or diphenhydramine (Benadryl) may be used for anxiety symptoms and sedation. Buspirone (BuSpar) is beneficial for patients with generalized anxiety syndromes. Less commonly, thioridazine (Mellaril), 25 to 50 mg daily as needed, may be used for the short-term treatment of severe anxiety and insomnia in addicted patients.

VI. Prescription drug problems.

Clearly, the most important risk factor for prescription drug abuse and dependence is the personal history of the individual. Patients with a history of substance abuse or dependence are at the highest risk for developing prescription drug problems. A family history of chemical dependency may also predict risk, but it is a less well-established risk factor than personal history. There are, however, clear-cut needs for these classes of medications in the general population.

A. Prescribing for recovering patients.

1. *Sedatives.*
   We believe that benzodiazepines and similar sedatives are contraindicated in the treatment of patients in recovery from an alcohol or sedative problem with few exceptions, including detoxification and treatment of an acute seizure. We caution alcoholic patients that benzodiazepines are like "booze in pill form."
2. *Opiates.*
   Opiates should be avoided in the long term, but in acute situations of pain, they can be used cautiously with close follow-up and built-in accountability with the patient's peers, treatment personnel, and the primary care provider. Exhaustion of all other pain-relieving modalities, such as nerve blocks, biofeedback, and physical therapy is preferred.

B. Prescribing for patients with unrecognized substance problems.

The primary care physician is more likely to encounter the patient with an undiagnosed or unrecognized substance abuse problem (which becomes apparent when the physician tries to wean or discontinue the prescription drug) than the abusing or dependent patient needing mood-altering drugs. Drugs should be tapered in a supportive way, with an emphasis on primary treatment or relapse treatment. The provider often feels betrayed and personally deceived, and this feeling can manifest in judgmental behavior or attitudes toward the dependent patient. Discontinuing treatment with the patient and telling the patient to go elsewhere "solves" the provider's, but not the patient's, problem.

C. Treating prescription drug problems in patients without usual risk factors.

Another common scenario involves the patient with no previous or family history of chemical dependency, who is prescribed benzodiazepines for a psychiatric disorder, a transient situational disturbance, or a temporary sleep disorder and then encounters difficulty discontinuing the drug. If the primary care physician prescribes these agents for more than 1 to 2 months, whether or not there is dose escalation, some patients will not be able to discontinue taking the medication for physiologic or psychological reasons. Treatment of a newly entertained primary psychiatric disorder with the appropriate drug is one solution. Slow weaning, frequent visits, and a contract can be used in this type of situation. Sometimes the drug involved can be used, but other times, the physician may instead prescribe a longer-acting drug in order to avoid the psychological dependency the patient may have developed.

Case Study

Mrs. K. is a 73-year-old woman who is new to the physician's practice. She is referred by her daughter, whom the physician has treated for hyperthyroidism. Mrs. K. has been under the care of a primary care physician and treated for reactive airways, hypertension, and an anxiety and sleep disorder. For the past 6 months, she has been taking increasing doses of alprazolam (Xanax) up to her current dose of 1 mg three times a day. In addition, she has been unable to get to sleep at night and temazepam (Restoril), 15 mg at bedtime, was added the previous month. She comes to the physician for ongoing care and because her symptoms are "breaking through."

Mrs. K. is not a drug seeker. She has never had a problem with sedatives or alcohol and has no apparent family history of substance disorders. She is in distress, however, and part of it is her possible underlying anxiety disorder and part of it may be iatrogenic benzodiazepine habituation. Over the next few months, the focus is on maintenance and trust building. Her antihypertensive agents and reactive airway medications are optimized. The nighttime benzodiazepine dose is discontinued, and the patient is given an intermediate dose of trazodone (Desyrel), to augment sleep and control her anxiety symptoms at night. Chest pain develops, which is finally determined to be caused by gastroesophageal reflux disorder. She is weaned off of the alprazolam by reducing the dose by 0.5 mg every 7 to 14 days.

She is seen biweekly to weekly, and paroxetine (Paxil) therapy is started. If her appointment interval is lengthened, she presents with chest pain or labile hypertension between appointments, so a regular interval of weekly visits is maintained. Finally, after 3 months, she is no longer taking the alprazolam and is stable on the paroxetine therapy and a low dose of clonazepam (Klonopin). Clonazepam was picked because it is longer acting than alprazolam, has less of an immediate effect than alprazolam, and is therefore less reinforcing. (Dependent, drug-seeking patients who abuse benzodiazepines report having relatively "no buzz" when comparing clonazepam with alprazolam.) The patient is currently taking paroxetine, 20 mg/d, clonazepam, 0.5 mg at night, and no "as needed" antianxiety agents. After sustained stabilization, gradual attempts to wean the clonazepam will be made (see Chapter 9 for specific approaches to the anxiety disorders).

The multitude of medical problems (gastroesophageal reflux disorder, hypertension, atypical chest pain, and reactive airways) makes the treatment of this patient painstakingly complex. Any one of these problems can flare during the weaning process. The target of avoiding the long-term use of short-acting benzodiazepines has to be an overall goal for successful treatment. There are many distractions when working with patients who have multiple problems, but the same goal has to be a focus even in less complex patients. This patient is now seen every 3 to 6 months and is doing very well.

Acknowledgment
The authors thank Mary Closser, DO, Michael Fleming, MD, and David Gorelick, MD, for their helpful reviews of the manuscript.

References

1. Anglin TM. Interviewing guidelines for the clinical evaluation of adolescent substance abuse. Pediatr Clin North Am 1987; 34:381–398. (True to its title, this is must reading for those seeing adolescents.)
2. Comerci CG. Office assessment of substance abuse and addiction. Adolescent Medicine: State of the Art Reviews, 1993; 4:277–293. (An excellent review of screening tools designed for use with adolescents as well as practical interview techniques.)
3. Physicians' Desk Reference, 51st Edition. Montvale, NJ: Medical Economics; 1997, p. 859.
4. Fleming MF, Barry KL. Addictive Disorders. St. Louis: Mosby-YearBook, 1992.

Suggested Reading

Alcoholics Anonymous. Third Edition. New York: Alcoholics Anonymous World Services; 1976. (The "big book" of AA explains the 12 steps that have helped more alcoholics recover than any other approach. This text is obtainable through the address in section IV.G.2.a.)

Alcoholism in the Elderly: Diagnosis, Treatment, and Prevention: Guidelines for Primary Care Physicians. Chicago: American Medical Association; 1995. (Booklet contains a copy of the Michigan Alcoholism Screening Test—Geriatric Version, as well as treatment and referral guidelines. Obtainable from Department of Geriatric

Health, American Medical Association, 515 North State Street, Chicago, IL 60610 [telephone: 312-464-5085]).

American Psychiatric Association. Diagnostic and Statistical Manual of Mental Disorders, 4th Edition (DSM-IV). Washington, DC: American Psychiatric Association; 1994.

Dufour MC, Archer L, Gordis E. Alcohol and the elderly. Clin Geriatr Med 1992; 8:127–141. (An excellent review of the topic for practitioners who work with this population.)

Fleming MF, Barry KL. Addictive Disorders. St. Louis: Mosby–Year Book; 1992. (An excellent, comprehensive, and practical textbook written from a family practice perspective.)

Galanter M, Kleber H, Editors. Textbook of Substance Abuse Treatment. Washington DC: American Psychiatric Press; 1994. (Focuses on specific treatments used in specialty settings, such as addiction medicine and psychiatry, but is succinct and clear.)

Miller WR, Rollnick S, Editors. Motivational Interviewing: Preparing People to Change Addictive Behavior. New York: Guilford; 1991. (Highly recommended for acquiring new techniques for motivating resistant patients. Filled with transcripts and concrete examples of what to say to patients who do not think that they have a problem.)

Morse RM, Flavin DK. The definition of alcoholism. JAMA 1992; 268:1012–1014.

NS Miller, Editor. Comprehensive Handbook of Drug and Alcohol Addiction. New York: Marcel Dekker; 1991.

Pearson TA, Terry P. What to advise patients about drinking alcohol: The clinician's conundrum. JAMA 1994; 272:967–968.

Project SAEFP Executive Committee: Project SAEFP Workshop Materials: Substance Abuse Education for Family Physicians. Kansas City, MO: The Society of Teachers of Family Medicine; 1991. (Available by calling 800-274-2237.)

Regier DA, Farmer ME, Rae DS, et al. Co-morbidity of mental disorders with alcohol and other drug abuse. JAMA 1990; 264:2511–2518.

Sullivan JT, Sykora K, Schneiderman J, et al. Assessment of alcohol withdrawal: The revised Clinical Institute Withdrawal Assessment for Alcohol scale (CIWA-Ar). Br J Addict 1989; 84:1353–1357.

National Institute on Alcohol Abuse and Alcoholism. The physicians' guide to helping patients with alcohol problems. Washington DC: US Department of Health and Human Services; 1995. NIH publication 95-3769. (Contains guidelines for alcohol screening and brief intervention by the primary care physician.)

The primary care setting: Recognition and care of patients with alcohol problems. Alcohol Health Res World 1994; 18:93–168. (Entire issue devoted to this topic with specific articles for the family physician, general internist, obstetrician/gynecologist, pediatrician, and trauma physician. Contains screening tests and a superb review of laboratory tests. May be purchased from the US Government Printing Office. Telephone: 202-783-3238.)

Worner TM. New strategies in treating the alcohol withdrawal syndrome. Hosp Med 1995; 31(3):54–63. (Contains detailed protocol for out-patient detoxification by the primary care physician.)

Appendix

Screening for Alcohol Problems

AUDIT (Alcohol Use Disorders Identification Test)*

An excellent and simple 10-question, patient-administered questionnaire for detecting alcohol problems. Patients simply circle the appropriate answer. Scoring is conducted by the examiner and involves some translation: questions 1 to 8 are scored 0, 1, 2, 3, or 4. Questions 9 and 10 are scored 0, 2, or 4 only. The response coding is summarized below.

The minimum score (for nondrinkers) is 0, and the maximum possible score is 40. A score of 8 or more indicates a strong likelihood of hazardous or harmful alcohol consumption.

Score	0	1	2	3	4
Question 1	Never	Monthly or less	2–4 times per month	2–3 times per week	≥4 times per week
Question 2	1 or 2	3 or 4	5 or 6	7 to 9	≥10
Questions 3–8	Never	< Monthly	Monthly	Weekly	Daily or almost daily
Questions 9 and 10	No		Yes, but not in the last year		Yes, during the last year

Patient Name ______________________________ Date ______________

AUDIT

Please circle the answer that is correct for you

1. How often do you have a drink containing alcohol?
   Never   Monthly or less   Two to four times a month   Two to three times a week   Four or more times a week
2. How many drinks containing alcohol do you have on a typical day when you are drinking?
   1 or 2   3 or 4   5 or 6   7 to 9   10 or more
3. How often do you have six or more drinks on one occasion?
   Never   Less than monthly   Monthly   Weekly   Daily or almost daily
4. How often during the last year have you found that you were not able to stop drinking once you had started?
   Never   Less than monthly   Monthly   Weekly   Daily or almost daily
5. How often during the last year have you failed to do what was normally expected from you because of drinking?
   Never   Less than monthly   Monthly   Weekly   Daily or almost daily
6. How often during the last year have you needed a first drink in the morning to get yourself going after a heavy drinking session?
   Never   Less than monthly   Monthly   Weekly   Daily or almost daily
7. How often during the last year have you had a feeling of guilt or remorse after drinking?
   Never   Less than monthly   Monthly   Weekly   Daily or almost daily
8. How often during the last year have you been unable to remember what happened the night before because you had been drinking?
   Never   Less than monthly   Monthly   Weekly   Daily or almost daily
9. Have you or someone else been injured as a result of your drinking?
   No   Yes, but not in the last year   Yes, during the last year
10. Has a relative or friend or a doctor or other health worker been concerned about your drinking or suggested you cut down?
   No   Yes, but not in the last year   Yes, during the last year

*Adapted from Saunders JB, Aasland OG. Babor TF, et al. Development of the Alcohol Use Disorders Identification Test (AUDIT): WHO collaborative project on early detection of persons with harmful alcohol consumption-II. Addiction 1993; 88:791–804.

MAST-G (Michigan Alcoholism Screening Test—Geriatric Version)*

The MAST-G is a geriatric version of the MAST questionnaire (for use in those ≥55 years). It is composed of 24 questions to which the patient answers "yes" or "no." A cut-off score of 5 or greater (i.e., five "yes" responses) indicates a strong possibility of a drinking problem, and more detailed questioning by the clinician is indicated.

Patient Name ____________________ Date __________

Michigan Alcoholism Screening Test—Geriatric Version (MAST-G)

Question		Yes	No
1. After drinking have you ever noticed an increase in your heart rate or beating in your chest?	1.	___	___
2. When talking with others, do you ever underestimate how much you actually drink?	2.	___	___
3. Does alcohol make you sleepy so that you often fall asleep in your chair?	3.	___	___
4. After a few drinks, have you sometimes not eaten or been able to skip a meal because you didn't feel hungry?	4.	___	___
5. Does having a few drinks help decrease your shakiness or tremors?	5.	___	___
6. Does alcohol sometimes make it hard for you to remember parts of the day or night?	6.	___	___
7. Do you have rules for yourself that you won't drink before a certain time of the day?	7.	___	___
8. Have you lost interest in hobbies or activities you used to enjoy?	8.	___	___
9. When you wake up in the morning, do you ever have trouble remembering part of the night before?	9.	___	___
10. Does having a drink help you sleep?	10.	___	___
11. Do you hide your alcohol bottles from family members?	11.	___	___
12. After a social gathering, have you ever felt embarrassed because you drank too much?	12.	___	___
13. Have you ever been concerned that drinking might be harmful to your health?	13.	___	___
14. Do you like to end an evening with a nightcap?	14.	___	___
15. Did you find your drinking increased after someone close to you died?	15.	___	___
16. In general, would you prefer to have a few drinks at home rather than go out to social events?	16.	___	___
17. Are you drinking more now than in the past?	17.	___	___
18. Do you usually take a drink to relax or calm your nerves?	18.	___	___
19. Do you drink to take your mind off your problems?	19.	___	___
20. Have you ever increased your drinking after experiencing a loss in your life?	20.	___	___
21. Do you sometimes drive when you have had too much to drink?	21.	___	___
22. Has a doctor or nurse ever said they were worried or concerned about your drinking?	22.	___	___
23. Have you ever made rules to manage your drinking?	23.	___	___
24. When you feel lonely does having a drink help?	24.	___	___

*From Blow FC, Brower KJ, Schulenberg JE, et al. The Michigan Alcoholism Screening Test—Geriatric Version (MAST-G): A new elderly-specific screening instrument. Alcohol Clin Exp Res 1992; 16:372.

Screening for Drug Problems

DAST-10 (Drug Abuse Screening Test)*

The DAST-10 is used for rapid screening of (nonalcohol) drug abuse. It is a 10-item, yes-no, self-administered questionnaire. It is a shortened version of the original 28-item DAST. Scoring ranges from 0 to 10. Guidelines for scoring are:

1–2 = low problem severity
3–5 = moderate severity
6–8 = substantial severity
9–10 = severe problems

Name ______________________ Date ______________

Drug Abuse Screening Test (DAST-10)

Drug Use Questionnaire (DAST-10)

The following questions concern information about your possible involvement with drugs *not including alcoholic beverages* during the past 12 months. Carefully read each statement and decide if your answer is "Yes" or "No." Then, circle the appropriate response beside the question.

In the statements "drug abuse" refers to (1) the use of prescribed or over-the-counter drugs in excess of the directions and (2) any non-medical use of drugs. The various classes of drugs may include: cannabis (marijuana, hashish), solvents, tranquilizers (e.g., Valium), barbiturates, cocaine, stimulants (e.g., speed), hallucinogens (e.g., LSD) or narcotics (e.g., heroin). Remember that the questions *do not* include alcoholic beverages.

Please answer every question. If you have difficulty with a statement, then choose the response that is mostly right.

These questions refer to the past 12 months.

	Circle Your Response	
1. Have you used drugs other than those required for medical reasons?	Yes	No
2. Do you abuse more than one drug at a time?	Yes	No
3. Are you always able to stop using drugs when you want to?	Yes	No
4. Have you had "blackouts" or "flashbacks" as a result of drug use?	Yes	No
5. Do you ever feel bad or guilty about your drug use?	Yes	No
6. Does your spouse (or parents) ever complain about your involvement with drugs?	Yes	No
7. Have you neglected your family because of your use of drugs?	Yes	No
8. Have you engaged in illegal activities in order to obtain drugs?	Yes	No
9. Have you ever experienced withdrawal symptoms (felt sick) when you stopped taking drugs?	Yes	No
10. Have you had medical problems as a result of your drug use (e.g., memory loss, hepatitis, convulsions, bleeding, etc.)?	Yes	No

*From Skinner HA. The Drug Abuse Test. Addict Behav 1982; 7:363–371.

Alcohol Withdrawal Severity Ratings

The Clinical Institute Withdrawal Assessment Scale for Alcohol—Revised (CIWA-Ar Scale)*

The CIWA-Ar scale can be used to determine the level of care and the need for pharmacologic detoxification. The 10-item scale takes 2 minutes to administer and can be readministered every 30 to 60 minutes as needed. One author uses the following scoring protocol:

0–8: no medications
8–15: medications as an out-patient
>15: medications as an in-patient

A less conservative scoring protocol follows:

0–10: no medications
10–20: may benefit from pharmacotherapy based on clinical judgment and assessment of other risk factors in section V.A.2.b
20–67: medication needed

*From Sullivan JT, Sykora K, Schneiderman J, et al. Assessment of alcohol withdrawal: The revised Clinical Institute Withdrawal Assessment for Alcohol scale (CIWA-Ar). Addiction 1989; 84:1353–1357.

Clinical Institute Withdrawal Assessment-Alcohol (CIWA-Ar)

Patient Name ______________________

Time: ______________ Date: ______________

Pulse: ______________ BP: ______________

Nausea & Vomiting: Ask "Do you feel sick to your stomach?" "Have you vomited?" Observation.
- 0 No nausea and no vomiting
- 1 Mild nausea with no vomiting
- 2
- 3
- 4 Intermittent nausea with dry heaves
- 5
- 6
- 7 Constant nausea, frequent dry heaves and vomiting

Tremor: Arms extended and fingers spread apart. Observation.
- 0 No tremor
- 1 Not visible, but can be felt fingertip to fingertip
- 2
- 3
- 4 Moderate, with patient's arms extended
- 5
- 6
- 7 Severe, even with arms not extended

Paroxysmal Sweats: Observation.
- 0 No sweat visible
- 1 Barely perceptible sweating, palms moist
- 2
- 3
- 4 Beads of sweat obvious on forehead
- 5
- 6
- 7 Drenching sweats

Anxiety: Ask "Do you feel nervous?" Observation.
- 0 No anxiety, at ease
- 1 Mildly anxious
- 2
- 3
- 4 Moderately anxious or guarded, so anxiety is inferred.
- 5
- 6
- 7 Equivalent to acute panic states, as seen in severe delirium or acute schizophrenic reactions

Agitation: Observation.
- 0 Normal activity
- 1 Somewhat more than normal activity
- 2
- 3
- 4 Moderately fidgety and restless
- 5
- 6
- 7 Paces back and forth during most of the interview, or constantly thrashes about

Tactile Disturbances: Ask "Have you any itching, pins & needles sensations, any burning, any numbness or do you feel bugs crawling on or under your skin?" Observation.
- 0 None
- 1 Very mild itching, pins & needles, burning or numbness
- 2 Mild itching, pins & needles, burning or numbness
- 3 Moderate itching, pins & needles, burning or numbness
- 4 Moderately severe hallucinations
- 5 Severe hallucinations
- 6 Extremely severe hallucinations
- 7 Continuous hallucinations

Auditory Disturbances: Ask "Are you more aware of sounds around you?" "Are they harsh?" "Do they frighten you?" "Are you hearing anything that is disturbing to you?" "Are you hearing things you know are not there?" Observation.
- 0 Not present
- 1 Very mild harshness or ability to frighten
- 2 Mild harshness or ability to frighten
- 3 Moderate harshness or ability to frighten
- 4 Moderately severe hallucinations
- 5 Severe hallucinations
- 6 Extremely severe hallucinations
- 7 Continuous hallucinations

Visual Disturbances: Ask "Does the light appear to be too bright?" "Is the color different?" "Does it hurt your eyes?" "Are you seeing anything that is disturbing to you?" "Are you seeing things you know are not there?" Observation.
- 0 Not present
- 1 Very mild sensitivity
- 2 Mild sensitivity
- 3 Moderate sensitivity
- 4 Moderately severe hallucinations
- 5 Severe hallucinations
- 6 Extremely severe hallucinations
- 7 Continuous hallucinations

Headache, Fullness in Head: Ask "Does your head feel different?" "Does it feel like there is a band around your head?" Do not rate dizziness or lightheadedness. Otherwise, rate severity.
- 0 Not present
- 1 Very mild
- 2 Mild
- 3 Moderate
- 4 Moderately severe
- 5 Severe
- 6 Very severe
- 7 Extremely severe

Orientation and Clouding of Sensorium: Ask "What day is this?" "Where are you?" "Whom am I?"
- 0 Oriented and can do serial additions
- 1 Cannot do serial additions or is uncertain about date
- 2 Disoriented for date by no more than 2 calendar days
- 3 Disoriented for date by more than 2 calendar days
- 4 Disoriented for place and/or person

Total Score: ______________________

Maximum Possible Score: 67

Rater's Name: ______________________

Al-Anon
Is It for You?

Millions of people are affected by the excessive drinking of someone close. The following twenty questions are designed to help you decide whether or not you need Al-Anon:

1. Do you worry about how much someone else drinks?
2. Do you have money problems because of someone else's drinking?
3. Do you tell lies to cover up for someone else's drinking?
4. Do you feel that if the drinker loved you, he or she would stop drinking to please you?
5. Do you think that the drinker's behavior is caused by his or her companions?
6. Are routines frequently upset or meals delayed because of the drinker?
7. Do you make threats, such as, "If you don't stop drinking, I'll leave you"?
8. When you kiss the drinker hello, do you secretly try to smell his or her breath?
9. Are you afraid to upset someone for fear it will set off a drinking bout?
10. Have you been hurt or embarrassed by a drinker's behavior?
11. Does it seem as if every holiday is spoiled because of drinking?
12. Have you considered calling the police for help in fear of abuse?
13. Do you find yourself searching for hidden liquor?
14. Do you often ride in a car with a driver who has been drinking?
15. Have you refused social invitations out of fear or anxiety?
16. Do you sometimes feel like a failure when you think of the lengths you have gone to control the drinker?
17. Do you think that if the drinker stopped drinking, your other problems would be solved?
18. Do you ever threaten to hurt yourself to scare the drinker?
19. Do you feel angry, confused, and depressed most of the time?
20. Do you feel there is no one who understands your problems?

If you have answered yes to three or more of these questions, Al-Anon or Alateen may help. You can contact Al-Anon or Alateen by looking in your local telephone directory or by writing to:

Al-Anon Family Group Headquarters, Inc.
1600 Corporate Landing Parkway
Virginia Beach, VA 23454-5617

18

DAVID S. ROSEN, MD, MPH

MARK A. DEMITRACK, MD

Eating Disorders and Disordered Eating

I. Epidemiology and pathophysiology.

A. Eating pathology—a spectrum of behavior.

Eating disorders are diseases of the developed world. Among the population of individuals with symptomatic disturbances of eating behavior, *two major, operationally defined eating disorders exist: anorexia nervosa and bulimia nervosa.* Prevalence estimates for these conditions have been established, with reasonable confidence, in the young female population, the group that is generally considered to be at highest risk for the development of these disorders. For anorexia nervosa, the prevalence is approximately 1%; for bulimia nervosa, estimates are slightly greater, at nearly 3%.

Some comments can be made about these figures and the definitions that underlie them. First, most studies would suggest that at least for bulimia nervosa, the prevalence of this illness has been increasing over the past few decades. Some of this increase may be accounted for by improved diagnosis, but sociocultural influences, especially the increasing emphasis in Western societies on thinness and physical beauty, are undeniably important determinants of this increase.

A more important factor is probably that these definitions circumscribe the most severe end of the continuum of a set of behaviors that exist in the general population. In our own studies of eating behavior in undergraduate women at the University of Michigan, more than 30% report that they regularly diet to lose weight, and at least 15% report that they habitually binge eat and regularly use strategies to counteract the effects of the binges, including vomiting or laxative or diuretic use. The frequency of these behaviors is slightly less than the stringent level required for the operationally defined eating disorders; nevertheless, their potential clinical consequences are alarming.

Given this information, it is our view that *eating disorders are not simply an idiosyncratic, uncommon disease of the subspecialist mental health practitioner but are a substantial medical concern from a primary care health perspective.* We feel this is so partly because of the sheer prevalence of eating-disordered behaviors in the general population. Moreover, emerging experience would suggest that early recognition of, and intervention with, individuals at risk may have an important influence on the course and the development of a full-blown eating disorder.

B. Etiology.

The etiology of the eating disorders is not completely understood. As in other psychiatric illnesses, contemporary research and clinical practice in eating disorders would suggest that a risk factor model provides the most information on the causes of these illnesses. From this perspective, the disease is conceptualized as resulting from the convergence of many factors, such as those intrinsic to the individual (e.g., genetic or acquired attributes), or extrinsic factors (e.g., psychosocial pressure for thinness).

Several areas are worthy of particular consideration in evaluations in routine practice. For instance, a family history of eating disorder, affective illness, or alcoholism in first-degree relatives is associated with an increased relative risk for the occurrence of an eating disorder in an individual. Other extrinsic factors that contribute to the development of the illness include occupational risk (e.g., in athletes, ballet performers, fashion models), personality characteristics (e.g., perfectionism, obsessionality, intolerance of error), and parental eating behavior and weight (e.g., family history of obesity, intense weight control or dieting practices, especially in the mother). Evidence is also accumulating that supports the view that physical or sexual abuse may play a role in the risk for eating disorders; however, it is still unclear whether this risk is specific to eating disorders or results in a general increase in vulnerability for the development of psychiatric disease.

C. Pathophysiology.

Fundamental to an understanding of the underlying pathophysiology of eating disorders is a determination of the relationship of measurable physiologic changes to the nutritional state of the individual. Because most research has been performed on ill or recovered populations, very little is known about physiologic abnormalities that may have existed before the overt expression of the eating disorder (i.e., predisposing factors). Of equal importance is the determination of whether particular state-associated physiologic events may themselves have significant behavioral consequences that then aggravate the disease process (i.e., perpetuating factors). Some current research has also focused on establishing the extent to which nutrition-induced physiologic changes may persist, despite short-term improvement in the nutritional status of the patient.

To date, numerous biochemical variables have been surveyed in patients with eating disorders. Several areas have attracted particular interest. For instance, studies of cerebrospinal fluid, plasma, and urine confirm abnormalities in the major monoamine neurotransmitter systems (i.e., noradrenergic, serotonergic, and dopaminergic function). In neuroendocrine systems, investigators have found disruptions in the hypothalamic-pituitary axes regulating adrenal, gonadal, and thyroid function; alterations in the secretion of antidiuretic hormone and consequent disruptions in fluid balance; and disturbances in the meal-related release of gut peptides, such as cholecystokinin. Abnormal regulation of the endogenous opioid system has also attracted significant research interest.

In most instances, these abnormalities resolve with restoration of normal nutritional status, although the time course to truly normal levels varies widely, depending on the system of study. However, the fact that these same neurochemical and neuroendocrine systems play important roles in the regulation of mood, cognition, and appetite suggests that during the active phase of the illness, the systems may have clinical significance. An understanding of these biochemical events also holds promise for the development of a more rational approach to pharmacotherapy for these conditions and may, in part, explain the utility of antidepressant medications in the treatment of some patients with eating disorders.

II. Evaluation and diagnostic overview.

A. Differential diagnosis.

1. *Medical disorders.*
   Many medical conditions can mimic the presentation of eating disorders. In the absence of an immediately obvious medical explanation, the diagnosis of an eating disorder is typically entertained when the presenting symptoms include loss of appetite, weight loss, or unexplained vomiting. However, in patients with eating-disordered behavior resulting from a primary medical illness, the attitudinal features of a primary eating disorder are usually absent (e.g., desire for thinness, body image distortion). In these patients, it is important to avoid ascribing the absence of these latter features to deception or denial on the part of the patient. A brief description of some important medical illnesses that may be included in the differential diagnosis of an eating disorder follow.
   a. *Inflammatory bowel diseases.* Patients with inflammatory bowel diseases may present with anorexia, weight loss, or vomiting. Diarrhea, abdominal pain, or both, are common but may be absent. Stool is often positive for gross or occult blood. *The erythrocyte sedimentation rate can nearly always discriminate between inflammatory bowel disease and eating disorders; erythrocyte sedimentation rate is increased in inflammatory bowel disease and is typically subnormal in eating disorders.*
   b. *Thyroid disease.* Hyperthyroidism causes weight loss despite adequate caloric intake. Anorexia, nausea, and vomiting may also occur. Patients generally appear to be anxious, and physical findings of hyperthyroidism are generally present, including heat intolerance, sweating, tremor, palpitations, and weakness. Goiter may or may not be appreciated.
   c. *Diabetes mellitus.* Weight loss despite polyphagia is the classic presentation of diabetes mellitus.
   d. *Central nervous system lesions.* A variety of central nervous system lesions, including tumors, may cause anorexia and weight loss because of effects on the satiety centers of the brain. Vomiting may occur when intracranial pressure is increased.
   e. *Malignancies.* Occult malignancies of any kind can cause significant unexplained weight loss, with or without accompanying anorexia.
   f. *Chronic infections.* Chronic infections, such as tuberculosis and acquired immunodeficiency syndrome, can cause weight loss and wasting.
2. *Psychiatric disorders.*
   a. *Mood disorders.* Loss of appetite and consequent loss of weight are cardinal features of depression. On the other hand, in a primary eating disorder, depression and other mood disturbances follow as a result of the malnutrition that is a defining feature of the eating disorder. *In patients presenting with both depressed mood and disordered eating, distinguishing between the primary diagnosis and the ensuing complications is sometimes difficult.* A detailed history that places the symptoms in temporal sequence may be helpful.
   b. *Obsessive-compulsive disorder.* Eating disorders are typically complicated by obsessional thinking and compulsive behavior. In some cases, however, anorexia, weight loss, or vomiting are epiphenomena of primary obsessive-compulsive disorder.

c. *Substance abuse.* Individuals with severe substance abuse problems are frequently malnourished and underweight. Undernourishment may be a direct effect of the substance use on appetite (e.g., amphetamines, cocaine) or may result from psychosocial factors.

d. *Psychotic disorders.* Frank psychosis of any cause can interfere with normal eating behavior.

B. Evaluation.

The initial evaluation of a potential eating disorder is aimed at establishing a firm diagnosis, assessing the severity of the disorder, determining the appropriateness of in-patient versus out-patient management, and identifying potentially serious medical complications.

1. *Diagnostic evaluation.*
A careful diagnostic interview should establish the presence or absence of criteria for eating disorders, including loss of weight, fear of weight gain, fat phobia, preoccupation with food, restrictive eating patterns or purging behaviors, body image distortion, out-of-control eating, and amenorrhea or menstrual irregularity. Some patients with disordered eating or eating disorders lack the capacity to accurately describe their behavior, making assessment more difficult. Additional information from family members and friends may illuminate an otherwise ambiguous case. When the typical features of eating disorders are absent, alternative medical or psychiatric diagnoses should be explored, and the possibility of denial or intentional deception should be considered. *All patients should be screened for risk of suicide, which can be present in any patient with disordered eating or eating disorders but which may be especially common in patients with bulimia nervosa.*

Other characteristics can help support the suspicion of an eating disorder: preference for eating alone, extremely limited food choices, unusual eating habits (e.g., preference for a certain spoon or bowl, eating of foods in particular order, unusual food combinations), excessive fluid intake, excessive chewing of ice or gum, or recent vegetarianism.

2. *Nutritional assessment.*
Information about eating and exercise patterns, history of weight changes or previous dieting practices, and purging behaviors should be elicited in the nutritional assessment. A careful diet history should be obtained; overall caloric intake and that of specific nutrients should be assessed. Calcium intake deserves special attention. Weight should be measured with the patient undressed and gowned. Height should be measured and body mass index calculated. *The body mass index (weight [in kilograms] divided by height [in meters] squared) more accurately reflects weight-height relationships than do traditional growth curves or standard height-weight tables, such as those provided by the Metropolitan Life Insurance Company.* Age-specific and gender-specific percentile tables for body mass index are available for adolescents and adults.

3. *Medical evaluation.*
Initial medical evaluation helps exclude other diagnoses and identifies the extent of systemic and organ-system dysfunction. Evidence of hemodynamic instability should be sought. Symptoms of orthostasis are relatively common, but syncope, presyncope, or palpitations should be viewed cautiously. Purging behaviors (vomiting, diuretic use, laxative use) all predispose to potentially dangerous electrolyte disturbances and should be quantified. Patients who deny purging should be examined for stigmata of vomiting which include parotid enlargement, soft palate lesions, dental erosions, or calluses of the knuckles (Russell's sign). *Occasional patients use syrup of ipecac to induce vomiting; this very dangerous practice, if present, must be recognized and immediately interrupted as it can very quickly lead to irreversible cardiomyopathy.*

Patients with eating disorders frequently complain of cold intolerance and cold distal extremities, fatigue, changes in mood, diminished concentration and memory, abdominal pain, and constipation.

The laboratory evaluation for patients with eating disorders contains three essential elements.

a. In patients with atypical presentations, the laboratory evaluation must be sufficient to rule out other diagnostic considerations. Depending on the specific symptoms and signs, this might include erythrocyte sedimentation rate, thyroid function studies, serum glucose level, serologic testing, or imaging studies of the head.

b. The initial laboratory evaluation should include measurement of serum electrolyte, calcium, magnesium, and phosphorus levels. Electrocardiography should be performed, and the primary care physician should look for evidence of a prolonged QT_c interval. Levels of serum protein and albumin may be depressed, but this finding offers no important therapeutic information.

c. In instances in which surreptitious vomiting is suspected, some investigators advocate the use of serum amylase determinations. Amylase levels are increased during active vomiting and return to normal within 72 hours after cessation of vomiting. When fractionated, a clear increase in the salivary isozyme is present.

III. General management guidelines.

A. Prevention.

For the primary care physician, prevention of eating disorders rests on recognizing and addressing early risk factors, screening at-risk patients, and providing prompt and effective interventions to patients identified with disordered eating before frank eating disorders supervene.

1. Early risk factors that are thought to be relevant to the development of disordered eating and eating disorders include low self-esteem, body image dissatisfaction, preceding trauma (including physical and sexual abuse), and a positive family history. Information on these risk factors should be sought routinely during health supervision visits. As noted in the beginning of this chapter, some evidence indicates that individual risk factors act cumulatively in the pathogenesis of disordered eating, making a higher index of suspicion appropriate when multiple risk factors are found.
2. Screening for symptoms of disordered eating and eating disorders should be a routine part of health supervision, particularly in at-risk patients. Formal tools are available for the assessment of eating behavior and eating attitudes; however, these are not typically used by primary care providers. Simple screening questions can help determine whether further evaluation is required (Table 18–1).
3. When early identification of disordered eating and eating disorders has resulted in appropriate intervention, better prognoses have been seen. Thus, concern over a patient's eating behavior should quickly lead to a coordinated plan that addresses the problem. "Wait-and-see" approaches are not indicated.

B. Coordinated approach.

The management of eating disorders requires an integrated, comprehensive approach that addresses the psychological, medical, and nutritional aspects of the disease. Psychiatric intervention is aimed at treating the underlying psychopathology, correcting distorted views of eating and body image, and identifying and managing comorbid psychiatric conditions. Nutritional intervention is required for assessing the current nutritional status and diet, for providing accurate nutrition information, and for providing structured dietary recommendations to patients whose own dietary judgment is nearly always severely compromised. Medical supervision is required for the identification and management of somatic disturbances of disordered eating; for guarding against life-threatening sequelae of starvation, malnutrition, and purging; and for anticipation and prevention of complications of refeeding.

1. *Team approach.*
   Ideally, the comprehensive array of services required for treating patients with eating disorders is delivered by an interdisciplinary team that includes physicians, mental health professionals, and nutritionists. In the in-patient setting, such services are best offered by eating disorder units or centers that include formal treatment protocols, especially trained nurses, and that create an overall therapeutic milieu. In the out-patient setting, similar therapeutic environments are occasionally found in day-treatment programs. More commonly, however, the team is decentralized, and patients see various providers individually who regularly communicate with each other.
2. *Limited resources.*
   In many communities, and especially in rural communities, comprehensive eating disorder programs, whether in-patient or out-patient, are unlikely to be present. In the absence of formal programs, patients are typically cared for by informal treatment teams that coalesce to care for individual patients. The composition of such ad hoc teams greatly depends on existing relationships, available community resources, local expertise, referral patterns, and reimbursement considerations. Nevertheless, *the general principles of comprehensive care and a team approach still apply and can be met through the close collaboration of local health care professionals, including the primary care provider.*

C. In-patient versus out-patient management.

The decision to hospitalize a patient for in-patient treatment of an eating disorder is influenced not only by clinical factors but also by the availability of local resources, insurance coverage, and patient or family preference. *Absolute indications for hospitalization include hemodynamic instability, significant hypovolemia, arrhythmias, congestive heart failure, cardiomyopathy, and suicidality.* Most specialists agree that once severe malnutrition has occurred, out-patient therapy is unlikely to be successful. Acute food refusal, uncontrollable binge eating or vomiting, and failure of appropriate out-patient therapy are

Table 18–1
Screening Questions for Disordered Eating or Eating Disorders

- What do you think of your weight right now? Do you think that you are too fat or that parts of your body are too fat?
- Over the past few months, has your weight been increasing, decreasing, or staying pretty much the same?
- Over the past few months, have you been on any diets or done anything else to try to control your weight?
- Have you ever felt that your eating was "out of control"?
- What do you think your perfect weight should be?
- What is the most you have ever weighed? The least?
- How would a 5-pound increase (or decrease) of weight affect you?

also indications for in-patient management. *For younger patients, early hospitalization may prevent the development of intractable symptoms and the need for repeated hospitalization.*

D. Behavioral management.

Patients with established eating disorders have dysfunctional eating habits that are deeply entrenched. These are frequently compounded by lack of insight, denial, and cognitive deficits that are attributable to malnutrition. Behavioral protocols, particularly in the in-patient setting, have been successfully used to overcome these challenges to the onset of therapy. These protocols usually include explicit written contracts, structured diets, and nutritional supplementation and activity restrictions, when necessary.

E. What to tell the patient and family.

1. Patients with eating disorders frequently resist the diagnosis and treatment recommendations, making the initial efforts of the primary care provider difficult and, at times, ineffective. The diagnosis must be stated as unambiguously as possible and supported with as much objective information as possible. Referring to standardized weight charts can be useful in calculating safe and appropriate weight for height with the patient. Explicitly connecting physical symptoms and signs to their causative malnutrition or purging can help patients overcome denial or minimization.
2. *Feelings of frustration, guilt, and helplessness often characterize families of patients with eating disorders.* Family members may blame themselves for a delay in diagnosis or for the disease itself. Family relationships may be strained because of well-intentioned but failed attempts by family members to manage the problem themselves. Some family members may be confused, frustrated, or angry with the patient for what they see is a lack of resolve or success in overcoming dysfunctional eating habits. On diagnosis, we offer families the advice listed in Table 18–2.

Table 18–2
Advice for Families

- Help to ensure that the patient receives the professional attention that he or she requires.
- Cooperate with the management plan that the professionals design.
- Once the patient is in the hands of professionals, back off! Avoid arguing, making recommendations, or getting into discussions about eating, food, or weight.
- Avoid power struggles.
- Be open, available, supportive, and a good listener. Do not make these characteristics contingent on eating or gaining weight.
- Be patient. Recovery is slow. Do not judge progress solely on the basis of eating or weight.
- Take care of yourselves. Do not let the eating disorder take over your lives too.

F. Return visits and follow-up care.

The management of eating disorders typically requires protracted efforts over a considerable period of time. Early in therapy, frequent visits are appropriate in order to foster a therapeutic alliance, to provide nutritional re-education, and to provide close medical surveillance. As progress is seen, the frequency of visits can be reduced to the level that meets the patient's psychological, nutritional, and medical needs. As treatment proceeds, it is important that members of the treatment team maintain contact with one another so that treatment barriers and setbacks can be recognized early and managed collaboratively and expectantly.

IV. Disordered eating.

A. Preclinical eating disorders and partial syndromes.

Case Study

S. is a 15-year-old high school sophomore who is brought to her primary care physician by her mother "for help with a diet." S. is of average weight for height but agrees that she would like to weigh 10 to 15 pounds less. She describes herself as not liking the way she looks and as having low self-esteem as a result. S. has tried numerous diets, has fasted for days at a time, and has recently attempted self-induced vomiting and the use of diet pills. Although she has lost 5 pounds in the past 2 months, she does not notice any difference in her appearance, nor does she feel a sense of accomplishment.

1. *Diagnosis and behavioral description.*
   Disordered eating that does not meet the criteria for formal eating disorders is both common and potentially serious. Partial syndromes resembling both anorexia nervosa and bulimia nervosa are seen. In some cases, disordered eating is simply the early presentation of a condition that will evolve into a full-blown eating disorder. In other cases, disordered eating is relatively static and does not progress in the short term. *Failure to meet criteria for anorexia nervosa or bulimia nervosa should not deter the primary care provider from offering early and aggressive intervention. This is especially true in younger patients, in whom earlier intervention is associated with a better long-term prognosis.*
2. *Risk factors.*
   The risk factors for preclinical eating disorders

are similar to those discussed under General Management Guidelines (see section III.A.1). Although less carefully studied than the risk factors for an eating disorder, the risk factors for disordered eating include body image dissatisfaction, excessive dieting, frequently skipped meals, and higher levels of overall psychological distress.

3. *Management.*
   a. *Medication.* Disordered eating is generally not treated with medication unless a primary mood or anxiety disorder complicates the clinical picture. For preclinical eating disorders that are rapidly progressive, the regimens are similar to those for anorexia nervosa and bulimia nervosa.
   b. *Counseling.* In patients with disordered eating, counseling addresses the abnormal behavior and its presumed pathogenesis. In patients with preclinical eating disorders, more intensive psychotherapy is indicated, with the intention of quickly arresting the progress of the disease.
   c. *Nutritional management.* Nutritional intervention may be particularly valuable in the patient with disordered eating whose knowledge of good nutrition is poor and whose eating behavior is still in the formative stages.

B. Athletes.

Case Study

M. is a 16-year-old runner who presents with amenorrhea. She has been running competitively for 2 years. She will compete in the state finals this year and is working toward a college scholarship in track. M. follows an increasingly strict training regimen. She has lost 12 pounds over the past 2 years and, with the encouragement of her coach, now wants to build her "lean muscle." M. had menarche at the age of 14 years but never established regular menstrual cycles. She has not had a menstrual period in over a year and wants to be sure nothing is "seriously" wrong.

1. *Diagnosis and behavioral description.*
   Success in activities and sports can be enhanced by maintenance of a lean body habitus, more so for elite participants. Carried to an extreme, some competitive athletes develop disordered eating as a functional behavior in an effort to excel. Disordered eating most typically resembles anorexia nervosa and is characterized by caloric and nutrient restriction and weight loss. Purging behaviors can also be seen.

2. *Risk factors.*
   Athletes who begin training earlier are at higher risk for disordered eating. Gymnasts, ballet dancers, runners, and wrestlers, particularly the most highly competitive, are especially vulnerable. Disordered eating may be triggered or reinforced when the expectations of parents, coaches, trainers, and peers exceed the current ability or performance of the individual. A sudden increase in training intensity may be a marker for individuals at higher risk to develop disordered eating.

3. *Management.*
   a. *Medication.* Pharmacologic therapy is generally not indicated, except in the management of comorbid psychiatric disease.
   b. *Counseling.* Athletic success must be placed in its proper context and not be accepted as legitimate grounds for dangerous eating behavior.
   c. *Nutritional management.* Nutritional counseling should be oriented toward providing a diet appropriate to the demands of the specific sport's activity level. The patient's drive to improve performance may improve receptivity to credible nutrition advice.

C. Young patients.

Case Study

K. is an 11-year-old girl who is brought to see her primary physician by her mother because of concerns about her eating. Over the past 8 months, K. has eaten fewer and fewer foods. She counts fat grams, has become vegetarian, and has developed a nearly obsessional preoccupation with "healthy eating." Her parents were supportive at first but became concerned over time as K.'s eating habits became more and more extreme. When interviewed, K. denies any weight and body image concerns or any intention to lose weight. She is defensive about her eating habits and finds it difficult to understand why others object to her healthy eating habits.

1. *Diagnosis and behavioral description.*
   The youngest patients with disordered eating—those who present prepubertally or peripubertally—usually present with an anorexia nervosa-like picture. They have proportionately lower weights and are more likely to be depressed. Bulimia nervosa is rare.

2. *Risk factors.*
   Pubertal onset seems to be the most consistent risk factor for disordered eating. It is hypothesized that these patients are more anxious about, and respond more negatively to, the normal changes in body habitus and fat distribution that occur with pubertal development.

3. *Management.*
   a. *Medication.* Little information exists to guide pharmacotherapy in this patient subgroup. Comorbid depression or anxiety disorders are treated with appropriate therapeutic regimens.
   b. *Counseling.* Special effort should be made to diagnose and treat patients early because this has been associated with a better prognosis. Family issues are likely to be especially im-

portant in younger patients, and hence, not unexpectedly, family therapy has been shown to improve long-term remission rates.

c. *Nutritional management.* Nutritional counseling is necessary in order to correct misinformation or misunderstanding and must be matched to the developmental abilities of the patient. Younger patients are liable to be more concrete in their thinking and to require and tolerate more structure in the implementation of dietary recommendations.

D. Male patients.

Case Study

M. is a 12-year-old boy being evaluated for persistent vomiting. Vomiting began when M. joined the swim team and was initially attributed to "nerves." However, vomiting continued once the swimming season ended. He has lost 9 pounds. A comprehensive medical assessment has failed to reveal any obvious organic explanation for M.'s symptoms. During the interview, M. confides how much better he thinks he looks as a result of his weight loss.

1. *Diagnosis and behavioral description.*
Although eating disorders are much more frequently seen in female patients (approximate female-to-male ratio of ≥ 10:1), *both anorexia nervosa and bulimia nervosa are seen in male patients as well.* In males, anorexia nervosa is far more common than bulimia nervosa, and in these patients, the syndrome resembles that seen in females. Overexercise is felt to be particularly common, as are binging and purging. Depressed mood and affective disorders are also common.

2. *Risk factors.*
Premorbid obsessional behavior is common. Parental psychopathology is also commonly noted. Some studies have indicated that homosexual men are at increased risk.

3. *Management.*
Because of the infrequency of eating disorders in male patients, establishing an unambiguous diagnosis is essential to proper management. The older the patient, the less likely it is that the eating disorder is the primary diagnosis. Relatively little is known about the treatment of male patients with eating disorders. Patients are treated empirically by use of the same protocols as in female patients, with special attention being paid to the role of overexercise.

V. Anorexia nervosa.

Case Study

E. is a 19-year-old woman who is seen by her primary care physician after a syncopal episode in the shower. E. began losing weight after beginning college and has lost nearly 40 pounds over the past 18 months. She is proud of her weight loss but still feels overweight and would like to lose 5 more pounds. Friends comment frequently on her thinness, but she has always considered these comments to be well-intentioned "white lies" designed to spare her feelings. On questioning, she reveals that symptoms of orthostasis have been present for months, and frequent presyncopal episodes have occurred. Confronted about the possibility of an eating disorder, E. is concerned that treatment of any kind will interfere with her studies and compromise her academic performance.

A. Diagnosis and behavioral description.

The hallmark clinical features of the patient with anorexia nervosa include refusal to maintain body weight at an appropriate level for age and height, coupled with an obsessive pursuit of thinness and a dramatic increase in physical activity, along with (in females) a cessation of menses. Associated symptoms include an irrational fear of gaining weight and a perception that one is grossly overweight, even though one is emaciated. A key psychological theme is often a struggle for personal autonomy, with the body remaining as the only area in which the patient feels successful in asserting himself or herself.

In current psychiatric nosology, two subtypes of anorexia nervosa are recognized: the restricting subtype and the binge eating/purging subtype. At present, nearly two thirds of most case series are represented by the latter form of anorexia nervosa, which may also present with more impulsive personality features and a higher risk for concurrent substance abuse and suicidality. In most cases, the age of onset is in adolescence, with a peak occurring during peripubertal years and again during the patient's first year away from home. The period of onset may influence the psychological themes that predominate (e.g., maturational avoidance versus separation issues).

In patients with anorexia nervosa, a range of concurrent psychopathology is commonly present that is sometimes persistent and severe enough to merit an additional diagnostic label. These associated psychiatric conditions may include major depression, anxiety disorders, obsessive-compulsive disorder (with evident obsessional activity in domains other than food and weight), and substance abuse. Proper identification of these disorders may be of particular use in treatment planning because strong evidence suggesting a true primary comorbid condition, as contrasted with malnutrition-induced psychiatric symptoms, may call for a more aggressive approach with pharmacotherapy early in treatment.

B. Risk factors.

The classic view of anorexia, which implicates a dysfunctional early relationship with the mother as the key underpinning for the development of the illness in later childhood and early adulthood, is now recognized as an oversimplification.

Anorexia nervosa is a multidetermined illness. Familial factors appear to play a role, and some of these factors are genetic. However, familial risk may increase with an impoverished psychosocial environment during early development and a history of physical or sexual trauma. As noted in previous sections, many of these familial factors may lead to an increased risk for psychiatric illness in general. Personality factors, such as perfectionism, obsessionality, or intolerance of ambiguity, appear to contribute to the patient's vulnerability. These personality attributes may be genetically determined, or may be encouraged by parental influence, or both. A poor feeding history is often obtained; however, the specific contribution of this factor to the ultimate development of the disorder is unknown. A family or personal history of obesity may increase the vulnerability. The contribution of occupational or athletic roles as risk factors for anorexia nervosa has been discussed elsewhere in this chapter (see section IV.B).

C. Management.

1. *Medication.*
   Many different medication classes have been tried, all unsuccessfully, as primary treatments for anorexia nervosa. These pharmacologic approaches have been driven by varying views of the relationship of anorexia nervosa to other known psychiatric illness. For instance, the avoidance of food and the distortions of body image perception may have a nearly delusional quality at times. Although antipsychotic drug therapy may consequently appear to make logical sense, little evidence suggests any sustained effect, aside from reduction of disabling anxiety symptoms in some instances. Similar reasoning underlies the use of antianxiety and antidepressant agents (i.e., because of the theory that eating disorders are variant forms of anxiety or depressive disorders). Indeed, in some instances, the use of medications may aggravate the symptomatic distress of the illness by increasing the patient's sense of loss of autonomy.

   Although no clearly efficacious medication therapy exists for this illness at present, investigators have recently shown interest in the use of the selective serotonin reuptake inhibitors (e.g., fluoxetine [Prozac], paroxetine [Paxil], sertraline [Zoloft]) as prophylactic agents for recurrence of symptoms after weight restoration. Further work is needed before specific treatment recommendations can be provided; therefore, the use of these medications must be seen as provisional at this time.

2. *Counseling.*
   Psychotherapeutic approaches are a mainstay of the treatment of anorexia nervosa. Two principal, and related, forms of psychotherapy have been evaluated in treatment studies: behavior modification and cognitive behavior therapy. The former is primarily used in the in-patient treatment of anorexia nervosa, and the latter can be adapted for use in both in-patient and out-patient settings. These psychotherapeutic approaches are specialized techniques that because of their labor-intensive nature, are usually not part of the strategies used by the primary care clinician. Nevertheless, several aspects of these techniques are relevant because they may inform a general attitude of dealing with the patient with an eating disorder. Both strategies fundamentally assume that the patient is interested in his or her own recovery, even though the patient may not always be conscious of this interest. In other words, it is important to meet the patient on his or her own terms in the recovery process. The treatment must be conducted in collaborative fashion. At the same time, another underlying assumption of these approaches is that for genuine progress to occur, the patient must be willing to challenge the fears and underlying distorted beliefs that facilitate the persistence of the illness. The patient must be willing to engage in new behaviors that may be frightening or overwhelming. An empathic, consistent posture on the part of the treating clinician is essential to the successful implementation of these approaches.

   Two other types of psychotherapeutic techniques have been studied in patients with anorexia nervosa. The first type is family therapy, which has been shown to be specifically useful in the younger patient who is still living at home with parents. The second type is group therapy. The latter technique can be particularly helpful in making it easier for patients to experiment with new ideas (e.g., that they are not, in fact, overweight) as they see others struggling with the same issues. Usually, unstructured forms of psychodynamic therapy are helpful only in the latter stages of treatment, when the patient's more disabling eating symptoms have been brought under control and the patient is prepared for these more sophisticated psychotherapy techniques.

3. *Nutritional management.*
   The ideal treatment arrangement for a patient with an eating disorder uses the early and aggressive involvement of a nutrition therapist. This individual is specifically skilled in the implementation of structured meal planning with defined caloric targets, nutrient selections, and weight restoration goals. This nutritionist is also familiar with the basic aspects of cognitive behavior therapy and uses these techniques to assist in changing the patient's dysfunctional eating behaviors. The ultimate goal of this intervention is to assist the patient in relearning normal eating habits. This is accomplished in a col-

laborative fashion with the patient, and the patient is empathically helped to eliminate abnormal eating behaviors and to replace them with appropriate eating habits. An exchange system of nutrient selection is frequently used to devise a working meal plan.

VI. Bulimia nervosa.

Case Study

Ms. S. is a 23-year-old dental student with a 5-year history of vomiting after meals. Her roommate recently disclosed Ms. S.'s behavior to her parents, and they have insisted that she make this appointment. Ms. S. describes frequent binge eating and eating that is "out of control." Her behavior causes considerable guilt, and she makes frequent self-deprecating comments throughout the interview. She expresses surprise when eating disorders are discussed because her weight is "normal."

A. Diagnosis and behavioral description.

The hallmark characteristics of a patient with bulimia nervosa are the presence of binge eating accompanied by strategies designed to rid the body of the unwanted calories ingested during the binge. Binge eating is a discrete behavior with definite period of onset and offset, usually less than 2 hours in duration. The binge has a distinctly uncomfortable and compulsive quality for the patient. The urge to binge is profound, and attempts to prevent it often lead to intolerable levels of anxiety and agitation. During the episode, the patient feels out of control of his or her behavior. Purging behavior may ensue nearly immediately after the binge ceases. One of the more common methods of purging is self-induced vomiting (e.g., manually induced or with the assistance of syrup of ipecac), but laxatives, diuretics, vigorous exercising, prolonged episodes of fasting, or enemas are also often used. A frequently reported pattern of behavior is sustained food restriction during the daytime hours, with binge eating occurring in association with attempts to eat a normal meal in the evening. In addition to these behaviors, a patient with bulimia nervosa is unduly concerned with body shape or weight for the maintenance of self-esteem.

B. Risk factors.

The most important proximate risk factor for binge eating and purging is dieting or restrained eating, particularly the reduction of dietary fat. Dietary fat is an essential signal for satiety. The absence of this input leads to a distorted regulation of hunger and satiety signals and leads to the increased urge to overeat or to frank binge eating behavior. Addressing this issue alone is of immense clinical value.

Bulimia nervosa shares many of the risk factors of anorexia nervosa. A history of obesity in the patient or family may arguably be of more significance as a risk factor for bulimia nervosa than for anorexia nervosa.

C. Management

1. *Medication.*
   Unlike in anorexia nervosa, several randomized controlled trials have clearly demonstrated the efficacy of antidepressant medications as adjuncts in the treatment of patients with bulimia nervosa. Both tricyclic antidepressants and the newer selective serotonin reuptake inhibitors are helpful. The crucial issue, however, is the word "adjunct." Without the implementation of a coherent and broad-based approach that addresses dysfunctional eating behaviors and distorted attitudes toward weight and body image, the effect of antidepressant medication is unlikely to be sustained beyond 6 to 9 months.
2. *Counseling.*
   The recommendations for therapy outlined earlier for anorexia nervosa can be echoed here as well. This type of counseling approach, if available, should be enthusiastically encouraged. Formal controlled trials of cognitive behavior therapy have clearly shown enduring success in the treatment of patients with bulimia nervosa. Specific targets for behavioral change are initially directed at normalizing eating behavior patterns in order to reduce the risk for binge eating episodes. Strategies directed at averting binge eating episodes may be used. Later in treatment, psychological issues related to body image, self-esteem, and weight may be usefully addressed.
3. *Nutritional management.*
   The recommendations for early and aggressive involvement of a nutrition therapist in the treatment of a patient with bulimia nervosa should be emphasized. As with the anorexic patient, a structured meal planning system is implemented, in the context of an overall program of cognitive behavior therapy.

VII. Medical complications.

A. General.

In most cases, the medical management of patients with eating disorders is the responsibility of the patient's primary care physician. Specialized eating disorder programs may have their own medical specialists, but only a small number of patients with disordered eating and eating disorders are cared for in such programs.

Medical complications are both common and potentially dangerous. Any organ system can be affected. Because patients with eating disorders are so often reluctant to reveal their symptoms, providers must be vigilant for early signs of organ system dysfunction or failure. Furthermore, many of the most serious medical complications of eating disorders may present suddenly and without warning—and sometimes with catastrophic consequences. A high index of suspicion and frequent and careful medical surveillance are essential.

B. Systemic.

Malnutrition leads to a decreased metabolic rate and an inability to maintain body temperature. Patients are intolerant to cold and report particularly having cold hands and feet. Their energy level is low, and they are chronically fatigued.

During refeeding, the calculated caloric requirement may in practice be excessive as a result of the lower resting metabolic rate.

C. Cognitive.

Cognitive impairment is demonstrable from formal neuropsychological testing and affects concentration, memory, problem solving, and motor function. Structural brain changes are seen with computed tomography. The causes of these changes are uncertain, but they presumably arise as a direct effect of malnutrition because they resolve with restoration of normal nutritional status. Depressive mood changes, irritability, and psychomotor retardation are also seen. A roughly linear relationship exists between the extent of malnutrition and the cognitive and affective changes; refeeding corrects these effects.

D. Cardiovascular.

Cardiovascular changes are nearly universal complications of anorexia nervosa. Bradycardia occurs as a consequence of decreased basal metabolic rate. Patients may remain asymptomatic despite heart rates in the 40s and 30s. Hypotension and orthostatic blood pressure changes are also common and also may not cause symptoms.

Electrocardiographic findings include prolongation of the QRS complex and the PR interval, and nonspecific ST segment changes. ST segment elevations that mimic myocardial ischemia are sometimes seen and are not associated with other evidence of ischemia. These resolve with refeeding. Patients with eating disorders who purge, especially those with hypokalemia or hypomagnesemia, *may have prolongation of the* QT_c *interval, which has been associated with an increased risk of sudden cardiac death.*

In anorexia nervosa, cardiac adaptation to diminished cardiac output may lead to a functional mitral valve prolapse with characteristic auscultory and echocardiographic findings.

During refeeding, congestive heart failure may be seen if rapid expansion of the circulating volume overwhelms the cardiovascular system's ability to adapt—the so-called *refeeding syndrome.* Irreversible cardiomyopathy may be caused by even limited use of syrup of ipecac to induce vomiting.

E. Gastrointestinal.

In patients who induce vomiting, gastroesophogeal reflux, upper gastrointestinal bleeding, and Mallory-Weiss tears of the esophagus may occur. In calorie-restricting patients, gastric emptying time and total gastrointestinal transit time both decrease, resulting in early satiety, bloating, and abdominal pain. Constipation is common. Although gastrointestinal symptoms usually improve with refeeding, their ultimate resolution lags well behind the restoration of normal body weight or the cessation of binge eating and purging. This is important to remember because persistent gastrointestinal discomfort may be a risk factor for early relapse.

Mild increases in serum transaminase levels are common. True hepatitis and pancreatitis can also occur but are rare.

Rare but lethal complications of refeeding include esophageal rupture and gastric rupture. Both are heralded by excruciating postprandial pain and signs of an acute abdomen. Mortality is high without immediate diagnosis and emergent surgical intervention.

F. Fluid and electrolyte levels.

Dehydration is common as a result of fluid restriction. Other patients drink excessive quantities of water, tea, or diet soft drinks in place of food, or they water load before medical visits so as to appear to weigh more than they do.

In patients who vomit, loss of hydrochloric acid results in a hypochloremic metabolic alkalosis. *Unexplained hypochloremia should alert the clinician to the likelihood of surreptitious vomiting.* In patients who abuse laxatives, loss of stool bicarbonate results in a hyperchloremic metabolic acidosis. In patients who purge by use of vomiting or laxatives, secondary hyperaldosteronism and renal compensatory mechanisms result in sodium retention at the expense of potassium, potassium depletion, eventual hypokalemia, and increased risk for cardiac arrhythmias. *Even mild serum hypokalemia already indicates significant total body potassium loss because of the likelihood of daily or near-daily purging.* Replacement therapy is required but should not be considered to be a substitute for treatment of the underlying eating disorder.

Hypomagnesemia and hypocalcemia are significant findings and also may necessitate replacement therapy. Hypophosphatemia is seen more often during refeeding of very underweight patients and may be life threatening.

G. Endocrinologic manifestations.

In anorexia nervosa, amenorrhea (primary or secondary) occurs as a result of hypothalamic dysfunction, loss of hormonal cycling, and hypoestrogenemia. The pattern of gonadotropin-releasing hormone secretion has been shown to revert to a prepubertal pattern, which is corrected by refeeding. In up to 20% of patients, amenorrhea precedes significant weight loss and may persist for some time after the underweight state is resolved. Hypoestrogenemia compromises skeletal mass, reduces bone mineral density, and increases risk for stress fractures.

Euthyroid sick syndrome occurs frequently in both underweight and normal weight patients with eating disorders and is characterized by decreased levels of thyroxine, decreased levels of triiodothyronine, increased levels of reverse thyroxine, and normal levels of thyroid-stimulating hormone. *Supplemental thyroid hormone therapy is not indicated.*

Growth hormone secretion declines during the active phases of the disease and, in younger patients, results in growth retardation. Growth resumes with refeeding, and catch-up growth is possible.

H. Integument.

Skin becomes dry and scaly and may develop "dirty skin dermatitis." Lanugo hair develops. Nails become brittle and crack and break. Vomiting produces caries on the lingual surfaces of teeth. The increase in caries occurs because gastric acid has a direct effect on the dental enamel and also because the persistent change in oral pH increases the relative proportion of cariogenic flora present in the mouth. Tongue, gingival, and other mucosal changes can be seen as a result of trauma (vomiting), malnutrition, or vitamin deficiencies.

VIII. When to refer.

Any patient who meets the criteria for an eating disorder, and for whom medical hospitalization is indicated, requires immediate referral. Once the acute medical situation has stabilized, care should continue to be provided by specialists in the care of eating disorders.

Any patient who meets the criteria for anorexia nervosa or bulimia nervosa should be referred to a specialist in the care of eating disorders. The primary care provider may continue to provide medical surveillance and manage medical complications, with consultation as appropriate.

Patients with disordered eating, especially those who are young, are vulnerable to progress to full-blown eating disorders. The decision to refer such patients is determined on a case-by-case basis, depending on the duration and the severity of the symptoms, the availability of resources, and the preferences of the provider, the patient, and the family.

IX. Prognosis.

Eating disorders are challenging illnesses to treat. The multisystem involvement of the diseases forces the clinician to think in an integrative fashion, and the initial resistance to therapeutic intervention may appear to be an insurmountable hurdle to the successful resolution of the illness. Nevertheless, when a treatment alliance can be formed early in the evaluation and sustained, collaborative effort is applied, the long-term outcome can be positive. However, even in the best of clinical hands, the relapse rate for these illnesses can be high. A more useful approach would be to acknowledge the reality of this risk and to aim to develop appropriate early responses to signs of disease recurrence rather than to give the patient an unrealistic view of the usual clinical course.

The key role for a primary care physician in the treatment of a patient with an eating disorder is underscored by the fact that early intervention is crucial. Ideally, if truly empathic and knowledgeable preventive strategies can be instituted before chronicity and entrenched dysfunctional eating behaviors develop, the long-term outcome may be encouraging.

Suggested Reading

American Dietetic Association. Nutrition intervention in the management of anorexia nervosa, bulimia nervosa, and binge eating. J Am Diet Assoc 1994; 94:902–907.

Fisher M, Golden NH, Katzman DK, et al. Eating disorders in adolescents. J Adolesc Health 1995; 16:420–437.

Society for Adolescent Medicine. Eating disorders in adolescents: Position paper. J Adolesc Health 1995; 16:476–480.

Yager J, Anderson A, Devlin M, et al. Practice guideline for eating disorders. Am J Psychiatry 1993; 150:207–228.

DAVID E. SCHTEINGART, MD

GLORIA J. EDWARDS, PhD

MONICA N. STARKMAN, MD

Obesity

Obesity is defined as an excess of body fat; this condition is associated with significant morbidity. Because of its prevalence, especially in the United States, obesity is a serious medical problem. Genetic, biologic, and behavioral factors contribute to its development.

The chief criteria for the classification of human obesity typically include age of onset and family history of obesity, degree of overweight, adipose tissue morphology, and distribution of body fat. Based on the age of onset of obesity and the characteristics of the adipose tissue, obesity is classified as juvenile-onset and adult-onset types. Patients with juvenile-onset obesity have increased cellularity of their adipose tissue, are likely to attain severe degrees of fatness, and are resistant to therapeutic intervention. In contrast, those with adult-onset obesity have hypertrophy of fat cells with mild or moderate obesity, or they have combinations of hypertrophy and hyperplasia if the obesity is severe. In addition, they are more likely to develop hypercholesterolemia, hypertriglyceridemia, and non–insulin-dependent diabetes. These patients are more able than those with juvenile onset obesity to lose weight and to maintain the weight loss for long periods. Based on the degree of overweight, people who are 20% to 40% overweight are considered to be mildly obese; those who are 41% to 100% overweight are moderately obese, and those more than 100% overweight are severely or morbidly obese. Based on the patients' somatotypes, obesity can be classified into abdominal, or upper body, and gluteofemoral, or lower body, types. Patients with abdominal obesity are at higher risk for metabolic and cardiovascular complications.

I. Evaluation and diagnostic overview.

The evaluation begins with a comprehensive clinical history:

A. Weight history.

Information should be obtained about the patient's weight milestones, including weight at birth: during early and late childhood; at the end of grade school, high school, and college; and at the beginning of marriage. In addition, knowledge of the patient's weight over the previous year determines if the obesity is in a stable or a dynamic phase.

B. Family history.

A strong family history of obesity may indicate genetic factors as well as social pressures for the patient not to lose weight because obesity is a factor of familial identity for some people.

C. Diet history.

A complete diet history involves assessment not only of the type of food consumed but also of the characteristics of the patient's eating habits. This information should be obtained by means of a diet diary. The diet is frequently excessive in calories, saturated fat, and refined sugars and is deficient in vitamins, calcium, and other micronutrients. Patients may fail to eat breakfast or lunch, eat large dinners, continue to snack through the evening or nibble between meals. Some patients engage in bingeing, at which time they consume large quantities of food. Information about the environment in which the patient eats may provide insight into the patient's eating habits that might be changed with appropriate behavior modification approaches. Alcohol may account for excessive caloric intake in patients who otherwise consume moderate amounts of food.

D. Weight reduction attempts.

The patient's previous weight reduction attempts should be described in detail, including the motivation to lose weight and the reasons for failure. Some patients are concerned about their appearance and social limitations and their ability to obtain employment and maintain satisfactory relationships, whereas others seek help because of family pressures to lose weight or because they have been advised by their physician to lose weight to improve their health.

E. Psychosocial history.

A brief psychosocial history should be obtained in order to determine if the patient has significant psychopathology that necessitates referral to a health care professional for further evaluation and management. In addition, some key information may help identify significant barriers for success with weight reduction and help assess the availability of a support system.

The patient's early experiences may be relevant, particularly when physical or emotional abuse, emotional deprivation, and disrupted family structure have occurred. In such cases, psychotherapy may be necessary. Major psychiatric illness, such as depressive disorder and anxiety, may provide a background in which the weight gain has occurred. Continued social and emotional dependence on family members may serve as indicators that weight loss may be difficult. Conversely, the patient's education, ability to gain employment, and ability to succeed in their personal lives give clues as to the patient's overall coping ability.

Obesity may provide advantages: a sense of power and an excuse from interpersonal involvement, from participation in challenging activities, and from sexual involvement. The balance between the disadvantages of being obese and the secondary gains derived from obesity determines the patient's successful involvement with a weight reduction effort.

The marital status or relationship with the partner should be explored. Particularly relevant are the partner's weight and the ability of the partner to encourage the patient's weight reduction effort. Occasionally, patients receive mixed signals from their partners, who may both look forward to the reduction yet fear that weight loss will cause changes in the marital relationship. Under these circumstances, the partner may sabotage the patient's attempts and induce the patient to eat by tempting the patient with fattening foods. A supportive family, in contrast, can greatly improve the patient's weight reduction effort.

An eating disorder, such as anorexia nervosa, with repeated episodes of severe dieting and starvation or bulimia, may be present and may influence the course of body weight.

F. Associated medical complications.

In evaluating the medical history of a patient with obesity, the primary care physician should assess whether (1) the obesity is a manifestation of an underlying medical or metabolic disease and (2) associated medical and metabolic complications exist. Obese patients who present with hypertension, diabetes, hirsutism, irregular menses or amenorrhea, and red striae should be investigated for Cushing's syndrome by appropriate laboratory procedures. Hypothalamic lesions, such as craniopharyngiomas, optic nerve gliomas, astrocytomas, pinealomas, eosinophilic granulomas, and pituitary tumors with suprasellar extension, may be associated with overeating without satiation and obesity. Usually, such patients exhibit other manifestations of hypothalamic disease, including diabetes insipidus, galactorrhea, hypopituitarism, sleep disturbance, vasomotor instability, and sham rage, as well as visual field impairment with involvement of the optic chiasm. Most obese patients do not have hypothyroidism, and most patients with hypothyroidism are not obese. If symptoms of hypothyroidism are present, patients should be evaluated with thyroid function tests, and if the diagnosis is confirmed, a trial of thyroxine for 3 months should precede any weight reduction program. A detailed history should be obtained in order to determine the presence of medical and metabolic complications, including hypertension, angina and myocardial infarctions, diabetes mellitus, insomnia, loud snoring, episodes of sleep apnea, upper abdominal pain, intolerance for fatty foods and previous evidence of gallbladder disease.

G. Physical examinations.

The degree of obesity should be determined by: (1) inspection; (2) measurement of height and weight, with calculation of body mass index (BMI); (3) measurement of skinfold thickness either by pinching with fingers or with calipers; and (4) estimation of body fat by techniques such as underwater weighing in a densitometric pool, bioelectric impedance plethysmography, ultrasound scanning, computed tomography, or dual-photon absorptiometry. These techniques require referral to specialized laboratories. BMI is calculated with the weight in kilograms and the height in meters by use of the following formula: weight/height^2. Based on the BMI at which risk of increased mortality begins to rise, a healthy weight should be associated with a BMI of less than 27.8 for males and less than 27.3 for females. A greater BMI is associated with an increasing risk. Skinfold thickness should be measured with calipers at four separate sites (usually the biceps, triceps, subscapular and suprailiac areas). Obesity is defined as triceps plus subscapular skinfold thickness of greater than 45 mm in males and greater than 69 mm in females. Measurement of the waist and hip circumference should be made in order to determine the waist-to-hip ratio, a value that is useful in determining the risk for metabolic and cardiovascular complications.

The examination of patients who are severely obese may be difficult. Auscultation of the lungs and heart frequently reveals distant sounds because of the subcutaneous fat. Examination of the abdomen may be difficult, and underlying pathology, such as hepatomegaly and palpable abdominal masses, may not be easily felt because of the large abdominal panniculus. Obese women commonly present with hirsutism and acne.

Hyperpigmentation of the skin over the neck and axilla may be present. In those areas, the skin may be thicker and have a velvet appearance consistent with acanthosis nigricans. Obese women often have intertriginous dermatitis under the breasts and abdominal panniculus. Candida infection can be detected in these sites. Large umbilical hernias are common and should be defined during the abdominal examination. Stasis dermatitis and stasis edema in the lower extremities are commonly noted. The skin is thick and hyperpigmented with superficial varicosities and hemosiderin staining. Measurement of blood pressure in obese patients may require special precautions. Large adult cuffs or thigh cuffs are needed for the accurate estimation of blood pressure in patients with an arm circumference that is at least 35 cm, with a BMI that is at least 34, or with a weight that is at least 95 kg. In these patients, the finding of high blood pressure or borderline hypertension is two times greater with standard cuffs than with a larger cuff. For patients with smaller dimensions, no significant difference appears to exist between measurements made with different cuffs. Large cuffs usually have dimensions of 15 × 43 cm, whereas the dimensions of standard cuffs are 12 × 35 cm. Not only may the diameter of the arm be large, but a conical shape also may make the fitting of the blood pressure cuff around the arm most difficult. Examination of genitalia in men may require that the prepubic fat tissue be pulled upward in order to bring out the penis, which is occasionally hidden within the surrounding prepubic fat. In women, pelvic examinations may be difficult, particularly when one attempts to define adnexal size.

H. Relevant laboratory orders.

A general biochemical evaluation should include a fasting blood glucose level and a 2-hour postprandial blood glucose; a glycosylated hemoglobin or a 3-hour glucose tolerance test. In patients with impaired glucose tolerance or mild diabetes who do not receive insulin or oral hypoglycemic agents, serum insulin levels are useful. The presence of normal or increased serum insulin levels with a peak response to oral glucose of greater than 60 μu/mL indicates substantial islet cell reserve and possible normalization of blood glucose levels with diet restriction and weight reduction. The biochemical studies should include measurement of serum levels of uric acid, hepatic enzymes, total cholesterol, high-density lipoprotein cholesterol, and triglycerides. Hormonal studies should be obtained if they are clinically indicated. In severely obese people, the physical examination may need to be supplemented with appropriate imaging procedures. Ultrasonography and computed tomography help define intra-abdominal pathology.

I. Assessment of health risk status for weight loss.

Assessment of health risk status for weight loss determines the need for medical supervision during weight reduction. Patients should be classified by health status into three categories:

1. *Low risk:* moderate obesity (< 100% greater than ideal body weight) with no known health problems that require medical monitoring or supervision during weight loss.
2. *Moderate risk:* Severe obesity (> 100% greater than ideal body weight) or medical conditions that could be aggravated or complicated during weight loss treatment. This may include drug therapy and conditions that limit the use of certain diets or physical exercise. Medical monitoring is recommended.
3. *High risk:* Severe, life-threatening conditions necessitating direct medical supervision during treatment. High-risk patients usually have morbid obesity complicated by cardiovascular, pulmonary, or metabolic disease.

II. Epidemiology and pathophysiology.

A. Prevalence.

A National Center for Health Statistics large-scale study in 1981 indicated that 26% of American adults (about 34 million) are considered to be overweight. Among these, approximately 12 million individuals are heavy enough to be classified as severely overweight.

The *incidence of obesity* in the United States is increasing, and particularly large increases are noted in children and adolescents. Gender, age, race, and poverty status influence the prevalence of obesity. Fewer men than women are obese, and in men, overweight increases up to 55 years of age and then declines. For women, the prevalence of obesity increases steadily up to 65 years of age and then levels off. Excess body weight is 7 to 12 times more common in women from lower social classes than in women from upper social classes. The prevalence of obesity at all ages is much higher in black women than in white women. Between the ages of 45 and 54 years, the prevalence of obesity in black women exceeds 60%, an amount double that of white women in the same age group. Across all age groups, the prevalence of obesity is slightly higher for men living above the poverty line than for those living below it. Independent of race, women living below the poverty line show a dramatically higher prevalence of obesity than those living above it.

B. Morbidity associated with obesity.

Hypertension is three to five times more likely to occur in obese than in nonobese individuals, hypercholesterolemia is twice more likely to occur, diabetes three times more likely, and endometrial cancer five times more likely. Atherosclerotic cardiovascular disease and gallbladder disease are also seen more commonly in obese patients than in nonobese patients. Although hypertension, hyperlipoproteinemia, and diabetes are risk factors for atherogenesis and increased prevalence of ischemic heart disease in obese people, obesity is by itself an independent risk factor, particularly in individuals who have been obese for more than 20 years. Cholelithiasis is more common in obese people, particularly in older women with multiparity and numerous episodes of weight loss and weight gain. Obese women experience endocrine abnormalities. Increased mortality from cancer is seen in obese people: colon, rectal, and prostate cancer in men; cancer of the gallbladder, breast, cervix, endometrium, uterus, and ovary in women. The regional pattern of fat distribution is also significant. A relationship exists between abdominal and visceral adiposity and insulin resistance and hyperlipoproteinemia.

Obese people frequently complain of pain in the lumbosacral area, hips, knees, and ankles. It has been assumed that excessive weight is a factor in promoting joint degeneration, and it is invariably recommended that obese patients with osteoarthrosis lose weight. The frequency and severity of symptoms of osteoarthrosis appear to be greatest in people with severe obesity.

Although obesity is associated with increased morbidity and mortality, weight reduction has a beneficial effect. It decreases blood pressure and levels of blood cholesterol and triglycerides, blood glucose, and uric acid. It has been estimated that if everyone were at ideal body weight, there would be a 25% lower incidence of coronary heart disease and a 35% lower incidence of heart failure and brain infarction. Weight reduction commonly improves complaints related to the musculoskeletal system because the mechanical stress on the weight-bearing joints can be significantly relieved, even by limited weight reduction.

C. Factors involved in the etiology of obesity.

Obesity is a condition of multifactorial etiology in which genetic, biobehavioral, and psychosocial factors contribute to energy imbalance. The relative significance of these factors likely varies widely among obese people.

Some studies suggest that family environment is far more important than heredity in determining the percentage of overweight in adults. Other studies, however, suggest that obesity is genetically determined. Treatment efforts should be directed to individuals with the highest genetic risk for developing obesity. For example, 80% of the offspring of two obese parents become obese, compared with no more than 14% of the offspring of two parents of normal weight. Combinations of diet control and increased physical activity may help control the weight of people with a genetic predisposition to obesity.

More recently, the gene responsible for obesity in genetically obese ob/ob mice has been identified. Normally, this gene, located in adipocytes, expresses a protein (leptin) that acts as a feedback signal on the brain to modulate the level of food intake. Genetically obese mice have a deficient expression of this protein. Leptin has also been found in human subjects, but the role it may play in human obesity remains to be determined.

Although excessive caloric intake must be a causal factor in obesity, epidemiologic survey data typically fail to show that within a population, those who are the most obese eat the most. It is likely that the techniques for obtaining these data are inaccurate and that the true caloric intake is higher than that reported by patients. Recent studies under controlled conditions have shown that obese people underestimate their calorie intake by at least 50%. If obese people overeat, the reasons are probably both biologic and psychological. On the one hand, the internal signals that govern hunger, satiety, and appetite operate automatically and may be abnormal in obesity. On the other hand, feeding behavior may be initiated voluntarily by external factors, including availability, preparation and palatability of foods, and social setting and pressures under which food is ingested. Direct observation in controlled settings indicates that obese people fail to decrease their food intake with age, fail to compensate their intake for changes in the caloric concentration of food ingested, and choose more food and eat more frequently and faster than nonobese people.

Alternatively, obese patients may suffer from diminished energy expenditure (thermogenesis), making a "normal" food intake excessive for that individual's caloric expenditure. A study of 24-hour energy expenditure shows that people with a tendency to gain weight have low values. The decreased thermogenesis observed in human obesity has not been clearly explained.

Psychosocial factors can be prominent in the development of obesity in some patients. Obese children have been found to be more emotionally disturbed than nonobese children and to have more disturbed relationships with their parents. Food may be offered to children for non-nutritional reasons, as an expression of affection and devotion. As a result of faulty learning experiences in childhood, children become unable to correctly identify internal signals that indicate hunger and satiety. Early associations between relief from emotional discomfort and food become firmly established. If a child is fed whenever he or she becomes restless or frightened, eating may become established as a component of social support, and feelings of security may become dependent on the eating situation. Receiving love and receiving nourishment may become confused with each other. More obese than nonobese patients come from homes in which food is associated with punishment and reward or where they report they had been given "too much" to eat. If parents are obese, an environment is often created in which everybody, obese or thin, is encouraged to eat. However, eating as a strategy for dealing with fear and anxiety can develop at any point in life. In obese adult patients, anxiety and depression are common triggers of excessive eating. Patients frequently report that they eat to diminish or prevent the experiencing of unpleasant affective states, such as boredom, guilt, anger, and frustration. Under periods of stress, many obese patients have significant weight gain. Although obese people may not differ from nonobese people in terms of general psychopathology, many obese persons do have emotional difficulties. Patients with childhood-onset obesity may be preoccupied with size and weight as a central issue that has been pervasive throughout their physical and emotional development. Patients with adult-onset obesity might have gained weight as a reaction to psychological stress and may have used overeating as a method for reducing dysphoria.

Social factors may also have an impact on the way obesity is perceived. In individuals from lower socioeconomic status groups, in which obesity is highly prevalent, being overweight represents less of a social stigma than in individuals from higher socioeconomic status groups. Obese people in this social context may not experience a significant amount of weight-related distress. Culturally, African Americans and some Hispanic Americans, depending on their socioeconomic status, may prefer body types that are different from the thin ideal that characterizes middle-class European Americans. Thus, differences in sociocultural background may determine a person's emotional response to being overweight.

III. Management guidelines.

A. Prevention.

Prevention is particularly important in children and adolescents from families with a high prevalence of obesity. Whether genetically predisposed to gain weight or psychosocially at risk, these youngsters are likely to become obese as they become adults. Childhood-onset obesity is particularly resistant to treatment and should be managed with proper counseling of the patients and their families. Emphasis should be on proper nutritional practices, physical activity, and resolution of family conflicts that are likely to affect the young person's behavior. Critical stages in a person's life may also be particularly susceptible to weight change and to development of eating disorders. These stages include puberty, pregnancy, medical or psychiatric illness, emotional crisis, and conflict in relationships. Counseling should be provided by a nutritionist or dietitian, an exercise trainer, and a social worker or psychologist, depending on the areas involved.

B. Weight reduction (Table 19–1).

After a medical, endocrine, psychiatric, social, and dietary history is obtained, the patient's evaluation should be completed with appropriate laboratory or radiographic procedures. When indicated, the evaluation should include the input of a dietitian and a psychosocial professional.

Weight loss programs should be designed to provide care appropriate to the patient's health-risk status, as defined earlier (Table 19–2). The objective is to cause weight loss with the highest possible fat to lean body mass ratio and to alter behavior in order to ensure long-term weight loss and maintenance of normal weight. Above all, weight loss should be safe. The basic components of these programs include (1) diet, (2) physical exercise, (3) psychosocial and eating behavior modification, and (4) anti-obesity drugs. It is clear that long-lasting weight reduction ultimately depends on the ability of patients to develop sustained control of their eating behavior. For patients with morbid obesity who have failed to respond to a well-structured medical management program, surgical approaches should be considered.

Table 19–1
Major Components of a Weight-Loss Program

Hypocaloric diets	
Low-risk patients:	1000–1200 kcal
Moderate-risk patients:	800–1000 kcal
High-risk patients:	<800–1200 kcal
Progressive intensity physical exercise	
Warm up and stretching	10 min
Aerobic progressive intensity exercise (target, 70% maximum heart rate)	20 min
Cool down—slow walking	5 min
Eating behavior modification	
Make the environment diet friendly	
Eat at specific times	
Eliminate any other concurrent activity (reading, watching television, arguing)	
Sit down at a table	
Use small dishes	
Take small bites; prolong chewing time	
Pace the meal	
Antiobesity medication (under medical supervision)	

Table 19–2
Management of Obesity: Suggested Treatment Protocol

Treatment	Health Risk Status		
	Low Risk	*Moderate Risk*	*High Risk*
Diet			
Moderate			
1000–1200 kcal	+	+	+
<800 kcal		+	+
Exercise	+	+	+
Behavior therapy	+	+	+
Medical monitoring		Recommended	Mandatory
Antiobesity drugs		With medical supervision	With medical supervision

The health-risk status should be determined by a physician before treatment is instituted. For low-risk patients who need to lose 20 to 30 pounds, diet counseling and eating behavior modification should be sufficient. The interventions can be easily implemented by dietitians and other health professionals with periodic monitoring by a physician. In contrast, in patients with medium-risk or high-risk status, who need to lose large amounts of weight and who have medical complications, combinations of properly selected therapies need to be administered by a trained multidisciplinary treatment team, often in the controlled environment of a hospital setting. The team should include a bariatric physician, a dietitian, a qualified exercise professional, and a mental health professional. Behavioral and psychosocial intervention by qualified professionals is a prerequisite for the attainment of long-lasting results.

1. *Diet.*
   The patient should be instructed regarding a hypocaloric diet. The level of caloric restriction suitable to a given patient should be determined. This level can vary between 600 and 1400 kcal/d. The diet should be moderately restricted in carbohydrate (40% of total calories); high in protein (30% to 35% of total calories), and low in saturated fat and should be divided into two or three meals daily. Some patients prefer to eat small meals several times daily, whereas others prefer to eat a larger single meal. If at all possible, patients should be encouraged to plan for multiple small meals. The diet should be supplemented with multivitamins and minerals in sufficient quantities to meet recommended dietary allowances. Usually, one capsule daily is sufficient to meet these requirements. Patients eating a hypocaloric diet must plan their meals in advance, and they must be instructed on how to calculate the composition and caloric value of various food items. Many books listing the calorie value of a large assortment of food items are available in most bookstores, and patients should be encouraged to use them when planning their menus. This method allows patients to avoid unstructured eating or finding themselves in situations where eating is out of control. Patients should be instructed on how to deal with social situations in which eating is involved so that their intake may remain within their dietary allowances even on those occasions. To receive proper and effective diet instruction, patients should work with a dietitian for an extended period. Printed diets alone handed out by physicians to patients are not likely to be effective. However, the physician should indicate the level of caloric restriction the patient should be given and the proportion of carbohydrate, protein, and fat the patient should eat.

   For most adults, diets of 1000 to 1200 kcal/d generally result in safe weight loss. However, the speed at which weight loss occurs varies considerably from patient to patient. Also variable is the patient's willingness and ability to remain on a diet long enough to achieve the desired weight goal. Drastic dietary restriction ranging from total fasting to nutrient-modified fast has become a popular means of achieving rapid weight loss in cases in which weight reduction is medically urgent or in which more liberal approaches have failed. If the diet is restricted to less than 800 cal/d, patients may develop mild ketonuria. Testing for urinary ketones (using Ketostix) several times daily provides both the patient and the physician with an objective measure of compliance to the diet program. Very low calorie diets (VLCDs) may be associated with dehydration. Thus, patients should be encouraged to drink at least 8 to 10 8-ounce glasses of water daily.

   Side effects observed during total fasting include ketosis; severe hypoglycemia; loss of electrolytes, especially potassium, sodium, calcium, magnesium and phosphate; and volume depletion and associated postural hypotension and arrhythmias, produced by degenerative myocardial fiber changes that can cause sudden death. Total fasting is therefore not recommended. Attempts have been made to correct the undesirable aspects of starvation by the use of semisynthetic nutrient supplements. Very low calorie semisynthetic or kitchen diets, when properly implemented and closely monitored, have been shown to induce large and continued weight loss with relative safety.

   Hypocaloric, 800- to 1200-kcal diets are safe and do not require medical supervision. In contrast, VLCDs may have side effects and should be monitored by health professionals experienced with these diet programs.

2. *Physical training.*
Physical training can increase caloric expenditure and cause beneficial metabolic effects. It improves sensitivity to insulin; improves glucose tolerance in obese patients with insulin resistance and mild diabetes; it decreases plasma triglyceride levels in obese patients with hypertriglyceridemia and decreases the degree of negative nitrogen balance associated with very restricted diets, thereby helping to preserve lean body mass. Although intense physical exercise can induce an increase in caloric expenditure of 1000 cal, more moderate exercise, as practiced by nonathletes, has a calorie cost of only 200 to 400 cal. The metabolic effects of physical training appear to depend on strenuous exercise and prolonged physical training and may not be apparent with lesser degrees of physical exercise. Physical exercise has also been used in weight reduction for its psychological effects. It can improve anxiety and self-esteem and may help patients adhere to a weight reduction program and to maintain weight loss once this has been achieved.

Before participating in an exercise program for weight reduction, patients should undergo a graded exercise test in order to determine their physical work capacity as well as the presence of underlying cardiovascular disease, which may limit their ability to exercise. Testing also helps patients overcome anxiety and gain confidence in their ability to exercise. A formal exercise prescription should be developed by an exercise counselor.

The most desirable type of exercise for obese patients is aerobic, progressive-intensity, endurance-type exercise (e.g., walking, jogging, swimming). The objective is for patients to exercise at 70% of their maximum heart rate for at least 30 minutes four times a week for optimal training effects to be achieved. However, it is useful to set up training protocols based on the performance of the patient during the exercise testing. Initially, patients should be encouraged to accomplish the goal of walking 2 miles at a speed faster than that required for leisure walking. The walk can be interrupted every 5 to 10 minutes with slower-speed walking. Over a 3- to 7-week period, patients may progress to the goal of two miles of continuous walking. Once obese patients are able to accomplish this goal, their fitness level reaches a point at which a more traditional approach to exercise training can begin. Aerobic exercise can then be instituted for achievement of 70% of the maximal heart rate response [$0.7 \times (220 - \text{age})$]. Safe exercise performance requires that the patient start the workout with a 10-minute period of warm-up and stretching and that the session be completed with a slower paced cool-down routine for 5 minutes. Comfortable footwear with good support is essential for safe exercise. Spinco-type inner soles help provide this support.

The combination of hypocaloric diets and exercise has been demonstrated repeatedly to provide an excellent vehicle for weight reduction. Patients can exercise vigorously, even while receiving a calorie-restricted diet.

3. *Psychosocial and behavioral management.*
Adherence to weight reduction programs and long-term success largely depend on the ability of patients to alter eating behavior. If serious psychosocial factors are present, the patient needs referral for psychotherapy in order to resolve underlying conflicts. Because environmental eating cues often contribute to overeating, teaching the patient to alter the environment in order to minimize these cues is prerequisite for a change in eating behavior. For example, patients should be advised to take such measures as eating only at a table with proper dishes and silverware; using small dishes when eating small portions; pacing themselves, taking longer to complete their meal; and not reading or watching television while eating. Without these changes, patients are likely to return to old patterns and to regain their weight. Behavior modification therapy, psychoanalysis, group psychotherapy, and peer support through self-help groups have all been reported to be relatively successful in the management of moderate obesity. Techniques used for behavior modification therapy generally include regular, weekly weighing; diaries of eating and other activities; changes in meal eating behavior; analysis of situations that lead to deviation from the prescribed diet; social support; and self-reinforcement. The magnitude of weight loss in most behavioral programs has been clinically significant, but long-term follow-up of patients who had initially lost weight while receiving behavior modification therapy indicates that many eventually regain their weight. However, behavior modification therapy as well as other methods of psychotherapy are helpful as adjunctive therapy within the context of a multidisciplinary approach to the treatment of obese patients. One of the essential aspects of a weight reduction program is the development of strategies for changing behavior. The following should be considered:
- Self-help programs: Take Off Pounds Sensibly (TOPS); Overeaters Anonymous (OA)
- Psychotherapy: individual or group
- Comprehensive behavior programs:
    - Self monitoring
    - Stimulus control

Modification of eating topography
Behavior reinforcement
Adjunctive behavioral strategies
Cognitive restructuring

Behavior reinforcement is based on a formal system of positive reinforcement, such as monetary refund, point systems, and other tangible rewards, to enhance adherence. Adjunctive behavioral strategies include social support from others, relaxation exercise for stress-related episodes, and assertiveness training on how to say "no." Cognitive restructuring techniques teach patients to identify negative monologues and to challenge negative thinking with constructive counterarguments: "I am not happy with my behavior, but I won't allow this minor setback to deter me from my long range goal." Take Off Pounds Sensibly and Overeaters Anonymous groups exist in most communities and can be found in the telephone directory. Many community hospitals offer group therapy for weight control and diet or fitness programs, which include nutritional and exercise counseling as well as stress management sessions.

4. *Anti-obesity medication.*
The addition of pharmacologic agents potentially allows more effective initial weight loss and long-term maintenance of weight reduction. Most of the drugs used for weight reduction decrease food intake by decreasing appetite and are chemical derivatives of β-phenylethylamine. Extensive double-blind therapeutic trials with some of these drugs show that compared with placebo, they produce an additional mean weight loss of approximately 0.5 pounds/wk for a limited period of time. Individual response to these drugs varies considerably, and some subjects lose substantially more than the mean weight loss. Once administration of the drug is discontinued, weight regain is the rule. Therefore, this type of drug therapy should be used only on a short-term basis, together with other long-term interventions. In some subjects, weight regain may be prevented by long-term administration of the drug, but the complications of this therapy have yet to be evaluated. Another pharmacologic approach is to interfere with the absorption of food from the gastrointestinal tract. Thyroid hormones have been frequently used in the treatment of obesity, but they should not be used in patients who are euthyroid, because the agents may need to be given in pharmacologic amounts that induce thyrotoxicosis, which causes loss of lean body mass. Several categories of pharmacologic agents are currently available for the treatment of obesity (Table 19–3):

Table 19–3
Anti-obesity Drugs

Serotonin agonists
- Fenfluramine (Pondimin): 20 mg PO, 3 times daily before meals
- Dexfenfluramine (Redux): 15 mg PO, 2 times daily before meals
- Fluoxetine (Prozac): 40–80 mg PO daily

Sympathomimetics
- Phentermine (Ionamin): 15–30 mg once daily
- Phenylpropanolamine: 75 mg, sustained release, once daily

Combined therapy
- Fenfluramine: 20 mg PO, 3 times daily
  +
  Phentermine: 15 mg PO once daily

Decrease fat absorption
- Orlistat: not yet commercially available

a. *Fenfluramine.* A *5-hydroxytryptamine,* non-A receptor agonist. Studies have been performed with fenfluramine over extended periods of time. A dose-related suppression of food intake and weight loss has been obtained with doses aimed at achieving plasma concentrations ranging from 100 to 200 ng/mL. Fenfluramine (Pondimin), a racemic mixture of the dextro- and levo- forms of the drug, is recommended in doses of 20 mg three times daily before meals. Dexfenfluramine (Redux), the dextro-isomer, is more active than the racemic mixture and has recently been approved as a prescription anti-obesity drug. It is recommended in doses of 15 mg twice daily.
b. *Fluoxetine (Prozac).* This agent is serotonin and dopamine agonist. Used as an antidepressant, it has been noted to have appetite suppressive effects. In double-blind, placebo-controlled studies, fluoxetine, given together with a weight reduction diet, caused greater weight loss than placebo. Fluoxetine also has been thought to decrease preference for sweet-tasting foods and to enhance consumption of protein. As an appetite suppressant, fluoxetine may need to be given in doses of 60 to 80 mg/d. These doses are much higher than those commonly used for the treatment of depression. Fluoxetine is a better antidepressant than appetite suppressant and it is not usually effective when used solely for weight reduction. However, because of its anorectic effect, fluoxetine should be a good choice for obese patients who need an antidepressant.
c. *Phenylpropanolamine, phentermine.* These agents are sympathomimetic drugs. Phenylpropanolamine is available in most of the over-the-counter appetite suppressants (e.g., Dexatrim), in doses of 75 mg sustained-release capsules. In at least three recent double-blind, placebo-controlled studies, phenyl-

propanolamine given together with a 1200-calorie diet induced greater weight loss than placebo over an 18-week period. The prescription drug phentermine (Ionamin), given in doses of 15 to 30 mg as a single dose in the morning, can also induce anorectic effects and greater weight loss than placebo. Sympathomimetic drugs may not only exert their effects through suppression of appetite, they may also have thermogenic effects. A postulated mechanism for diminished thermogenesis in obesity has been decreased sympathetic nervous system activity. Thus, sympathomimetic drugs could correct this abnormality and increase thermogenesis. Possible side effects, such as hypertension, palpitations, and increased nervousness, may be observed with these drugs.

Combinations of appetite suppressants with different mechanisms of action have been tested for their effectiveness and safety in long-term weight control. In a multimodal intervention study, fenfluramine, 60 mg daily, plus phentermine, 15 to 30 mg daily, added to a program of calorie restriction, exercise, and behavior modification, caused greater weight loss than when placebo was added to this regimen (14.2 kg, or 15.9% of initial body weight versus 4.6 kg or 4.9% of initial body weight; $P < .001$). This differential effect continued for 34 weeks. During an extended follow-up, patients who continued to take medication were able to maintain weight loss for up to 3 years.

d. *Thyroxine, triiodothyronine.* Most obese patients are not hypothyroid, and treatment with physiologic doses of thyroid hormones is not effective. Pharmacologic doses are likely to induce thyrotoxicosis, with its associated clinical side effects and morbidity. Weight loss occurs with increased breakdown of protein and calcium loss from bone. Triiodothyronine levels decrease with VLCDs. It has been suggested that treatment with triiodothyronine may enhance weight loss under these circumstances, but the resulting loss may be at the expense of body protein.

e. *Drugs that inhibit food absorption.* The most promising inhibitor is orlistate (Xenical), which has just completed a phase III clinical trial for the treatment of morbid obesity. Inhibition of intestinal lipase activity is the main mode of action. This lipase plays a key role in the hydrolysis of the bulk of dietary triglycerides within the intestinal lumen. Orlistat also inhibits gastric lipase, thus reducing the hydrolysis of dietary triglycerides during the gastric phase of digestion. In clinical studies, orlistat decreases fecal fat absorption by about one third of the amount of ingested fat over a broad range of doses. Tolerability of the drug is related to the amount of fat in the diet and, therefore, the amount of fat excreted in stool. In a double-blind, randomized, placebo-controlled study of 45 obese patients, at week 12, patients who received orlistat lost an average of 1.57 kg more than the patients who received placebo. The orlistat-treated group lost approximately 0.5 kg per month more than the placebo-treated group. The most common adverse events with orlistat included fatty oil evacuation, abdominal pain, soft stools, nausea, and oily spotting.

Anti-obesity drugs have the potential for improving the effect of diet, exercise, and behavioral interventions in the treatment of obese patients. Although these drugs have been approved for short-term use, the long-term benefit and safety for available and newly developed drugs is still being determined. Thus, long-term use of these anti-obesity drugs cannot yet be recommended.

5. *Surgical management.*
Because of the high failure rate of medical treatment and the high incidence of recidivism in the management of obesity, surgical procedures have been developed to interfere with the ability of patients to eat or absorb food. Surgical treatment for obesity should be considered only for patients whose weight has been greater than 100% above ideal body weight for at least 10 years, who have complications such as hypertension, diabetes, hyperlipidemia, osteoarthrosis, or sleep apnea, and who have failed to respond to a well-supervised medical treatment. The most commonly used procedures are subtotal gastrectomy and vertical banded gastroplasty. They are designed to reduce the size of the proximal stomach to a 50-mL pouch and to limit the ability of the patient to ingest large volumes of food at any one time.

C. Special considerations in prescribing a weight reduction program.

Treatment of the obese patient is difficult. Patients fail to lose weight and drop out of weight reduction programs in large numbers; fewer than 5% of patients maintain their weight loss and rapidly regain it, to begin another equally frustrating cycle. As a result of these experiences, obese patients are frequently a captive audience for those who promote "rapid and effective" cures for their weight problems. Many methods of weight reduction that are offered to the public are ineffective and costly. Other methods may induce weight loss but are dangerous. Patients need to be educated on how to recognize the relative value and risks of such programs.

The type of weight reduction program to be selected for any given patient depends on several considerations regarding the patient's obesity. These considerations include the patient's age, the reasons for wanting to lose weight, the age of onset of obesity, the degree of obesity, and the patient's previous experience with weight reduction.

1. *Children and adolescents.*
   Children and adolescents should not be given VLCDs, because these diets may seriously interfere with the patient's growth and development. Children are particularly susceptible and may suffer long-term consequences from very severe diets. In these young people, the weight reduction program should emphasize moderate caloric restriction, physical training, restructuring of eating patterns, and psychiatric therapy and counseling of both patients and their families. Family issues and interpersonal relationships within the family should be closely scrutinized.
2. *Elderly.*
   Severe caloric restriction should be used with caution in the elderly. In this group of patients, aging may be associated with catabolic changes, which may be greatly exaggerated by VLCDs. It is important for the older patient to maintain nitrogen balance and to prevent the development or progression of osteoporosis or aggravation of underlying medical diseases.
3. *Limiting conditions.*
   Underlying cardiovascular disease, hypertension, diabetes, and osteoarthrosis may impose limitations in the ability of obese elderly patients to exercise. The exercise prescription needs to be modified in order to protect these patients from injury or complications of an underlying disorder. The level of motivation for weight reduction in patients who are retired, single, and with limited economic means is often low. Group activities and strategies that can help these patients with the development of an effective social support system may be important in achieving long-lasting weight management.

D. Motivation for weight loss.

Before instituting a weight reduction program, the primary care physician should understand the patient's motivation for weight loss. Patients attempt weight reduction for various reasons. Some are concerned about their appearance, social limitations, and inability to obtain employment. Others initiate a weight reduction effort because of medical conditions for which weight reduction is essential. The latter are frequently motivated to lose weight and undertake weight reduction programs with greater effort and success. Frequently, patients who have experienced a myocardial infarction, onset of diabetes mellitus requiring insulin therapy, or severe disability with osteoarthrosis are persuaded of the need to undertake weight reduction. As patients lose weight, attention must be given to means for improving the person's physical appearance, especially in terms of dress and deportment. Group therapy activities aimed at increasing social skills and vocational training programs directed at improving the patient's ability to obtain employment are important components of the weight reduction program. As patients lose weight, the motivation for weight reduction is reinforced by these strategies. In contrast, patients may quickly abandon their effort and regain their weight if they lose weight but do not make progress in the areas of major concern. Family pressure to lose weight is not an effective inducement for obese patients to undertake a weight reduction program. Although patients may request evaluation and start a weight reduction program under pressure from concerned family members, they are likely to quickly abandon the effort if they have not shared the same need for being thinner.

The degree of obesity is a strong consideration for the selection of treatment strategies. Patients with mild-to-moderate obesity, 15% to 100% above ideal body weight (BMI, 28 to 40 kg/m^2), benefit from ambulatory programs, whereas those with severe obesity (> 100% above ideal body weight, BMI > 40 kg/m^2) may require inpatient or residential medical treatment programs or surgical approaches.

The patient's previous experience with weight reduction determines the patient's enthusiasm and ability to engage in the treatment program. Patients who previously have not attempted weight reduction or have not been involved with a professionally directed program are likely to be more successful in their effort than those who have lost and regained weight on multiple occasions. For these patients, the specific factors contributing to the obesity must be evaluated and treated before a new weight reduction effort is instituted.

IV. Success rate with various treatment approaches.

Medical treatment represents the first line of care in the management of obesity. However, these approaches produce only a moderate amount of weight loss, frequently, a 10% reduction in body weight. In addition, the lower weight is not well maintained over the long term.

Commercial weight control programs using low-calorie diets produce average losses of 10 to 20 pounds, but the significance of such reduction is minimized by high rates of attrition (80% over a 1-year period) and poor maintenance of weight loss in those who complete treatment. Self-help groups also have a high dropout rate and very modest initial weight loss.

Low-calorie diets administered by health care professionals on an out-patient basis appear to result in average weight losses of about 18 pounds, with only 25% of patients losing 20 pounds or more. Little information is available about the long-term efficacy of low-calorie diets, but available data suggest that weight loss is not well maintained.

Comprehensive behavioral interventions produce either weight loss of 20 pounds, or a 10% reduction in body weight. Attrition rates are relatively low (< 15%), and negative side effects of treatment are virtually nonexistent. In the year after treatment, patients regain about 40% of their initial weight loss. A combination of behavior therapy and psychotherapy seems to impair rather than enhance maintenance of weight loss.

The use of appetite-suppressing drugs in conjunction with dieting enhances the rate of weight loss by about 0.5 pounds/wk over 132 weeks. However, drug-induced weight loss is rapidly regained when the drug therapy is withdrawn.

Under proper medical supervision, VLCDs safely produce large and rapid reductions in weight. The magnitude of these losses (33 to 55 pounds) exceeds all conservative treatments for obesity. Unfortunately, VLCD-induced weight loss is poorly maintained: during the year after treatment, patients often regain 2/3 of their end-of-treatment weight loss.

Combining the use of VLCD with behavior therapy increases initial weight loss and fosters better maintenance of weight loss during the year after treatment. Nonetheless, long-term results with VLCDs with or without behavior therapy are discouraging. Follow-up of 2 to 5 years shows that most patients treated with VLCDs regain the entire amounts of weight initially lost with treatment.

V. Special situations: treatment-insensitive patients.

Patients with severe obesity and multiple medical complications should be considered for in-patient treatment or residential treatment under close medical supervision and in the context of a structured therapeutic environment. The support of a multidisciplinary group of health professionals with expertise in nutrition, physical exercise, and behavioral and psychological therapy under the guidance of a physician could help such patients achieve marked weight loss in relatively short periods of time. This is usually accompanied by a marked improvement in the medical complications that necessitated the weight reduction. Patients with medical complications commonly show improvement in these complications with moderate weight loss. There appears to be a threshold weight at which the complications develop and below which these complications do not develop. Getting people with severe obesity to lose weight to a functional level may be a realistic approach to patients with chronic obesity. A functional weight level is that at which most of the medical complications have been minimized and patients are able to maintain a reasonably normal life and gainful employment.

Obesity is a chronic condition for which a cure is not available. An obese patient's weight can be controlled as long as patients maintain long-term involvement with a weight reduction program and continue to engage in the strategies designed for weight reduction and maintenance. If obese patients and physicians consider obesity to be a chronic condition that is similar to such conditions as diabetes, it is clear that acute weight loss without ongoing chronic treatment will not ensure permanent weight maintenance in the same way that temporary glucose control in a diabetic patient does not imply that the diabetes has been cured. Only patients who can make permanent changes in lifestyle, alter the way that they respond to psychosocial stress, and improve personality characteristics that put them at risk for overeating and weight gain are most likely to benefit from weight reduction programs, minimize the hazards of being obese, minimize the morbidity associated with obesity, and maximize the life expectancy.

VI. Important management guidelines.

A. Obesity is a chronic condition that requires continuous care and a long-term approach.

B. Management should be planned in multiple stages spanning long periods of time.

C. Health care professionals need to offer patients lifelong assistance to meet the challenge of a relentless biologic and psychosocial tendency to gain weight. Most patients cannot independently sustain the substantial degree of psychological control necessary to override these social and biologic challenges.

D. Patients need a multicomponent program that includes ongoing professional contact, skills training, social support, and physical activity.

E. Patients need an initial weight-loss treatment program and a long-term post-treatment maintenance program to reinforce the self-control strategies learned in treatment. The longer patients remain in contact with health care professionals, the longer they will be able to sustain the eating and exercise habits necessary for the maintenance of weight loss.

F. The use of a problem-solving approach can provide health care professionals with a conceptual framework to assist patients in coping with the challenges of the post-treatment period.

G. Treatment should be geared to the stages of a person's life. For example, a person may have an easier time maintaining weight loss as a single, young adult than as an older, married mother.

H. **Develop strategies for relapse prevention:**

1. Identify situational factors that pose a high risk for an initial slip or lapse in control, such as negative emotional experiences, interpersonal conflicts, and social pressures.
2. Teach patients to set up an early warning system to signal potential backsliding and train them to gain coping skills for handling high-risk situations, thereby enhancing both their effectiveness and their confidence. This strategy could include developing a behavioral contract that allows patients to recognize when a lapse has occurred. For example, a weight gain of 3 pounds may call for reinforcement of diet and increase in exercise.
3. Reframe the problem: lapse versus relapse—patients should recognize the difference. A lapse or slip is only a temporary disruption in self-regulation. Under these circumstances, patients should be able to reframe or relabel the event as a learning experience that does not predict future problems.
4. Relapse rehearsal: use imagery to help patients rehearse; they should place themselves in possible high-risk situations and practice coping techniques.
5. For those in the social support system:
   - Keep the house and family relaxed.
   - Ask the dieter how they can help.
   - Learn to ignore and forgive lapses.
   - Exercise with the dieter.
   - Do not hide food from the dieter.
   - Do not lecture, criticize, or reprimand.
   - Do not expect perfection or 100% recovery.

VII. Caregiver assistance.

In treating obesity, it is important to develop treatment strategies that are congruent with the patient's cultural background. In that background, the primary care physician should include the patient's family, the patient's belief about the cause of his or her illness, and the social acceptance or rejection of the patient's weight. Attention to cultural differences is particularly important in regard to diet prescriptions, behavior counseling, and suggestions for changing of lifestyles. In this context, the physician should not assume that the patient represents the general culture, and efforts should be made to understand the special background characteristics and to adapt recommendations accordingly.

VIII. What to tell the patient at the beginning of treatment.

After completing the evaluation and planning treatment, the doctor might state something like the following:

Mr. [or Mrs.] A., Obesity is a chronic condition with potential serious medical complications. Although many diets are usually recommended by the medical profession as well as the lay press, long-term compliance with a diet necessary to achieve a good result is not always forthcoming. It is important to understand that you will need to devote significant effort and long-term commitment to controlling your weight. This does not mean that you will need to starve yourself or to restrict your diet indefinitely. Once you have achieved your desired weight loss, a maintenance program will need to be instituted. Although your dietary intake will need to be monitored and controlled on an ongoing basis, you will not need to necessarily remain on a reduction diet. *It is most important to consider the fact that at the present time, obesity is not curable but that it can be controlled.* The main purpose of losing weight is to improve your physical health and to make you feel more comfortable in your interpersonal and social relationships. This may not mean losing to an ideal body weight. What is frequently necessary for success to be achieved is a change in lifestyle. This change involves not only structuring your diet better, such as avoiding high-calorie-density foods, but also engaging in physical activity that you can perform several times a week, if possible, in the company of other people engaged in the same activity. Finally, what will really make a difference in your ability to succeed is an effort to understand the situations that trigger overeating and to seek help in changing these situations. We are ready to help you with information regarding referral to a nutritionist for diet instruction, physical training programs in which you can safely participate, and counseling resources in the community for services in which you will be able to participate. Drugs to help you lose weight can sometimes be added to your weight reduction program, but they need to be prescribed and monitored by your doctor.

Suggested Reading

Anderson T, Astrup A, Quaade F. Dexfenfluramine as adjuvant to a low-calorie formulae diet in the treatment of obesity: A randomized clinical trial. Int J Obes Relat Metab Disord 1992; 16:35–40.

Atkinson RL. Low and very low calorie diets. Med Clin North Am 1989; 73:203–215.

Bray GA. Complications of obesity. Ann Intern Med 1985; 103 (Suppl.):1052–1062.

Brolin RE. Results of obesity surgery. Gastroenterol Clin North Am 1987; 16:317–338.

Brownell KD, Kramer FM. Behavioral management of obesity. Med Clin North Am 73:185–201, 1989.

Ferguson JM, Feighner JP. Fluoxetine-induced weight loss in overweight nondepressed humans. Int J Obesity 1987; 11(Suppl. 3):163–170.

Health Implications of Obesity. National Institutes of Health Consensus Development Conference. Ann Intern Med 1985; 103(Suppl.):977–1077.

International Symposium on Nutrition and Obesity. The state of the science. Special Supplement. Med J Aust 1985; 142(Special Suppl.).

Kissebah AH, Vydelingum N, Murray R, et al. Relation of body fat distribution to metabolic complication of obesity. J Clin Endocrinol Metab 1982; 54:254–260.

Lampman RM, Schteingart DE, Foss ML. Exercise as a partial therapy for the extremely obese. Med Sci Sports Exerc 1985; 18:19–24.

Mabee TM, Meyer P, DenBesten L, Mason EE. The mechanism of increased gallstone formation in obese human subjects. Surgery 1976; 79:460–468.

Peiser J, Lavie P, Ovnat A, Charnuzi I. Sleep apnea syndrome in the morbidly obese as an indication for weight reduction surgery. Ann Surg 1984; 199:112–115.

Pi-Sunyer FX. Dietary practices in obesity. Bull NY Acad Med 1982; 58:263.

Ravussin E, Lilioja S, Knowler WC, et al. Reduced rate of energy expenditure as a risk factor for body weight gain. N Engl J Med 1988; 318:467–472.

Schteingart DE. Effectiveness of phenylpropanolamine in the management of moderate obesity. Int J Obes Relat Metab Disord 1992; 16:487–493.

Segal RR, Pi-Sunyer FX. Exercise and obesity. Med Clin North Am 1989; 73:217–236.

Silverstone T. Appetite suppressant drugs in the management of obesity: Current view. Int J Obesity 1987; 11(Suppl. 3):135–139.

Stunkard AJ, Sorensen TIA, Hanis C, et al. An adoption study of human obesity. N Engl J Med 1986; 314:193–198.

Petersmark KA, Editor. Toward Safe Weight Loss. Recommendations for Adult Weight Loss Program in Michigan. Michigan Health Council, The Center for Health Promotion, Michigan Department of Public Health; December 1990.

Weintraub M, Sunderasan PR, Madan M, et al. Long term weight control. Clin Pharmacol Ther 1992; 51:581–646.

Welle SL, Campbell RG. Decrease in resting metabolic rate during rapid weight loss is reversed by low-dose thyroid hormone treatment. Metabolism 1986; 35: 289–291.

Willbanks OL. Gastric restrictive procedures: Gastroplasty. Gastroenterol Clin N Am 1987, 16:273–281.

20

A. E. EYLER, MD, MPH

Sexuality Issues and Common Sexual Dysfunctions: Evaluation and Management in the Primary Care Setting

I. Overview and basic concepts of sexual medicine.

A. Introduction.

Sexuality is a fundamental aspect of human self-concept in both health and illness. Issues regarding sexual functioning present commonly in both in-patient and out-patient primary care practice. However, unlike impairments of other basic human activities, such as difficulties with eating or elimination, patient reports of sexual dysfunction are often dismissed by health care providers without a full evaluation. Physicians in the primary care and mental health disciplines are well situated to evaluate and treat most common sexual dysfunctions and to offer patients basic information regarding human sexuality and sexual health. This chapter describes the basic principles of the evaluation of sexual dysfunctions, with emphasis on basic sexuality interviewing and communication skills. Clinical management of less complex disorders is included, as are guidelines for referral of more complicated cases.

Physicians who do not include sexual medicine in their clinical practices often cite lack of training in this discipline, potential patient embarrassment, or fear of uncovering situations that they would be unable to manage effectively as reasons for this exclusion. However, the basic sexual history can be mastered by any clinician familiar with medical interviewing methods. Patients usually reflect the level of comfort in discussing sexual matters that their physicians demonstrate, and appropriate referral services for more complicated cases can be obtained through reputable sex counselors and therapists. In addition, patients are often grateful for the recognition of their sexual personhood that the inclusion of sexuality questions in the medical history implies.

Case Study

Ms. T. is a 37-year-old teacher who presents for routine annual gynecologic care. A brief review of her medical history indicates that she underwent right breast lumpectomy and radiation therapy for malignancy 2 years ago. She received follow-up chemotherapy and faces a guarded prognosis at this time. As the interview proceeds, questions are asked regarding social and sexual relationships, sexual functioning, and potential contraceptive needs. Suddenly, Ms. T. begins to weep. Fearing offense, her physician begins to apologize but is interrupted by the patient. She explains that she has no intimate relationship at this time but hopes to again in the future. For the most part, she is deeply touched at being treated as a "whole" person: "This is the first time in over 2 years that anyone has indicated that they thought I might be dating. I'm so tired of being seen as just a 'breast cancer case.'"

B. Diagnosis: Sexuality, sexual functioning, and relationship dynamics.

Sexual dysfunctions can result from physical pathology (e.g., diabetic neuropathy), psychological factors (e.g., anxiety), or a combination of both. In addition, disturbances in the partnered relationship can present as sexual problems, or conversely, sexual difficulties may be interpreted (by both patients and their physicians) as being caused by marital or relationship stress when, in fact, an undiagnosed illness or medication reaction is responsible. Certain diagnoses, such as orgasmic dysfunction, are frequently multifactorial in etiology. When the relative contribution is unclear or when diagnostic testing is prolonged, it is often helpful to proceed with behaviorally oriented treatment of the dysfunction, supportive counseling as indicated, and close clinical follow-up. *It is important to avoid assigning psychological or interpersonal causes to sexual dysfunctions that are the result of physical illness.* Adequate attention to the history and physical examination minimizes this possibility.

Sexual functioning affects couple and marital satisfaction and individual perception of health and is in turn influenced by other physiologic and disease processes. In addition, physical and sexual disabilities have psychological consequences, which must be recognized and treated. A list of medical illnesses that commonly affect sexual functioning is found in Table 20–1. Inclusion of (at least) a basic sexual history as a routine part of patient care often yields additional clinical benefits (Table 20–2).

Table 20–1
Illness and Sexual Functioning*

Arthritis	Pain may interfere with sexual activity. Hip involvement may make intercourse difficult (or impossible) and may impair other types of genital stimulation. Hand involvement may severely impair sexual expression.
Asthma	Sexual arousal may precipitate (or become associated with) attacks.
Cardiovascular disease	Angina and fear of pain or infarction may interfere with sexual desire and all phases of the sexual response cycle. Medication side effects can also cause dysfunction.
Depression	Depression often inhibits sexual desire. Some antidepressant medications may interfere with orgasm.
Diabetes mellitus	Impairment of excitement and orgasmic phases is common, especially erectile dysfunction in men. Desire (libido) usually remains intact.
Hypertension	Many phases of the sexual response cycle can be affected by antihypertensive medications and by vascular damage.
Multiple sclerosis	All phases of the sexual response cycle can be affected by demyelination or inflammation. Genital anesthesia can occur in advanced cases. Incontinence may also interfere with sexual expression.
Neurologic injury	Sexual consequences depend on the level and completeness of the injury as well as on psychological adjustment.
COPD (emphysema)	Breathing difficulties may interfere with plateau and orgasmic phases of the sexual response cycle. An upright (sitting) posture may facilitate breathing during intercourse. Diaphragmatic breathing and relaxation exercises may be helpful.
Sleep apnea	Fatigue, depressed mood, loss of sexual desire, and other dysfunctions are common.
Vascular disease	Impairments of excitement and orgasmic phases (especially erectile dysfunction) often accompany significant vascular disease of the lower extremities.

Data from Comfort A, Editor. Sexual Consequences of Disability. Philadelphia: George F. Stickley Co.; 1978.

*Many aspects of female sexual functioning have not been adequately researched. Medical conditions that inhibit erection or male orgasm may also cause sexual dysfunction in women.

COPD = chronic obstructive pulmonary disease.

C. Sexual self-concept: Sexual orientation and gender identity.

Human beings can seek sexual gratification or release without a partner, with persons of their own sex, with members of the other sex, or with animals. The apparently inherent and often lifelong attraction that individuals feel toward same-sex or opposite sex partners (or both) is referred to as *sexual orientation.* Although many cultures do not have specific terms to describe such concepts as homosexuality and heterosexuality or do not consider sexual orientation to be an important part of personal identity, contemporary Western culture places a great deal of emphasis on this aspect of human sexual self-concept, behavior, and fantasy.

There is no medical evidence that *heterosexuality* (orientation exclusively toward opposite-sex partners), *homosexuality* (orientation exclusively toward same-sex partners), or *bisexuality* (orientation toward partners of both sexes) is, per se, psychologically unhealthy or harmful. Clinical principles related to sexual orientation are discussed in section VI of this chapter.

Western culture also conceptualizes *sex* (male or female, as determined by chromosomes or by genital phenotype) as being synonymous with *gender* (internal self-perception of masculinity, femininity, or other related characteristics). Many other cultures (including many Native American and African groups) do not regard gender as being determined by sex, and they either provide an accepted role for persons for whom these aspects are not congruent or recognize more than two genders. Section VII of this chapter discusses transsexualism and related phenomena in greater detail. The concepts of sexual orientation and gender identity have been introduced here because portions of the sexual history and the initial evaluation of sexual disorders depend on an understanding of patient self-perception in these respects.

Table 20–2
The Sexual History: Clinical Benefits

- Provides information regarding patient's level of physical and emotional functioning
- May provide insight into other aspects of patient's mental health
- Offers a more complete social/family health assessment
- Offers the opportunity to discuss patient's concerns
- Demonstrates to the patient that he or she is respected as a complete, autonomous human being
- Provides an opportunity for preventive medicine
- Can clarify treatment goals in chronic illness

D. Sexual physiology and functioning: The sexual response cycle.

The clinical evaluation of sexual difficulties requires an understanding of normal sexual physiology and functioning. Regardless of the nature of the sexual episode (alone or with a mate or casual partner) or method of stimulation used, both women and men experience a characteristic series of physiologic stages as they approach orgasmic release. The human *sexual response cycle* (SRC) was first described by Masters and Johnson in 1966.[1] Understanding of the SRC makes possible the description, diagnosis, and treatment of sexual dysfunctions.

Masters and Johnson conceptualized the human SRC as consisting of four phases: *excitement*, *plateau*, *orgasm*, and *resolution*. The physiologic changes associated with the SRC are described in Table 20–3 and represented graphically in Figure 20–1. Masters and Johnson focused on the physical components of sexual functioning and obtained their information from interviews with, and observations of, healthy volunteers. Singer-Kaplan subsequently investigated sexual responsiveness from a more subjective, psychologically oriented perspective.[2, 3] She described the SRC as consisting of three phases: *desire*, *excitement*, and *orgasm*. *Orgasm* is described similarly in the two versions of the SRC. However, Singer-Kaplan combined excitement and plateau into a single phase because most people do not subjectively distinguish the two components, and she eliminated resolution as being a "nonphase," or a portion of the SRC that is not clinically relevant, because no known dysfunctions occur during it. She also added desire as the initial phase of sexual responsiveness. Desire is defined as "libido . . . the specific psychoneurological sensations that lead people to seek out sexual experiences, feel 'sexy' or sexually interested, or restless."[2] For medical purposes, either schema is acceptable, as long as it can accommodate the clinical data. For example, dysfunctions that affect sex-

Table 20–3
The Human Sexual Response Cycle

Excitement

Women
- Onset of vaginal lubrication
- Engorgement of vaginal walls
- Swelling of the glans clitoris; increase in shaft diameter
- Swelling of the labia minora
- Nipple erection; increase in breast size
- Muscle tension; sex flush (possible)

Men
- Increase in length and diameter of penis
- Elevation of testes
- Nipple erection (possible)
- Muscle tension; sex flush (possible)

Plateau

Women
- Further engorgement of the outer vagina and labia
- Retraction of the clitoris, under the clitoral hood
- Further nipple engorgement
- Increase in muscle tension; sex flush (possible)
- Marked increase in heart rate, respiration, BP

Men
- Slight increase in glans area; color change (possible)
- Increase in testicular size; rotation and further elevation
- Cowper's gland secretion
- Further increase in HR, RR, BP, muscle tension, sex flush (possible)

Orgasm

Women
- Strong muscular contractions in the outer vagina
- Contractions of uterus, anal sphincter
- Peak intensity of sex flush
- Strong, diffuse muscular contractions
- Doubling of HR, RR (possible)
- BP increase (as much as ⅓ > normal)
- Vocalization (possible)

Men
- Contractions of the testes, epididymis, vas deferens, seminal vesicles, prostate, urethra, penis, anal sphincter
- Ejaculation (3–4 contractions)
- General loss of voluntary motor control
- Peak testicular elevation, HR, RR, sex flush
- Vocalization (possible)

Resolution

Women
- Quick dispersion of vaginal engorgement
- Return to usual color, size, position of vagina, labia, clitoris
- Gradual decrease of breast and nipple size
- Disappearance of sex flush
- Return to normal of HR, RR, BP
- Muscular and psychological relaxation
- Sweating reaction (possible)

Men
- Return of penis to usual size
- Testicular descent
- Loss of nipple erection
- Disappearance of sex flush
- Return to normal of HR, RR, BP
- Muscular and psychological relaxation
- Sweating reaction (possible)

Data from Masters WH, Johnson VE. Human Sexual Response. Boston: Little, Brown & Co.; 1966.
BP = blood pressure; HR = heart rate; RR = respiratory rate.

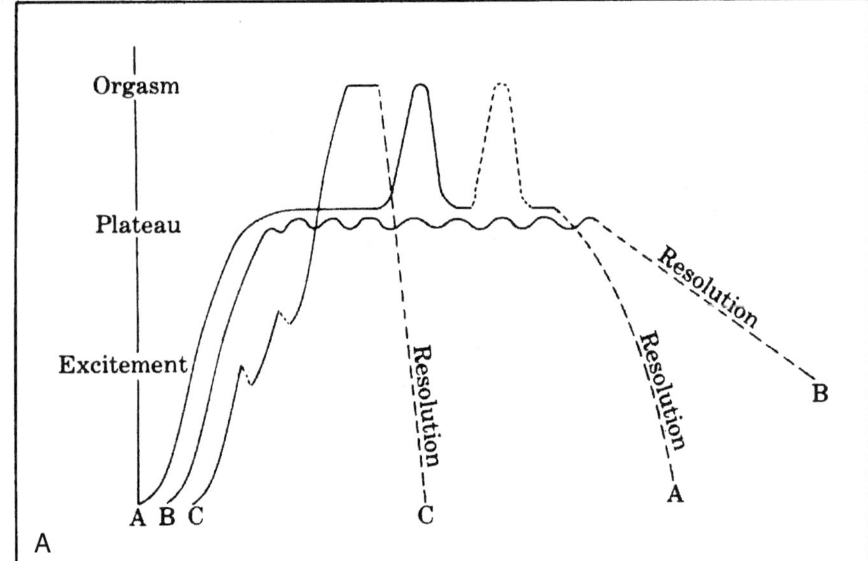

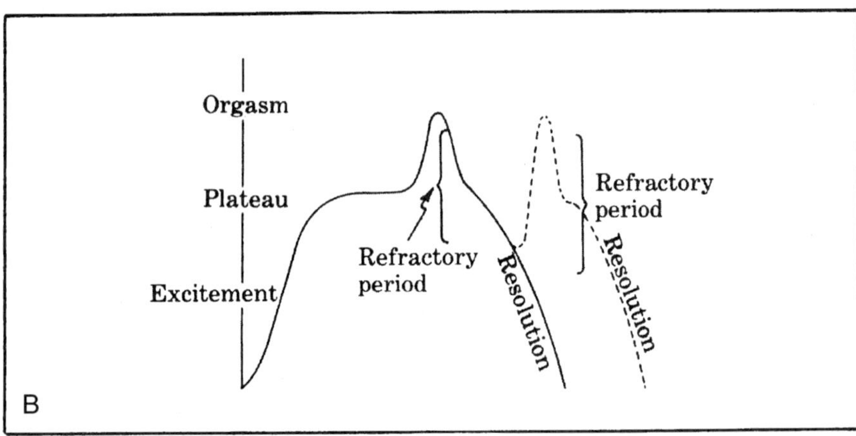

Figure 20–1
The female *(A)* and male *(B)* sexual response cycles. The phases of the response cycle are arbitrarily defined and differ considerably across individuals. Before the beginning of the response cycle is the phase of desire; this phase is not illustrated. The three illustrated phases are excitement, plateau, and orgasm. The length of the plateau phase is variable. For men with premature ejaculation, the plateau phase is usually quite brief; for women, a brief plateau phase may precede a very intense orgasm (illustrated by cycle C). Women may have multiple orgasms without dropping below the plateau phase. Most women are not multiorgasmic. Directly after ejaculation, most men enter a refractory period, when ejaculation is impossible. The male refractory period may last from minutes to hours. Women have no refractory period. The resolution phase for women is characterized by considerable variability. (Adapted from Kolodny RC, Masters WH, Johnson VE. Textbook of Sexual Medicine, Fourth Edition. Boston: Little, Brown & Co.; 1979, pp. 7–18.)

ual desire or the plateau phase should be described in those terms. Many clinicians prefer to combine these two descriptions of the SRC for general use.

Case Study
Ms. J. is a 28-year-old doctoral student who presents for an annual gynecologic examination and renewal of her prescription for oral contraceptives. A routine screening sexual history reveals that she has one male partner (her fiance), with whom she has lived for the past 2 years. Their relationship has always been positive and mutually supportive, although a bit strained since they both have been working on their dissertations. Her only sexual complaint is that during the past few months, she has required more time to reach orgasm. She states that this is not a "huge" problem ("I have a very patient lover"), but that it is fatiguing and annoys her. Medically, she is very healthy, eats a nutritious diet, exercises, and does not smoke. Her only problem has been an increase in migraine headaches, for which she has been taking prophylactic fluoxetine (Prozac), 20 mg daily. She uses no other medications except oral contraceptives, drinks minimal alcohol, and does not use other drugs.

Further discussion characterizes Ms. J.'s sexual difficulties as a prolongation of the plateau phase of the sexual response cycle, which is a common side effect of fluoxetine. Options for treatment include changing her medication regimen, using additional methods of sexual stimulation (e.g., using a clitoral vibrator during intercourse) in order to achieve orgasm more quickly, or doing nothing because this medication effect usually attenuates with time.

Case Study
Mr. L. is a 56-year-old widower who is raising his 8-year-old granddaughter. He has come to the primary care physician's office for a hypertension check-up and prescription refill. Overall, he feels well, but he has a lot less energy than he used to and seems "down" a lot. In response to routine sexual history questions (included in the review of systems for all patients with hypertension), he reports that he is not in a relationship currently, thinks that he would like to be, but just does not seem to have the energy to be more social. He awakens in a state of arousal occasionally but does not masturbate because he "just doesn't feel like it."

Further discussion reveals that Mr. L. is suffering from previously undiagnosed clinical depression, which is detectable on interview as loss of libido, a desire phase dysfunction. He is successfully treated with supportive counseling and pharmacotherapy, resulting in a more positive life outlook, an improved relationship with his granddaughter, and an (eventual) return of normal sexual desire and social impulses.

II. Epidemiology and pathophysiology.

Because of a lack of specific research data, estimating the prevalence of sexual dysfunction in contemporary society is difficult. However, most clinicians who routinely include questions about sexual functioning in the medical history (particularly the review of systems) find that substantial numbers of patients benefit from detection and treatment of sexual dysfunctions that, because of embarrassment or lack of knowledge about treatment possibilities, they would not have reported without being asked. The data that are available support this clinical impression. For example, Frank and colleagues[4] found that in 100 couples, most of whom were well educated, 40% of the men had experienced erectile or ejaculatory dysfunction, and 63% of the women had experienced difficulties with arousal or orgasm; however, none had received any medical attention or therapy for these problems.

Sexual dysfunctions can result from physical impairments, psychological disorders or stress, unsatisfactory relationship dynamics, or a combination of factors. In addition, sexual "normality" is in many respects a culturally defined phenomenon; many behaviors that are considered abnormal or unusual in contemporary North American society are (or have been) commonplace elsewhere. *Behaviors and preferences that are unusual but not harmful to the patient or partner should not be regarded as dysfunctional.* Furthermore, physicians must be aware that many sexual attitudes and behaviors are more common than is often believed and that obtaining a sexual history sometimes reveals unexpected answers. *It is extremely important not to express shock, disbelief, judgment, or disgust, regardless of any conflicts that may exist between the values of the patient and the physician.* If these concerns are sufficiently problematic as to prevent providing the patient with appropriate medical care, then the patient should be referred to another physician.

For example, in a recent survey of American sexual attitudes and behavior, in which the sample population conformed to the population distribution of the United States (as reported by the United States Bureau of the Census) with respect to age, gender, marital status, income, region, and education, the following findings were reported:[5]

- Among participants who described themselves as "very religious," more than 30% admitted having extramarital sexual relations at least once, and more than 70% had had premarital sexual experience. Overall, more than 25% of female respondents and more than 33% of male respondents reported having had at least one extramarital affair.
- Seventeen percent of women and 22% of men reported having had at least one homosexual experience.
- Eight percent of middle-income women reported having had sex for money. Twenty percent of men reported having paid money for sex; this proportion was the same across all income levels.
- Eleven percent of women and 14% of men reported having some personal experience with sadomasochism.

In order to be effective in the clinical setting, the physician must avoid making assumptions regarding past or current sexual experience based on the appearance, profession, marital status, or social standing of the patient. Techniques for clinical interviewing and discussion of sexuality concerns are described in the following section.

Case Study

Dr. J. is a 32-year-old house officer in a surgical subspecialty. He has presented repeatedly for testing for sexually transmitted diseases. Despite his high levels of anxiety, none of the work-ups have revealed the presence of disease. After an initial reticence from the patient in discussing his risk behaviors, the physician elicits a complete sexual history, which reveals the following information: having received a very strict upbringing, religiously and socially, Dr. J. believes that nonmarital intercourse is wrong. His first intercourse experience occurred at the age of 26. He has lived with two women, one of whom he became engaged to, but he experienced orgasmic dysfunction frequently, often avoided sex altogether, and "managed to sabotage" both relationships. Since the dissolution of his engagement, he has begun having sex with prostitutes because this seems "less wrong somehow." Despite the use of "safer sex" precautions, he is strongly fearful of acquiring sexually transmitted disease, which he would regard as punishment for his misbehavior. He is also worried about the possibility of anyone finding out about his contacts with prostitutes because this is completely at odds with his professional image, and he asks that this information not be recorded in the medical record. It is clear that his difficulties exceed sexual dysfunction per se and are related to fundamental issues of self-perception, life choices, and substantial intrapsychic conflicts. The seriousness of this situation is discussed, and Dr. J. is referred for in-depth psychotherapy. In addition, safer sex measures are explored and reviewed. He is reassured regarding doctor-patient confidentiality and is praised for his honesty in this clinical situation. A follow-up appointment is also scheduled.

III. General management guidelines.

A. Physician training and level of intervention.

All practicing physicians in the primary care and mental health fields can provide a needed service to their patients by routinely inquiring about sexual concerns, sexual functioning, and sexual goals. However, clinicians who choose not to become knowledgeable in the field of sexual medicine may decide to limit their practice in this area to detection and referral rather than providing treatment. Nonetheless, patients often perceive the mere recognition that sexuality is considered to be an important part of life, and that sexual dysfunctions are a legitimate medical concern, as therapeutic in itself. This is referred to as the *permission* step in the *P-LI-SS-IT* model of sex therapy: validating that sexual concerns are important and reasonable and giving the patient permission to discuss them. The other steps in the PLISSIT model are *limited information, specific suggestions,* and *intensive therapy,* which should be provided only by clinicians specifically trained in this area. The PLISSIT model is presented in Table 20–4 and is discussed further in the management of specific disorders.

B. Patient focus: Individual and dyad.

Although sexual dysfunctions are clinical entities with definitional criteria, the primary focus in sexual medicine is on the goals and the expectations of the patient and partner or partners rather than on the personal values of the physician or on the meeting of any arbitrary standard of sexual health. For example, a patient who is experiencing medication-induced orgasmic dysfunction may find this very bothersome or may not be at all concerned. Conversely, a man who can postpone ejaculation for "only" 45 minutes during intercourse may consider this to be unacceptable premature ejaculation if his usual experience is of being able to maintain erectile control for one hour or more. When evaluating sexual concerns, it is crucial to include discussion of the perceptions, goals, and sexual plans of the patient and couple, especially if change (resulting from progressive illness or other circumstances) is expected.

During the sexuality portion of the medical interview, it is also important to clarify the circumstances that surround sexual dysfunction. For example, is the difficulty chronic (or related to fundamental questions of sexual orientation or gender identity) or does it manifest only with a particular partner or under certain circumstances? Details in this regard are often significant in the diagnosis and treatment of sexual dysfunctions.

Case Study

Mr. R. is a 29-year-old engineer who is being evaluated for erectile dysfunction. When asked when he first experienced this problem, he replies, "March 15th, at 8:00 a.m." Further discussion reveals that Mr. R. and his wife have been attempting conception for 2 years, without success, and are in the process of undergoing a medical work-up for infertility. On the morning of March 15th, they were to have had intercourse at 8 a.m., so that a postcoital test could be performed at the medical office at 9:00 a.m. Mr. R. was not able to sustain an erection at that time and has been unable to achieve an erection sufficient for intercourse since then, although he awakens with morning erections and is able to masturbate to orgasm. Given this important historical information, his fears and concerns regarding the possibility that he is "responsible" for the infertility and that he will never be able to father a child can be addressed, and a costly and time-consuming search for physiologic causes for erectile dysfunction can be avoided.

C. Complete history and examination.

1. *History.*
   a. *Technique.* When obtaining the medical-sexual history or discussing sexuality concerns, the primary care physician should adopt a nonjudgmental attitude and a calm, relaxed appearance. Patients must be given appropriate assurances of confidentiality and provided with sufficient opportunities to ask questions. Physicians should also avoid using labels when discussing sexual behaviors, especially those that are unclear or pejorative (e.g., "frigidity" for orgasmic dysfunction or "impotence" for erectile dysfunction). Physicians must be prepared to indicate the medical reason behind each question (not simply curiosity), to admit ignorance regarding unusual sexual practices or in-depth therapy techniques (if this is the case), and to make appropriate referrals. It is very helpful to keep in mind the level of intervention (PLISSIT model) that one is pursuing and to remember that clinicians can provide medical information and treatment options but that giving direction regarding sexual life choices is inappropriate, as well as unlikely to be helpful or well received.

      Three particularly useful interviewing techniques are *inclusion, normalization,* and *universalization.* In the *inclusive approach,* patients are reassured that questions regarding sexual-

Table 20–4
The PLISSIT Model

- Permission: validating that sexual concerns are important and reasonable; giving permission to discuss them.
- Limited Information: can be provided regarding sexual functioning and health.
- Specific Suggestions: regarding the sexual concern or complaint, without engaging in more intensive interventions (e.g., suggesting a change in preferred coital position for a patient who has developed respiratory disease or arthritis).
- Intensive Therapy: may be provided by health professionals with sufficient training and experience.

Adapted from Annon JS, Robinson CH. The use of vicarious learning models in treatment of sexual concerns. In: LoPiccolo J, LoPiccolo L, Editors. Handbook of Sex Therapy. New York: Plenum Publishing Corp.; 1978.

ity are a routine part of clinical practice and preventive care. For example, when interviewing an adolescent patient, the physician can introduce the sexual history by explaining: "I'm going to ask you a few questions that I ask all my young adult patients about their health and relationships." A patient of any age can be reassured that "sexual functioning is an important part of health. I ask all my patients about it." In *normalization*, the clinician introduces subjects that may be emotionally laden or difficult by communicating to the patient that these experiences are (unfortunately) prevalent and that he or she is not alone: "Many people have been sexually abused or molested as children. Did you have experiences like that when you were young?" *Universalization* assumes that "everyone has done everything" and thereby makes answering in the affirmative easier in potentially sensitive questions. For example, patients can be asked, "How often do you masturbate?" instead of, "Do you masturbate?"

b. *Content.* The sexual history contains basic medical information, such as prior illnesses, injuries, hospitalizations, and surgeries; chemical and toxin information, including medication use, nonprescription drug use, industrial and employment exposures, alcohol and recreational drug use; relationship history (current and past); social history, including childhood sexual experiences and physical or sexual abuse; self-concept (gender identification and desired role or roles, sexual orientation); information about sexual functioning, including the onset, nature, and context of sexual dysfunctions, sexual functioning in other contexts (including masturbation); and sexual plans and goals.

Two formats for the sexual history are presented in Tables 20–5 and 20–6. Table 20–5 represents a basic sexual history, which can be incorporated into clinical encounters with patients of any age, including routine office visits and health maintenance examinations. The history presented in Table 20–6 is much more detailed and can be used in the comprehensive evaluation of sexual problems. Portions of the longer history can be used in the evaluation of more limited dysfunctions.

Even when it is understood that the clinical interview should address particular issues, specific phrasing can be problematic. The following questions are therefore offered as particularly useful alternatives:

Table 20–5
The (Screening) Sexual History

This is a very basic screening sexual history that can be routinely included in clinical encounters. Key questions include:

1. Sexual activity (type and frequency).
2. Sexual partners, if any, and their relationship to the patient.
3. Sexual orientation.
4. Satisfaction with sexual functioning as well as the existence and nature of any problem with sexual functioning.
5. Understanding of the health issues relevant to his or her sexual behavior and whether the patient has taken precautions (if applicable) to prevent injury, transmission of infection, or undesired pregnancy.
6. Conversely, understanding of the implications of the patient's sexual functioning for his or her physical condition or therapeutic regimen.
7. Any anxieties, misconceptions, or questions that the patient may be willing to share about sexual issues or sexual functioning.
8. Any relevant past events, especially emotional, physical, or sexual abuse.

Data from Cheadle MJ. The screening sexual history. Clin Geriatr Med 1991; 7:9–13.

- *General questions:* "What questions or concerns do you have about sex or sexual functioning?"
  (To adolescents): "What questions do you have about your body or your health? about relationships?"
- *Introductory relationship questions:* "Do you have a spouse or partner?" "Are you currently in an intimate relationship?" "Is this relationship exclusive, or do you have other partners?" (Avoid using terms or pronouns that imply a heterosexual relationship. These may be interpreted as indicating a judgmental attitude and can interfere with the accuracy of the interview.)
- *Introductory questions about sexual behavior:* "Are you sexually active?" "Have your sexual partners been men, women, or both?"
- *Preventive/screening questions:* "What questions do you have about AIDS and other sexually transmitted diseases?" "Do you think that you may be at risk?" "Why/why not?" "Are you using contraception currently?" "What are your pregnancy plans?"
- *Questions regarding the goals/satisfaction with sexual relationship:* "How satisfied are you with your sexual relationship ("sex life," and so on)? If you could magically change your sexual relationship to be just the way you wanted it, what would that be?"

Note:

If the patient does not understand usual

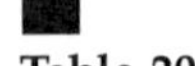

Table 20–6
The (Longer) Sexual History

Background information: age, employment, education, finances, substance use, etc.

Relationship history:

1. Who lives at home with you presently? How are those relationships?
2. Do you have an ongoing sexual relationship or current partner (or partners)?
3. How long have the two of you been together?
4. During that time, when were you the happiest?
5. How has your relationship changed over time? What influenced that change?
6. What are one or two things that seem most satisfying in your relationship?
7. What are one or two things that are most dissatisfying in your relationship?
8. How do you think your partner/spouse perceives your relationship?

Sexual history:

1. What was your earliest sexual experience? (Explore affect: pleasant? unpleasant? frightening?)
2. Do you remember how you learned about sex?
3. What were the attitudes of your family about sex? How were you prepared for puberty? Marriage? Sexual relationship(s)?
4. How were you prepared for changes in your body as you became a teenager?

Men:

- How old were you when your body began to change?
- What were your feelings about these body changes and voice changes?
- What reactions did your parents, friends, and siblings have to these changes?
- How old were you when you had your first erection?
- How old were you when you had your first nocturnal emission (wet dream)?
- Who told you about wet dreams?
- How many sexual partners have you had in your lifetime?
- Have your sexual partners been women, men, or both?
- Were you ever sexually molested, abused, or mistreated as a child? (What happened?)

Women:

- How old were you when your breasts began to develop?
- How old were you when you began menstruating (having periods)?
- What were your feelings about these physical changes?
- What reactions did your parents, friends, siblings have to these changes?
- Did you have any problems related to your periods (too heavy, irregular, etc.)?
- Who prepared you for menstruation?
- How old were you when you first learned about your clitoris?
- How old were you when you first experienced orgasm?
- Have you experienced orgasm alone (in masturbation)? With other partners (same sex, opposite sex)?
- How many sexual relationships have you had in your lifetime?
- In what situations do you find orgasm difficult?
- Were you ever sexually molested, abused, or mistreated as a child? (What happened?)

Attitudinal development and self-concept:

1. How attractive did you feel in comparison to others when you were a child, adolescent, and adult?
2. How attractive do you feel now?
3. Are you pleased with your body?
4. What would you change if you could?
5. How attractive are you to your partner?
6. Are you satisfied with your masculinity/femininity?
7. When you were growing up, how did your religious views influence your attitudes about sexuality? Currently?
8. What influences did your family have on your sexual attitudes and development?
9. Was your ethnic background important?
10. Were your parents' political views important?
11. How did your peer group act with regard to sexual issues and behavior?
12. Who provided you with sexuality education?
13. Was it adequate?

Masturbation:

1. How old were you when you began to masturbate?
2. Did you feel guilty?
3. Have you discussed masturbation with your partner(s)?

Contraception (omit if patient has never experienced a heterosexual relationship):

1. What methods of contraception have you used?
2. Did they cause any difficulties for you? (medically? sexually?)
3. Did they ever fail to protect you/a partner from pregnancy?
4. Who do you think should be responsible for contraception?

Sexually transmitted disease (STD) exposure and prevention:

1. Have you ever been treated for a sexually transmitted disease?
2. What concerns do you have about STDs/HIV?
3. What measures do you take to protect yourself from STDs/HIV?
4. Are you knowledgeable about HIV and AIDS?

Present sexual relationship(s):

1. How would you describe your affectional or sexual life now?
2. What activity gives you the most pleasure?
3. What activity is most satisfying?
4. In this relationship, what changes have there been in the way you want yourself or your partner to perform?
5. How often do you and your partner have sex? Who usually initiates these experiences?
6. What are ways the two of you express tenderness?
7. Do you talk to each other about your relationship? About sex?
8. What other ways do you have for meeting your sexual needs?
9. If you could magically change your sex life so that it would be just the way you would like it, how would it be?
10. What other questions and concerns do you have about sex or sexual activity?

Data from Foley S, Adler J, Marszalek-Gaucher E. Unpublished data, 1981.

medical-sexual terminology, it may be helpful to substitute other terms. However, the use of slang should be avoided because it can easily be interpreted by the patient as a change in professional boundaries. The patient should be asked to explain anything that the physician does not understand.

2. *Physical examination.*
Diagnosis of many sexual dysfunctions can be made through the interview alone. Nonetheless, in the absence of diagnostic certainty, a complete physical examination should also be performed. Areas of particular relevance to sexual functioning include the thyroid gland; cardiovascular and pulmonary systems; nervous system, including the sensory organs and mental status; genital, rectal, and urologic areas; and dermal integrity.
Disturbances in sexual functioning are often indicative of other systemic illnesses (Table 20–1), and the physician should be alert for signs of previously undiagnosed physical pathology.

3. *Diagnostic studies.*
There is no "sexuality panel" or standard set of diagnostic studies that should be performed at the beginning of the evaluation of a sexual dysfunction. Laboratory work should address any evidence of endocrine, cardiac, or other physical pathology that is detected during the history and physical examination. Elderly or physically disabled patients may also require functional studies, such as pulmonary function tests and cardiac stress testing. Tests that may be useful in specific sexual dysfunctions are discussed later in this chapter.
"Routine" tests should not be ordered for the evaluation of sexual pathology.

D. Treatment.

The common sexual dysfunctions are listed in Table 20–7.

General principles for treatment of any sexual dysfunction involve appropriate guidance (*limited intervention* or *referral*) and close clinical *follow-up.* In general, the *PLISSIT model* is helpful in determining the level of nonreferral treatment that can be provided in each clinical situation. In many cases, offering validation of the individual's sexuality and *permission* to discuss sexual issues and functioning (as in the case of Ms. T., section I.A) is sufficient. Many clinical cases in primary care practice can be managed with *limited information* or *specific suggestions,* as is illustrated subsequently.

Table 20–7
Sexual Dysfunctions

Etiology
Drugs
Neurogenic
Vascular
Endocrine
Disability/illness/degenerative diseases
Psychological/social
Classification
Sexual desire disorders
Sexual arousal disorders
Orgasm disorders
Sexual pain disorders
Sexual dysfunction, not otherwise specified

Data from American Psychiatric Association. Diagnostic and Statistical Manual of Mental Disorders. Washington DC: American Psychiatric Association; 1994.

Case Study

Mr. S. is a 55-year-old metal worker who is brought to medical attention by his wife, with her chief complaint of his unwillingness to have intercourse with her. Their sexual relationship was reportedly satisfactory until her recent hysterectomy; since the surgery, they have continued to cuddle and kiss but have not engaged in any form of genital touching, at his unexplained insistence. Further inquiry reveals that he believes that without the uterus to "hold it open," her vagina may collapse and "trap" his penis. After receiving the limited information that the vagina is a muscular organ that retains its shape and strength after hysterectomy, he is reassured and able to resume mutually satisfactory intercourse.

Other common clinical situations in which the provision of limited information regarding sexuality and sexual functioning can prove helpful include times of physiologic change, such as menopause, pregnancy, and the elder years.

Examples of treatment involving *specific suggestions* include offering advice regarding alternative positions for intercourse following cesarean section (to take the pressure off the scar) or in cases of advanced rheumatoid arthritis (to maintain sexual functioning), or advising couples whose sexual relationships are becoming impaired due to one or both partners' progressive COPD that having intercourse in a large rocking chair may provide some of the needed motion and allow increased sexual participation with limited respiratory capacity.

It is important for primary care physicians and mental health professionals to locate appropriate referral resources for individuals and couples whose sexual dysfunctions require continued behavioral counseling (*intensive therapy,* which should not be provided without specific training in this discipline). For example, a patient of either gender who experiences orgasmic dysfunction after a sexual assault would be best served by referral to a therapist skilled in both sex therapy and survivor recovery issues. The certifying body for sex therapists in the United States is the American Association of Sex Educators, Counselors, and Therapists (AASECT). Physicians who practice in communities without resources in this professional discipline can contact AASECT for referral information.

Follow-up in cases of sexual dysfunction is also important. Even if the intervention consists of the provision of limited information, further discussion at a later time is often helpful. Scheduled follow-up is especially useful when a referral has been made. Patients may be more likely to follow through with the referral appointment if the personal physician expresses interest in integrating sexual health with other aspects of physical and mental well-being on an ongoing basis. In addition, such an expression of interest may provide an opportunity to address any problems that have been encountered with the referral process and to offer further support as the patient confronts potentially sensitive issues. However, physicians should be alert to the possibility that a patient may attempt to circumvent the treatment process (e.g., he or she may avoid keeping the referral appointment because, "I can't talk to anyone but you about this") and must stay within the limits of their professional expertise.

The treatment of many of the common sexual dysfunctions is discussed in the following two sections. However, sexual medicine is a broad clinical discipline, and this text is not comprehensive. Clinicians who are interested in obtaining further information or training are advised to consult the references listed at the end of this chapter. *Human Sexuality and its Problems*[6] is an excellent general reference.

IV. Female sexual dysfunctions.

A. Organismic dysfunction.

Orgasmic dysfunction refers to the inability to reach orgasm when desired. This condition is further divided into *primary inhibited orgasm,* in which the patient has never (yet) experienced orgasm, and *secondary inhibited orgasm,* in which the dysfunction manifests after previous satisfactory orgasmic functioning. Not included in this disorder is the inability to reach orgasm with vaginal intercourse because fewer than 50% of women are orgasmic without additional clitoral stimulation. Although their male partners may desire primarily vaginal intercourse, many women prefer simultaneous vaginal and clitoral stimulation, oral-genital sex, or clitoral stimulation alone for sexual satisfaction.

1. *Causes.*
   Common causes for primary inhibited orgasm include lack of knowledge regarding female sexual anatomy and functioning; lack of prior self-stimulation; guilt feelings about sexuality, sexual fantasies, and sexual behavior (which occurs frequently in women who have been raised with negative messages regarding sexuality or strict religious or cultural prohibitions, even if their behavior never violates these principles); and physical or sexual abuse. Secondary inhibited orgasm can be caused by other medical and psychological illnesses, lack of personal or partner knowledge regarding sexual functioning or technique, relationship problems, stressful life circumstances or preoccupations, substance abuse, dyspareunia, and abuse.

2. *Evaluation.*
   The clinical history in cases of secondary inhibited orgasm should focus on the patient's perception of this dysfunction: time and circumstances of onset, possible causes, effect on relationships, treatment goals, and physiologic functioning during sexual stimulation, including adequacy of lubrication and ability to sustain states of high arousal. In addition, contributing factors (e.g., fatigue, depression, postpartum physical and social changes, preoccupation with other life issues, substance abuse, other medical illnesses) and relationship issues (e.g., lack of tenderness or interest in nonintercourse stimulation or foreplay by the partner, early ejaculation, contraceptive responsibility, lack of privacy) should be explored.

   When orgasmic dysfunction is primary, it is also important to ascertain that the patient is knowledgeable regarding the nature of orgasm. In males, orgasm is usually accompanied by ejaculation, which serves as a reference point and milestone during adolescence. In women, no such "marker" is present. Portrayals of female orgasm in novels and films are often overstated or misleading. The question, "Do you experience rhythmic contractions of your vagina followed by a feeling of physical and psychological relaxation?" may be helpful in assessing the experience of orgasm.

   In both primary and secondary inhibited orgasm, the physician should ask about past or current experiences of violence and victimization, including emotional (psychological), physical, and sexual abuse.

   In most cases of orgasmic dysfunction, no specific physical examination or laboratory testing is necessary. Neurologic, gynecologic, or other examination may be suggested by the clinical history.

3. *Treatment.*
   Treatment of orgasmic dysfunction usually involves increasing knowledge and sexual options for the patient and partner. Women experiencing primary inhibited orgasm often benefit from receiving information about female sexual anatomy and function. *For Yourself: The Fulfillment of Female Sexuality*[7] is an ex-

cellent book to recommend for women who have not yet experienced orgasm. Masturbation is also frequently helpful because it provides information about sexual responsiveness and preferred stimulations, which can then be transferred to sexual situations with the partner. Many people who have been discouraged from masturbation for religious reasons are not opposed to participating in this behavior in order to improve their orgasmic functioning or marriage relationship. Partner education is usually important, especially with regard to the importance of clitoral stimulation and adequate preintercourse love-making. Changing the focus of the relationship from intercourse to mutual pleasuring, spontaneity, and satisfaction can be crucial. Referral for more in-depth therapy is indicated if the evaluation reveals significant relationship dysfunction, past abuse as an etiologic factor, or other severe medical or psychosocial complications.

Case Study
Ms. J. is a 21-year-old retail worker who presents for annual gynecologic examination and refill of oral contraceptive prescription. When asked about sexual functioning, she replies that she has never experienced orgasm and attributes this to two rapes, which she suffered early in life, the first at age 6 years and the second at 12. She received no counseling or treatment after either assault and was afraid of sexual contact for many years, but she now has a boyfriend with whom she has an enjoyable sexual relationship. She would like to experience orgasm and also wonders if she is "normal" because she enjoys intercourse but is never orgasmic. Further discussion focuses on the other benefits that she experiences in her sexual relationship (increased closeness and affection), the fact that many women (and some men) enjoy intercourse without reaching orgasm, and options for treatment (because she would like to experience orgasm). She chooses to begin with reading For Yourself: The Fulfillment of Female Sexuality[7] and also accepts a referral for counseling regarding her abuse experiences.

Case Study
Mrs. D. is a 36-year-old clerical worker and mother of three children who presents for annual gynecologic care. When asked about sexual functioning, she replies that she experiences orgasm with her husband much less frequently than she would like to. Further history reveals that her husband very often reaches orgasm before she does and that love-making ceases at that time. She masturbates occasionally and believes that she can begin to share information regarding her preferred types of stimulation with her husband, so that he can continue to pleasure her after his orgasm. However, at a follow-up visit, she reports that she was informed by her husband that he regards sex with her as being for his own pleasure and that he has no interest in continued lovemaking after he is satisfied. This revelation was disappointing but seems consistent with his nonhelpful stance regarding child care and other aspects of the relationship. She declines a referral for counseling at this time but states that she has "a lot to think about."

B. Vaginismus.

Vaginismus is an involuntary, usually painful, spastic contraction of the pelvic musculature surrounding the outer third of the vagina. It may be complete (precluding intercourse, tampon insertion, or other vaginal penetration), partial (resulting in dyspareunia or difficulty with other forms of vaginal penetration, including speculum examination), or situational (e.g., occurring when intercourse is anticipated).

1. *Etiology.*
   Vaginismus may be idiopathic. In many cases, however, its onset follows an episode (or episodes) of pelvic trauma, such as painful intercourse, sexual assault, rough gynecologic examination, complicated episiotomy, vaginal infections or pelvic inflammatory disease, pelvic congestion, or pelvic surgery. Childhood or adolescent sexual abuse may also lead to vaginismus during adulthood.

2. *Diagnosis.*
   The diagnosis of vaginismus is generally made on the basis of history. Patients report being unable to engage in vaginal intercourse or to use tampons or vaginal contraceptives, or they experience pain and difficulty with intercourse, digital vaginal stimulation, or pelvic examination. The physical examination may occasionally be revealing. Patients who demonstrate visible contraction of the pelvic floor musculature with anticipated speculum examination should be asked about dyspareunia, previous pelvic trauma, and other sexual concerns. Physical examination can also detect pertinent anatomic abnormalities, such as vaginal septa.

3. *Treatment.*
   True vaginismus is not under the conscious control of the sufferer, and *therapy must be directed at restoring this control under conditions that respect the autonomy of the patient and maintain safety from further trauma.* At no time should the patient be encouraged to participate in activities that she perceives as uncomfortable, stressful, painful, or upsetting, regardless of the expectations of her partner. Furthermore, if the patient expresses fear or anxiety (either verbally or physically), the pelvic examination may be deferred until a subsequent visit, at which time she can be accompanied by a supportive friend. In severe cases, sedation may be necessary, even for routine gynecologic examination.

Any physical abnormalities detected on pelvic examination, such as infections, should first be treated. After this, the patient may begin self-treatment with size-graded vaginal dilators, gradually teaching her vagina to remain relaxed and to receive nonpainful, self-controlled penetration. Warmth and lubrication are helpful. The initial dilator used should be of very small diameter (usually smaller than a tampon) in order to avoid triggering vaginal spasm. Referral to a sex therapist is often helpful, and treatment of post-traumatic stress disorder and other sequelae of past trauma may be crucial. Follow-up over time is necessary.

Case Study

Ms. M. is a 19-year-old student who presents with the chief complaint of inability to have intercourse. She is currently involved in her first dating relationship involving genital intimacy. She and her boyfriend (for whom this is also a first sexual relationship) attempted intercourse twice during the past weekend but were unsuccessful because of the tight spasticity of her vagina. She is able to use tampons and to enjoy manual-genital stimulation to orgasm, both alone and with her boyfriend. She is concerned that there is "something wrong" anatomically. Physical examination reveals a somewhat thickened but normal hymen and no vaginal septum, sign of infection, or other abnormality except for contraction of her pelvic musculature before examination with a pediatric speculum. Further discussion reveals some ambivalence about intercourse, resulting from her family background and (now questioned) religious beliefs, and also concerns regarding contraception. She is referred to a sex therapist with experience in treating vaginismus and seen in follow-up by her personal physician. After a program of self-controlled vaginal dilation, personal values clarification, and contraceptive protection, she is able to begin having satisfactory sexual intercourse.

Case Study

Mrs. J. is a 42-year-old secretary who has sought sex therapy because she has never been able to have intercourse at any time during the 22 years of her marriage. She sought medical assistance 2 months after her wedding, and despite giving a history classic for vaginismus, was told that she just "needed to relax" and that the ability to have intercourse would come with time. A few years later, another physician dismissed her questions with the statement that she should "consider herself lucky that her husband had stayed with her." Recently, she has read more about sex therapy and would like to find out if any treatment is available for her problem. She is referred to a qualified sex therapist. After approximately 6 months of cognitive therapy (around issues of childhood abuse and adult autonomy) and self-directed vaginal dilation, she is able to begin having intercourse with her husband. No further problems are detected in follow-up.

C. Dyspareunia.

Dyspareunia refers to pain experienced immediately before, during, or after intercourse by either women or men.

1. *Etiology.*
   Dyspareunia can be caused by anatomic or physiologic factors (e.g., vaginal septa, partial vaginismus, and inadequate lubrication), relationship difficulties, poor sexual technique, or a rough or abusive partner. Emotional factors (e.g., religious conflicts and the sequelae of childhood abuse) may also contribute.
2. *Diagnosis.*
   Diagnosis of dyspareunia is made by history and physical examination. Useful questions include the onset, duration, and circumstances in which this problem occurred, the location of the pain (e.g., superficial, deep, unilateral, bilateral), and whether it is specific to a particular partner or practice. In addition to evidence of infection, vaginismus, or anatomic abnormality, physical examination may reveal evidence of trauma, such as introital fissuring and bruising of the medial thighs, because some women experiencing dyspareunia are in relationships with husbands or boyfriends in which tolerance of sexual roughness and insensitivity is expected.
3. *Treatment.*
   Treatment of dyspareunia depends on determination of its cause and usually requires clinical follow-up. Treatment of physiologic causes, such as atrophic or infectious vaginitis, is often straightforward. The clinical management of vaginismus was discussed earlier in this chapter. In some cases, providing information regarding the importance of clitoral stimulation and adequate sex play before intercourse, as well as the option of using supplemental water-based lubrication may be sufficient, especially if the pain is located in the proximal vagina or introitus. "Deep" dyspareunia is often caused by overvigorous penetration or excess cervical pressure and may respond to limited educational interventions. For example, many people do not realize that both penises and vaginas vary in length, and that in cases in which the former is longer, the vagina may not stretch to accommodate full penile engulfment; attempts to do so, however, cause deep dyspareunia. Changing position to allow the woman to control the amount of cervical pressure may also be of crucial importance.

   In cases in which partner roughness or poor sexual technique is a factor, it is important to stress that no one should be required to tolerate sexual pain (and that this can lead to medical complications, e.g., vaginismus) and to clarify the patient's goals for the relationship. In some cases, referral for sex therapy for the couple may prove helpful; in other cases, the patient may be able to bring about change in the sexual relationship with sufficient information and assertiveness. If dyspareunia is the result of deliberate carelessness or abuse by the partner, ending the relationship may be the only viable option. (Chapter 21 of this text gives information regarding the medical management of domestic violence and partner abuse.)

V. Male sexual dysfunctions.

A. Erectile dysfunction.

Erectile dysfunction is the most common reason for which men consult sex therapists in North America. Erectile dysfunction consists of the inability to obtain or sustain an erection and is analogous to insufficient lubrication in women (both of which are excitement phase disorders). Erectile dysfunction is preferred over the older term, *impotence,* which is vague and demeaning to the patient. Very occasional or isolated episodes of erectile dysfunction are common and do not usually require treatment. The evaluation and treatment of more consistent or problematic erectile dysfunction is discussed below.

1. *Etiology.*
Erectile dysfunction can be caused by physiologic impairments, psychological dysfunction, or a combination of both. Physiologic causes include trauma (e.g., T12 spinal cord injury or serious genital injury), neurovascular disease (as often accompanies diabetes mellitus), degenerative disorders (e.g., multiple sclerosis), Peyronie's disease (which can make erection painful), and postpriapism erectile dysfunction. Psychological causes include depression, anxiety, fear of failure, guilt, previous physical or sexual abuse, conflict regarding sexual orientation or gender identity, intrusive nonsexual thoughts or preoccupation with other aspects of life, stress, fatigue, and relationship difficulties. Both women and men who are experiencing sexual dysfunction often develop problems as a result of the *spectator effect*: fear of recurrent failure or difficulty causes part of the attention to be focused on self-performance (as a "spectator") rather than on pleasuring and enjoyment; this phenomenon further decreases arousal.

2. *Evaluation.*
Evaluation and diagnosis of erectile dysfunction are usually based on the history. As with other sexual dysfunctions, it is important to ask about the onset, duration, and circumstances of the dysfunction, as well as the patient's opinion regarding possible causes and the significance to his sexual relationship or relationships. Psychosocial interviewing should also be conducted. In addition, the presence or absence of nocturnal penile tumescence is of crucial diagnostic importance (NPT). If NPT is occurring with regularity, the cause of the erectile dysfunction is unlikely to be primarily physical. Various means of testing for NPT have been developed, including nocturnal monitors and the "postage stamp test." In the latter, the penis is encircled with a single thickness of paper that is joined with a stamp. If the stamp is intact after sleep, erection has not occurred. Although some patients may benefit from more specific evaluation, the history alone is often sufficient. The patient should be asked whether he awakens with early morning erections.
Physical examination may be revealing if evidence of endocrine dysfunction, infection, neurologic or vascular disease, or the calcifications of Peyronie's disease are present. In most cases, physical examination is normal. If needed, specific testing of the penile vasculature can be carried out by a urologist.

3. *Treatment.*
Successful treatment of patients with erectile dysfunction depends on correct etiologic identification and appropriate follow-up. Underlying medical causes should be treated aggressively, and referral care (e.g., urology, vascular surgery) should be obtained as appropriate. Ongoing emotional support of the patient and partner may be helpful, even if the treatment of the dysfunction itself falls within the domain of another specialty. In addition, some adjunctive treatments may be beneficial. For example, men with vascular disease leading to erectile dysfunction may ultimately require surgical therapy, but they may experience temporary relief with the application of 1 to 2 cm of a transdermal nitroglycerin ointment to the skin of the scrotum 10 minutes before intercourse. Precautions pertinent to this therapy are the same as when topical nitrates are applied to other parts of the body. Patients with erectile dysfunction that is not otherwise remediable may benefit from external suction devices or surgically placed penile implants (semirigid or inflatable).
Patients for whom erectile dysfunction has a primarily or exclusively psychological cause may benefit from individual cognitive or pharmacologic therapy. Survivors of physical or sexual abuse may require long-term therapy and support with a therapist experienced in this area. In addition, attention must be paid to the relationship context, as illustrated in the following case study.

Case Study

Mr. M. is a 24-year-old accountant who has presented to a sex therapist for evaluation of erectile dysfunction. He and his fiancee live in different cities and can spend only one weekend per month together. They have been in an exclusive relationship for about 3 years and began having intercourse 6 months ago. During their past few visits, he has been unable to get an erection and is concerned that something is "wrong." Further history reveals that Mr. M. is in excellent health, takes no medications, does not abuse alcohol or other drugs, and frequently awakens with early morning erections. He can maintain an erection sufficient to achieve orgasm when masturbating, although he does so rarely. This is the first sexual relationship involving intercourse for both partners. They are not using contraception because they lack knowledge about contraceptive methods and are embarrassed about procuring them. Mr. M. is worried that his fiancee will become pregnant (which would be a major embarrassment for both partners) and feels that their sexual relationship was much more satisfying in the past, when they regularly had manual-genital sex but no intercourse. When the therapist points out that he has done the "gentlemanly thing" by stopping intercourse (albeit through refusal to obtain an erection), his affect brightens considerably, and he is able to list options that would be satisfactory, including postponing intercourse and obtaining appropriate contraception. Follow-up reveals no recurrence of the dysfunction.

B. Premature ejaculation.

Premature ejaculation refers to the occurrence of male ejaculation (usually with orgasm) before this is desired by the individual, his partner, or both. Attempts to quantify "averages," such as the number of thrusting movements accomplished before ejaculation, and to compare the behavior of individuals complaining of premature ejaculation to these "norms," have not proved useful.

1. *Etiology.*
Men who are young, sexually inexperienced, or having intercourse infrequently are most likely to experience premature ejaculation. In some cases, premature ejaculation (followed by immediate cessation of sexual activity) may be a means of expressing hostility toward the partner or of practicing self-punishment. In addition, premature ejaculation is somewhat situationally defined: short duration of intercourse is valued by women (and men) who do not enjoy sex and by those in commercial sex situations.

2. *Evaluation.*
Evaluation of premature ejaculation is based on the patient's history. Onset, circumstances, and (personal and relationship) meaning of the dysfunction should be explored, as should pertinent past sexual experiences. For example, young men whose first sexual experiences were rushed (e.g., because of fear of discovery or participation in commercial sex settings) may later have difficulty establishing ejaculatory control in more relaxed contexts. Masturbation experience may also be important: can the patient prolong his erection while masturbating? In addition, information regarding level of sexual knowledge and partner expectations may be significant, as in the following case study.

3. *Treatment.*
Several options are available for the treatment of premature ejaculation; these can be selected and combined by the patient and the partner: the *squeeze technique*, the *stop and start* technique, masturbation training, and non–intercourse-based pleasuring. In situations without underlying relationship difficulties, the prognosis is excellent. More complicated cases should be referred to a sex therapist. Physicians and therapists who are not experienced in this area should facilitate referral to another professional.

In the squeeze technique, the partner places her or his thumb on the ventral surface of the penis, either at the frenulum or at the base, and her or his first two fingers on the dorsal side (Fig. 20–2). The application of firm (squeezing) pressure for 3 to 5 seconds, followed by quick release, temporarily relieves the need to ejaculate. The couple can resume penile stimulation when the sensation of impending ejaculation has subsided and can use the squeeze technique repeatedly as needed. The advantage to this technique is that rather than attempting to improve ejaculatory control, the patient can rely on his partner for assistance and be relieved of the anxiety created by the ejaculatory dysfunction. The squeeze technique was developed by Masters and Johnson and is described in further detail in their basic text.

"Stop and start" refers to the process of learning to stop or reduce penile stimulation when ejaculation is approaching, but not imminent, and resume when arousal has partially dissipated. The patient can continue to pleasure his partner by other means during this interval. Masturbation training aimed at increasing ejaculatory control may also be useful, and changing the focus of the relationship from achieving partner orgasm with intercourse to mutual pleasuring (as described in the following case) often results in an improved sexual relationship, regardless of immediate success in prolonging ejaculation.

Case Study

Mr. L. is a 19-year-old retail worker who presents for a complete physical. His past medical and surgical histories are unremarkable. His stated reason for the examination is "just to be sure everything's okay." His physical examination is completely within normal limits. After he has been reassured that he is medically normal, he volunteers his real concern: he is involved in his first sexual relationship, including intercourse, with a woman his own age. He is very much in love and wants to do everything he can to please her. However, when they have intercourse, she sometimes experiences orgasm and sometimes does not. He is shy in discussing their sex life with her, but he did ask his 25-year-old cousin about

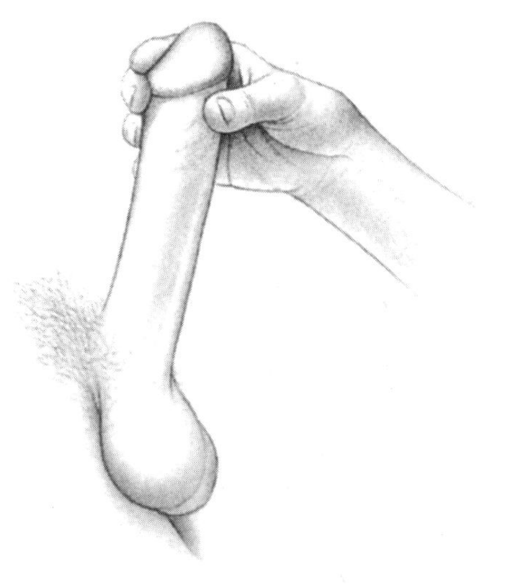

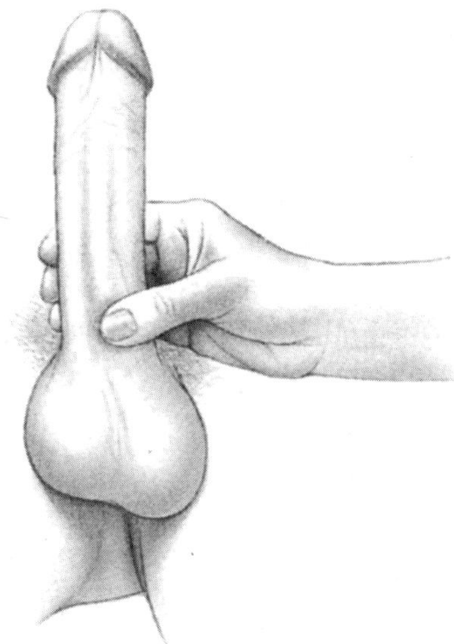

Figure 20–2
The squeeze technique, which can be applied either at the corona *(left)* or at the base of the penis *(right)*, is useful for the treatment of premature ejaculation. (From Allgeier AR, Allgeier ER: Sexual Interactions, Fourth Edition. Lexington, MA, D.C. Heath and Company, 1995, p. 225. Reprinted with permission of Houghton Mifflin Company.)

women's orgasms. His cousin told him that he and his wife "climax together about 90% of the time" and that he "just has to get the hang of it." Further discussion reveals that before intercourse was added to their sexual relationship, both Mr. L. and his girlfriend had no difficulty in reaching orgasm through manual-genital and oral-genital sex and were not concerned about whose orgasm occurred first. After learning that most couples do not orgasm simultaneously with 90% frequency and that it is fine to continue to pleasure a partner manually or orally after ejaculation, rather than relying on intercourse alone for the partner's orgasm, he is much relieved and is able to resume a less pressured and mutually satisfying sexual relationship.

C. Dyspareunia.

The definition of dyspareunia is gender neutral (see section IV). However, men experience dyspareunia much less often with vaginal-penile intercourse than do women. In discussing dyspareunia, it is important to specify the site of the discomfort and the sexual activity involved (i.e., whether the male patient is the inserting or is the anally receptive partner).

1. *Etiology.*
Dyspareunia in men is often the result of concurrent medical illness, such as Peyronie's disease or neuropathy, although relationship dynamics and poor sexual technique may also cause sexual discomfort, such as when the penis is extended too far caudally during intercourse with the female partner on top. Anal dyspareunia in men and women is usually the result of insufficient lubrication or spasm of the anal musculature.
2. *Evaluation.*
Evaluation consists of the history and physical examination. As with most sexual dysfunctions, onset, context, and patient perceptions regarding possible causes and impact on the patient's relationship or relationships are important. Physical examination may reveal evidence of neuropathy, urethritis, epididymitis, Peyronie's disease, prostatitis, anal fissures, hemorrhoids, or other pertinent findings.
3. *Treatment.*
Treatment of dyspareunia involves correction of underlying physical pathology, counseling regarding sexual technique, and referral of complicated cases to a urologist or sex therapist, as indicated.

VI. Sexual orientation issues.

A. The sexual orientation spectrum.

Sexual orientation is a social construct. Many nonhuman primates and other mammals engage in sexual stimulation with members of both sexes. Among humans, "normality" with regard to which sexual acts are acceptable, with whom, and under what circumstances has varied enormously in different cultures and eras. For example, no word for homosexuality existed in ancient Greece because it was assumed that most males (and some females) would have sex with both women and men. However, modern Western cultures, including the United States, have until the past few decades regarded same-sex sexual partnerships as immoral or as evidence of medical or psychological illness. (Homosexuality was removed from the roster of mental disorders by the American Psychiatric Association in 1974.) Current theories regarding the determinants of sexual orientation favor genetic, or a combination of genetic and social factors, rather than developmental impairment or maladaptation.

Furthermore, until the publication of *Sexual*

Behavior in the Human Male[8] by Kinsey and colleagues in 1948, it was generally assumed that homosexual behavior was uncommon. Kinsey, a zoologist, hypothesized that sexual orientation might be found along a continuous spectrum, from exclusive heterosexuality through exclusive homosexuality, and might vary across the lifespan in different individuals. His theories proved correct and generated the *Kinsey Scale* (Table 20–8), which is a useful tool for discussing sexual orientation issues with patients and clinicians.

B. Prevalence of homosexuality, bisexuality, and heterosexuality.

For at least 130 years, researchers have attempted to measure the prevalence of homosexuality and bisexuality, assuming heterosexuality as a "norm," with varying degrees of success and resultant controversy. Some of the milestones of this research follow:

In 1864, Karl Heinrich Ulrichs estimated that one German male in 500 was homosexual, based on his social observations. Critics stated that this figure was far too high.

In 1903–1904, Magnus Hirschfeld surveyed approximately 3000 students and 5700 metal workers. Based on a response rate of 49%, he concluded that 94.3% of German men were heterosexual, 2.3% were homosexual, and 3.4% were bisexual. He was fined 200 Deutschmarks on the grounds that impressionable young men could have been led toward "perverse tendencies" as a result of his survey.

In 1948, Kinsey and coworkers[8] concluded that for the total white male population, approximately 37% had had at least some homosexual experience; 25% had had more than incidental experience for at least 3 years; 18% had been at least as homosexual as heterosexual in behavior and/or attractions for at least 3 years; 13% had been more homosexually than heterosexually oriented for at least 3 years; 10% had been mostly homosexually oriented for at least 3 years; 8% had been exclusively homosexual for at least 3 years; and 4% had been exclusively homosexual all their lives. (The Kinsey team attempted to recruit participants of varying racial identities but were able to reach statistical significance only for the white population.) In 1953, Kinsey and coworkers[9] published *Sexual Behavior in the Human Female,* which estimated that in the total white female population, approximately 13% had at least some overt, postpubertal homosexual experience and that 3% to 8% of unmarried women aged 20 to 35 years were more homosexually than heterosexually oriented. Contrary to prevailing societal beliefs at that time, this research also discovered that of the 142 participants with the most lesbian experience 50% were without regrets, and that 68% of women in long-term lesbian relationships were usually or always orgasmic, as opposed to 40% of their married counterparts.

Further sexuality research (e.g., Laumann et al., 1994) has found lower prevalences of homosexuality than those found by Kinsey and colleagues, usually in the range of 1% to 4%. However, many report same-sex encounters at some time in life, although they currently identify as heterosexual. It is possible that Kinsey and coworkers and their more modern colleagues are measuring the same human sexual behaviors and orientations but interpreting the data differently. Until people lack the legal or discrimination-based incentive to conceal (and under-report) their same-sex sexual experiences, it is likely that this question will remain unresolved. In the 1990 United States Census, 88,200 homosexual male households and 69,200 lesbian households were reported.

Because many gay, lesbian, and bisexual patients do not share information regarding sexual orientation with their physicians (especially if a sexual history is not obtained), it is likely that most physicians greatly overestimate the number of heterosexual patients in their clinical practices.

Table 20–8
Sexual Orientation: The Kinsey Scale

0: *Exclusively heterosexual* throughout post-puberty life. "Their socio-sexual contacts and responses are exclusively with individuals of the opposite sex."

1: *Incidental homosexual experience* which has involved physical contact or psychic response. "Such homosexual experiences as these individuals have may have occurred only a single time or two, or at least infrequently in comparison to the amount of their heterosexual experience."

2: *More than incidental homosexual experience,* and/or "if they respond rather definitely to homosexual stimuli."

3: *As homosexual as heterosexual.* "Individuals rated 3 stand midway on the heterosexual-homosexual scale. They are about equally homosexual and heterosexual in their overt experience and/or their psychic reactions."

4: *More homosexual than heterosexual.* "Individuals are rated as 4's if they have more overt activity and/or psychic reactions in the homosexual, while still maintaining a fair amount of heterosexual activity and/or responding rather definitely to heterosexual stimuli."

5: *Almost entirely homosexual.* "Individuals are rated 5's if they are almost entirely homosexual in their overt activities and/or reactions . . . [but] they do have incidental experience with the opposite sex and sometimes react psychically to individuals of the opposite sex."

6: *Exclusively homosexual* "both in regard to their overt experience and in regard to their psychic reactions."

Data from Kinsey AC, Pomeroy WB, Martin CE. Sexual Behavior in the Human Male. Philadelphia: WB Saunders Co.; 1948.

C. General clinical considerations in the care of gay, lesbian, and bisexual patients.

In general, all patients have the same medical needs and expectations, regardless of sexual orientation, such as accurate diagnosis and treatment and respectful physician-patient (and physician-family) communication. However, because of the legal and social risks currently associated with homosexuality, the following considerations are especially important for the care of gay, lesbian, and bisexual patients.

1. *Confidentiality.*
"Sodomy" and "crimes against nature" statutes in many states specifically criminalize certain sexual behaviors, especially anal intercourse and fellatio. However, these laws are rarely enforced against heterosexuals, especially married people. Because mention in the medical record of these behaviors may amount to documentation of illegal activity, it is extremely important to maintain record confidentiality, including the keeping of a separate file for sexuality-related information. This may be of benefit in the care of heterosexual patients as well. In addition, as long as sexual orientation–based discrimination and violence continue, a homosexual or bisexual orientation should not be documented in the medical record without the full permission of the patient.

2. *Avoid "heterosexual assumptions."*
Many clinicians assume that individuals are heterosexual until the clinicians are given evidence to the contrary, which can interfere with physician-patient communication and the provision of quality medical care. For example, in the Michigan Lesbian Health Survey,[10] respondents reported having encountered the following problems in their medical care experiences: 61% stated that medical providers assumed that they were heterosexual; 46% had had it assumed that they were part of a "traditional" family; 20% felt that their concerns had not been taken seriously; 9% had had experiences in which their partner was not allowed to stay with them in the medical setting; and 6% reported having encountered physicians who tried to "cure" them of their lesbianism. It is often helpful to phrase introductory questions in a gender-neutral form while getting to know new patients. For example, asking, "Are you in a partnered relationship?" as opposed to "Are you married?" and "What are your plans regarding pregnancy?" rather than "What form of contraception do you use?" provides an opportunity for the patient to openly communicate his or her life circumstances and health concerns.

3. *Insurance needs, violence, and social stress.*
Patients in same-sex couples are generally not eligible for spousal health insurance benefits and are therefore less likely than their heterosexual counterparts to be adequately insured. This is especially true for lesbians, because women in this country generally earn lower wages than men do. Children born or adopted into lesbian or gay families may also be without insurance, if their biologic or legally adopting parent chooses to forego formal employment in order to fulfill child care responsibilities. One quarter of the respondents in the Michigan Lesbian Health Survey reported having foregone needed health care because of financial limitations.
In addition to facing social and employment discrimination, lesbians and gay men are frequently targets of violence. Hate crimes against lesbian and gay persons, including beatings and murder, are on the increase in this country. It is believed that this increase represents a true increase in violent acts rather than simply improved reporting.[11] Depression, anxiety, and substance abuse are common sequelae of physical and emotional abuse. When treating gay people with these psychiatric conditions, the physician must ask about previous and recent abuse experiences.

D. Gay, lesbian, and bisexual youth.

1. *Barriers to healthy development.*
In addition to the psychological challenges faced by all adolescents, gay, lesbian, and bisexual youth encounter further barriers to the development of a healthy adult self-concept and positive interpersonal relationships. These barriers include social sanctions by peers; being barred from social organizations, such as the Boy Scouts; awareness of new discrimination after internalization of prejudices and stereotypes regarding homosexuality during childhood; and lack of positive role models and knowledge about healthy relationships.
Gay, lesbian, and bisexual adolescents also experience increased difficulty in obtaining needed medical services, because of fear of rejection, judgment, ridicule, or breaches of confidentiality by medical providers. Furthermore, because parents can consent for mental health services on behalf of their minor children, some homosexual youth receive inappropriate psychiatric therapy, including in-patient treatment, with the goal of changing their sexual orientation or gender identity. The National Coalition for Lesbian Rights maintains a toll-free hotline for teens who find themselves in this situation: (800) 528-NCLR.

2. *Sexuality issues and mental health care.*
Adolescence is a time of experimentation. Concurrent heterosexual and homosexual feelings and attractions are common, and a single same-sex sexual encounter (or a small number of such experiences) is not necessarily pre-

dictive of a gay, lesbian, or bisexual identity as an adult. However, predominantly homosexual attractions during the teen years are unlikely to change with time. Although there are anecdotal reports of individuals who, through psychotherapy or other means, were able to "give up" their homosexual orientation, *there is no reasonable medical evidence that "sexual reorientation therapy" is consistently successful in changing homosexuals into heterosexuals, or vice versa.* In fact, efforts to change sexual orientation may seriously interfere with self-acceptance, intensify feelings of shame or guilt, and lead to serious sequelae. Adolescents should be given the time and psychological freedom they need for self-exploration and should be reassured by their families and physicians that they will continue to be accepted, regardless of the ultimate direction that their adult sexuality may take. (Parents seeking information or informal support may be referred to Parents and Friends of Lesbians and Gays, 1101 14th St. N.W., Suite 1030, Washington, DC 20005.)

Drug and alcohol experimentation is also common during the teen years and may be used by gay and lesbian adolescents to numb fears regarding sexual orientation or to make heterosexual encounters (which are often undertaken in an effort to prove that the individual is not homosexual) less unpleasant. Unfortunately, substance use also interferes with judgment regarding personal safety, contraception, and safer sex precautions and should be sympathetically discouraged. It is also a risk factor in teen suicide.

Across the life span, suicide risk is greatest among adolescents and the elderly. Furthermore, although no differences in American suicide rates are detectable between heterosexual and homosexual adults, suicide appears to be most common among gay and lesbian youth. Remafedi[12] found that 41 of 137 homosexual adolescents surveyed had attempted suicide and that a majority of these episodes were of moderate to severe lethality. An estimated 30% of successful suicides involve sexual orientation issues. In addition, gay, lesbian and bisexual youth are at much higher risk than are heterosexual teens for family rejection and subsequent homelessness. Physicians who care for adolescents, especially gay youth, should be alert to the possibility of depression, suicide, family stresses, and sexual health risks.

E. Preventive services and health maintenance.

In general, the needs of gay men and lesbians for health promotion and preventive services are the same as those of their heterosexual counterparts. However, several distinctions exist.

Health maintenance services, including clinical breast examination, mammography, and cervical cancer screening, are frequently associated with contraceptive, prenatal, and postpartum visits and are therefore less likely to be obtained by "nonreproductive" women, including celibate women and many lesbians. This disparity is compounded by the differences in insurance coverage and provider acceptance that are often experienced by heterosexual and lesbian women. In addition, although no known physiologic differences exist between lesbian and heterosexual women, their health risk profiles are often dissimilar. Lesbians are less likely to have internalized the female thinness standard of Western culture and are more likely to be nulliparous; therefore, compared with heterosexual women, they are often at lower risk for osteoporosis but at higher risk for cancers of the breast, endometrium, and ovary. Data regarding cardiovascular risks are lacking. Conversely, female-female transmission of sexually transmitted diseases (including human immunodeficiency virus [HIV]) is much less efficient than male-female transmission, and lesbians are at very low risk for unplanned pregnancy and its complications.

Gay men are more likely to exercise regularly and less likely to be obese than are heterosexual men, although (as with sexual behavior) individual variation is substantial. Gay men report having occasional difficulty obtaining adequate health care (because of provider prejudices and fear of HIV) and the clinician bias that "everything is due to HIV," and that HIV testing should be ordered whenever a gay man presents with unusual symptomatology, even when it is not at all suggestive of HIV or acquired immunodeficiency syndrome. Although HIV spread rapidly among urban gay men in the early days of the epidemic, subsequent reduction in sexual risk taking has been substantial. At present, risk-reduction practices should be reinforced with sexually active patients of all orientations.

VII. Gender identity.

A. The spectrum of gender identity and expression.

Western culture has traditionally assumed that biologic sex (male or female) is concordant with gender (internal self-perception of masculinity and femininity), although in many other parts of the world, these facets of human existence are not seen as being necessarily related. Furthermore, many non-Western cultures recognize the existence of more than two genders and have different expectations for persons who do not fit either the men's or the women's role. Throughout Western history, some individuals have lived "cross-gendered" and been perceived throughout all or part of adult life as belonging to the gender opposite their biologic sex. Currently, many people are seeking medical assistance in changing their gender, either through the hormonally mediated acquisition of gender-opposite characteristics or through sex reassignment surgery.

A *cross-dresser*, or *transvestite*, is a person who at times dresses as the opposite sex, either to be publicly perceived as such, or for sexual pleasure. Contemporary fashions allow for substantial overlap in men's and women's clothing, and people who incorporate "gender-opposite" elements that are within the realm of current fashion should not be referred to as cross-dressers. A *transgender* individual is one who seeks to take on the social role of the other gender, either full time or part time, often with the assistance of hormonal therapy, but who does not desire genital surgery. *Transsexuals* usually desire full sex-reassignment surgery. Together, people in these groups are referred to as the *gender community*. In addition, recent years have seen the recognition of persons who do not perceive themselves as being "fully male" or "fully female" and who seek to create new gender identities, similar to those found in other parts of the world. Like sexual orientation, gender identity is best represented as a continuum, one schematic example of which is presented in Table 20–9.

Members of the gender community are individuals and should be referred to in the manner that they indicate is appropriate. Reliable population prevalence estimates for transgender and transsexual people are not yet available; however, the complete gender community, including cross-dressers and gender-blended individuals, may exceed 1% of the adult population.

Table 20–9
Gender Self-Perception

Female	I have always considered myself to be a woman (or girl).
Female with maleness	I currently consider myself to be a woman, but at times I have thought of myself as really more of a man (or boy).
Gender-blended—female predominant	I consider myself gender-blended because I consider myself (in some significant way) to be both a woman and a man, but somehow more of a woman.
Othergendered	I am neither a woman or a man, but a member of some other gender.
Ungendered	I am neither a woman, a man, or a member of any other gender.
Bigendered	I consider myself bi-gendered because sometimes I feel (or act) more like a woman and other times more like a man, or sometimes like both a woman and a man.
Gender-blended—male predominant	I consider myself gender-blended because I consider myself (in some significant way) to be both a man and a woman, but somehow more of a man.
Male with femaleness	I currently consider myself to be a man, but at times I have thought of myself as really more of a woman (or girl).
Male	I have always considered myself to be a man (or boy).

From Eyler AE, Wright K. Gender identification and sexual orientation among females with gender-blended self-perception in childhood and adolescence. XIV Harry Benjamin International Gender Dysphoria Symposium. Sept. 9, 1995, Kloster Irsee, Bavaria, Germany.

B. Primary care.

Transsexuals who have completed sex reassignment are often indistinguishable from other members of their new gender and may obtain medical services without routinely revealing their preoperative history. *Male-to-female* (MTF) sex-reassignment surgery is currently technically advanced; individuals who have undergone male-to-female sex-reassignment surgery are often not identified as such, even on cursory gynecologic examination. *Female-to-male* (FTM) surgery is less perfect; even so, it may not be easily identifiable. However, both FTM and MTF patients require ongoing hormonal supplementation, which can be managed by the primary care physician. In addition, transsexuals need routine health promotion and preventive services. The general rule is that any intact organ should be cared for (e.g., a woman with a prostate gland needs routine prostate screening). Similarly, screening mammography guidelines do not distinguish between genetic women and MTF women.

Cross-dressers and transgenderists often encounter more difficulty in obtaining adequate medical services. Cross-dressers frequently make modifications to the appearance that are not easily explained to nonsympathetic health care providers. For example, a man who has performed extensive body hair removal for cosmetic purposes can either wait several months between medical appointments, in order to let the chest and extremity hair regrow (with resultant body image distress and physical discomfort) or face questioning about presumed unusual sexual practices or a potential endocrine disorder. Transgender persons who are receiving hormones (and electrolysis, if male-to-female) can present an unusual blend of gender-associated physical characteristics, which they can be understandably reluctant to reveal in a nonsupportive environment.

It is usually best to ask cross-dressed or

trangendered patients how they would like to be addressed and, if a legal name change has not been finalized, to file the medical chart under both names. Transgender persons are also at risk for hate crime violence; the same precautions regarding confidentiality as were discussed in the sexual orientation section of this chapter should be followed.

C. Multidisciplinary care and referrals.

The initiation of hormonal therapy for gender modification, and sex reassignment surgery are life-changing medical interventions that should be undertaken only for patients who have completed a rigorous screening process and are in supportive mental health care. The Harry Benjamin International Gender Dysphoria Association has developed guidelines that have been successfully implemented and thoroughly evaluated worldwide. In general, patients undergoing gender transformation receive concurrent care from (at a minimum) a mental health professional with special training in this area and a family physician, internist, or endocrinologist who is knowledgeable about hormonal reassignment and general medical care. Additional professionals in urology, gynecology, plastic surgery, and nursing are consulted when needed, with ongoing communication occurring between members of the medical team whenever a treatment change is planned. Physicians with a strong interest in care of transsexual, transgendered, or cross-dressing persons, or who wish to provide gender reassignment services, are advised to contact the Harry Benjamin International Gender Dysphoria Association, P.O. Box 1718, Sonoma, California 95476.

Summary

Sexuality is a core aspect of personal identity, and, along with mobility, feeding, elimination, and self-care, sexual functioning is a basic activity of daily living and a common concern of patients in primary care and mental health practices. Knowledge regarding human sexual behavior in health and illness enables the clinician to provide appropriate care to patients who are experiencing sexual difficulties. Many sexual dysfunctions can be treated by the family physician or primary psychiatrist. Referral to a certified sex therapist should be pursued in more complicated cases.

References

1. Masters WH, Johnson VE. Human Sexual Response. Boston: Little, Brown & Co.; 1966.
2. Kaplan HS. Disorders of Sexual Desire and Other New Concepts and Techniques in Sex Therapy. New York: Simon & Schuster; 1979.
3. Kaplan HS. The New Sex Therapy: Active Treatment of Sexual Dysfunctions. New York: Times Books; 1974.
4. Frank E, Anderson C, Rubinstein D. Frequency of sexual dysfunction in "normal" couples. N Engl J Med 1978; 299:111–115.
5. Janus SS, Janus CL. The Janus Report on Sexual Behavior. New York: John Wiley & Sons; 1993.
6. Bancroft J. Human Sexuality and Its Problems. Third Edition. London: Churchill Livingstone; 1996.
7. Barbach LG. For Yourself: The Fulfillment of Female Sexuality. New York: Anchor Doubleday; 1976.
8. Kinsey AC, Pomeroy WB, Martin CE. Sexual Behavior in the Human Male. Philadelphia: WB Saunders Co.; 1948.
9. Kinsey AC, Pomeroy WB, Martin CE, Gebhard PH. Sexual Behavior in the Human Female. Philadelphia: WB Saunders Co.; 1953.
10. National Organization for Women, Michigan. The Michigan Lesbian Health Survey, 1991.
11. Herek GM, Berrill KT. Hate Crimes: Confronting Violence Against Lesbians and Gay Men. Thousand Oaks, California: Sage Publishing; 1992, pp. 19–77.
12. Remafedi G. Death by Denial: Studies of Suicide in Gay and Lesbian Teenagers. Boston: Alyson Publications; 1994.

Suggested Reading

Allgeier AR, Allgeier ER. Sexual Interactions. Fourth Edition. Lexington, MA: D.C. Heath & Co.; 1995.

Annon, JS. The Behavioral Treatment of Sexual Problems: Brief Therapy. New York: Harper & Row Publishers; 1976.

Annon JS, Robinson CH. The use of vicarious learning models in treatment of sexual concerns. In: LoPiccolo J, LoPiccolo L, Editors. Handbook of Sex Therapy. New York: Plenum Publishing Corp.; 1978.

Cheadle, MJ. The screening sexual history. Clin Geriat Med 1991; 7:9–13.

Comfort A, Editor. Sexual Consequences of Disability. Philadelphia: George F. Stickley Co.; 1978.

Eyler, AE, Wright K. Gender identification and sexual orientation among genetic females with gender-blended self-perception in childhood and adolescence. XIV Harry Benjamin International Gender Dysphoria Symposium. Sept. 9, 1995, Kloster Irsee, Bavaria, Germany.

Herdt G, Editor. Gay and Lesbian Youth. New York: Harrington Park Press; 1989.

Kolodny RC, Masters WH, Johnson VE. Textbook of Sexual Medicine. Boston: Little, Brown & Co.; 1979.

Lehmann EO, Gagnon JH, Michael RT, Michael S. The Social Organization of Sexuality. Chicago: The University of Chicago Press, 1994.

Ross MW, Channon-Little LD. Discussing Sexuality: A Guide for Health Practitioners. Antarmon, Australia: MacLennan & Petty Pty; 1991.

21

A. E. EYLER, MD, MPH

MARIAN COHEN, MSW

MARTHA O. KERSHAW, MD

Domestic Violence and Abuse

General Principles

I. Evaluation and diagnostic overview.

Although largely under-reported, interpersonal violence and abuse, especially between relatives and domestic partners, is a leading cause of morbidity and mortality in the United States and the world. Physicians in primary care and mental health disciplines must deal with both acute presentations and chronic sequelae of this epidemic on an ongoing basis. This chapter describes the diagnosis and management of three principal forms of interpersonal violence: child abuse and neglect, partner abuse, and elder abuse.

A. Physician avoidance of assessing for violence and abuse.

Despite the substantial morbidity and mortality that result from interpersonal violence and abuse, many clinicians avoid asking their patients about experiences of violence and victimization and do not recognize signs of abuse when they are present. Because specific instruction about this common health hazard has only recently begun to be included in medical school curricula, continuing medical education is often needed. Consequently, physicians commonly assert that their training has provided insufficient preparation for managing these issues. Clinicians frequently fear "opening Pandora's box" by inquiring about physical and sexual violence; they think that by asking about these issues, they will create a situation in which the office routine is disrupted, the patient becomes agitated or depressed, or "more harm than good" is accomplished. Some clinicians even fear becoming a target of the abusive partners or spouses of patients or expending inordinate amounts of clinical time and effort with minimal results.

Dealing with the medical aspects of interpersonal violence and abuse can be emotionally demanding for the clinician and can, in the short run, require significant investment of professional energy. Nonetheless, *diagnosing and intervening in cases of abuse can increase patient health and satisfaction, decrease health care costs and lost work time, and save lives.* For example, a woman who lives with a violent husband or partner is substantially more likely to die from physical abuse than from cervical cancer. If she presents to the primary care physician's practice for a health maintenance examination, the inclusion of a brief violence history as part of the clinical encounter is more likely to save her life than is the Papanicolaou test, and with practice, the violence history is just as easy to perform. Similarly, asking children who present for pre-Kindergarten check-ups about fears, inappropriate touching, and so on requires very little extra effort and may prevent a lifetime of chronic physical and psychological morbidity. Indeed, interpersonal violence and abuse are common causes of morbidity and mortality in the United States; if even 10% of cases were detected early and managed appropriately, national health care expenditures and costs to industry attributable to injury and absenteeism would be significantly reduced.

For clinicians who are not experienced in managing cases involving abuse, it is important to remember that *this is an area of practice in which multidisciplinary problem solving is often crucial and that assistance is frequently available.* It is far easier to provide medical intervention and treatment successfully if other, more experienced professionals are involved; these professionals include social workers from Child Protective Services (CPS) or a domestic violence shelter, law enforcement officers and legal aid workers. Timely, appropriate intervention can be provided much more easily if community resources are identified in advance. With a few telephone calls, the clinician can assemble a set of community-based resources that are available to help. In small communities, such agencies may be limited; accordingly, national "hotline" numbers can be substituted. Even very small outreach activities, such as placing posters that offer the telephone numbers of the local domestic violence intervention services in the women's restroom, can result in "silent referrals" for patients in need, which can be life saving.

This chapter provides an overview of the practical aspects of managing clinical cases involving violence, abuse, and victimization. Additional sources of information are provided at the end of the chapter. *Child abuse, adult battering, sexual violence, and elder abuse are common causes of misery, disability, and death that can be prevented or reduced through astute clinical practice and timely intervention.*

B. Definitions.

The American Medical Association diagnostic and treatment guidelines on domestic violence state that, "Family violence usually results from the abuse of power or the domination and victimization of a physically less powerful person by a physically more powerful person.[1]" Other factors that create or maintain a power differential, such as unequal financial resources, family connections, or health status, can also foster a situation in which the more powerful individual can exert inappropriate control or intimidation over the less powerful individual. All such misuses of power, especially those that involve physical violence or psychological intimidation, constitute *abuse*. Diagnosis and management vary, depending on the status of the victim: child, spouse or partner, or dependent elder.

Neglect refers to the failure of the responsible individual to provide for the basic needs and safety of a dependent, whether that person is a minor child, an elderly parent, a disabled spouse, or other family member.

A *perpetrator* is an individual who performs or permits the actions that constitute abuse or neglect. The term *batterer* refers more specifically to a perpetrator who engages in physical violence.

C. Differential diagnosis.

In all cases of suspected abuse or neglect, it is necessary to distinguish between inflicted injury (or the withholding of needed goods and care) and other conditions that would mimic the consequences of such actions. For example, a long bone fracture in a child may be the result of parental battering, accidental injury, or a constitutional disorder, such as osteogenesis imperfecta. An elderly person who presents with wasting may be experiencing caretaker neglect, physiologic decline, degenerative disease, or some combination of these factors. In all cases, a careful history and examination, followed by consistent, appropriate follow-up, are necessary for diagnostic accuracy and effective management.

II. Epidemiology and etiology.

Family violence and neglect are pervasive hazards with certain common etiologic features.

A. Epidemiology.

The full magnitude of the morbidity and mortality caused by abuse and neglect is not known. Survey research indicates that most instances of family violence never come to medical or legal attention. Nonetheless, recent estimates indicate that on a global scale, victimization is responsible for one of every five healthy days of life lost to women of reproductive age.[2] In the United States, women are more likely to be beaten, raped, or killed by a male partner (husband, ex-husband, current or ex-boyfriend) than by all other assailants combined. Men are injured or killed by female partners, although much less commonly: approximately 90% to 95% of batterers are men, and women are more likely to commit acts of violence in self-defense. Violence also exists in gay male and lesbian relationships, although the epidemiology of this aspect of interpersonal violence has not been adequately studied. *It is clear that domestic violence occurs in heterosexual and homosexual relationships and in all racial, ethnic, religious, and socioeconomic groups.* In addition, approximately 1.5 to 2 million American adults older than 60 years are abused every year, usually by family members and caretakers. Over 1 million instances of child neglect are reported annually, although the true incidence is probably much higher. At least 1000 children die from injuries caused by family members each year. With regard to the relative risk of dying, many Americans live in homes that are more dangerous than many war zones.

B. Etiology.

Although victimization is often dismissed as "human nature" (and therefore not preventable or remediable), cross-cultural research demonstrates that this is not the case. Societies exist in which violence is rare and gender-based violence is virtually nonexistent. Low-violence cultures share certain key characteristics, which are presented in Table 21–1. Circumstances and stressors that may precipitate all forms of abuse and neglect are also listed in Table 21–2. *These risk factors for abuse do*

Table 21–1
Characteristics of Low-Violence Societies

Strong sanctions against interpersonal violence
Community support for victims
Flexible gender roles for women and men
Equality in decision making and resources in the family
Cultural ethos that condemns violence as a means of resolving conflict
Female power and autonomy outside the home

Adapted from Heise LL. Gender-based abuse: The global epidemic. In Dan AJ, Editor. Reframing Women's Health, Multidisciplinary Research and Practice. Thousand Oaks, California: Sage Publications; 1994; pp. 233–250, with permission.

Table 21–2
Factors Increasing Risk for Violence

Alcoholism and/or substance abuse
External stressors
Poverty or financial difficulties
Losses
Family disruption
Work stress
Life cycle changes
Rigid or conflicted family roles or rules
Past history of abusive relationship
Mental or physical disability in family
Social isolation

not constitute excuses for violent behavior; they are presented as guidelines for early recognition and intervention by health professionals.

III. General management guidelines.

Specific intervention strategies applicable to cases of child abuse and neglect, partner violence, and elder abuse are presented in the pertinent sections of this chapter. General principles for the medical response to all forms of family violence are discussed later and summarized in Table 21–3.

A. Physician/health care professional response.

Providers of primary care and mental health services can best respond to the family violence epidemic by *routinely asking about experiences of abuse, especially when risk factors are present.* Interpersonal violence should be considered as a possible cause of all bruises and other injuries. Patients should be asked about this specifically, and in private whenever possible, because they may otherwise feel uncomfortable telling the primary care physician about what really happened. All reports of violence must be taken seriously and documented. Above all, *a prompt response, by the primary care physician, in concert with other disciplines,* including social support services and the legal system, must be made in order to *ensure the safety of the victim from further abuse.*

Table 21–3
The Medical Management of Abuse

Be alert to signs of abuse or neglect
Conduct a thorough evaluation and search for injuries
Document historical and physical findings in the medical record
Believe the victim (take all reports of violence and abuse seriously)
Maintain patient confidentiality
Refer patient to appropriate community resources
Provide support for patient and family, when possible
Provide close follow-up
Report to authorities (Child or Adult Protective Services) as required by state laws
Work on management of countertransference and other emotional responses

B. Documentation.

All reports of violence and accompanying physical findings must be recorded in the medical record, including the emergency department report, counseling notes, and the general office record. Family violence, neglect, and other forms of abuse should be noted in the problem list. Photographs should be obtained when possible; otherwise, the pertinent physical findings should be sketched or diagrammed (Table 21–4). The medical record is often the only documentation of injuries and abuse. It is therefore critical to provide sufficient detail that it will be usable in later months, after the physical injuries have healed. Statements made by victims and caregivers, observed behaviors, descriptions and photographs of injuries, diagnostic tests, and an assessment as to whether the injuries could be reasonably explained by the given history should all be documented, especially in cases involving child abuse.

C. Consultation.

The primary care physician should obtain consultation from experts in interpersonal violence and victimology and should work cooperatively with appropriate support services, in a timely fashion. Child Protective Services (CPS), Adult

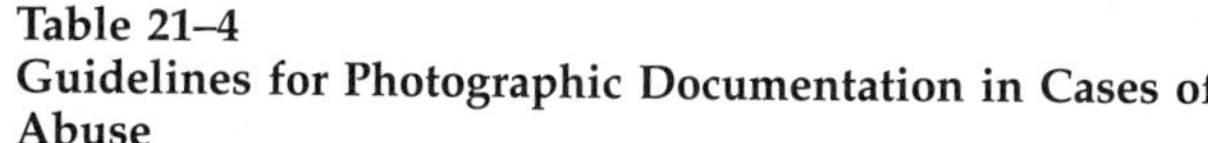

Table 21–4
Guidelines for Photographic Documentation in Cases of Abuse

Take photographs before altering the appearance of the injury through medical treatment, if possible.
Photograph bites in both color and black and white, if available. Color photography is best for all other injuries. Use a color standard (true color bar), if possible.
Photograph the injury close-up, from a distance (for body perspective), and from different angles. Include the victim's face in at least one exposure. Obtain 2 or more photos of each specific injury. Carefully document the location of each injury.
Use a coin or a ruler to provide perspective about injury size.
Carefully document the date, the victim's name, the photographer's name, and the names of others who are present. Do this in such a fashion that it will be clear and accessible at a later date.

Adapted from Berkowitz C, Bross DC, Chadwick DL, et al. American Medical Association diagnostic and treatment guidelines on child physical abuse and neglect. Arch Fam Med 1992; 1:187–197.

Protective Services (APS), shelters for victims of domestic violence, and physicians, social workers, and other professionals who specialize in the evaluation of suspected abuse and neglect can greatly increase the effectiveness of the primary care provider in resolving clinical situations involving family violence and in protecting vulnerable individuals from additional threat and injury. *The primary care physician must become familiar with local resources and reporting procedures on a prospective basis, and keep this information readily available.*

D. Confidentiality.

Competent adults who are experiencing intimidation, violence, or other abuse may present for medical treatment but choose not to leave their living situations or to take legal action. Given the potential for further violence resulting from, for example, a failed separation attempt, and the right of adults to make decisions in their own interests, confidentiality must be respected. A nonjudgmental, supportive stance toward adult victims of violence and an ongoing clinical relationship may eventually enable the patient to take more definitive action to ensure her (or his) future security.

E. Legal requirements.

Although competent adults may decide not to take action against an assailant or abuser, state laws require health professionals to report suspected abuse or neglect of children, elderly dependents, and mentally incapacitated adults. Many states also require physician reporting of injuries afflicted by dangerous weapons such as firearms and knives.

F. Follow-up.

All experiences of victimization are traumatic, and survivors often experience a psychological disorganization that makes following through with treatment plans difficult. In addition, further violence may make decisive action impossible. Whenever abuse or neglect is suspected, appropriate clinical follow-up must be arranged, and patients who do not keep appointments must be contacted in order to ensure their safety. The primary care physician should stress the importance of follow-up and should give patients the telephone numbers needed to contact both the physician and any other resources that might be helpful. Also, when possible, the primary care physician should obtain a telephone number or address at which the patient feels it would be safe for her (or him) to be contacted, if it becomes necessary.

G. Management of personal responses.

Transference and countertransference between the patient and the physician are well known to practicing clinicians. Dealing with cases involving violence or neglect frequently elicits strong emotions on the part of the health professionals involved. These reactions range from rage against the perpetrator ("I'd like to kill the animal who did this!") to identification with the batterer ("He's not such a bad guy. If she doesn't like it, why doesn't she leave him?"). People who routinely evaluate abuse cases are also at risk for professional burnout. All professionals are strongly advised to find appropriate means to deal with personal emotional responses, including Balint groups (collegial discussion/support groups) and individual therapy, in order to maintain personal health and professional effectiveness.

H. Prevention.

Prevention of abuse and neglect depends on early recognition of risk and timely, appropriate response. Health care professionals can prevent suffering, serious injury, and death by remaining alert to the possibility of abuse and neglect when evaluating health risks during routine practice. Furthermore, the acute abuse episode often carries the potential for further violence. Violence escalates with time, and the batterer may kill during his next rage, even if the initial injury was not medically serious. Children who are physically or sexually abused often become perpetrators as adults and inflict this suffering on the next generation. Early intervention by the health care team may prevent these later sequelae. In addition, efforts by health care professionals and other concerned individuals to increase societal awareness about domestic violence, to highlight the unacceptability of interpersonal violence as a means for resolving conflict, and to provide alternative strategies for dealing with frustration in family relationships may eventually decrease the incidence of domestic abuse and its medical complications.

IV. Sequela of abuse experiences.

Acute consequences of abuse include serious injury, disability, and death. Among both adult and pediatric survivors, long-term sequelae include depression, difficulties with interpersonal relationships, perpetration of abuse on others, return to violent relationships, sexual dysfunction, eating disorders, post-traumatic stress disorder, and suicide. Extreme dysfunction may result, and most patients with borderline personality disorder and dissociative identity disorder have histories of severe premorbid childhood abuse. Early supportive counseling may lessen the risk of these long-term complications. When patients present with complaints that suggest these disorders, the physician should ask about past or current abuse.

Child Abuse and Neglect

I. Definition and scope of problem.

Although often misdiagnosed and under-reported, child abuse and neglect are major causes of morbidity and mortality among infants, children, and adolescents. More than 600,000 cases of physical abuse are reported in the United States each year, resulting in at least 1000 deaths. Physical abuse that does not result in significant injury is usually not reported. Nonetheless, at least 10% of injuries seen in emergency departments are the result of abuse. More than 500,000 cases of child sexual abuse are reported annually; most cases are never reported. Surveys of adults indicate that approximately 30% of girls and 20% of boys are sexually assaulted by the age of 18 years. An estimated 1.3 to 1.5 million cases of child neglect are reported each year. It is not possible to determine the number of pediatric deaths that result from neglect.

A. Neglect.

Failure to provide for the basic needs of a minor (nutrition, shelter, clothing, supervision, and a safe environment, including protection from injury caused by peers) constitutes child neglect. Eviction of an adolescent from the family home is another form of neglect.

B. Physical abuse.

Any nonaccidental physical injury to a child or adolescent by any adult or older child with responsibility for the minor's care constitutes physical abuse.

C. Sexual abuse.

Because of the differential in power and ability to consent, any sexual activity between an adult and a minor constitutes sexual abuse. (For married minors, sexual expression is an exception to this definition. The legal age for marriage varies by state. However, nonconsensual sexual activity within a marital relationship also constitutes sexual assault.)

1. *Incest.*
   In more than 90% of cases of child sexual abuse, the minor and the perpetrator are related biologically or by marriage. The general term for this behavior is *incest.* Fewer than 10% of perpetrators are women. In at least 50% of cases, the perpetrator is the child's father or stepfather. The remainder of cases involve uncles, brothers, stepbrothers, grandfathers, and other male relatives (including common law relatives, such as the mother's boyfriend). Most men who sexually abuse boys have consensual sexual relationships with adult women and self-identify as heterosexual.
2. *Molestation.*
   Sexual abuse in which the child or adolescent and the perpetrator are not related is called *molestation.* Fewer than 10% of all cases fit this pattern, and in most cases, the perpetrator is known to the victim. Perpetrators include neighbors, family friends, teachers, clergy, doctors, and health professionals. Assault by strangers is rare.

II. Risk factors.

General risk factors for family violence are listed in Table 21–2. *Children are easy targets for sexual, physical, and emotional abuse because they are vulnerable and dependent, emotionally and physically, on the people taking care of them.* Additional situational characteristics that are associated with child abuse and neglect follow.

A. Bonding difficulties.

Infants born prematurely, who require initial intensive care, or who are born after a pregnancy complicated by medical or social stressors are more often mistreated than are their healthy, full-term peers.

B. Challenging child.

Children with physical, emotional or developmental disabilities, chronic illnesses, or ongoing requirements for special care are at risk for abuse and neglect. Poor physical or emotional health of the caretaker or caretakers can compound this problem.

C. Caretaker stresses.

People at the highest risk for becoming perpetrators of child mistreatment include those who are inexperienced or immature (regardless of chronologic age), were themselves abused, have unrealistic expectations for children at particular developmental stages, or lack alternative strategies for responding to the challenges of child care. Child abuse is often a self-reinforcing behavior pattern because it is an effective short-term strategy: *it immediately relieves parent frustration and extinguishes the behavior that the parent wants to stop.* However, the long-term consequences to the child, family, and future generations can be devastating.

D. Parental/caretaker absence.

Children who are abused sexually often live in situations in which one or both parents (or primary caregivers) is unavailable. They may be physically absent because of illness, death, family conflict, divorce, excessive work hours, or other disruptive circumstances. "Emotionally absent" parents may be home with their children but fail to protect them from sexual abuse, especially by another member of the family. For example, a mother who has chronic depression may be home with her children full time but may fail to "notice" or intervene when her husband initiates sexual contact with their daughter. Conversely, sexual abuse in day care settings is rare.

III. Diagnosis.

Child abuse and neglect are detected through careful history, examination, and laboratory and radiographic evaluation. Some questions regarding abuse should be routinely included as part of periodic well child care. Children who present with acute injuries should be evaluated more thoroughly. Because the parent or caregiver often does not initially admit to the true cause of an injury, abuse is not detected unless members of the health care team keep this possibility in mind during routine patient care and ask appropriate diagnostic questions.

A. History.

Abused and neglected children often present with physical complaints that are seemingly unrelated to their abuse experience, such as abdominal pain and sleep disturbances. In addition, certain characteristic behaviors are common in abused children. These are summarized in Table 21–5. Detection of abuse and neglect in routine clinical situations depends on clinician alertness. The following approach can be incorporated into general medical practice.

1. *Routine assessment.*
An assessment for current or potential abuse can be routinely included in adult and pediatric health maintenance visits. Parents should be asked questions about current family stressors, discipline, child behavior, and home safety. It is also important to inquire about current or past abuse of the parent and to refer parents and caregivers who have abuse histories to parenting education or support groups, or more in-depth counseling, as needed. These questions can be included as part of the medical history or social history during health assessments or can be asked in an abbreviated fashion during other office visits.
Children should be asked open-ended questions about their perception of their own safety, such as:
   - Are you afraid of anyone?
   - Does anyone ever hurt you?
   - Does anyone make you keep secrets?

The primary care physician should make an effort to interview older children (greater than 10 years of age) in private. Parents usually respond positively to the clinician's observation that "kids this age need a little privacy. I'll ask you to return to the waiting room so we can finish the physical examination; then I'll come and get you so that we can discuss follow-up plans."

2. *Developmental monitoring.*
Many abusing or neglectful parents lack knowledge regarding normal child development. The primary care physician should be alert for statements that indicate unrealistic expectations or inappropriate responsibilities for a child, precocious sexual knowledge, or violent childhood behavior. For example, many parents overestimate their children's ability to learn to avoid hazards and do not understand the need to "child proof" the child's environment. A 6-month-old infant cannot be expected to learn not to grasp at bright, shiny objects, such as earrings or eyeglasses. Similarly, a 3-year-old child who is responsible for more than minimal household chores may be experiencing mistreatment in other ways as well. Although it is appropriate for a 5-year-old child to have basic information about sex and reproduction, all first-person references to sexual acts warrant investigation. Children who hurt or bully others are likely to be experiencing abuse themselves.

3. *Symptom and injury investigation.*
Abuse should be considered as a possible cause for all childhood injuries and suggestive symptoms (Table 21–5). The child should be asked about his or her safety:
   - Are you afraid of anyone?
   - Does anyone ever hurt you?
   - Does anyone make you keep secrets?

The physician should follow-up positive responses with more open-ended questions:
   - What happened?
   - When did that happen?
   - Who did that?

The primary care physician should try to get as much of the history in the child's own words and avoid asking leading questions about specific actions or perpetrators. The physician should try to learn and use the child's own

Table 21–5
Childhood Behaviors Associated with Abuse

Fears/mistrust
Social withdrawal
Regression from previous developmental milestones
Secondary enuresis or encopresis
Accident proneness
Sleep disturbances
Destruction of objects or property
Abusiveness toward other children
Poor school performance
Running away
Sexual display/acting out/excessive or public masturbation
Pseudomaturity (adult interests, especially sexual, or responsibilities, e.g., child care)
Promiscuity

vocabulary for body parts and behaviors. Having an anatomically correct doll available and asking the child to tell the physician what he or she calls body parts can help the physician clarify what the child is describing.

In these situations, children who are able to communicate verbally should be interviewed in private, if possible. Parents may initially object to being asked to wait in the reception area, but they usually cooperate if the importance of this procedure is emphasized. If the parent, rather than the child, is the main person objecting to the private interview, the physician's concern about possible abuse should heighten, and consideration should be given to referring the family to a child protection team.

Many injuries are accidental; further investigation is probably not needed if the child's account matches that of the caregiver, the mechanism of the injury and the physical findings are compatible, the parent seems appropriately concerned, and the child seems comfortable with the adult. *A full evaluation by experts in child protection should be strongly considered whenever the injury seems unlikely to have resulted from the stated accident or whenever a delay has occurred in the seeking of medical attention, especially if the victim is an infant.* For example, a fall from the couch is highly unlikely to explain a fracture in a 4 month old. A splash burn on the front of a toddler who "pulled soup off the stove" and whose mortified parent seeks immediate medical treatment may prompt some investigation into safety and accident prevention training but would cause much less suspicion about abuse than would burns on both feet or hands of a toddler who "got into a hot tub too soon," especially if there had been any delay in seeking treatment or if the child was blamed for the injury because "the child should have known better."

Table 21–6
Physical Signs of Child Abuse

Bruises and welts
- Forming a regular pattern
- Resembling the instrument (hand, belt buckle, cord, chain, teeth)

Burns
- Cigar or cigarette burns (especially soles, palms, back, buttocks)
- Immersion burns (stocking/glove pattern, no splashes, donut-shaped burns on buttocks or genitalia)
- Patterned burns resembling an electrical appliance (iron, grill, coil)

Lacerations and abrasions
- Rope burns (wrist, ankles, neck, torso)
- Sensitive or protected areas (palate, mouth, gums, lips, eyes, ears)
- External genitalia (internal genital lacerations less common)

Fractures
- Skull, ribs, long bones, metaphyses

Abdominal injuries
- Bruises of the abdominal wall
- Intramural hematoma of duodenum or proximal jejunum
- Intestinal perforation
- Ruptured liver or spleen
- Ruptured blood vessels
- Kidney or bladder injury
- Pancreatic injury

Central nervous system injuries
- Subdural hematoma (often resulting from blunt trauma or violent shaking)
- Retinal hemorrhage
- Subarachnoid hemorrhage (often resulting from shaking)
- Cerebral edema and secondary cerebral infarction

Sexual organs
- Abrasions or bruises of the inner thighs or external genitalia (labia, scrotum or penis)
- Distortion or thinning of the hymen; enlarged hymenal opening
- Alteration of anorectal tone (marked laxity or spasm)
- Sexually transmitted diseases (syphilis and gonorrhea diagnostic, others highly probable)
- Pregnancy

Other injuries
- Chemical abuse
- Munchausen's syndrome by proxy (i.e., illness induced by caretaker to gain attention, e.g., insulin injections to produce hypoglycemia, laxatives to produce diarrhea)
- Suffocation

Adapted from Berkowitz C, Bross DC, Chadwick DL, et al. American Medical Association Diagnostic and Treatment Guidelines on Child Physical Abuse and Neglect. Arch Fam Med 1992;1:187–197. Copyright 1992, American Medical Association; Berkowitz C, Bross DC, Chadwick DL, et al. American Medical Association Diagnostic and Treatment Guidelines on Child Sexual Abuse. Arch Fam Med 1993; 2:19–27.

B. Examination.

Findings suggestive of child abuse are often present on routine pediatric examinations, although they are usually dismissed or overlooked by clinicians who do not consider the possibility of abuse in children of intact and seemingly functional families. In addition, well child examinations frequently omit portions of the complete physical examination. The external genitalia and skin should be examined routinely. Significant information is missed if the child is not fully undressed. Additional physical findings suggestive of child abuse and neglect are presented in Tables 21–6 and 21–7.

The child's behavior often provides additional clues regarding abuse and neglect. Many children are shy, especially about genital examinations, but children who are unusually fearful or exhibitionistic should be evaluated more closely for other evidence of abuse. For example, a child who pulls his or her underwear down before being asked may just be being playful, but this

Table 21–7
Physical Findings in Child Neglect

Undernutrition
  Apparent on physical examination
  Detectable on age-appropriate growth curves

Poor hygiene
  Unusually dirty (relative to other children)
  Severe diaper rash

Development delay

Severe dental caries

Untreated medical illnesses

Adapted from Berkowitz C, Bross DC, Chadwick DL, et al. American Medical Association Diagnostic and Treatment Guidelines on Child Physical Abuse and Neglect. Arch Fam Med 1992; 1:187–197. Copyright 1992, American Medical Association.

behavior should prompt questioning about the possibility of abuse. Conversely, neglected children often seem unconcerned about the absence of the parent or caretaker and respond unusually positively to anyone who offers them attention. The primary care physician should observe for and document unusual behavior during all pediatric encounters.

C. Diagnostic tests.

Diagnostic tests should be performed as appropriate to the injury or suspected abuse, including x-ray studies and genital cultures. A generous radiographic evaluation of injured infants should be obtained, including full-body radiographs in order to evaluate for previous fractures, if suspected. A positive result on gonorrhea culture or serologic test for syphilis, or the presence of semen or sperm, is de facto evidence of child sexual abuse. Positive cultures for other sexually transmitted diseases are suggestive but not diagnostic. Candidal vaginitis alone does *not* typically suggest abuse.

IV. Management.

The goal of all intervention in cases of suspected child abuse and neglect is protection of the child from further harm, identification of risks and appropriate solutions, and compliance with legal reporting requirements. In most cases of suspected abuse or neglect, the child can be left in the custody of his or her parent or parents or guardian while an investigation is conducted. In cases involving more severe injury or serious threat of further abuse, the child should be hospitalized and immediate legal intervention sought.

A. Reporting requirements.

All states require that people who work with children, including physicians, nurses, social workers, teachers, and child care providers report all cases of suspected child abuse or neglect. A clinical algorithm for decision making in cases of possible sexual abuse is provided in Table 21–8. Immunity from liability is provided for all reports made in good faith, even if the abuse is not confirmed. Each state provides a contact telephone number, usually through the department of social services or the police department. Many states also require health providers to file a written report within a specified period of time. The National Child Abuse Hotline (1-800-422-4453) can be used by anyone needing more information about child abuse and neglect or about reporting mechanisms and requirements. The primary care physician should locate the contact numbers for pertinent local agencies in advance and have this information available in the office. If the primary care physician is in doubt about whether or not a

Table 21–8
Guidelines for Making the Decision to Report Suspected Sexual Abuse

Data Available			Response	
History	*Physical Examination*	*Laboratory*	*Level of Concern*	*Action*
None	Normal findings	None	None	None
Behavioral changes	Normal findings	None	Low (worry)	+/− report follow-up
None	Nonspecific	None	Low (worry)	+/− report follow-up
Nonspecific (or parent only)	Nonspecific	None	Possible (suspect)	+/− report follow-up
None	Specific	None	Probable	Report
Clear statement	Normal findings	None	Probable	Report
Clear statement	Specific	None	Probable	Report
None	Normal, nonspecific or specific	Positive (GC culture, VDRL, semen, sperm)	Definite	Report
Behavioral changes	Nonspecific	Other STDs	Probable	Report

GC = gonococcus; VDRL = Venereal Disease Research Laboratory; STD = sexually transmitted disease; +/− report = a report may or may not be indicated (the decision to report should be based on discussion with Child Protective Services personnel or other expert consultation).

Adapted from Berkowitz C, et al. Guidelines for the evaluation of sexual child abuse. Pediatrics 1991; 87:254. Reproduced by permission of Pediatrics, copyright 1991.

report should be filed, CPS can usually be consulted by telephone and asked about what action is appropriate before a report is filed.

B. Family management.

Whenever possible, parents or guardians should be informed that a CPS referral has been made. This can be handled gently by explaining that reporting is required by law "whenever this type of injury takes place" or whenever the suspicion of abuse has been raised. Although many adults react negatively to this information, some also experience relief, which may be expressed at a later time. Often families believe that a CPS referral means that their child will be taken away from them. In fact, CPS focuses on family preservation and removes the child from the family home as a last resort. Most parents want their children to be safe and do not want to harm them. However, caring for children can be extremely challenging, and adults resort to violence generally out of frustration or a lack of alternative strategies.

The goal of any protective intervention should be to keep the child safe and to identify appropriate solutions to problems and dangers. The primary care physician should frame the intervention in this manner when presenting it to the family. Also, the physician should remain as neutral and supportive as possible, even when the injury brings out strong emotions on the part of the health care team. The job of the medical professional is to report suspected abuse and neglect and to ensure the immediate safety of the child, not to retaliate against or prosecute the suspected perpetrator.

C. Documentation.

Documentation is crucial in cases of suspected child abuse and neglect. All pertinent findings, including the child's and caretakers' statements, signs of undernutrition, bruises, welts, abrasions, lacerations, burns, and other injuries, must be carefully documented in the chart. Photographs are best for documenting physical injuries, but free-hand drawings and measurements are also helpful. Whenever possible, the physician should consult with an expert in child abuse and neglect.

V. Risk identification and family support.

Early identification of familes at risk can help prevent child abuse. Parents who are experiencing family stress, who have a poor understanding of nonviolent discipline techniques, or who lack information about normal child development can be given information and provided with alternative child-rearing strategies. Health care professionals who work with children can be instrumental in helping adults find the resources they need to parent well. In addition to providing anticipatory guidance regarding developmental milestones and age-appropriate disciplinary techniques at well child visits, offering information about community resources for parents *before* a child protection report becomes necessary can be a life-saving service.

Partner Abuse

I. Definition and scope of problem.

Partner abuse involves the physical or emotional intimidation or violation of one member of a presently or previously intimate couple by the other. The abuse may involve physical battering; sexual coercion or assault; psychological intimidation; physical restraint; financial exploitation; prevention of employment, education, or visits with relatives or friends; threats against the victim or others; or any other form of intimidation, coercion, exploitation, or assault. Specific forms of partner abuse are summarized in Table 21–9. The abuser is usually either physically stronger than the victim or in financial control of the relationship. The most common constellation is the current or ex-husband or boyfriend as perpetrator and the wife or girlfriend as victim. However, partner abuse also occurs in gay male and

Table 21–9
Presentation of Partner Abuse

Psychological abuse
Threatening harm
Physical or social isolation
Displaying extreme jealousy or possessiveness
Degrading, intimidating partner
Belittling, criticizing, insulting, name calling, ongoing verbal harassment
False accusations, blaming partner for everything
Ignoring, dismissing, ridiculing partner's needs; deprivation
Lying, breaking promises, destroying trust
Putting partner in dangerous situations, such as by driving recklessly
Physical and sexual abuse
Pushing, shoving, slapping, punching, kicking, choking
Holding, tying down, or restraining partner
Abandoning partner in a dangerous place
Refusing to help when partner is sick or injured
Assaulting with a weapon
Pursuing sexual activity when partner is not fully conscious, is not asked, or is afraid to say no
Using verbal sexual intimidation, criticism, sexually degrading names
Forcing or attempting unwanted sexual acts
Coercing partner to have sex without contraception
Coercing partner to have sex without protection against sexually transmitted disease, including human immunodeficiency virus
Hurting partner during sex, including genital assault or the use of weapons for oral, anal, or vaginal penetration

lesbian relationships and in heterosexual relationships in which the victim is male. Like other forms of domestic violence, *partner abuse is a crime.*

Partner violence accounts for approximately one third of emergency department visits by women for injuries of any kind. Most patients do not disclose this information without sympathetic and direct questioning, and most patients are not asked. Nearly one quarter of women are abused by a current or former partner at some time during their lives. Federal Bureau of Investigation statistics indicate that more than half of female murder victims are killed by a current male partner or ex-husband. Rape is a common form of assault in violent relationships; 14% of ever-married women report having experienced marital rape or sexual assault by an ex-husband. Clinical experience suggests that partner violence against heterosexual men, gay men and lesbians is relatively less common; however, good-quality, large-scale survey research has not been conducted. Data are also lacking regarding the true incidence of dating violence and rape, although some evidence suggests that it may be similar in incidence and character to marital violence. In addition, many women in violent marriages report having been abused in previous relationships.

The main issue in all abusive relationships is *control.* Batterers may limit victims' access to money, resources, family, friends, and other relationships. Verbal abuse is a universal precursor to battering. Over time, one partner in the relationship is made to feel inferior, worthless, inadequate, or helpless. Apologies for violence are often accompanied by accusations or statements about how the abuse could have been avoided if the victim had behaved differently. Many abusive partnerships involve a *cycle of violence,* in which the perpetrator promises reform after an assault, the couple reconciles, and the abuse continues at a later time. Experiences of genuine intimacy or mutuality may occur, but this does not change the fact that *the context of the relationship is violent and that further battering is likely to occur in the future* (Fig. 21–1).

II. Risk factors.

Characteristics and circumstances associated with an increased risk of all forms of domestic violence are listed in Table 21–2. Factors that are specifically related to partner abuse include a *power differential* in the relationship, in which one partner is financially or emotionally dependent on the other; temporary or permanent *disability,* including pregnancy; a *force orientation,* that is, the belief on the part of the perpetrator that violence is an acceptable solution to conflicts and problems; and a *past history or family history of abuse.* Children who are abused, or who witness domestic violence, are at high risk for becoming perpetrators (or victims) in adulthood and for experiencing lasting psychological effects (see General Principles, section IV).

III. Prevention.

Clinicians frequently report that dealing with domestic violence is a frustrating experience. People who have been abused are often not "ideal" patients: they miss appointments, request tranquilizers, offer vague somatic complaints, do not follow through with treatment, and do not leave their batterers. In contrast, perpetrators are often articulate, interesting community figures who present themselves more favorably. In order to deal most effectively with the problem of partner abuse and to maintain a balanced perspective, health professionals must also focus on violence prevention through the early detection of risks and patient education. One suggested approach follows.

A. Routine assessment.

Relationship and sexual histories should be included in the medical interview on a routine basis. The primary care physician should focus on childhood experiences:

- Was the patient ever abused, physically or sexually, as a child?
- Was she or he a witness to parental or other violence in the family home?
- Has he or she been threatened or attacked in a previous relationship during adulthood?

Patients with previous histories of abuse or who have been witnesses to violence may benefit from counseling or further education regarding domestic violence and healthy relationships.

B. Review of present relationship.

Questions regarding child bearing and contraception are routine aspects of the annual gynecologic examination. In addition, both women and men can be asked more specific questions regarding present partnerships as part of routine health maintenance.

- Can the patient rely on his or her partner for emotional support?
- What is the level of mutuality in the partnership?
- Is the sexual relationship satisfying and mutually acceptable?
- Does she or he feel safe with the partner at all times, even if the partner has been drinking?

Any uncertainty should be pursued. Many people do not identify abusive relationships as such until the level of violence becomes severe. Routine questioning can uncover potentially dangerous situations and enable intervention to take place before major injuries occur.

C. Education.

Coercion and violence are not a normal part of marriage or other relationships, and they need not be tolerated. No one has the right to force another person to have sex, or to have unprotected sex, even if the two participants are married. Occasional conflict is a universal feature of close rela-

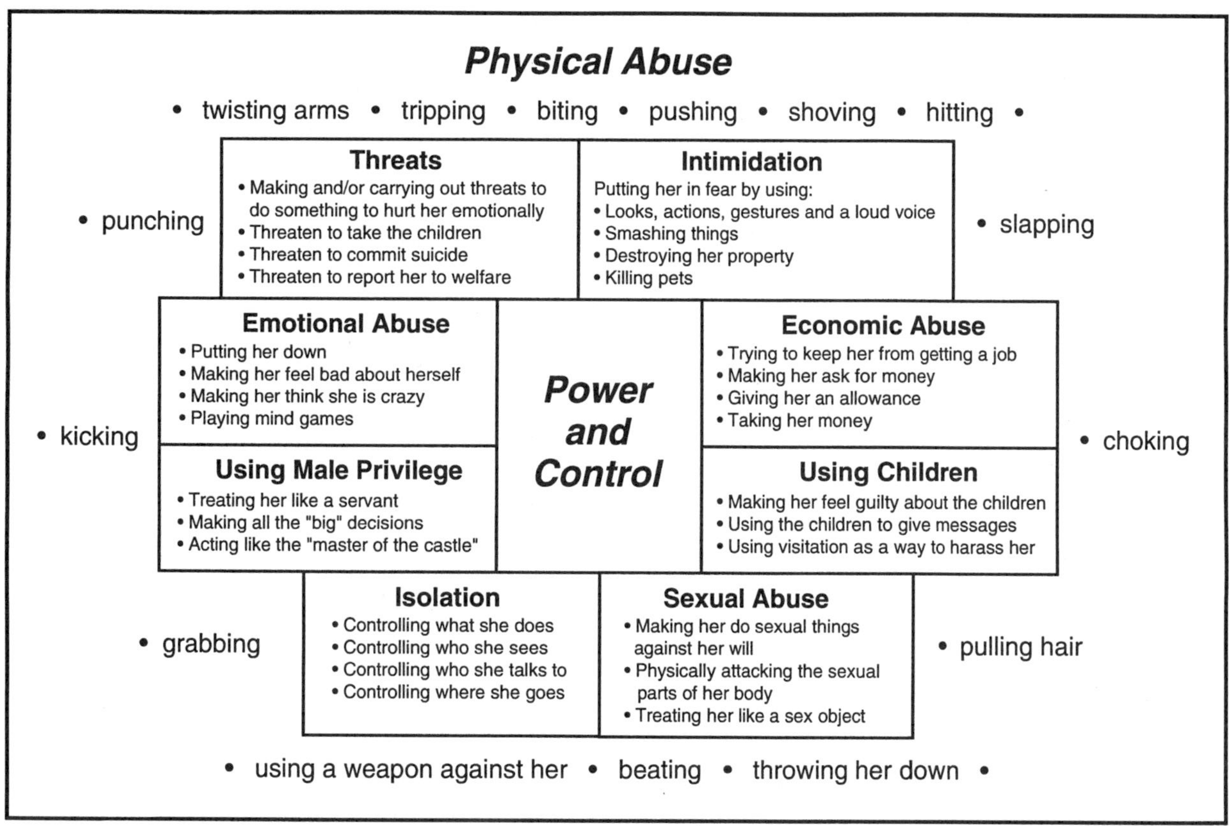

Figure 21–1
The cycle of violence. An assault occurs, and the recipient protests (e.g., "I'm leaving!"). The perpetrator then promises reform; the couple reconciles, the abuse continues at a later time, and the cycle of violence continues. Although the perpetrator may use primarily one means to gain power and control (e.g., economic abuse), often several are used. (Adapted from a figure developed by the Domestic Abuse Intervention Project, Duluth, Minnesota.)

tionships, including marriage. However, there are many ways of dealing with conflict that do not involve violence, intimidation, or domination of one person by the other. Domestic violence is a criminal offense. Patient education regarding these straightforward facts, during one-to-one clinical encounters, through written materials, and via timely referral, can be life saving.

IV. Diagnosis.

Partner abuse is diagnosed through clinician alertness, careful interviewing and examination techniques, and appropriate follow-up of suggestive clinical presentations.

A. History.

Suggested diagnostic questions are presented in Table 21–10. The primary care physician should inquire routinely about current living arrangements and significant relationships, including problems and overall safety. The physician should *ask* about the causes of injuries and infections. *The physician should not assume that sexual behavior is consensual.* For example, if a female patient indicates that the bruises on her thighs were caused by her boyfriend or husband "getting a little carried away," ask about what happened and whether this was enjoyable, upsetting, or frightening for her. The physician should always observe the patient's affect; and be alert for signs of depression, belittling of the self, and so on. *The physician should interview each patient alone, or at least with the partner absent.* This is especially important in the emergency department setting or when an injury has occurred. Batterers are often very solicitous of their victims after the assault has occurred. Unless the injured person is asked specifically about what happened, in private, the abuse often goes undetected. Common medical complications of violence are listed in Table 21–11. The primary care physician should maintain a high index of suspicion for abuse in these situations and in others that suggest the possibility of violence, such as excessive work loss, sleep disturbances, substance abuse, somatization or "bad nerves," sexual dysfunction, depression, and frequent injuries or "accident proneness."

Table 21–10
Interviewing for Partner Abuse

Does your partner physically hurt or threaten you? Have you ever been in a relationship in which you were hurt or threatened? Are you or have you been treated badly in other ways?

Has your partner ever destroyed things you cared about or stolen your things?

Has your partner ever threatened or abused your children?

Has your partner ever forced you to have sex when you did not want to or made you do something sexually that you did not like?

We all get into arguments. What happens when you and your partner fight at home?

Do you ever feel afraid of your partner?

Has your partner ever prevented you from leaving the house, getting a job, seeking friends, or continuing your education?

How does your partner act when he or she has been drinking or using other drugs?

Are there guns or other weapons in your home? Has your partner or anyone else ever threatened to use them?

Table 21–11
Common Medical Complications of Partner Violence

Acute
- Contusions, lacerations, fractures
- Blunt abdominal trauma
- Closed head injury, concussion
- Oral, pharyngeal, vaginal, anal trauma, some requiring surgical repair
- STDs, including hepatitis B and HIV
- Unwanted pregnancy: 5% of heterosexual assault victims become pregnant (single episode)
- Obstetric complications: preterm labor, stillbirths, low birth weight infants, miscarriage
- Depression, PTSD, suicide

Chronic
- Increased use of the medical care system, including number of surgeries
- Chronic pain syndromes: headache, back pain, TMJ pain, pelvic pain
- Chronic gastrointestinal disorders
- Negative health behaviors: alcoholism or drug use, eating disorders, sexual risk taking
- Psychiatric: depression, chronic anxiety, PTSD, relationship/sexual difficulties, somatization disorders, suicide

STD = sexually transmitted disease; HIV = human immunodeficiency virus; PTSD = post-traumatic stress disorder; TMJ = temporomandibular joint.

B. Physical examination.

The primary care physician, should inquire about, evaluate, and document injuries (e.g., bruises, abrasions) noted on routine physical examinations. The examination should be especially thorough if the injury involves the pelvic or sexual organs, including the anus, or occurs during pregnancy. Patients who experience discomfort, difficulty, or anxiety with pelvic or rectal examinations should receive gentle and supportive treatment and should be asked about current and past abuse. *The physician should be alert to any discrepancy between an injury and its proposed mechanism.* Injuries resulting from battering are often attributed to a fall down stairs or some other household accident. In such cases, the patient should be asked to describe the accident in more detail or asked about precipitating factors (e.g., "Were you pushed?").

C. Diagnostic tests.

Ancillary tests should be obtained as indicated for the specific injury or infection. The primary care physician should be especially alert for pregnancy complications and for sexually transmitted infections, including human immunodeficiency virus, in patients who have been battered. Sexual assault often accompanies other forms of domestic violence, and the pregnant woman is frequently a target for battering.

V. Management.

General management guidelines for cases involving domestic violence are summarized in Table 21–3. *The immediate goal is protection* of the patient and the patient's dependents (children and elderly relatives) from further harm, as well as follow-up until the situation is resolved. Early referral to community resources (e.g., domestic violence shelters and legal aid) can be crucial. Encouraging the victim to call the police or to involve sympathetic family members or friends can stop the isolation that often accompanies domestic violence and help prevent retaliation. All interventions should be conducted in a supportive atmosphere with *confidentiality* assured. The primary care physician should ask the patient whether it is safe for her to take home written materials that pertain to domestic violence. If it is not safe, the physician should offer important telephone numbers on plain stationery or a prescription sheet. As a part of safety planning, the primary care physician should arrange for a safe way to follow up with the patient by phone. For instance, if the physician's identifying himself or herself as a doctor might arouse suspicions in the batterer, the physician could agree in advance to say that he or she is calling from some local business. The physician should ask the patient in advance for the names of friends that could be contacted as a way of reaching the patient, if necessary. The physician might also ask the patient if the police can be called if he or she is unable to contact the patient and believes that the patient might be in immediate danger.

Many people who have been abused, especially if the intimidation or violence has been long term, are not psychologically or practically able to leave their batterers immediately and are not helped by physician insistence that they do so. Conversely, any suggestion that the victim precipitated, caused, or "must like" the abuse (because the patient is staying in a potentially dangerous situation) can be extremely damaging. Most physicians have considerably more financial resources, self-esteem, and practice at autonomous problem solving than do the victims of violence whom they treat. Supportive activities for physicians, such as Balint groups (collegial support/discussion groups), may help to manage countertransference and avoid projection of personal viewpoints onto patients who have suffered violence and psychological abuse.

Batterers

I. Definition and scope of problem.

Battering is defined as a pattern of abusive behavior which includes physical assault, threats, and intimidation, emotional abuse, sexual abuse and isolation of the victim.[3] Approximately 85% to 95% of perpetrators of domestic violence are men. Identified batterers are usually in their 20s and 30s but may be older. Men are less likely to report abuse when a woman is the perpetrator. Violence occurs in both heterosexual and homosexual relationships. This section focuses primarily on male abuse of female partners because that is the constellation that is most common and the area about which the most information is available. Batterers come from various ethnic, racial, and occupational backgrounds, although those who are identified most frequently are from lower socioeconomic groups.

II. Risk factors.

Studies have not identified any consistent psychiatric diagnoses in batterers, but abusive men frequently have common characteristics. These are listed in Table 21–12. Some, but not all, batterers meet the Diagnostic and Statistical Manual of Mental Disorders[4] criteria for personality disorders or depression. Most researchers believe that abusive behavior is the result of multiple factors, including individual characteristics, family history of violence, and cultural beliefs that violence is an acceptable means by which problems can be solved and that violence toward women is acceptable or tolerated.

III. Diagnosis.

Batterers are more difficult to identify in primary care because they usually do not present with symptoms that suggest problems with violence. They may sometimes present with injuries related to the violent episode, such as hand fractures, lacerations, and eye injuries. The physician can screen for violent behavior by asking about it during routine history taking. An approach called the *funneling technique,* developed by Ambuel and Hamberger,[5] is described in Table 21–13. The inquiry should begin with less threatening questions and progress to questions about more serious violence, depending on the patient's responses. Batterers often minimize or deny the abuse, and the questioning may not result in identification of violent behavior. Nevertheless, this approach allows the physician to broach the subject and may sometimes provide the opportunity for a patient who is troubled about his or her violent behavior to begin to talk about it and seek help.

Table 21–12
Who Are the Batterers?

Rigid sex-role stereotypes
Low self-esteem, depression
High need for power and control
Tendency to minimize and deny problems or violence
Tendency to blame others for their behavior
Violence in family of origin, particularly witnessing of parental violence
Drug and alcohol abuse (not causative but often associated)

Adapted from Hamberger LK. Identifying and intervening with men who batter. In: Hendricks-Matthews M, Editor. Violence Education: Toward a Solution, Kansas City, MO: Society of Teachers of Family Medicine; 1992, p. 58.

IV. Intervention.

A. Approach to the patient.

After recognition of violent behavior by a patient, the physician can discuss the negative consequences of this for the patient as well as the patient's partner and their children. Discussion can include legal and economic ramifications (paying fines, going to jail), and emotional costs to the family, including the batterer, such as loss of the family unit through separation or divorce. These consequences may include "anxiety, depression, chronic stress, and (among children) school difficulties and problems with peers," as well as low self-esteem.[6] *Men who batter often do not recognize the cascade of emotional harm that their violence causes. The physician can tell the patient that violence is never appropriate or justified and is illegal and can encourage the patient to seek help in order to stop his pattern of violence.* Ultimately, the batterer is in danger of losing his or her partner, children, and property. Physicians should become familiar with the local laws regarding battering and restraining orders and discuss these with their

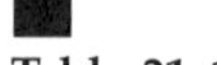

Table 21–13
Funneling Technique for Assessing Current Partner Violence

The goal of the funneling technique is to move from general, open-ended questions to specific, direct questions that help the primary care physician thoroughly assess violence in a relationship. This technique can also be applied to assessing past partner violence by asking about past relationships.

1. "Tell me about your relationship with your partner."
2. "People have different ways of showing disagreement or anger in relationships. Sometimes people talk loudly, shout, threaten, hit, or use weapons. How do you show anger and disagreement to your partner?"
   a. Wait for response, then ask "Anything else?" or "And then what happens?" Repeat until patient offers nothing else.
   b. Probe for specific types of violence.
      "Have you ever yelled at them?"
      "Have you ever demeaned or berated them?"
      "Have you ever threatened them, their children, or someone else?"
      "Have you ever destroyed their property or other things?"
      "Have you ever forced unwanted physical or sexual contact?"
      "Have you ever tried to control their movements and activities?"
      "Have you ever pushed or hit them?"
      "Have you ever threatened them with a weapon?"
      "Have you ever hurt them with a weapon or object?"

From Ambuel B, Hamberger L. K. Family Peace Project, Family and Community Medicine, Medical College of Wisconsin (unpublished report).

patients. Societal recognition of female-to-male violence and battering within same sex relationships is just beginning, and formal programs for victims and batterers are extremely rare. *The primary care physician should consult with local antiviolence projects for additional suggestions.*

Counseling programs designed specifically for batterers are more effective than other forms of counseling, but even these have limited success. Education about anger control and alternatives to violent behavior is a crucial component of the rehabilitation of batterers. Group sessions are frequently used to break through patients' denial and justification of their behavior. If a good relationship exists between the doctor and the patient, the doctor can provide continued support and encourage the patient to follow through on recommendations for counseling.

The physician can also confront the batterer's rationalizations. For example, one patient dismissed his wife's injuries with the statement "she bruises easily." This provided an opportunity for the physician to explain that any level of partner violence, no matter how minimal, is unacceptable and illegal, and that any blow that is hard enough to leave a bruise is harmful and potentially dangerous.

Conjoint therapy sessions with the couple are not advised until the batterer's violent behavior is under control. However, a separate meeting with the partner, if the patient gives permission, can be helpful in reinforcing the recommendations and can give the physician an opportunity to encourage the abused partner to seek help for herself or himself. Only rarely can a relationship involving violence be salvaged. Usually, the couple must separate for the safety of the victim. After rehabilitation and counseling, both partners may be able to initiate other, nonviolent relationships. If depression and/or substance abuse are part of the patient's or the partner's difficulties, treatment for these diagnoses should be recommended as well.

B. Documentation.

Documentation in the medical record of the discussion with the patient and of all findings, including psychosocial data, is important for substantiation of legal intervention, if that becomes necessary.

C. Notification.

Most states do not have a requirement for physicians to report domestic violence when the parties involved are competent adults. However, the state may have laws regarding a duty to warn a potential victim if the physician believes that the victim's life may be in danger. If child abuse is identified in the course of the interview, that information must be reported to the appropriate authorities (see Child Abuse and Neglect section).

Elder Abuse

I. Definition and scope of problem.

Elder abuse or maltreatment may include "physical, psychological, financial abuse or neglect, and it may be intentional or unintentional."[7] The specific presenta-

Table 21–14
Presentations of Elder Abuse

- Physical abuse
  - Pushing, striking, pinching
  - Force feeding
  - Incorrect positioning
  - Improperly using restraints or medications
  - Sexual coercion or assault
- Physical neglect
  - Withholding adequate meals or hydration, physical therapy, or hygiene
  - Failing to provide physical aids (eyeglasses, hearing aids, dentures)
  - Failing to provide safety precautions
- Psychological abuse
  - Verbal berating, harassing, or intimidating
  - Threatening punishment or deprivation
  - Treating older person like an infant
  - Isolating older person from family, friends, or activities
- Psychological neglect
  - Leaving older person alone for long periods of time
  - Ignoring or giving older person the "silent treatment"
  - Failing to provide companionship, changes in routine, news, or information
- Financial or material abuse
  - Denying the older person a home
  - Stealing money or possessions
  - Coercing the older person into signing contracts, assigning durable power of attorney, purchasing goods, or making changes in a will
  - Failing to use available funds necessary to sustain or restore health of older person (neglect)
- Self-neglect
  - Failing to maintain adequate meals or hydration
  - Failing to maintain a safe environment
  - Failing to use physical aids (eyeglasses, hearing aids, dentures)
- Violation of personal rights
  - Denying older person's right to privacy
  - Denying older person right to make decisions regarding: health care or other personal issues (marriage, divorce, companionship)
  - Forcibly evicting and/or placing elderly person in a nursing home

tions of elder mistreatment are listed in Table 21–14.[8] A 1991 congressional report indicated that 1.5 to 2 million older adults (older than 60 years) are abused annually. This number includes adults living alone, those living with family members or others, and those living in institutions. Often, the spouse or adult child of the older person is the perpetrator of the abuse or neglect, but paid or informal caregivers may also be responsible. Elder abuse occurs in men and women of all racial, ethnic, and socioeconomic groups. Suspected self-neglect by an older person who is cognitively or physically unable to take care of himself or herself also requires evaluation.

II. Risk factors.

Risk factors for elder abuse include those listed previously in Table 21–2. In addition, any situation in which an older adult is dependent on a caregiver because of cognitive or physical deficits must be evaluated for the potential for abuse or neglect. If unsafe conditions in the home or inadequate housing are suspected, these possibilities must also be assessed.

III. Diagnosis.

Elder abuse is most often detected through medical interview and physical examination, usually as part of the routine out-patient care of elderly persons.

A. History.

Suggested questions about abuse or neglect that can be included in the patient interview are listed in Table 21–15.[9] The physician should emphasize his or her interest in the well-being of the patient and the family. The physician should avoid approaching the patient or family from an accusatory or judgmental stance. Basic questions regarding abuse should be asked routinely, as part of the normal preventive care of elderly persons. The older person should be interviewed separately from the caregiver. Another source may be needed if the patient is cognitively impaired or unable to provide information. Other sources may include other family members, neighbors, clergy, and friends.

Table 21–15
Interviewing for Elder Abuse

- Ask the patient direct questions:
  - Has anyone at home ever hurt you?
  - Has anyone ever touched you without your consent?
  - Has anyone ever made you do things you did not want to?
  - Has anyone taken anything that was yours without asking?
  - Has anyone scolded or threatened you?
  - Have you ever signed any documents that you did not understand?
  - Are you afraid of anyone at home?
  - Are you alone a lot?
  - Has anyone ever failed to help you take care of yourself when you needed help?
  - Any questions answered affirmatively should be followed in order to determine how and when the mistreatment occurs, who perpetrates it, and how the patient copes with it.

Adapted from Elder Mistreatment Guidelines for Health Care Professionals: Detection, Assessment and Intervention, Mount Sinai/Victim Services Agency Elder Abuse Project, New York, 1988.

B. Physical examination.

The physical examination should focus on evaluation of unexplained injuries, assessment of functional decline or poor nutritional status, and evidence of depression. As is the case in child abuse, injuries due to accidental trauma generally occur on extensor surfaces, and bruises or lacerations on other areas of the body warrant more careful evaluation. Diagnostic tests, such as x-ray studies, should be ordered as indicated.

IV. Management.

Physician intervention in cases of suspected (or potential) elder abuse consists of immediate protection of the patient, reporting to the governmental agency responsible for further investigation, careful documentation, risk factor identification and caregiver support. Medical management steps are summarized in Table 21–3.

A. Protection of the patient.

If the older person seems to be in immediate danger, APS should be notified, and safety plans, such as hospital admission, a court protective order, or a safe home placement, should be considered. If the older person is not in immediate danger, there is more time for a comprehensive assessment and for implementation of supportive services aimed at alleviating some of the factors that may be contributing to the risk of abuse or neglect.

B. Reporting requirements.

APS in each state has the legal responsibility for investigation and intervention when elder abuse and neglect are suspected. In most states, physicians and other health care professionals are required to report cases of suspected adult abuse to APS. The reader is referred to his or her local health department and the Department of Social Services for further information.

C. Documentation.

Careful documentation in the medical record of all findings, including psychosocial data, is essential in order to facilitate legal intervention if that becomes necessary. The patient's statements, behavior, and appearance should all be documented. If the potential for abuse is detected but no evidence of actual mistreatment is present, documentation of available information should accompany further assessment.

D. Risk factor identification and caregiver support.

If basic risk factors for elder abuse or neglect are attended to at an early stage and if the caregiver is open to receiving assistance and support, prevention of the abuse or of more severe abuse may be possible. The health care team can provide education and emotional support to the caregiver and to the patient. Providing assistance for the caregiver in locating added support through family, friends, and community resources is also essential. The patient and/or family members can be referred for social work, counseling services, legal assistance, and advocacy.

Primary prevention of domestic violence and abuse

Domestic violence is a criminal activity that results in premature death, excess morbidity, lost productivity, family disruption, psychological disability, obstetric complications, poor childhood development, unnecessary medical expenditures, and profound human misery. Family violence and abuse are preventable.

Health care professionals can reduce the incidence of domestic abuse through timely diagnosis and treatment (to prevent further violence) and through primary prevention activities. Suggested interventions are listed below.

I. Community education and awareness activities.

Physicians should place informational literature regarding family violence in medical offices, emergency departments, and other high-volume health facilities. Posters should be placed in hospital elevators and waiting rooms, and public service announcements should be sponsored on radio and local television. The physician should use available resources to increase community awareness regarding domestic abuse. *Family violence is unacceptable; help is available.*

II. Parent and caretaker support.

The primary care physician should identify local resources for parenting education, caretaker respite, and other support services. The physician should discourage the use of physical punishment and intimidation as preferred modes of discipline. Instead, parents should be encouraged to learn methods that rely on communication, rewards for positive behavior, and consistent limits with nonviolent consequences, such as time out and withdrawal of privileges. The physician should refer at-risk families for preventive intervention before the situation at home becomes explosive. Information about community resources should be made easily available to patients through handouts, wallet cards, and other avenues that encourage self-referral.

III. Legal policies.

The most effective means of decreasing repeat episodes of partner violence has been the mandatory arrest law.

In communities with these statutes, the batterer is arrested whenever police intervene in situations of family violence, whether the victim presses charges or not. Thus, the perpetrator receives a criminal record, even if he or she is able to intimidate the victim into dropping criminal charges. In Ann Arbor, Michigan, police cars have bumper stickers that inform the community that "Domestic Violence is a Crime." Primary care physicians should work with local law enforcement agencies to spread this message and should investigate and work to improve local statutes regarding family violence.

IV. Emergency resources.

Effective intervention in cases involving violence and abuse is much more difficult without adequate community resources, such as temporary shelters for victims of partner violence, available foster care placements, CPS, and APS. The primary care physician should support the creation and maintenance of these crucial services.

V. Violence prevention training.

Alternatives to violence in child rearing, elder care, and intimate relationships exist. Physicians should support parenting preparedness training, conflict resolution education, and other violence prevention activities in schools, religious organizations, and community groups and should also re-evaluate their family, community, and medical practices in light of the characteristics of low-violence societies listed in Table 21–1. *Violence, except for self-defense or for the protection of another person, is never justified.*

References

1. Flitcraft AF, Hadley SM, Hendricks-Matthews MK, et al. Diagnostic and Treatment Guidelines on Domestic Violence. American Medical Association. Chicago: Ill, 1992.
2. Heise LL. Gender-based abuse: The global epidemic. In: Dan AJ, Editor. Reframing Women's Health, Multidisciplinary Research and Practice. Thousand Oaks, California: Sage Publications; 1994, pp. 233–250.
3. Abrams M, Shah R, Keenan-Allyn S. Sexual abuse in children and adolescents: A detection and management guide. Female Patient 1988;13:17–33.
4. American Psychiatric Association. Diagnostic and Statistical Manual of Mental Disorders. Washington, DC: American Psychiatric Association; 1994.
5. Ambuel B, Hamberger K. Family Peace Project, Family and Community Medicine. Medical College of Wisconsin (unpublished report).
6. Hamberger LK. Identifying and intervening with men who batter. In: Hendricks-Matthews, Editor. STFM Violence Education: Toward a Solution. Kansas City, MO: Society of Teachers of Family Medicine; 1992, pp. 55–62.
7. Aravanis SC, Adelman RD, Breckman R, et al. Diagnostic and treatment guidelines on elder abuse and neglect. Arch Fam Med 1993; 2:371–388.
8. Payne T, et al. Reach Out: Intervening in elder abuse, The Michigan Health Professional's Reference Guide to Elder Abuse, Michigan State Medical Society Task Force on Family Violence. Michigan State East Lansing, MI: Michigan State Medical Society; 1995.
9. Elder Mistreatment Guidelines for Health Care Professionals: Detection, Assessment and Intervention, Mount Sinai/Victim Services Agency Elder Abuse Project, New York, 1988.

Suggested Reading

Berkowitz C, Bross DC, Chadwick DL, et al. American Medical Association diagnostic and treatment guidelines on child physical abuse and neglect. Arch Fam Med 1992; 1:187–197.

Berkowitz C, Bross DC, Chadwick DL, et al. American Medical Association diagnostic and treatment guidelines on child sexual abuse. Arch Fam Med 1993; 2:19–27.

Chell D. Who are the batterers? Iowa Med 1995; 85:28.

McNeese M. When to suspect child abuse. Am Fam Physician 1982; 25:190–197.

IV

The Information Highway

22

MILTON P. HUANG, MD

THOMAS CARLI, MD

NORMAN E. ALESSI, MD

The World Wide Web as a Psychiatric Information Source for the Primary Care Physician

Four major sections form this chapter. Basic overview material about the Internet and the World Wide Web comprise the chapter's first three sections. "Useful Web sites" is the last section; it contains addresses for sites with information for primary care physicians. Experienced "web surfers" may wish to begin with this chapter's last section.

The fastest-growing source of new information on psychiatry is the Internet. More and more academic institutions, publishers, and commercial groups are putting information into electronic form. The most popular place for adding such information to the Internet is the World Wide Web. The Web is an Internet based information source that makes documents containing text, images, and other media accessible through a computer.

I. Internet basics.

A. What is the Internet?

The Internet is a worldwide computer network. The term *network* simply means that the different computers are connected and can communicate because they share the following:

1. *Physical connections.*
   Physical connections include telephone wires or fiber optic cable. Sometimes, these connections are mediated through devices such as modems, which create an interface between a computer and a telephone line.
2. *Shared protocols.*
   These are agreements between computers about how communications occur. Many types of communications are possible over the Internet, such as electronic mail (e-mail) messages or even video conferencing.

B. How does it work?

All computers on the Internet use a common protocol called *transmission control protocol/internet protocol* (TCP/IP). Each computer has a unique IP address that identifies it on the network. When someone wants to communicate, the following steps occur:

1. *Digitization.*
   The message is converted from voice, text, or picture into computer binary code and put into a digital packet.
2. *Transmission.*
   The packet is labeled with the target IP address and sent out on the network. The network directs it to the target computer in the same way that United States mail routes a letter using the zip code.
3. *Reconversion.*
   The target computer converts the digital packet back into the original voice, text, or picture.

It is essential for the sender and receiver to be using the same protocol for correct digitization and reconversion to take place.

C. What is the World Wide Web?

The World Wide Web is a part of the Internet that agrees to communicate using hypertext transfer protocol (http).

1. *Web documents.*
   Web documents are composed of text and graphics, like the pages of a book.
2. *Hypertext.*
   Hypertext consists of highlighted words that link a particular Web document to other Web documents. If the computer user is reading a Web document on his or her computer screen and clicks on a hypertext work by use of a mouse, a new page or document is displayed.
   The Web of documents, or Web pages, are created by these links, which provide access to World Wide Web information from computers all around the world.

D. How does it work?

1. *Client server.*
   All Web documents are stored on computers known as *servers.* The purpose of the server is to send a specified document when it receives a request from a "client" computer.

2. *Web browser.*
The Web browser is the software on a client computer that sends the request for a document, receives the document back from the Internet, and converts and displays it as the desired text and graphics.

3. *Uniform Resource Locator* (URL).
The URL is the means by which a desired document is specified. If the user types in an appropriate URL into his or her Web browser (e.g., http://www.psych.med.umich.edu/web/UMpsych/index.htm), the browser knows which server and which document it should ask for from the Internet. The URL has three basic parts. The first part (http) specifies the Web protocol (hypertext transfer protocol). The second part (between the "//" and the first "/") is the server name. In this case, "www.psych.med.umich.edu" is a computer located in the psychiatry department in the medical area of the University of Michigan. The subsequent parts specify which document should be retrieved from the server. In this case, the requested file is "index.htm" in the "UMpsych" directory in the "Web" directory. If all the aforementioned steps work correctly, this is all the information the browser needs to get the document from the Web. If the computer user already has a document on his or her screen, the process is much simpler; the computer user needs only click on the hypertext because these terms already contain URL information.

II. Connecting to the Internet.

In order to connect to the Internet the computer user must have the correct equipment and establish a connection through an Internet service.

A. Equipment.

Three types of equipment are necessary for an Internet connection.

1. *Computer.*
Any computer can be connected to the World Wide Web as long as it can support a modem/network hardware and Web browsing software (discussed later). Because every computer cannot support every speed of network connection or every type of browser, the purchase of preconfigured systems can simplify the set-up.

2. *Network hardware.*
This is the device that connects the computer to the network. The three most commonly available types of connection are the telephone line, integrated services digital network (ISDN), and ethernet.
   a. *Telephone line.*
   Modems are the devices that connect computers through a telephone line. Modems are relatively slow; higher-speed modems (14.4 or 28.8 kilobytes per second) are preferable.
   b. ISDN *Integrated services digital network.*
   The ISDN is a type of digital line that is becoming more widely available. This line can provide communications at speeds of 56 to 64 kilobytes per second. A digital modem is necessary for connecting a computer to such a line.
   c. *Ethernet.*
   This is a standard for high-speed communications in local area networks (LAN), as might exist within an institution. A computer needs an ethernet card and cable to hook up to the rest of the network. Such installations are best discussed with the person in charge of local network administration.

3. *Software.*
Computers need software in order to implement all the necessary communication protocols. Three main types are required:
   a. *Internet software.*
   This allows the computer to communicate using IP. Examples include WinSock or MacTCP. This software is usually included in the operating system (OS) that comes with the computer.
   b. *Connectivity software.*
   This allows the computer to use the network hardware described in section II.A. One example is MacPPP, which operates a modem to connect two computers through a telephone line. This functionality is included in WinSock and Windows 95, although it is not part of the standard installation. If it is not included in the operating system, such software can usually be obtained from the organization providing internet service (see section II.B.).
   c. *Web browser software.*
   This software requests and displays World Wide Web documents. The most popular Web browser software is Netscape Navigator. Other examples include Microsoft Internet Explorer, Spry Mosaic, or America On-Line web browser. Each browser has different capabilities and displays documents differently. Browser software can be purchased in stores or downloaded over the Internet.

B. Internet Service.

A connection to the Internet can be obtained in several ways.

1. *Internet service providers* (ISPs).
These organizations sell direct connections to the Internet. They work with or are companies that lay cable for people needing high-speed connections. They also can hook up people wanting low-speed connections by providing

dial-in lines for modems. Some of these providers are local and offer low monthly rates. Others, such as ANS, PSI, UUNet, and The Well, operate nationally. Lists of telephone numbers for such services can be found in books about the Internet, or on the World Wide Web itself at http://theList.com.

2. *Institutions.*
   Many institutions sign contracts with an ISP in order to provide Internet services to their members. If the computer user belongs to an academic institution or a local or national medical or professional society, he or she may be eligible for such a connection. These organizations have information regarding the availability of this connection.

3. *On-line service providers.*
   These organizations have their own dial-in information networks and often provide access to the Internet through their network at an hourly charge. Examples include Compuserve, America OnLine, and Prodigy. Although much more expensive than an ISP, on-line service providers usually furnish substantial help to members who have difficulties with connecting.

III. Using the World Wide Web.

A. Using a browser.

Every browser is different, but they all generally share characteristics that can make them easier to use.

1. *Home.*
   When a browser starts up, it opens with a particular World Wide Web page. This is the home page for the browser (or the manufacturer's company). It has links to help users start Web exploration and can usually be returned to at any time by pressing a "home" button. Browsers have provisions for changing this home site to a Web page of the user's own choice.

2. *Navigation.*
   As the computer user moves from page to page, the browser keeps track of all the pages visited. A "back" button returns the user to the previous page. A menu of all visited sites is usually available for more rapid return to a previously seen page.

3. *Bookmarks.*
   The list of visited pages is not remembered after the program is stopped. A bookmark facility (also known as "hotlist" or "favorites") is used to save the URL of a page. The bookmark list is saved when the computer is turned off and provides rapid access to favorite sites without requiring that the URL be retyped each time.

B. World Wide Web tools.

The World Wide Web is vast, and particular Web pages serve as tools for helping users find pages of interest.

1. *Web indices.*
   These are pages that create a hierarchical list of subjects, identifying particular pages as appropriate for the learning of certain topics. This tool is for beginners or people who like to browse through different topics in a bookstore. One example is the Medical Matrix page (http://www.slackinc.com/matrix/), which divides a list of Web sites into 55 specialties, each of which is further subdivided. Examples of indices that cover all topics (not just medicine) include Yahoo and Excite (see section IV).

2. *Search engines.*
   Search engines are Web pages that allow the user to type in a term of interest. A computer then searches a database for all the pages it can find that contain the search term. This tool is for people who can exactly specify the topic on which they desire information. Examples of search engines include Alta Vista, Infoseek, and Lycos (see section IV). Many index pages include search engines.

C. Precautions.

The World Wide Web is new and was little used before 1993. Some precautions must be taken when this new technology is used.

1. *Lack of review.*
   Anyone can add information to the World Wide Web. There is currently little review of information to establish standards of veracity, as compared with that used in the publication of information in paper journals. Information cannot always be trusted, and false rumors abound, some of which circulate repeatedly.

2. *Rapid changes.*
   Many documents change, information is not always available in the same place twice because many URLs become outdated when organizations update their equipment or stop funding projects.

3. *Time investment.*
   The World Wide Web takes up a lot of time, not only for learning all of the aforementioned technology described but also for other reasons.
   a. Information can be hard to find or not available. Powerful search engines may return too many possible sites.
   b. Waiting times for pages to appear can be long, especially with a slower modem connection.
   c. People who enjoy having a wealth of information lose track of time.

IV. Useful Web sites.

World Wide Web addresses constantly change, so the URLs listed in this section may be incorrect by the time this text is published. For a limited time after the publication of this book, this section of this chapter will be maintained on the World Wide Web as a Web page with updated links. This page is located at http://www.psych.med.umich.edu/web/primcare/ and will simplify exploration. Finally, the inclusion of a site on the list below does not indicate that these are the "best" sites or even that the content of the sites is accurate.

A. General medical sites.

1. *Medical Matrix.*
   http://www.slackinc.com/matrix/
   This is an extensive listing that organizes links to medical information, online continuing medical education courses, patient education material, medical software, medical employment opportunities, and more. The "quick" list of links to specialty information at http://www.slackinc.com/matrix/SPECIAL.HTML includes more than 1700 resources in categories ranging from addiction medicine and bariatrics to travel medicine and urology. All links are well organized and have brief annotations.
2. *MedWeb: Adam's Guide to Medical Resources on The Internet.*
   http://www.mcs.com/~ablock/www/medweb.html
   Seventy-four links provide the starting point for those interested in a broad range of general specialities in medicine, including psychiatry, and general diseases within medicine, such as oncology and multiple sclerosis. It is a starting point for users familiar with internet protocols to start their explorations.

B. General psychiatry.

1. *Internet Mental Health.*
   http://www.mentalhealth.com/
   An encyclopedia of mental health information on mental disorders, treatments, research, medications, software, and other internet links. Created by Canadian Phillip Long, MD, it is vast in content and visionary in its intent to be the Internet resource for mental health.
2. *Online Psychological Services: Mental Health Information Link.*
   http://www.onlinepsych.com/treat/mh.htm
   Contains more than 350 links to various aspects of mental health, organized around 25 topics ranging from aging and attention-deficit disorder to sexual abuse and suicidology.

C. Psychopharmacology.

1. *United States Department of Justice Drug Enforcement Administration.*
   http://www.usdoj.gov/deal/deahome.htm
   Excellent resource for anyone using medications, especially concerning issues of abuse and illegal use of medications.
2. *Psychopharmacology Tips.*
   http://uhs.bsd.uchicago.edu/~bhsiung/tips/tips.html
   Very popular Web site run by Ivan Goldberg, MD, and edited by Robert Hsiung, MD. "Tips" are posted by members of the *Interpsych* psychopharmacology discussion list and include practical recommendations about prescribing, indications, interactions, tapering, and so on.
3. *Psychiatry and Psychopharmacology.*
   http://www.onlinepsych.com/tour/psypharm.htm
   This site provides lists of articles, journals, Web links, list servers, discussion groups and newsgroups, and training and professional organizations related specifically to psychiatry and psychopharmacology.

D. Specific psychiatric topics.

1. *Depressive disorders.*
   a. *Internet Depression Resources List.*
      http://earth.execpc.com~corbeau/depress.html
      A comprehensive list concerning issues about affective disorders, including depression, bipolar illness, panic disorder, and suicide.
   b. *Depression in Primary Care. Volume 1. Detection and Diagnosis.*
      http://text.nlm.nih.gov/ftrs/dbaccess/ahcpr
      This is Volume 1 of a two-volume set of clinical practice guidelines developed by the Agency for Health Care Policy and Research (AHCPR), a part of the United States Department of Health and Human Services. The clinical practice guideline statements contained in *Depression in Primary Care* were developed to assist patients and primary care practitioners in the detection and diagnosis of depressive conditions and in the treatment of major depressive disorder. The "Depression Guideline Report" contains more than 3500 relevant references.
   c. *Depression in Primary Care. Volume 2. Treatment of Major Depression.*
      http://text.nlm.nih.gov/ftrs/dbaccess/ahcpr
      This is Volume 2 of the clinical practice guidelines developed by the AHCPR. This volume covers the treatment of major depressive disorder, including acute phase, maintenance, and strategic planning.
   d. *Seasonal Affective Disroder.*
      http://www.mentalhealth.com/book/p40-sad.html
      This site provides a summary of an important presentation of depression. This

home page contains information about the definition, presentation, epidemiology, and treatment of depression.

e. *Suicide Awareness and Voices of Education (SA/VE).*
http://www.save.org/
This Web site is maintained by Suicide Awareness and Voices of Education, an organization whose mission is to educate about suicide and to speak for suicide survivors. This site is extremely well organized and brings information to its readers concerning the presence of depression and suicide. Very useful.

2. *Anxiety disorders.*

a. *The Panic-Anxiety Page.*
http://www.algy.com/anxiety/index.html

> The Panic-Anxiety Page is an individual effort by Steve Ward of Murfreesboro, Tennessee. The aim of the page is to: Provide visitors with the most current and comprehensive index and archive of anxiety-related information on the web; Connect users with self-help and professional resources in their community; Cultivate and maintain a variety of online support forums; and, Educate users about anxiety's causes and treatments.

This site does a good, thorough job.

b. *Anxiety Disorders.*
http://www.mentalhealth.com/book/p41-anx.html
This site, which was created by the American Psychiatric Association, Joint Commission on Public Affairs, and provides a general overview of all the anxiety disorders, theories about etiology, and treatment. It is comprehensive, brief, and to the point. This site includes a bibliography.

c. *Anxiety Disorders.*
http://www.nimh.nih.gov/publicat/anxiety.htm
This is a complete patient handout created by the National Institute of Mental Health, written by Marilyn Dickey, a freelance writer in Washington, DC. The handout covers all the anxiety disorders and describes how patients may find help. This site provides vignettes that help illustrate the nature of these disorders.

3. *Psychoses and schizophrenia.*
http://w3socpsy.med.rug.nl/@?docs/schizx.htm
This page covers general research on the topic of schizophrenia from the Department of Psychiatry at the University of Groningen. It includes topics of diagnosis, etiology, and treatment as well as excellent papers on the subjective and cognitive aspects of schizophrenia.

4. *Problems of children and adolescents.*

a. *Facts for Families.*
http://www.aacap.org/web/aacap/factsFam/
"To educate parents and families about psychiatric disorders affecting children and adolescents."
This award-winning Web site was created and is maintained by the American Academy of Child and Adolescent Psychiatry (AACAP). This multilingual (French and Spanish) Web site contains information on 53 topics of interest to parents and others who know or have children and adolescents with emotional and behavioral disorders or problems. These pages can be downloaded and distributed to the parents of patients.

b. *Teen Suicide.*
http://www.aacap.org/web/aacap/factsFam/suicide.htm
Taken from the AACAP Web site, "Facts for Families," this page provides pertinent information concerning teen suicide.

c. *Living with ADHD.*
http://www.inet.net/adopt/issues/emot5.html
This page is excerpted from "Living with the Very Active Child," by Freda Wise. This Web site is short but raises interesting issues concerning dealing with children with attention-deficit hyperactivity disorder.

d. *Nocturnal Enuresis and Encopresis.*
http://vh.radiology.uiowa.edu/Providers/Lectures/Conferences/CPS/40Nocturnal.html
This is a nice site with pertinent information concerning the management of enuresis and encopresis. It provides a good review of psychopharmacology studies.

e. *Panic Disorders in Children and Adolescents.*
http://www.aacap.org/web/aacap/factsFam/panic.htm
This page is taken from the AACAP Web site, "Facts for Families."

f. *The Anxious Child.*
http://www.aacap.org/web/aacap/factsFam/anxious.htm
Taken from the AACAP Web site, "Facts for Families."

g. *Methylphenidate.*
http://www.usdoj.gov/dea/pubs/methyl/contents.htm
Drug Enforcement Agency site dealing with the most frequently prescribed psychoactive medication in children. Pros and cons are explored as well as trends that may influence the use of these drugs in children and adolescents.

5. *Common neurologic disorders.*

a. *Alzheimer's Disease.*
http://werple.mira.net.au/~dhs/ad2.html
The Alzheimer's Web site contains information aimed at physicians and researchers interested in Alzheimer's disease, as well as links to recent research and electronic discussion groups.

b. *Parkinson's Web.*
http://neuro-chief-e.mgh.harvard.edu/parkinsonsweb/Main/PDmain.html
This page was created by physicians at the Massachusetts General Hospital Department of Neurology. It contains links to patient information and links to diagnosis, surgical treatment, medications, behavioral interventions, support groups, and bibliographic references.

c. *HIV/AIDS-Journal of the American Medical Association (JAMA) site.*
http://www.ama-assn.org/special/hiv/hivhome.htm
This is an extensive resource maintained by JAMA, including several practice guidelines, news reports, patient information and support groups, and search capabilities of JAMA articles and the National Library of Medicine database.

d. *HIV/AIDS: HIV/AIDS Treatment Information Service.*
http://text.nlm.nih.gov/ftrs/pick?collect=atis&ftrsK=0
This is an index to acquired immunodeficiency virus (AIDS)-related documents created by the AHCPR. This site includes their clinical practice guideline for the evaluation and management of early human immunodeficiency virus (HIV) infection, morbidity and mortality weekly reports, and patient materials on HIV and HIV in children.

e. *Post Stroke Rehabilitation.*
http://text.nlm.nih.gov/ftrs/pick?ftrsK=0&collect=ahcpr&dbName=psrc
This site provides clinical practice guidelines for poststroke rehabilitation developed by the AHCPR. The site includes sections on epidemiology, etiology, assessment methods, rehabilitation management, and transitioning to the community.

6. *Sleep disorders and insomnia.*
http://www.njc.org/MSUhtml/MSU_sleep.html
This site provides a thorough overview of the topic of sleep disorders. This site is ideal for the medical professional who wants a textbooklike presentation with accompanying style and references. It is produced by the National Jewish Center for Immunology and Respiratory Medicine.

7. *Chronic fatigue syndrome and fibromyalgia.*

a. *Chronic Fatigue Syndrome.*
http://www.iacnet.com/health/13874775.htm
This is a useful pamphlet written by Jean M. Carey for the American Council on Science and Health, giving general information on diagnosis, criteria, course, and treatment.

b. *Fibromyalgia Resources.*
http://www.hsc.missouri.edu/fibro/index.html
This site is maintained by the Missouri Arthritis Rehabilitation Research and Training Center and provides information for patients and physicians. Articles in this site cover diagnosis, etiology, and treatment, including medication management.

8. *Chronic pain.*

a. *The Integrated Approach to the Management of Pain.*
http://text.nlm.nih.gov/nih/cdc/www/55txt.html
This site provides The National Institutes of Health Consensus Development Conference Statement on "The Integrated Approach to the Management of Pain." It contains recommendations for physicians about the assessment of pain and pharmacologic and nonpharmacologic treatment.

b. *Pain Control.*
http://www.healthtouch.com/level1/leaflets/102.429/102429.htm
This site has a series of patient oriented leaflets by the National Institute of Neurological Disorders and Stroke that covers general issues of chronic pain, pain control techniques, postsurgical pain, and cancer pain.

c. *Chronic Pain Assessment and Treatment.*
http://home.navisoft.com/aapa/pain.htm
This site provides a summary sheet of psychological considerations in chronic pain management. It was written by Alan Brandis, PhD, of Atlanta Area Psychological Associates. This site includes a patient-oriented list of frequently asked questions on types of therapy, including psychotherapy, family therapy, stress reduction training, biofeedback training, hypnosis, and medication.

9. *Nicotine and smoking.*

a. *NO SMOKE software for Windows.*
http://www.autonomy.com/smoke.htm
This smoking cessation site has links to every anti-smoking page on the World Wide Web and Smoke No More Forum so that people and organizations can share ideas.

b. *Smoking and Health: A Physician Responsibility.*
http://www.chestnet.org/smoking.html
This site provides a Statement of the Joint Committee on Smoking and Health (American College of Chest Physicians, American Thoracic Society, Asia Pacific Society of Respirology, Canadian Thoracic Society, European Respiratory Society, International Union Against Tuberculosis and Lung Disease). The site gives an interesting overview of the perils of smoking and the responsibilities that doctors have with their patients to implement cessation.

10. *Alcohol- and drug-related problems.*

a. *National Clearinghouse for Alcohol and Drug Information.*

http://www.health.org/
This is the home page of the National Clearinghouse for Alcohol and Drug Information. This site contains a list of referral resources on and off the Internet and an extensive collection of links to publications aimed at community leaders, educators, family and friends, health professionals, and clinicians.

b. *National Institute on Alcohol Abuse and Alcoholism.*
http://www.niaaa.nih.gov/
This site is the home page of the National Institute on Alcohol Abuse and Alcoholism, one of the institutes of the National Institutes of Health. This site contains pointers to research monographs, patient pamphlets, news alerts, research databases, and statistical data. "The Physicians' Guide to Helping Patients with Alcohol Problems" at http://www.niaaa.nih.gov/publications/physicn.htm is a step-by-step manual.

11. *Eating disorders.*
   a. *Lucy Serpell's Eating Disorders Resources.*
   http://www.psyc.nott.ac.uk/~les/eat.htm
   This is a neatly organized page of various Web sites relevant to eating disorders, including conferences, self-help pages, treatment centers, and research.
   b. *Serotonin and Eating Disorders.*
   http://www.pharminfo.com/pubs/msb/seroton.html
   This site is an article from the *Medical Sciences Bulletin* that discusses the use of serotonergic drugs in the treatment of eating disorder and obesity. The site includes citations.

12. *Obesity.*
   a. *Understanding Obesity and Weight Loss.*
   http://www-med.stanford.edu/MedCenter/MedSchool/DGIM/Teaching/Modules/obesity.html#RTFToC5
   This site contains a teaching module written by Robert B. Baron MD, MS, for the University of California at San Francisco Division of General Internal Medicine. It discusses etiology, patient selection, diet therapy, exercise, behavior modification, medication treatment, and surgery.
   b. *Patient Information Documents on Nutrition and Obesity.*
   http://www.niddk.nih.gov/NutritionDocs.html
   This site gives patient information on dieting, weight loss, and exercise from the National Institute of Diabetes and Digestive and Kidney Diseases of the National Institutes of Health.
   c. *Focus On . . . Obesity.*
   http://pharminfo.com/pubs/msb/obesity.html
   This site contains an article on the medical treatment of obesity. The article is extremely biased toward drug treatment.

13. *Sexuality issues and common sexual dysfunctions.*
   a. *Sexual Disorders.*
   http://www.cityscape.co.uk/users/ad88/sex.htm
   This article lists all sexual disorders from the *Diagnostic and Statistical Manual of Mental Disorders, Fourth Edition,*[1] and provides brief information on prevalence, treatment, and self-auditing of physician practice.
   b. *Impotence.*
   http://text.nlm.nih.gov/nih/cdc/www/91txt.html
   This is the site for the National Institutes of Health Consensus Development Conference Statement on Impotence. The site discusses psychological and cultural factors, physiology, diagnostic assessment and testing, and treatment and treatment efficacy.

14. *Domestic violence and abuse.*
   a. *Screening for Violent Injuries.*
   http://cpmcnet.columbia.edu/health.sci/.gcps/gcps051.html
   This article from the Columbia-Presbyterian Medical Center describes the problems of abuse, the efficacy of screening, and recommendations for clinical intervention.
   b. *Domestic Violence Resources.*
   http://marie.az.com/%7Eblainn/dv/family/
   This site contains a set of articles taken from the Academic Family Medicine Mail-list. It covers the topics of counseling battered women, taking care of yourself while working with women on the edge of crisis, domestic violence training project true/false quiz, becoming a source for battered women, signs of the batterer, and assessing whether batterers will kill.
   c. *Women's Mental Health & Domestic Violence.*
   http://www.healthtouch.com/level1/leaflets/101810/102031.htm
   This series of well-written patient information pamphlets was created by the National Coalition Against Domestic Violence. Topics include statistics on domestic violence, verbal and emotional abuse, predictors of domestic violence, the abusive partner, and more.

E. World Wide Web sites for organizations.

1. *American Medical Association.*
   http://www.ama.assn.org
2. *American Psychiatric Association.*
   http://www.psych.org
3. *National Institutes of Health.*
   http://www.nih.gov/
4. *National Institute of Mental Health.*
   http://www.nimh.nih.gov/

5. *National Alliance for the Mentally Ill.*
   http://www.nami.org
   NAMI is a grassroots, self-help support and advocacy organization of families and friends of people with serious mental illness, and those persons themselves. NAMI's mission is to reduce stigma and mental illness and to improve the quality of life for those who suffer from severe brain disorders such as schizophrenia, depression, manic depression, panic disorder, and obsessive-compulsive disorder.

6. *American Medical Informatics Association.*
   http://www.amia.org/
   The AMIA serves as an authoritative body in the field of medical informatics and represents the United States in the informational arena of medical systems and informatics in international forums.

7. *Psychiatric Society for Informatics.*
   http://www.psych.med.umich.edu/web/psi/
   This organization is dedicated to promoting the understanding and use of informatics and information technology in psychiatry.

F. World Wide Web indices and search engines.

1. *Yahoo.*
   http://www.yahoo.com
   One of the original indices, Yahoo collects thousands of Internet sites and organizes them according to topic. It also has news updates, weather, maps, and other useful information.

2. *Alta Vista.*
   http://altavista.digital.com
   Alta Vista is one of most comprehensive search engines; it evaluates a database of millions of Internet sites.

3. *Infoseek.*
   http://www.infoseek.com
   Infoseek is one of most sophisticated search engines; it is organized to help users find desired sites efficiently by identifying desired areas of interest.

Reference

1. American Psychiatric Association. Diagnostic and Statistical Manual of Mental Disorders, ed 4. Washington, DC: American Psychiatric Association; 1994.

Suggested Reading

December J, Randall N. The World Wide Web Unleashed. Second Edition. Indianapolis, IN: SAMS net; 1995.

Eager B. Using the World Wide Web. Indianapolis, IN: QUE; 1994.

Hogarth M, Hutchinson D. An Internet Guide for the Health Professional. Sacramento, CA: New Wind Publishing Company; 1996.

V

Appendices

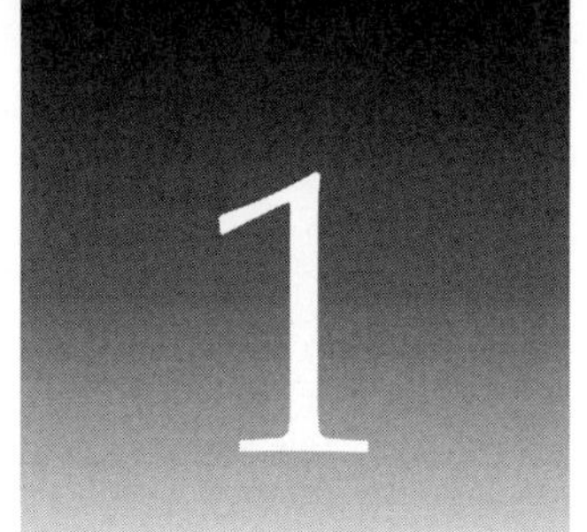

MICHAEL D. JIBSON, MD, PhD

Medication Fact Sheets: Patient Handouts Describing the Major Side Effects of Psychotropic Drugs

Informed consent for the use of psychotropic medication is essential. In general, psychotropic medications require a higher standard of informed consent than do other medications. Some legal venues require that patients be given written information regarding these medications, including the reason they are being prescribed, their expected benefits, and their most common and serious side effects. The following psychotropic medication fact sheets are guidelines for the information that should be presented to patients and families before treatment. This information is presented using language that is appropriate for patients and families. *These descriptions do not include every reported side effect of the medications listed but instead represent a reasonable summary of the most important issues.* The degree of detail included may be adjusted to meet the needs of the individual patient.

Accordingly, *the fact sheets are not to be used as mere handouts;* they should be used as part of a verbal discussion about the psychotropic medication being recommended. This method reinforces the central idea that the doctor and the patient are partners in care, provides an opportunity to stress the importance of compliance, describes why it is necessary to continue the drug even if symptoms improve, and makes patient education an intrinsic part of the care process. Patients tend to remember primarily the information they receive directly from the doctor. Without a verbal exchange, the handout becomes a mere procedural requirement and is less likely to be a source of useful information for the patient. The doctor should identify and highlight those items on the fact sheet that deserve emphasis for the particular clinical situation. The fact sheet then serves as a reminder and becomes a resource for future reference.

The verbal exchange should include a statement like:

> *The fact sheet I am giving you describes what most patients experience with this medicine. You may experience one or more of these side effects, but it is extremely unusual for any individual to experience all of them. You might also experience a rare side effect not listed on the sheet. Keep the fact sheet handy; if you do experience a problem, you may want to see if it is a problem that is listed. Please call me at my office if you experience anything unusual or troubling or if you have any questions as we proceed with treatment.*

For the pregnant patient, the fact sheets need to be used in conjunction with "Information for the Pregnant Patient and Family" (see Chapter 2). Contained in that section is information relevant to psychotropics administration while breast feeding. Also in Chapter 2, Table 2–5, "Common Psychotropic Drugs and Risk Categories During Pregnancy," provides useful information.

Antidepressant

Bupropion

Medications in This Class Include
Bupropion (Wellbutrin)
Sustained-release Bupropion (Wellbutrin SR)

This Medication Is Used to Treat the Following Psychiatric Conditions:
Depressed mood
Dysthymia
Attention deficit disorders

Other Uses of Bupropion
None

What to Expect from Bupropion
This medicine is intended to improve mood, increase attention span, or decrease hyperactive behavior. The medicine must be taken for 3 to 6 weeks for its full effects to be seen. It may be continued after the symptoms have disappeared in order to prevent them from returning.

Side Effects
As with any medication, bupropion may cause side effects. Most of these are minor and improve or disappear after a short time on the medicine. If side effects are especially troubling or interfere with your ability to function, notify your doctor.

Common Side Effects	Uncommon Side Effects
Tremor	*Allergic reaction
Constipation	*Seizure
Agitation	Blurred vision
Dry mouth	Hypertension
Dizziness	Confusion
Sweating	Headache
Insomnia	Menstrual complaints
Nausea/vomiting	Palpitations
	Cardiac arrhythmia
	Anxiety
	Increased appetite
	Sexual dysfunction
	Stomach upset

Consequences of Long-Term Use
None

Special Considerations
Risk of seizure is directly related to the dose of this medication, therefore Wellbutrin should not be taken in individual doses larger than 150 mg. Wellbutrin SR has a lower risk of seizure, and may be taken in larger individual doses.

*Notify your doctor promptly if this side effect occurs.

Antidepressant

Mirtazapine (Remeron)

This Medication Is Used to Treat the Following Psychiatric Conditions:
Depressed mood
Dysthymia

Other Uses of Mirtazapine
None

What to Expect from Mirtazapine
This medicine is intended to improve depressed or dysthymic mood. The medication must be taken for 3 to 6 weeks for its full effects to be seen. It may be continued after the symptoms have disappeared in order to prevent them from returning.

Side Effects
As with any medication, mirtazapine may cause side effects. Most of these are minor and improve or disappear after a short time on the medicine. If side effects are especially troubling or interfere with your ability to function, notify your doctor.

Common Side Effects	Uncommon Side Effects
Sedation	*Allergic reaction
Increased appetite	Muscle aches
Weight gain	Weakness
Increased cholesterol and triglycerides	Swelling
Dry mouth	Confusion
Constipation	Tremor
Dizziness	Abdominal pain
	Agitation
	Anxiety
	Hypertension
	Nausea/vomiting
	Thirst

Consequences of Long-Term Use
None

Special Considerations
Rare cases of agranulocytosis and severe neutropenia (low levels of white blood cells) have been reported during clinical trials.

*Notify your doctor promptly if this side effect occurs.

Antidepressants

Monoamine Oxidase Inhibitors (MAOIs)

Medications in This Class Include
Phenelzine (Nardil)
Tranylcypromine (Parnate)

These Medications Are Used to Treat the Following Psychiatric Conditions:
Depression
Anxiety
Panic attacks
Agoraphobia

Other Uses for MAOIs
None

What to Expect from an MAOI
This medicine is intended to improve mood, reduce anxiety, reduce the frequency and intensity of panic attacks, and reduce unreasonable fear of public places or social situations. The medicine must be taken for 3 to 6 weeks for its full effects to be seen. Its administration may be continued after the symptoms have disappeared in order to prevent them from returning.

Dietary and Medication Restrictions
MAOIs may cause a dangerous increase in blood pressure (hypertensive crisis) in the presence of certain foods or medicines. Symptoms of a hypertensive crisis may include severe headache, cold sweat, change in heart rate, pounding heart, fever, stiff neck, chest pain, and enlarged pupils. If this occurs, seek emergency treatment immediately.

Foods to Avoid
Aged cheese
Liver
Pickled meat and fish
Smoked meat and fish
Dry sausage
Sauerkraut
Pea and bean pods
Meat tenderizer
Caviar
Canned figs
Yeast extract
Meat extract
Red wine
Sherry
Liqueurs

Foods to Limit
Yogurt
Processed cheese
Sour cream
Avocados
Raisins
Bananas
Chocolate
Soy sauce
Cola drinks
Coffee
Tea
Beer (including nonalcoholic)

Medicines to Avoid
Other antidepressants
Meperidine (Demerol)
Decongestants
Cold medicines
Cough medicines
Allergy medicines
Stimulants
Tryptophan
Parkinsonism medicines

Side Effects
As with any medication, MAOIs may cause side effects. Most of these are minor and improve or disappear after a short time on the medicine. If side effects are especially troubling or interfere with your ability to function, notify your doctor.

Common Side Effects
Dizziness
Lightheadedness
Headache
Drowsiness
Insomnia
Constipation
Dry mouth
Stomach upset
Weight gain
Sexual dysfunction
Fatigue or weakness
Tremor
Twitching
Edema (water retention)

Uncommon Side Effects
*Allergic reaction
*Hypertensive crisis
Decreased appetite
Nervousness
Difficulty urinating
Blurred vision
Confusion

Consequences of Long-Term Use
None

*Notify your doctor promptly if this side effect occurs.

Antidepressants

Selective Serotonin Reuptake Inhibitors (SSRIs)

Medications in This Class Include
Fluoxetine (Prozac)
Fluvoxamine (Luvox)
Paroxetine (Paxil)
Sertraline (Zoloft)

These Medications Are Used to Treat the Following Psychiatric Conditions:
Depression
Dysthymia
Anxiety
Panic attacks
Obsessive-compulsive disorder
Bulimia

Other Uses for SSRIs
None

What to Expect from an SSRI
This medicine is intended to improve mood, reduce anxiety, and reduce the frequency and intensity of panic attacks, obsessive-compulsive behaviors, and binging and purging behaviors. The medicine must be taken for 3 to 6 weeks for its full effects to be seen. Its administration may be continued after the symptoms have disappeared in order to prevent them from returning.

Side Effects
As with any medication, SSRIs may cause side effects. Most of these are minor and improve or disappear after a short time on the medicine. If side effects are especially troubling or interfere with your ability to function, notify your doctor.

Common Side Effects	Uncommon Side Effects
Dry mouth	*Allergic reaction
Nausea	Decreased appetite
Diarrhea	Fatigue
Tremor	Nervousness
Insomnia	
Sexual dysfunction	
Drowsiness	
Dizziness	
Sweating	
Stomach upset	

Consequences of Long-Term Use
None

*Notify your doctor promptly if this side effect occurs.

Antidepressants

Serotonin/Norepinephrine Reuptake Inhibitors

Medications in This Class Include
Nefazodone (Serzone)
Trazodone (Desyrel)

These Medications Are Used to Treat the Following Psychiatric Conditions:
Depression
Insomnia
Anxiety
Severe agitation
Irritability

Other Uses for These Medications
None

What to Expect from These Medications
This medicine is intended to reduce symptoms of depression, assist with sleep, or reduce anxiety, agitation, or irritability. This medicine is immediately effective for sleep but must be taken for 3 to 6 weeks for its other effects to be seen. Administration of the medicine may be continued after the symptoms have disappeared in order to prevent them from returning.

Side Effects
As with any medication, these may cause side effects. Most of the effects are minor and improve or disappear after a short time on the medicine. If side effects are especially troubling or interfere with your ability to function, notify your doctor.

Common Side Effects	Uncommon Side Effects
Drowsiness	*Allergic reaction
Dizziness	Confusion
Lightheadedness	Poor coordination
Fatigue	Tremor
Headache	Blurred vision
Constipation	*Prolonged painful erection (rare)
Nausea	
Dry mouth	

Consequences of Long-Term Use
None

*Notify your doctor promptly if this side effects occurs.

Antidepressants

Tricyclic and Heterocyclic Antidepressants

Medications in This Class Include
Amitriptyline (Elavil, Triavil)
Amoxapine (Asendin)
Clomipramine (Anafranil)
Desipramine (Norpramine)
Doxepin (Sinequan)
Imipramine (Tofranil)
Maprotiline (Ludiomil)
Nortriptyline (Pamelor)
Protriptyline (Vivactil)
Trimipramine (Surmontil)

These Medications Are Used to Treat the Following Psychiatric Conditions:
Depressed mood
Dysthymia
Anxiety
Panic attacks
Obsessive-compulsive disorder
Attention-deficit disorder
Eating disorders
Other conditions as described by your doctor

Other Uses for Tricyclic Antidepressants
Migraine headache
Chronic pain
Bed wetting

What to Expect from a Tricyclic Antidepressant
This medicine is intended to improve mood, reduce anxiety, reduce the frequency and intensity of panic attacks, improve concentration, and reduce obsessive-compulsive behaviors. The medicine must be taken for 3 to 6 weeks at optimal doses for its full effects to be seen. It may be continued after the symptoms have disappeared in order to prevent them from returning.

Side Effects
As with any medication, tricyclic antidepressants may cause side effects. Most of these are minor and may improve or disappear after a short time on the medicine. If side effects are especially troubling or interfere with your ability to function, notify your doctor.

Common Side Effects	Uncommon Side Effects
Dry mouth	*Allergic reaction
Drowsiness	*Difficulty urinating
Blurred vision	*Irregular heartbeat
Constipation	Changes in menstrual cycles
Dizziness or lightheadedness	Numbness or tingling
Weight gain	Skin sensitivity to light
Headache	Tremor
Sweating	
Increased heart rate	
Sexual dysfunction	

Consequences of Long-Term Use
Dental caries due to dry mouth

*Notify your doctor promptly if this side effect occurs

Antidepressant

Venlafaxine (Effexor)

This Medication Is Used to Treat the Following Psychiatric Conditions:
Depression
Dysthymia

Other Uses of Venlafaxine
None

What to Expect from Venlafaxine
This medicine is intended to reduce symptoms of depression. The medicine must be taken for 3 to 6 weeks for its full effects to be seen. Its administration may be continued after the symptoms have disappeared in order to prevent them from returning.

Side Effects
As with any medication, venlafaxine may cause side effects. Most of these are minor and improve or disappear after a short time on the medicine. If side effects are especially troubling or interfere with your ability to function, notify your doctor.

Common Side Effects	Uncommon Side Effects
Nausea	*Allergic reaction
Headache	Tremor
Drowsiness	Agitation
Insomnia	High blood pressure
Dry mouth	
Dizziness	
Constipation	
Nervousness	
Sweating	
Weakness or fatigue	
Sexual dysfunction	
Loss of appetite	

Consequences of Long-Term Use
None

*Notify your doctor promptly if this side effect occurs.

Antipsychotic

Clozapine (Clozaril)

This Medication Is Used to Treat the Following Psychiatric Conditions:
Delusions
Hallucinations
Disorganized thinking or behavior
Severe mood swings

Other Uses of Clozapine
In some instances clozapine has been used to treat tardive dyskinesia.

What to Expect from Clozapine
This medication is intended to reduce symptoms of psychosis (delusions, hallucinations, disorganized thinking) or severe mood swings. It must be taken for at least 6 weeks for its full effects to be seen. Its beneficial effects tend to increase with time. It may be continued after the symptoms have disappeared in order to prevent them from returning.

Side Effects
As with any medication, clozapine may cause side effects. Most of these are minor and improve or disappear after a short time on the medicine. If side effects are especially troubling or interfere with your ability to function, notify your doctor.

Common Side Effects	Uncommon Side Effects
Sedation	*Allergic reaction
Excessive salivation	*Seizure
Tachycardia (racing heart)	Weight gain
Dizziness	Tremor
Constipation	Sweating
Urinary problems	Fainting
Hypotension	Restlessness
Headache	Slow, rigid movements
Nausea/vomiting	Agitation
Fever	Confusion
	Weakness/Fatigue
	Jerking movements/spasms
	Sexual dysfunction

Special Considerations
Clozapine is associated with a decreased number of white blood cells in about 2% of patients. This side effect is potentially fatal if not detected early. For that reason, weekly monitoring of white blood cells is required when clozapine is administered.

*Notify your doctor promptly if this side effect occurs.

Antipsychotic

Olanzapine (Zyprexa)

This Medication Is Used to Treat the Following Psychiatric Conditions:
Delusions
Hallucinations
Disorganized thinking or behavior
Severe agitation

Other Uses of Olanzapine
None

What to Expect from Olanzapine
This medicine is intended to reduce symptoms of psychosis (delusions, hallucinations, disorganized thinking) or agitation. It must be taken for 3 to 6 weeks for its full effects to be seen. It may be continued after the symptoms have disappeared in order to prevent them from returning.

Side Effects
As with any medication, olanzapine may cause side effects. Most of these are minor and improve or disappear after a short time on the medicine. If side effects are especially troubling or interfere with your ability to function, notify your doctor.

Common Side Effects	Uncommon Side Effects
Sedation	*Allergic reaction
Constipation	Headache
Dizziness	Stomach upset
Agitation	Muscle rigidity
Restlessness	Lightheadedness
Weight gain	Tremor
Dry mouth	Racing heart
Nasal congestion	Swelling
	Speech difficulty

Consequences of Long-Term Use
Tardive dyskinesia (involuntary rolling movements of the fingers, rhythmic movements of the jaw or tongue, or movements elsewhere in the body) is more likely to occur as the dose and time on the medicine increases. In rare instances it may continue after administration of the medicine is stopped.

*Notify your doctor promptly if this side effect occurs.

Antipsychotic

Risperidone (Risperdal)

This Medication Is Used to Treat the Following Psychiatric Conditions:
Delusions
Hallucinations
Disorganized thinking or behavior
Severe agitation
Mood swings

Other Uses for Risperidone
None

What to Expect from Risperidone
This medicine is intended to reduce symptoms of psychosis (delusions, hallucinations, disorganized thinking), agitation, or mood instability. It must be taken for 3 to 6 weeks for its full effects to be seen. It may be continued after the symptoms have disappeared in order to prevent them from returning.

Side Effects
As with any medication, risperidone may cause side effects. Most of these are minor and improve or disappear after a short time on the medicine. If side effects are especially troubling or interfere with your ability to function, notify your doctor.

Common Side Effects	Uncommon Side Effects
Drowsiness	*Allergic reaction
Restlessness	*Arm, leg, neck, or jaw cramps
Lightheadedness	*Difficulty swallowing
Anxiety	Slow, shuffling movements
Stiff muscles	Masklike face
Constipation	Insomnia
Nausea	Rapid heartbeat
Nasal congestion	Upset stomach
	Dizziness
	Seizures

Consequences of Long-Term Use
Tardive dyskinesia (involuntary rolling movements of the fingers, rhythmic movements of the jaw or tongue, or movements elsewhere in the body) is more likely to occur as the dose and time on the medicine increase. In rare instances, it may continue after administration of the medicine is stopped.

*Notify your doctor promptly if this side effect occurs.

Antipsychotics

Typical Neuroleptics

Medications in This Class Include
Chlorpromazine (Thorazine)
Fluphenazine (Prolixin, Permitil)
Haloperidol (Haldol)
Loxapine (Loxitane)
Mesoridazine (Serentil)
Molindone (Moban)
Perphenazine (Trilafon)
Pimozide (Orap)
Prochlorperazine (Compazine)
Thioridazine (Mellaril)
Thiothixene (Navane)
Trifluoperazine (Stelazine)

This Medication Is Used to Treat the Following Psychiatric Conditions:
Delusions
Hallucinations
Disorganized thinking or behavior
Severe agitation
Tourette's syndrome
Mood swings

Other Uses for Typical Neuroleptics
Nausea
Intractable hiccups

What to Expect from a Typical Neuroleptic
This medicine is intended to reduce symptoms of psychosis (delusions, hallucinations, disorganized thinking), agitation, and mood instability, or to control the tics of Tourette's syndrome. This medicine must be taken for 3 to 6 weeks for its full effects to be seen. Administration of the medicine may be continued after the symptoms have disappeared in order to prevent them from returning.

Side Effects
As with any medication, typical neuroleptics may cause side effects. Most of these are minor and improve or disappear after a short time on the medicine. If side effects are especially troubling or interfere with your ability to function, notify your doctor.

Common Side Effects	Uncommon Side Effects
Stiff muscles	*Allergic reactions
Restlessness	*Arm, leg, neck, or jaw cramps
Slow, shuffling movements	*Difficulty swallowing
Masklike face	*Difficulty urinating
Dry mouth	Dizziness or lightheadedness
Drowsiness	Changes in menstrual cycles
Blurred vision	Swollen or painful breasts
Constipation	Inappropriate secretion of milk
Tremor	Irregular heartbeat
Sexual dysfunction	

Consequences of Long-Term Use
Tardive dyskinesia (involuntary rolling movements of the fingers, rhythmic movements of the jaw or tongue, or movements elsewhere in the body) is more likely to occur as the dose and time on the medicine increase. In rare instances, it may continue after administration of the medicine is stopped.

*Notify your doctor promptly if this side effect occurs.

Anxiolytic

Buspirone (BuSpar)

This Medication Is Used to Treat the Following Psychiatric Conditions:
Anxiety
Agitation

Other Uses of Buspirone
None

What to Expect from Buspirone
This medicine is intended to reduce symptoms of generalized anxiety or agitation. It is not usually effective for panic attacks. It must be taken for 3 to 6 weeks for its full effects to be seen. It may be continued after the symptoms have disappeared in order to prevent them from returning.

Side Effects
As with any medication, buspirone may cause side effects. Most of these are minor and improve or disappear after a short time on the medicine. If side effects are especially troubling or interfere with your ability to function, notify your doctor.

Common Side Effects	Uncommon Side Effects
Dizziness	*Allergic reaction
	Drowsiness
	Nervousness
	Lightheadedness
	Agitation
	Nausea
	Headache
	Numbness
	Weakness

Consequences of Long-Term-Use
None

*Notify your doctor promptly if this side effect occurs.

Anxiolytics/Sedatives/Hypnotics

Benzodiazepines

Medications in This Class Include
Alprazolam (Xanax)
Chlordiazepoxide (Librium)
Clonazepam (Klonopin)
Clorazepate (Tranxene)
Diazepam (Valium)
Estazolam (ProSom)
Flurazepam (Dalmane)
Hydroxyzine (Atarax)
Lorazepam (Ativan)
Oxazepam (Serax)
Quazepam (Doral)
Temazepam (Restoril)
Triazolam (Halcion)
*Zolpidem (Ambien)

These Medications Are Used to Treat the Following Psychiatric Conditions:
Anxiety
Panic attacks
Agitation
Insomnia
Irritability

Other Uses for Benzodiazepines
Alcohol withdrawal
Muscle relaxation
Seizures

What to Expect from a Benzodiazepine
This medicine is intended to reduce symptoms of anxiety, to reduce the frequency and intensity of panic attacks, to help with sleep, and to decrease tension, agitation, and irritability. The effects of this medicine are usually seen within 30 to 60 minutes of each dose. Administration of the medicine may be continued after the symptoms have disappeared in order to prevent them from returning.

Side Effects
As with any medication, benzodiazepines may cause side effects. Most of these are minor and improve or disappear after a short time on the medicine. If side effects are especially troubling or interfere with your ability to function, notify your doctor.

Common Side Effects	Uncommon Side Effects
Drowsiness	†Confusion
Additive effect with alcohol	†Hallucinations
Difficulty walking	Dizziness
Difficulty concentrating	Memory problems

Consequences of Long-Term Use
This medicine is habit forming and has potential for abuse and dependency. For this reason, it is often used for only a short time. In some conditions, however, longer-term use is appropriate. If administration of the medicine is stopped after several weeks or more, it must be decreased slowly so that withdrawal symptoms are avoided.

*Not chemically related to benzodiazepines but included because its actions are very similar to those of benzodiazepines.
†Notify your doctor promptly if this side effect occurs.

Mood Stabilizers

Anticonvulsant Mood Stabilizers

Medications in This Class Include
Valproic acid (Depakene)
Divalproex sodium (Depakote)
Carbamazepine (Tegretol)

These Medications Are Used to Treat the Following Psychiatric Conditions:
Mood swings
Manic episodes
Refractory depression
Refractory psychosis
Severe agitation

Other Uses for These Medications
Seizure disorders
Trigeminal neuralgia

What to Expect from a Mood Stabilizer
This medicine is intended to reduce mood swings. It may also be used together with an antidepressant to treat severe depression, or with a neuroleptic to treat psychosis. It must be taken for 3 to 6 weeks for its full effects to be seen. Administration of the medicine is generally continued after the symptoms have disappeared in order to prevent them from returning.

Blood levels of these medicines must be monitored throughout their use.

Side Effects
As with any medication, mood stabilizers may cause side effects. Most of these are minor and improve or disappear after a short time on the medicine. If side effects are especially troubling or interfere with your ability to function, notify your doctor.

Common Side Effects	Uncommon Side Effects
Drowsiness	*Allergic reactions
Dizziness	Confusion
Difficulty walking	Poor coordination
Nausea	Blurred vision
Headache	Hair loss
Tremor	Low white blood cell count (carbamazepine)
Weight gain (valproic acid)	

Consequences of Long-Term Use
Rarely, liver damage (especially with valproic acid and divalproex)

Special Considerations
Use of anticonvulsant mood stabilizers during pregnancy may be associated with damage to the fetus, particularly spinal cord abnormalities.

*Notify your doctor promptly if this side effect occurs.

Mood Stabilizer

Lithium

Medications in This Class Include
Lithium carbonate (Eskalith, Lithonate, Lithotabs, Lithobid)
Lithium citrate

This Medication Is Used to Treat the Following Psychiatric Conditions:
Mood swings
Manic episodes
Severe depression
Refractory psychosis

Other Uses for Lithium
Low white blood cell count

What to Expect from Lithium
This medicine is intended to reduce the frequency and severity of mood swings. It may be used together with antidepressants or neuroleptics to increase their action against depression or psychosis. Lithium must be taken for 3 to 6 weeks for its full effects to be seen. Treatment is generally continued after the symptoms have disappeared in order to prevent them from returning.

Blood levels of this medicine must be monitored throughout its use.

Side Effects
As with any medication, lithium may cause side effects. Most of these are minor and improve or disappear after a short time on the medicine. If side effects are especially troubling or interfere with your ability to function, notify your doctor.

Common Side Effects	Uncommon Side Effects
Nausea	*Difficulty walking
*Vomiting	Metallic taste
Diarrhea	Acne
Weight gain	Hair loss
Tremor	*Abnormal heartbeat
Increased thirst	Congestive heart failure
Frequent urination	*Confusion
Drowsiness	

Consequences of Long-Term Use
Decrease in thyroid function
Alteration in kidney function

Special Considerations
Excessively high blood levels of lithium may cause severe nausea, vomiting, severe diarrhea, inability to walk, severe tremor, confusion, and seizures.

Use of lithium during pregnancy may be associated with damage to the fetus, particularly heart abnormalities.

*Notify your doctor promptly if this side effect occurs.

Psychostimulants

Medications in This Class Include
Dextroamphetamine (Dexedrine)
Methylphenidate (Ritalin)
Pemoline (Cylert)

These Medications Are Used to Treat the Following Psychiatric Conditions:
Attention-deficit hyperactivity disorder
Narcolepsy
Severe depression

Other Uses for Psychostimulants
None

What to Expect from a Psychostimulant
This medicine is intended to increase attention span and focused activity, reduce symptoms of depression, or reduce excessive sleepiness. This medicine begins to be effective 30 to 60 minutes after each dose. Administration of the medicine may be continued after the symptoms have disappeared in order to prevent them from returning.

Side Effects
As with any medication, psychostimulants may cause side effects. Most of these are minor and improve or disappear after a short time on the medicine. If side effects are especially troubling or interfere with your ability to function, notify your doctor.

Common Side Effects	Uncommon Side Effects
Anxiety	*Allergic reaction
Irritability	Twitching
Decreased appetite	Abnormal movements
Insomnia	Dry mouth
Agitation	*Delusions
Moodiness	*Hallucinations
Nausea	
Rapid heartbeat	
High blood pressure	

Consequences of Long-Term Use
This medicine is habit forming and has potential for abuse and dependency. For this reason, it is sometimes used for only a brief period. For some conditions, however, longer-term use is appropriate. If administration of the medicine is stopped after several weeks or more, it must be decreased slowly to avoid withdrawal symptoms.

This medicine may cause slowed or reduced growth in children.

*Notify your doctor promptly if this side effect occurs.

2

PATRICIA MARES MILLER, RN, MS, CS

DAVID J. KNESPER, MD

THOMAS CARLI, MD

Guide to Self-Help Books About Primary Care Psychiatry Problems

Self-help books are often an important addition to a patient's overall treatment plan. By providing self-help materials and asking such questions as "What did you learn from the reading I suggested?" during subsequent meetings, physicians encourage patients to be partners in their own health care. Accordingly, health care providers should become familiar with several books that they can recommend.

As is to be expected, this guide is incomplete, and real treasures may be omitted. The reverse is true; we may have included materials that some may feel should have been omitted. We have not had an opportunity to review every book listed; some are listed because they have been recommended highly to us. Suggestions can be sent by United States mail to *Primary Care Psychiatry,* University of Michigan Medical Center, 1500 East Medical Center Drive, Room B1C204, Box 0020, Ann Arbor, MI 48109-0020, or by e-mail to primepsyc@umich.edu.

Abuse: Emotional, partner, physical, sexual, and verbal

Bass E, Davis L. The Courage to Heal: A Guide for Women Survivors of Child Sexual Abuse. New York: Harper & Row Publishers; 1988 (paperback, $22.50). Clear, direct source of information for the survivor in the recovery process. Extensive resource guide.

Evans P. The Verbally Abusive Relationship: How to Recognize it and How to Respond. Holbrook, MA: Bob Adams; 1992 (paperback, $9.95). Identifies and shows the effects of verbal abuse and gives suggestions to therapists and patients.

Haden ES. You Can't Say That To Me: Stopping the Pain of Verbal Abuse—An Eight-Step Program. New York: John Wiley & Sons; 1995 (paperback, $12.95).

Island D, Letellier P. Men Who Beat the Men Who Love Them: Battered Gay Men and Domestic Violence. New York: Harrington Park Press; 1991 (paperback, $17.95). Defines violence. Explores issues specific to men, both batterers and victims.

Jones A, Schechter S. When Love Goes Wrong: What to Do When You Can't Do Anything Right. New York: Perennial; 1992 (paperback, $11.00). Personal vignettes to illustrate abuse. Checklists help identify control issues, abuse, and substance abuse. Helpful and informative.

Lobel K, Editor. Naming the Violence: Speaking out about Lesbian Battering. Seattle: Seal Press; 1986 (paperback, $12.95). Articles, essays, and personal stories provide information about woman abuse.

Martin D. Battered Wives. New York: Volcano Press; 1981 (paperback, $5.99).

NiCarthy G. Getting Free: You Can End Abuse and Take Back Your life. Second Edition. Seattle: Seal Press; 1986 (paperback, $12.95). A widely used book that covers such issues as getting emergency help from doctors, police, and prosecutors and protecting children.

NiCarthy G. The Ones Who Got Away: Women Who Left Abusive Partners. Seattle: Seal Press; 1987 (paperback, $12.95). Describes the experiences of many women who have rebuilt their lives.

Norwood R. Women Who Love Too Much. New York: Pocket Books; 1985 (paperback, $6.99). Case histories illustrate why women choose the wrong men. Offers hope and a recovery plan.

Rendetti C. Violent Behavior: Partner Abuse in Lesbian Relationships. Newberry Park, CA: Sage Publications; 1992 (paperback, $24.00).

White EC. Chain Chain Change: For Black Women Dealing with Physical and Emotional Abuse. Seattle: Seal Press; 1985 (paperback, $5.95). Examines the influences of racism and sexism in domestic violence.

Zambrano MJ. Mejor Sola Que Mal Accompanada: Para la Mujer Golpeada/For the Latina in an Abusive Relationship. Seattle: Seal Press; 1985 (paperback, $10.95).

Acquired immunodeficiency syndrome

Eidson T, Editor. The AIDS Caregiver's Handbook. Revised edition. New York: St. Martin's Press; 1993 (paperback, $14.95). Practical book about all aspects of the problem for patients, partners, and families.

King MB. AIDS, HIV and Mental Health. New York: Cambridge University Press; 1993 (paperback, $21.95). Guide through comorbidity of psychiatric symptoms, with the clinical and political aspects of acquired immunodeficiency syndrome.

Pinsky L, Douglas P. The Essential HIV Treatment Fact Book. New York: Pocketbooks (a division of Simon and Schuster); 1992 (paperback, $7.00). Concise factual information, including risk-reduction guidelines and insurance and legal aspects.

Alcohol, addictions, and substance-related disorders

Black C. My Dad Loves Me; My Dad has a Disease. Denver: Mac Publishing; 1982 (paperback, $9.50). Alcoholism from a child's viewpoint.

Knapp C. Drinking: A Love Story. New York: Doubleday Delacorte Press; 1991 (hardback, $22.95). Articulate, ruthless confrontation of the author's love of alcohol and its impact throughout her life.

McGovern G. Terry: My Daughter's Life and Death Struggle With Alcoholism. New York: Villard; 1996 (hardback, $21.00). Straightforward parents' account of years of daughter's addiction, treatment attempts, and finally death. Family drama of love and loss.

Washton A, Boundy D. Willpower Is Not Enough: Understanding and Recovering from Addictions of Every Kind. New York: Harper-Perennial; 1990 (paperback, $11.00). Presents clear message that recovery means making lifestyle changes as well as stopping the behavior.

Alzheimer's disease and dementia

Mace N, Rabins P. The 36-Hour Day. Baltimore: Johns Hopkins University Press; 1981 (paperback, $8.95). Everyone's recommendation.

Sherman B. Dementia with Dignity: A Handbook for Carers. New York: McGraw-Hill Book Co.; 1991 (paperback, $23.95). Written for nursing home staff in Australia, this short book describes the skills every caregiver needs, regardless of nationality.

Robinson A, Spender B, White L. Understanding Difficult Behaviors: Some Practical Suggestions for Coping with Alzheimer's Disease and Related Illnesses. Ann Arbor: Geriatric Education Center of Michigan; 1988 (paperback, $12.00). A local classic. Highly recommended, but it is not available at the local bookstore. Can be obtained by writing to Alzheimer's Association of South Central Michigan, P.O. Box 1713, Ann Arbor, MI 48106 or by calling 1-800-782-6110.

Anxiety

Griest J, Jefferson J, Marks I. Anxiety and Its Treatments: Help is Available. Washington DC: American Psychiatric Press; 1984 (hardback, $18.50). Older book but still frequently recommended.

Marshall JR. Social Phobia: From Shyness to Stage Fright. New York: Basic Books; 1994 (hardback, $23). Describes the problems and considers possible etiology and current treatment options.

Rapoport J. The Boy Who Couldn't Stop Washing. New York: NAL/Dutton; 1989 (paperback, $10.95). A classic book offering insights into the origins and trauma of obsessive-compulsive disorder.

Ross J. Triumph Over Fear. New York: Bantam; 1995 (paperback, $12.95). Helpful book discussing diagnosis and treatment of anxiety, panic attacks, and phobias.

Attention-deficit hyperactivity disorder

Barkley RA. Taking Charge of ADHD. New York: Guilford Press; 1995 (paperback, $16.95). Highly recommended.

Hallowell EM, Ratey JJ. Driven to Distraction: Recognizing and Coping with Attention Deficit Disorder from Childhood through Adulthood. New York: Pantheon Books; 1994 (paperback, $12.00). Readable, thoughtful, informative, and practical book about understanding and living with attention-deficit disorder.

Silver LB. Attention Deficit–Hyperactivity Disorder and Learning Disabilities Booklet for Parents. Summit, NJ: Ciba-Geigy Corp; 1990. Available free by calling The Learning Disabilities Association of America at 412-341-1515 or Ciba-Geigy at 800-742-2422.

Assertiveness

Brower SA, Brower GH. Asserting Yourself: A Practical Guide for Positive Change. Updated Edition. Reading, MA: Addison-Wesley Publishing Co.; 1991 (paperback, $11.95). Unlike many one-message books on the subject, this book provides a more comprehensive approach and sample scripts.

Carter J. Nasty People: How to Stop Being Hurt by Them Without Becoming One of Them. Chicago: Contemporary Books; 1989 (paperback, $5.95). Written for victims of "invalidation" and those who invalidate others.

Chenevert M. STAT: Special Techniques in Assertiveness Training. Fourth Edition. St Louis: Mosby–Year Book; 1994 (paperback, $17.95). Written especially for nurses, but the techniques have wide application.

Brain-behavior relationships

Ornstein R. The Roots of the Self: Unraveling the Mystery of Who We Are. San Francisco: Harper Collins; 1995 (paperback, $12). Clear writing and some humor are used to review development, genetics, brain organization, and current personality theory.

Damasio AR. Descartes' Error: Emotions, Reason, and the Human Brain. New York: G.P. Putnam's Sons; 1994 (hardback, $24.95). The mind-body problem is revisited with new insights by a leading neurologist-neuroscientist. This is a clearly written book about a tough subject.

Children and adolescents

Hibbs ED, Jensen PS, Editors. Psychosocial Treatments for Children and Adolescents: Empirically Based Strategies for Clinical Practice. Washington, DC: American Psychological Association; 1996 (hardback, $59.95 [nonmembers]; $44.95 [members]). This is a meaty text that tries to bridge the gap between research and clinical practice.

Chronic fatigue

Kenny T. Living With Chronic Fatigue Syndrome: A Personal Story of the Struggle for Recovery. New York:

Thunders Mouth Press; 1994 (hardback, $12.95). Intense, thoughtful personal account of chronic fatigue syndrome by a broadcaster.

Cognitive therapy

Burns DD. The Feeling Good Handbook. New York: Plume/Penguin Group; 1990 (paperback, $17.95). A practical, readable book that teaches cognitive therapy skills and applies them to depression, anxiety, fears, marital conflict, and more.

Hawton K, Salkovskis PM, Kirk J, Clark D, Editors. Cognitive Behaviour Therapy for Psychiatric Problems: A Practical Guide. Oxford, England: Oxford University Press; 1989 (paperback, $37.50). More of a practitioners' textbook. Packed with information. Helpful for motivated patients.

Counseling and psychotherapy

Albow KR. To Wrestle With Demons: A Psychiatrist Struggles to Understand His Patients and Himself. Washington DC: American Psychiatric Press; 1992 (paperback, $9.95). In a series of essays, a psychiatrist shares the personal impact of patients' problems.

Basch MF. Understanding Psychotherapy: The Science Behind the Art. New York: Basic Books; 1990 (paperback, $15.00). Vignettes describe psychotherapy and its helpfulness.

Fishman KD. Behind the One-Way Mirror: Psychotherapy and Children. New York: Bantam Books; 1995. Psychotherapy described as collaborative problem solving benefiting children, adolescents, and families.

Death

Nuland SB. How We Die. New York: Knopf/Random House; 1994 (paperback, $13.00). Won 1994 National Book Award; Nuland, who is a surgeon and professor of medical ethics at Yale, considers allowing patients to die in peace and dignity.

Depression

Bloomfield HH, McWilliams P. How to Heal Depression. Los Angeles: Prelude Press; 1994 (paperback, $5.95). Direct, clear, and compassionate book. Written in brief, one-page informative sections with quotations on the opposite page. Recommended to us by our patients.

Manning M. Undercurrents: A Therapists's Reckoning with Depression. San Francisco: Harper Collins; 1995 (hardback, $20.00). Relates diary entries made as the author candidly faces multiple failed therapies for her severe clinical depression and finally the effective use of electroconvulsive therapy.

Rosenthal N. Winter Blues: Seasonal Affective Disorder. What It Is and How to Overcome It. New York: Guilford Press; 1993 (paperback, $14.95). Information presented in a readable style from director of light therapy studies at the National Institute of Mental Health.

Thompson R. The Beast: A Reckoning with Depression. Kirkwood, NY: Putnam Publishing Group; 1995 (hardback, $23.95). Personal account of life-long battle with mental illness and realization of the impact the patient's illness had on other people.

Evolutionary biology, darwinian medicine

Nesse RM, Williams GC. Why We Get Sick. New York: Times Books; 1994 ($24.00). When is it best to let a fever run its course? The very foundations to questions like this are explored in ways that might revolutionize the practice of medicine.

Grief and suicide

Kuklin S. After a Suicide: Young People Speak Up. New York: G.P. Putnam's Sons; 1994 (paperback, $9.95). Clearly written. Its purpose is to help survivors and to encourage people who are suicidal to seek help and better solutions.

Viorst J. Necessary Losses. New York: Simon & Schuster; 1986 (paperback, $5.95). Practical thoughtful, humorous message that loss is part of the life cycle and not only part of death.

Westberg G. Good Grief. Philadelphia: Fortress Press; 1971 (paperback, $5.00). Short book that addresses stages of grief that occurs with the loss of an important someone or something. Also available in large print.

Eating disorders

Fairburn CG. Overcoming Binge Eating. New York: Guilford Press; 1995 (paperback, $14.95). Self-help program for binge eating.

Siegel M, Brisman J, Weinshe M. Surviving an Eating Disorder: Strategies for Family and Friends. New York: Harper Perennial; 1988 (paperback, $12.50). For all the important people in the lives of persons with eating disorders.

Elder care and abuse

Cohen SZ, Gans, BM. The Other Generation Gap: The Middle-Aged and Their Aging Parents. New York: Dodd, Mead & Co.; 1988. Strategies for the "sandwiched generation." (This book is no longer in print.)

Lustbader W, Hoyman N. Taking Care of Your Aging Family Members. New York: Free Press, Division of MacMillan Publishing Co.; 1986 (paperback, $14.95). Revised and expanded. Practical book. Comprehensive, multiple examples and suggested resources. Boxed areas highlight such issues as driving, memory loss, and bladder control.

Pilemar K, Wolf RS, Editors. Elder Abuse: Conflict in the Family. Westport, CT: Greenwood Publishing; 1986 (paperback, $16.95).

Silverstone B, Hymen HK. You and Your Aging Parents: The Modern Family's Guide to Emotional, Physical and Financial Problems. New York: Pantheon Books; 1982 (paperback, $16.00).

Factitious disorders (getting sick on purpose)

Feldman MD, Ford CV. Patient or Pretender: The Strange World of Factitious Disorders. New York: John Wiley & Sons; 1994 (paperback, $14.95). Written for physicians, but patients seem to benefit.

Learning Disabilities

Levine M. Keeping A Head in School: A Student's Book about Learning Abilities and Learning Disorders. Cambridge, MA: Educators Publishing Services; 1991 (paperback, $25.50; cassette [set of six; read by Dr. Levine], $27.85). To obtain, call publisher at 617-547-6706. Gives practical advice, hope, study strategies, and creative methods, as well as an overview of learning disabilities and related problems.

Novich BZ, Arnold MM. Why is My Child Having Trouble at School? A Parent's Guide to Learning Disabilities. Kirkwood, NY: Plenum Publishing Corp: 1995 (paperback, $12.95). Step-by-step guide through the process of identifying and getting help for biologically based learning problems.

Bipolar disorder

Jamison KM. Touched with Fire: Manic-Depressive Illness and the Artistic Temperament. New York: Free Press; 1993 (hardback, $24.95). Considers the lives of the famous and advocates the use of medication while preserving the artistic personality. The author is a researcher who knows first hand what it means to be "touched with fire."

Marital and relationship problems

Gray J. Men are from Mars, Women are from Venus. New York: HarperCollins; 1992 (hard cover, $25.00). For men who are still from Mars. Women who have moved on will find this book somewhat out-of-date.

Markman H, Stanley S, Blumberg S. Fighting for Your Marriage. San Francisco: Jossey-Bass Publishers; 1994 (paperback, $14.00). Teaches and builds skills that serve to strengthen relationships.

Tannen D. You Just Don't Understand: Women and Men in Conversation. New York: Ballantine Books; 1991 (paperback, $12.50). If miscommunication between couples is the problem, this book is the answer.

Mental illness

Spitzer RL, Gibbon MG, Skodol AE, et al., Editors. DSM-IV Case Book. Washington DC: American Psychiatric Press; 1994 (paperback, $32.50). Case vignettes and discussion describing the common mental disorders. Appendix D provides an index of cases by diagnosis.

Parenting and child development

Brazelton TB. Infants and Mothers: Differences in Development. Revised. New York: Dell Publishing; 1983 (paperback, $16.95). Start here and then go on to read Brazelton's other books.

Clark L. The Time-out Solution: A Parent's Guide for Handling Everyday Behavior Problems. Chicago: Contemporary Books; 1989 (paperback, $10.95). Help during difficult times.

Comer J, Poussaint A. Raising Black Children. New York: Plume; 1992 (paperback, $12.95). Question-and-answer format. Parenting issues focusing on raising a black child in a white-dominated culture. Comprehensive.

Dodson F. How to Discipline with Love from Crib to College. New York: Signet; 1977 (paperback, $5.99). Practical strategies focusing on developmental needs. Addresses range of families: single, blended, two parent.

Elium J, Elium D. Raising a Daughter. Berkeley: Celestial Arts; 1994 (paperback, $12.95). Practical. Gives developmental stages. Discusses parenting concerns in today's world. Authors' first book, Raising a Son, equally relevant.

Faber A, Mazlish E. How to Talk so Kids Will Listen and Listen so Kids Will Talk. New York: Avon Books; 1980 (paperback, $12.00). Builds on Ginott's work. Gives exercises to increase skills and gives examples.

Ginott H. Between Parent and Child. New York: Avon Books; 1956 (paperback, $5.99). Concise and positive. Emphasizes skills used to increase effective communication between parents and children or any adult involved with children.

Gordon T. P.E.T., Parent Effectiveness Training. New York: Peter Plume; 1970 (paperback, $12.95). A classic, and still current. Gives program to increase clear parent-child communication with techniques for conflict resolution.

Orvin GH. Understanding the Adolescent. Washington, DC: American Psychiatric Press; 1995 (hardback, $21.95). Highly recommended.

Multiple sclerosis

McFarlane EB. Legwork. New York: Charles Scribner's Sons; 1995 (hardback, $22.00). Outstanding and inspiring first-person account of multiple sclerosis; suitable for patients and families dealing with any chronic illness.

Schapiro R. Symptom Management in Multiple Sclerosis. Second Edition. New York: Demos Publications; 1995 (paperback, $19.95).

Wolf JK. Mastering Multiple Sclerosis. Second Edition. Rutland, VT: Academy Books; 1987 (paperback, $22.95).

Parkinson's disease

Lieberman A, Williams F, Imke S, et al. Parkinson's Disease: The Complete Guide for Patients and Caregivers. New

York: Simon & Schuster; 1993 (paperback, $11.00). For patients who want to know, this book tells it like it is. A current favorite.

Schizophrenia

Schiller L, Bennett A. The Quiet Room. New York: Warner Books; 1994 (paperback, $10.99). Moving personal story of woman's struggle with schizophrenia and eventual recovery through acceptance of illness, supports, and medication.

Torrey EF. Surviving Schizophrenia: A Manual for Families, Consumers and Providers. Third Edition. New York: Harper Perennial; 1995 (paperback, $14.00). Clear information about schizophrenia.

Sexuality

Barbach LG. For Yourself: The Fulfillment of Female Sexuality. New York: Penguin; 1976 (paperback, $5.99).

Hacker S, Hacker R. What Every Teenager Really Wants to Know About Sex. New York: Carroll & Graf Publishers; 1993 (paperback, $10.95). Question-and-answer format. Organized by topic. First two chapters are for parents.

Kirk S, Rothblatt M. Medical, Legal and Workplace Issues for the Transsexual. Watertown, MA: Together Lifeworks; 1995 (paperback, $18.95).

Reinisch JM. The Kinsey Institute New Report on Sex: What You Must Know To Be Sexually Literate. New York: St. Martin's Press; 1990 (paperback, $7.99). Factual. Provides diagrams. Question-and-answer format.

Sleep disorders

Kavey NB. Practical Book of Remedies: 50 Ways to Sleep Better. Lincolnwood IL: Publication International; 1995 (paperback, $9.98). A joint effort by the editors of *Consumer Guide* and The Sleep Disorders Center at Columbia-Presbyterian Medical Center for adults and children. Can be obtained by calling 800-745-9299.

Stress

Kabat-Zinn J. Full Catastrophe Living: Using the Wisdom of Your Body and Mind to Face Stress, Pain, and Illness. New York: Dell Publishing; 1991 (paperback, $12.95). Guide to mindfulness meditation aimed at patients with pain and other physical problems that can be improved by behavioral medicine interventions.

McWilliams P. You Can't Afford the Luxury of a Negative Thought. Los Angeles: Prelude Press; 1995 (paperback, $5.95). Dealing with negative thinking and its impact, subtle and obvious, on a person's life.

Sapolsky RM. Why Zebras Don't Get Ulcers. New York: W.H. Freeman & Co., Publishers; 1995 (paperback, $14.95). Modern medicine deals with chronic diseases that have causes and consequences heavily related to personality and life's accumulation of stress.

Reference

La Rossa J Jr, Editor. The first annual resource guide to psychiatric books and journals. Prim Psychiatry 1995;2:20–75.

3

PATRICIA MARES MILLER, RN, MS, CS

Resource Service Catalogues Listing Numerous Handouts for Primary Care Patients

This appendix attempts to provide a list of resource service catalogues that are useful in the care of patients in the primary care setting. Some important resource services may have been omitted, and listings of other organizations may have changed since the publication of this text. Information regarding organizations and telephone numbers that should be added or deleted can be sent by United States mail to *Primary Care Psychiatry*, University of Michigan Medical Center, 1500 East Medical Center Drive, Room B1C204, Box 0020, Ann Arbor, MI 48109-0020, or by e-mail to primepsyc@umich.edu.

A Mental Illness Awareness Guide for Physicians and Other Health Care Professionals

Purpose: The purposes are to educate about mental illness, provide assistance with recognizing mental illness in patient groups, and increase knowledge of resources, treatment methods, compliance, and psychiatric referral techniques.

Contents: Contents are divided into sections that are designed for photocopying. Sections are "Mental Illness in the Primary Care Setting," "Referrals and Consultation," "Education," "Resources" (including an extensive bibliography), "Organizations," "Local APA Contacts," "Program Materials," 12 different "Let's Talk About Mental Illness" columns, and "Warning Signs and Knowledge Quizzes."

Cost: The catalogue is free. The requester may require the name of an American Psychiatric Association member to obtain materials.

Ordering: American Psychiatric Association, Division of Public Affairs, 1400 K Street, NW, Washington, DC 20005. Telephone: 202-682-6000

Consumer Information Center Catalogue

Purpose: The purpose is to provide a list of free and low-cost federal publications of consumer interest.

Contents: Publications from approximately 40 government agencies are divided into broad topic sections containing lists of publication titles, a brief description of each publication, length, and cost. Mental health publications are included under the "Health" section. An example is: "What to Do When a Friend is Depressed."

Cost: The catalogue is free. Up to 25 different free booklets can be ordered at one time. Discounts may apply for quantity orders (≥100). A low-cost service fee is requested when materials are ordered.

Ordering: The Consumer Information Catalogue, Consumer Information Center, P.O. Box 100, Pueblo, CO 81002.

National Institutes of Health, National Institute of Mental Health Publications

Purpose: The purpose is to provide the public with information about mental illness, treatment, and research.

Contents: A user-friendly format contains titles and some descriptions of NIMH publications. The publication is divided into the following sections: "Specific Mental Disorders," "General Information," "Plain Talk Series," "Research," "Destigmatization," "Spanish Language Publications," and "Professional Publications." Most publications are legally reproducible.

Cost: The catalogue is free. Each requester is allowed 10 free single copies from the catalogue.

Ordering: Information Resources and Inquiries Branch, Room 7C-02, Office of Scientific Information, National Institute of Mental Health, 5600 Fishers Lane, Rockville, MD 20857. Telephone: 301-443-4513 (Monday to Friday, 8 a.m. to 5 p.m.).

Patient Information Guide for Neurology, 1997 Edition

Purpose: The purpose is to help physicians and others locate patient-oriented materials and services for patients with neurologic disorders.

Contents: This is an easily readable resource for patient information materials and services in the field of neurology. Under each diagnosis, beginning with acoustic neuroma and including rare disorders, is a national organization address and telephone number, publications, and other services.

Cost: The catalogue costs $10.00.

Ordering: American Academy of Neurology, 221 University Avenue SE, Suite 335, Minneapolis, MN 55414. Telephone: 612-623-8115; fax: 612-623-3504; e-mail: aan@aan.com.

4

PATRICIA MARES MILLER, RN, MS, CS

Guide to Organizations Dedicated to Specific Primary Care Psychiatry Problems

This appendix lists some hotlines and help lines; organizations are other important sources for relevant books, pamphlets, newsletters, catalogues of educational materials, cassettes, videos, networking, workshops, and so on. This not an exhaustive list, and listings of some organizations may have changed since the publication of this text. Information about organizations and telephone numbers that should be added or deleted can be sent by United States mail to *Primary Care Psychiatry,* University of Michigan Medical Center, 1500 East Medical Center Drive, Room B1C204, Box 0020, Ann Arbor, MI 48109-0020, or by e-mail to primepsyc@umich.edu.

Abuse and Domestic Violence

Child Help USA (National Child Abuse Hotline). Telephone: 800-422-4453. Answers 24 hours a day with a recording that offers menu selections.

National Council on Child Abuse and Family Violence. 1155 Connecticut Avenue, NW, Suite 400, Washington DC 20036. Telephone: 202-429-6695.

National Family Violence Helpline. Telephone: 800-222-2000. Recorded menu or operator assistance regarding child, partner, spouse, or elder abuse.

Nationwide Crisis Hotline. Telephone: 800-999-9999. Targets groups younger than 21 years and their families. Recording gives directions.

Acquired Immunodeficiency Syndrome (AIDS) and Human Immunodeficiency Virus (HIV)

AmFAR (American Foundation for AIDS Research). 733 Third Avenue, Twelfth Floor, New York, NY 10017. Telephone: 800-39-AmFAR. AmFAR publishes the *AIDS/HIV Treatment Directory,* a free quarterly listing of clinical research.

Centers for Disease Control and Prevention, National AIDS Clearinghouse. P.O. Box 6003, Rockville, MD 20849-6003. Telephone: 800-458-5231, 9 a.m. to 7 p.m. Eastern Standard Time. Bilingual Spanish and English materials available.

Mundo. P.O. BOX 11535, Oakland, CA 94611. Monthly newsletter on women and HIV/AIDS; available in Spanish or English.

National AIDS Hotline. Telephone: 800-342-AIDS.

Positive Woman. P.O. Box 33061, Washington, DC 20033. Telephone: 202-745-1078. A bimonthly newsletter about treatment options for HIV-positive women.

Treatment Issues. Gay Men's Health Crisis, Department of Medical Information, 129 West 20th Street, New York, NY 10011. Telephone: 212-337-1950. A free newsletter about experimental AIDS therapies.

Alcohol and Substance Abuse

Alcoholics Anonymous World Headquarters. 475 Riverside Drive, New York, NY 10115. Telephone: 212-870-3400.

Al-Anon World Service. 1372 Broadway, New York, NY 10018. Telephone: 212-302-7240.

National Clearinghouse for Alcohol and Drug Abuse. NCADI, P.O. Box 2345, Rockville, MD 20852. Telephone: 301-468-2600.

Alzheimer's Disease

Alzheimer's Association. 70 E. Lake Street, Suite 600, Chicago, IL 60601. Telephone: 800-621-0379. Provides 24-hour inquiry and information services.

Anxiety Disorders

Anxiety Disorders Association of America (AADA). 6000 Executive Boulevard, Suite 200, Rockville, MD 20852. Telephone: 301-231-9350.

Panic Disorder Education Network Program, National Institute of Mental Health, Parklawn Building, Room 7-99, 5600 Fishers Lane, Rockville, MD 20857. Telephone: 800-64-PANIC.

Autism

Autism Society of America. 7910 Woodmont Avenue, Suite 650, Bethesda, MD 20814. Telephone: 800-3-AUTISM.

Chronic Fatigue

The Chronic Fatigue and Immune Dysfunction Syndrome Association of America. P.O. Box 220398, Charlotte, NC 28222. Telephone: 800-442-3437.

The National CFS Association. 919 Scott Avenue, Kansas City, KS 66105. Telephone: 913-321-2278.

National Chronic Fatigue Syndrome and Fibromyalgia Association. 3521 Broadway, Suite 222, Kansas City, MO 64111. Telephone: 816-931-4777.

Depression

National Depressive and Manic Depressive Association (NDMDA). 730 N. Franklin, Suite 501, Chicago, IL 60610. Telephone: 312-642-0049.

National Foundation for Depressive Illnesses. Telephone: 800-248-3444.

Eating Disorders

Bulimia, Anorexia & Self-Help, Inc. (BASH). 6125 Clayton Ave., Suite 215, P.O. Box 39903, St. Louis, MO 63139. Telephone: 800-762-3334.

National Association of Anorexia Nervosa and Associated Disorders (ANAD). Box 7, Highland Park, IL 60035. Telephone: 708-831-3438. An advocacy organization that offers free educational support and networking services to patients and their families.

Learning Disabilities/Attention-Deficit Disorder

Attention Deficit Disorder Association (ADDA). P.O. Box 972, Mentor, OH 44061. Telephone: 800-487-2282.

Children and Adults with Attention Deficit Disorder (CHADD). 499 NW 70th Avenue, Suite 308, Plantation, FL 33317. Telephone: 305-587-3700.

Learning Disabilities Association of America (LDA). 4156 Library Road, Pittsburgh, PA 15234. Telephone: 412-341-1515.

Mental Illness

National Mental Health Services Knowledge Exchange Network, P.O. Box 42490, Washington, DC 20015. Telephone: 800-789-2647.

National Alliance for the Mentally Ill (NAMI). 2101 Wilson Blvd., Suite 302, Arlington, VA 22201. Telephone: 800-950-NAMI.

Self-Help Clearing House. St. Claire's Riverside Medical Center, Pocono Road, Denville, NJ 07834. Telephone: 201-625-9565. Provides local and national referral services. Carries support group listings.

Multiple Sclerosis

National Multiple Sclerosis Society. 733 Third Avenue, New York, NY 10017. Telephone: 800-FIGHT MS (800-344-4867).

National Multiple Sclerosis Society Job Raising Program. Information can be obtained by dialing 800-FIGHT MS and selecting 1. Callers are automatically connected to the multiple sclerosis chapter in the state from which the caller is calling.

Schizophrenia and Depression

National Alliance for Research on Schizophrenia and Depression (NARSAD). 60 Cutter Mill Road, Suite 200, Great Neck, NY 11021. Telephone: 516-829-0091.

Sexuality

American Association of Sex Educators, Counselors, and Therapists (AASECT). P.O. Box 238, Mount Vernon, IA 52314. Telephone: 319-895-8407. This telephone is initially answered at a doctor's office; the caller needs to indicate that he or she is seeking AASECT.

Gay/Lesbian Medical Association. 273 Church Street, San Francisco, CA 94114. Telephone: 415-255-4547.

Harry Benjamin International Gender Dysphoria Association. P.O. BOX 1718, Sonoma, CA 95476. Telephone: no known listing.

International Foundation for Gender Education. P.O. Box 367, Wayland, MA 01778. Telephone: 617-899-2212.

Lesbian, Gay, Bisexual People in Medicine (Standing Committee of the American Medical Student Association). 1890 Preston White Drive, Reston, VA 22091. Telephone: 800-767-2266. This telephone is answered by the American Medical Student Association. The caller must ask the operator to connect him or her with someone from this group. The caller may connect with voice mail.

National Advocacy Coalition on Youth and Sexual Orientation. c/o Hetrick-Martin Institute, Two Astor Place, New York, NY 10003. Telephone: 212-674-2400.

Parents Families and Friends of Lesbians and Gays (PFLAG). 1101 14th Street, NW, Suite 1030, Washington, DC 20005. Telephone: 202-638-4200.

5

PATRICIA MARES MILLER, RN, MS, CS

Referral Information from Mental Health Professional Associations

This appendix provides a list of several mental health professional associations that may be useful to patients and primary care physicians. Additional groups of services providers, with which we are too unfamiliar to list, surely exist. Information about mental health services provider groups that should be added because readers have found them meaningful healthcare participants can be sent by United States mail to *Primary Care Psychiatry,* University of Michigan Medical Center, 1500 East Medical Center Drive, Room B1C204, Box 0020, Ann Arbor, MI 48109-0020, or by e-mail to: primepsyc@umich.edu.

Mental Health Professionals

American Psychiatric Association (APA). 1400 K Street, NW, Washington, DC 20005. Telephone: 202-682-6000. The caller must state the request for a name and telephone number of a psychiatrist in his or her area. The caller is given the name and number of a psychiatrist, or the number for the state psychiatric association, or both.

American Psychological Association (APA). 750 First Street, NE, Washington, DC 20002-4242. Telephone: 800-374-2721. The caller must request the Practice Directory component; the caller receives the telephone number for the state association that, in turn, gives the names and telephone numbers of area psychologists.

National Association of Social Workers (NASW). 750 First Street, NE, Washington, DC 20002. Telephone: 800-638-8799. The caller must request the Clinical Register component and then receives the name, telephone, field of practice, and work setting of area social workers. The number for the state chapter is available too.

Allied Mental Health Professionals

American Association for Marriage and Family Therapy (AAMFT). 1100 17th Street, NW, 10th Floor, Washington, DC 20036. Telephone: 202-452-0109.

American Counseling Association (ACA). 5999 Stevenson Avenue, Alexandria, VA 22304. Telephone: 703-823-9800.

American Nurses Association (ANA). 600 Maryland Avenue, SW, West 100, Washington, DC 20024-2571. Telephone: 800-274-4262.

Association for the Advancement of Behavior Therapy (AABT). 15 West 36th Street, New York, NY 10018. Telephone: 212-279-7970.

Index

Note: Page numbers in italics indicate figures; those with a *t* indicate tables.